ESSENTIALS OF DENTAL RADIOGRAPHY

FOR DENTAL ASSISTANTS AND HYGIENISTS

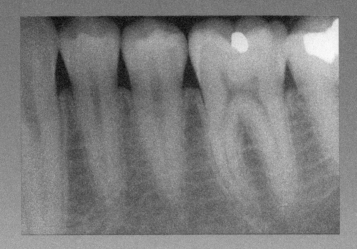

TENTH EDITION

Evelyn M. Thomson, BSDH, MS
Gene W. Hirschfeld School of Dental Hygiene
Old Dominion University
Norfolk, Virginia

Orlen N. Johnson, BS, DDS, MS
College of Dentistry
University of Nebraska Medical Center
Lincoln, Nebraska

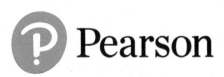

330 Hudson Street, NY NY 10013

Notice: The author and the publisher of this volume have taken care that the information and technical recommendations contained herein are based on research and expert consultation, and are accurate and compatible with the standards generally accepted at the time of publication. Nevertheless, as new information becomes available, changes in clinical and technical practices become necessary. The reader is advised to carefully consult manufacturers' instructions and information material for all supplies and equipment before use, and to consult with a health care professional as necessary. This advice is especially important when using new supplies or equipment for clinical purposes. The author and publisher disclaim all responsibility for any liability, loss, injury, or damage incurred as a consequence, directly or indirectly, of the use and application of any of the contents of this volume.

Vice President, Health Science and TED: Julie Levin Alexander
Assistant to Vice President: Sarah Henrich
Director, Portfolio Management: Marlene McHugh Pratt
Executive Portfolio Manager: John Goucher
Managing Content Producer: Melissa Bashe
Portfolio Management Assistant: Lisa Narine
Development Editor: Danielle Doller
Director of Marketing: David Gesell
Executive Marketing Manager: Brittany Hammond
Manager of Digital Production: Amy Peltier

Digital Developer: William Johnson
Production Editor: Karen Berry, SPi Global
Operations Specialist: Mary Ann Gloriande
Creative Digital Lead: Mary Siener
Cover Designer: Laurie Entringer
Composition: SPi Global
Printer/Binder: LSC Communications
Cover Image: Evelyn Thomson, Orlen Johnson, *Essentials of Dental Radiography for Dental Assistants and Hygienists*, 10e, 9780134460741, © 2018. Pearson Education, Inc., New York, NY.

Library of Congress Cataloging-in-Publication Data

Names: Thomson, Evelyn M., author. | Johnson, Orlen N., author.
Title: Essentials of dental radiography for dental assistants and hygienists
  / Evelyn M. Thomson, Orlen N. Johnson.
Description: Tenth edition. | New York, NY: Pearson, 2017. | Includes
  bibliographical references and index.
Identifiers: LCCN 2016043133| ISBN 9780134460741 | ISBN 013446074X
Subjects: | MESH: Radiography, Dental | Dental Assistants | Dental Hygienists
Classification: LCC RK309 | NLM WN 230 | DDC 617.6/07572--dc23
LC record available at https://lccn.loc.gov/2016043133

24 2021

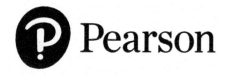

ISBN-10: 0-13-446074-X
ISBN-13: 978-0-13-446074-1

Thank you to my husband, Hu Odom, for your loving patience, support, and encouragement.

—Evie

CONTENTS

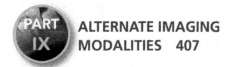

PREFACE

Dental radiography plays an integral role in comprehensive preventive oral heath care. Mastery of skills needed to perform radiographic examinations competently and safely requires an understanding of theoretical concepts and a committed adherence to radiation protection principles. *Essentials of Dental Radiography for Dental Assistants and Hygienists* presents a clear link between theory and practice, to prepare dental assistants and dental hygienists for roles as members of the oral health care team who can produce diagnostic quality radiographs in a variety of situations and circumstances, and who can assist in the interpretation of images for the benefit of patients. The tenth edition of *Essentials of Dental Radiography for Dental Assistants and Hygienists* retains core fundamentals presented in earlier editions that focus on an in-depth study of key principles, while expanding and incorporating new concepts that reflect technological advancements in the field of oral and maxillofacial radiography.

Organization

Essentials of Dental Radiography for Dental Assistants and Hygienists is divided into nine sections that take a reader from radiation basics and the fundamentals of dental radiographic techniques, to management of special needs and an introduction to alternate imaging modalities. Each chapter is student centered, beginning with an outline that provides a ready reference to the topics presented, a list of key terms that are defined within the text, and an introduction that provides a realistic rationale to pique interest for learning the material. Learning objectives that are tested by study questions allow a student to assess learning outcomes. The objectives and study questions are written in the same order that the material appears in the chapter, guiding the reader through assimilation of chapter content. Procedure features highlight and simplify critical steps of complex techniques, and serve as a handy reference in laboratory and clinical settings. Practice Points call student attention to possible use of theory in real-life situations, and provide a "mental break" by illustrating how that theory is applied. Meaningful case studies relate directly to radiological applications presented in the chapter and challenge students to apply knowledge gained from the reading to real-life situations through decision-making activities.

New to This Edition

Changes made to the tenth edition of *Essentials of Dental Radiography for Dental Assistants and Hygienists* reflect the expanding body of knowledge and evidence-based practice advances that influence the prescription, delivery, and evaluation of radiographic examinations. A complete and thorough revision and a reorganization of topic presentation have produced a coherent and intelligible resource for learning. Augmenting readability is the transition to color figure images that enhance and highlight key points. Figure images have been updated to reflect advancements in technology and practice—for example, illustrating radiographic techniques using digital image receptors and recommended rectangular collimation. Other outstanding features of this edition include:

- **Integration of digital imaging throughout all chapters.** Digital imaging has become a requisite part of oral health care practice prompting the need to make digital imaging a fundamental component of study throughout the book.
- **Enhancement of the chapter on digital imaging.** A thorough revision has produced an in-depth explanation of digital image acquisition technology to assist the reader in gaining a higher level of understanding befitting what would be expected of a dental assistant and dental hygienist.
- **Consolidation of the chapters on dental x-ray film and film processing.** In response to the diminishing use of film-based imaging, these two chapters were streamlined to reflect essential knowledge, and incorporated into one concise chapter. Film-based imaging is an established standard of care, and licensing board examinations continue to require oral health care professionals to demonstrate a working knowledge of its use so important subject matter has been kept intact.
- **Expansion of the chapter on legal and ethical responsibilities.** In response to the increasing adoption of electronic patient records, considerable information has been added to prepare dental assistants and dental hygienists for the responsibilities and challenges encountered with the electronic transfer and storage of digital radiographic images.
- **Revision and change in order of presentation of the chapter on panoramic imaging.** A panoramic examination plays an essential, rather than supplemental, role in oral and maxillofacial imaging, and, as such, its introduction has been moved up from the end of the book to better fit within the section on radiographic techniques. The interpretive discussion now forms the foundation for a new chapter on recognizing normal radiographic anatomy on panoramic images, which has been placed immediately following the chapter on recognizing anatomy on introral images.
- **Repurposed chapters on interpretation.** The radiographic appearance of dental materials and foreign objects is more clearly presented in its own chapter;

and a new instructional focus was given to the chapter on recognizing radiographic anomalies and lesions for the purpose of developing skills needed to describe, rather than definitively diagnose, conditions observed.

- **Consolidation of the chapters on quality control and environmental safety.** The combination of these interrelated topics helps establish a link between the attainment of quality for both image production and for the ecological impact associated with image production.
- **Reorganization of the section on radiographic techniques for specific needs.** The chapters on pediatric radiography, radiography for special needs, and for specific oral conditions represent a reorganization of a plethora of technique modifications into a cohesive, orderly presentation that enhances clarity to aid in learning how and when to apply a multitude of technique variations. Some of the material has been determined to be better presented with supplemental and

extraoral techniques as part of the alternate imaging modalities section.

- **New chapter on three-dimensional imaging.** The volume of references in the literature describing potential uses for three-dimensional imaging for oral and maxillofacial diagnoses and treatments warrants a new chapter to introduce the reader to cone beam computed tomography (CBCT).

Whereas *Essentials of Dental Radiography for Dental Assistants and Hygienists* is written primarily for dental assisting and dental hygiene students, practicing dental assistants, dental hygienists, and dentists may also find this book to be a helpful reference, particularly when preparing for a relicensing examination. Additionally, *Essentials of Dental Radiography for Dental Assistants and Hygienists* may be a valuable study guide for on-the-job-trained oral health care professionals who may be seeking radiation safety certification credentials.

ACKNOWLEDGMENTS

Thank you to Orlen Johnson and all of the coauthors of the previous nine editions of *Essentials of Dental Radiography for Dental Assistants and Hygienists* who provided the foundation upon which is the success of this tenth edition. It is a privilege to be associated with a textbook with this long-standing history. Thank you to everyone at Pearson for their direction and patience. I particularly want to express appreciation to John Goucher, Portfolio Manager, for his expert guidance and caring counsel; Melissa Bashe, Managing Content Producer, and Nicole Ragonese, Program Manager, who both worked tirelessly with me, once again, on another edition; and Danielle Doller, Development Editor, for her expert feedback and kind advocacy. Also, thank you to Karen Berry, Full Service Project Manager, and the team at SPi Global for putting everything together. The support and guidance from Dale A. Miles, DDS, MS is also greatly appreciated. The quality of this edition reflects the input from my colleague Ann M. Bruhn, BSDH, MS, Assistant Professor at Gene W. Hirschfeld School of Dental Hygiene, Old Dominion University, Norfolk, Virginia, who enthusiastically accepted the challenge of contributing author.

Evie Thomson

CONTRIBUTING AUTHOR
TO THE TENTH EDITION

Ann M. Bruhn, BSDH, MS
Gene W. Hirschfeld School of Dental Hygiene
Old Dominion University
Norfolk, Virginia

REVIEWERS OF THE TENTH EDITION

Patricia Belmonte, MSHA
College of Dupage
Glen Ellyn, Illinois

April Catlett, PhD
Central Georgia Technical College Macon Campus
Macon, Georgia

Kerri H. Friel, RDH, COA, CDA, MA
Community College of Rhode Island
Warwick, Rhode Island

Anna Marie Hauser, RDH, MBA
Idaho State University, Clinical Practice
Pocatello, Idaho

Mary Jacobs RDH, Ed.M.
The College of Lake County
Grayslake, Illinois

Jessica Kiser, RDH, BS, MS
Cape Fear Community College
Wilmington, North Carolina

Lori Schmidt, CDA, RDH
Kaskaskia College
Centralia, Illinois

Karen Siebert, BSDH, MA
The College of Lake County Dental Hygiene Program
Grayslake, Illinois

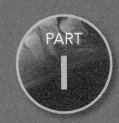

PART

I

Radiation Basics

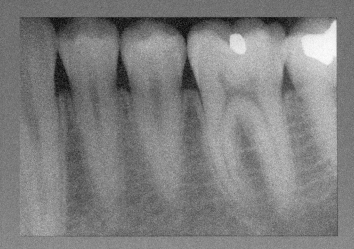

① Dental Radiography: Historical Perspective and Future Trends

CHAPTER OUTLINE

OBJECTIVES

Following successful completion of this chapter, you should be able to:

1. Define the key terms.
2. State when x-rays were discovered and by whom.
3. Trace the history of radiography, noting the prominent contributors.
4. List two historical developments that made dental x-ray machines safer.
5. Explain how rectangular PIDs reduce patient radiation exposure.
6. Identify the two techniques used to expose dental radiographs.
7. List five uses of dental radiographs.
8. Become aware of other imaging modalities available for use in the detection and evaluation of oral conditions.

KEY TERMS

Bisecting technique
Cone
Cone beam computed tomography (CBCT)
Digital imaging

Oral radiography
Panoramic radiography
Paralleling technique
Position indicating device (PID)
Radiograph
Radiography

Radiology
Roentgen ray
Roentgenograph
Sensor
X-ray
X-ray film

Introduction

Technological advancements continue to affect the way we deliver oral health care. Although new methods for diagnosing disease and treatment planning comprehensive care have been introduced, dental radiographs, the images produced by x-rays, remain the basis for many diagnostic procedures and play an essential role in oral health care. **Radiography** is the making of radiographs by exposing an image receptor, either film or digital sensor. The purpose of dental radiography is to provide the oral health care team with radiographic images of the best possible diagnostic quality. The goal of dental radiography is to obtain the highest quality radiographs while maintaining the lowest possible radiation exposure risk for the patient.

Dental assistants and dental hygienists meet an important need through their ability to produce diagnostic quality radiographs. The basis for development of the skills needed to expose, process, mount, and evaluate radiographic images is a thorough understanding of radiology concepts. All individuals working with radiographic equipment should be educated and trained in the theory of x-ray production. The concepts and theories regarding x-ray production that emerged during the early days of x-radiation discovery are responsible for the quality health care available today. This chapter presents a historical perspective that recognizes the contributions of the early scientists and researchers who supplied us with the fundamentals on which we practice today and advance toward the future.

Discovery of the X-ray

Oral **radiology** is the study of x-rays and the techniques used to produce radiographic images. The study begins with the history of dental radiography and the discovery of the x-ray. The x-ray revolutionized the methods of practicing medicine and dentistry by making it possible to visualize internal body structures noninvasively. Wilhelm Conrad Roentgen's (pronounced "rent'gun"; Figure 1–1 ■) experiment in Bavaria (Germany) on November 8, 1895, produced a tremendous advance in science. Roentgen's curiosity was aroused during an experiment with a vacuum tube called a Crookes tube (named after William Crookes, an English chemist). Roentgen observed that a fluorescent screen near the tube began to glow when the tube was activated by passing an electric current through it. Examining this strange phenomenon further, he noticed that shadows could be cast on the screen by interposing objects between it and the tube. Further experimentation showed that such shadow images could be permanently recorded on photographic film (Figure 1–2 ■).

In the beginning, Roentgen was uncertain of the nature of this invisible ray that he had discovered. When he later reported his finding at a scientific meeting, he spoke of it as an **x-ray** because the symbol *x* represented the unknown. For his work, Roentgen was awarded the first Nobel Prize for physics in 1901. After his findings were reported and published, fellow scientists honored him by calling the

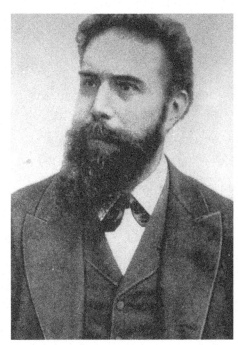

FIGURE 1–1 **Wilhelm Conrad Roentgen (1845–1923).** (Courtesy of Radiology Centennial, Inc.)

invisible ray the **roentgen ray** and the image produced on photosensitive film a **roentgenograph**. Because a photographic negative and an x-ray film have basic similarity and the x-ray closely resembles the radio wave, the prefix *radio-* and the suffix *-graph* were combined into **radiograph**, the term used by health professionals today.

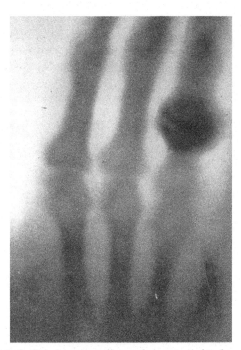

FIGURE 1–2 This famous radiograph, purported to be of Roentgen's wife Bertha's hand, was taken on December 22, 1895. (Courtesy of Radiology Centennial, Inc.)

Important Scientists and Researchers

A few weeks after Roentgen announced his discovery, German physicist Otto Walkhoff first exposed a prototype of a dental radiograph. This was accomplished by covering a small, glass photographic plate with black paper to protect it from light and then wrapping it in a sheath of thin rubber to prevent moisture damage during the 25 minutes that he held the film in his mouth. A similar exposure can now be made in 0.10 second. The resulting radiograph was experimental and had little diagnostic value because it was impossible to prevent film movement during the long exposure time, but it did prove that the x-ray would have a role in dentistry. The length of the exposure made the experiment a dangerous one for Walkhoff, as the dangers of overexposure to radiation were unknown at the time.

It is not known conclusively who made the first dental radiograph in the United States, but, as early as 1896, C. Edmund Kells, a New Orleans dentist, was credited with putting the radiograph to practical use in dentistry. Kells made numerous presentations to organized dental groups and was instrumental in convincing many dentists that they should use **oral radiography** as a diagnostic tool. At that time, it was customary to send the patient to a hospital or physician's office on those rare occasions when dental radiographs were prescribed.

Because x-rays are invisible, scientists and researchers working in the field of radiography were not aware that continued exposure produced accumulations of radiation effects in the body and, therefore, could be dangerous to both patient and radiographer. When radiography was first put to use in treatment diagnoses, it was common practice for the dentist or dental assistant to help a patient hold the film in place while making the exposure. These oral health care professionals were exposing themselves to unnecessary radiation. Frequent repetition of this practice endangered their health and may have led to permanent injury or death. Beginning in 1901 William Herbert Rollins, a dentist and physician, recognized these dangers with publications alerting the profession to the need for radiation protection. Unfortunately, his advice was not taken seriously by many of his fellow practitioners for some time. Fortunately, although the hazards of prolonged exposure to radiation are not completely understood, scientists have learned how to reduce them drastically by proper use of fast film and digital sensors, safer x-ray machines, and strict adherence to safety protocol.

A significant advancement in the goal of reducing radiation exposure came in 1913 when William David Coolidge, working for General Electric Company, introduced the hot cathode tube. The x-ray output of the so-called Coolidge tube could be predetermined and accurately controlled, greatly reducing the amount of radiation exposure to the patient. To further promote the safe use of radiation in the diagnoses of oral disease, Howard Riley Raper, at Indiana Dental College, wrote the first dental radiology textbook, *Elementary and Dental Radiology,* to assist practitioners in developing prudent use of radiation. Raper is also credited with having introduced the profession to the bitewing radiographic technique in 1925.

Table 1–1 ▪ lists noteworthy scientists and researchers and their contributions to dental radiology.

Dental X-ray Machines

Today, it can be assumed that every dental office in the United States that offers comprehensive oral health care to patients will have safe x-ray equipment. It is worth noting that initially few hospitals and only the most progressive physicians and dentists possessed x-ray equipment. This limited use of dental radiography can be attributed to the fact that the early equipment was primitive and sometimes dangerous. X-rays were sometimes used for entertainment purposes by charlatans at fairgrounds, so people often associated them with quackery. Resistance to change, ignorance, apathy, and fear delayed the widespread acceptance of radiography in dentistry for years.

Dental x-ray machines manufactured before 1920 were an electrical hazard to oral health care professionals because of open, uninsulated high-voltage supply wires. A few years after his introduction of the Coolidge tube, Coolidge and General Electric introduced the Victor CDX shockproof dental x-ray machine. The x-ray tube and high-voltage transformer were placed in an oil-filled compartment that acted as a radiation shield and electrical insulator. Modern x-ray machines use this same basic construction. Variable, high-kilovoltage machines were introduced in the mid-1950s, allowing increased target–image receptor distances to be used, which in turn increased the use of the paralleling technique.

Major progress has been made in restricting the size of the x-ray beam. One such development was the replacement of the pointed **cone** through which x-rays pass from the tube head toward the patient by open cylinders. When the pointed cones were first used, it was not realized that the x-rays were scattered through contact with the material of the cones. Because cones were used for so many years, many still refer to the open cylinders or rectangular tubes as cones. The term **position indicating device (PID)** is more descriptive of its function of directing the x-rays, rather than of its shape. A further improvement has been the introduction of rectangular lead-lined PIDs. This shape limits the size of the x-ray beam that strikes the patient to the actual size and shape of the image receptor (Figure 1–3 ▪).

Panoramic radiography was introduced in 1948, but didn't become popular until the 1960s with the introduction of the panoramic dental x-ray machine. Panoramic dental x-ray machines are capable of exposing the entire dentition and surrounding structures on a single image. Most oral health care practices today have a panoramic x-ray machine.

Practice Point

Never hold the film packet or digital sensor in the patient's oral cavity during the exposure. If the patient cannot tolerate placement of the image receptor or hold still throughout the exposure, the patient's parent or guardian may have to assist or an extraoral radiograph may have to be substituted. The parent or guardian should be protected with lead or lead equivalent barriers such as an apron or gloves when they will be in the path of the x-ray beam.

Table 1–1 Noteworthy Scientists and Developments in Dental Radiography

Name	Event	Year
W. C. Roentgen	Discovered x-rays	1895
O. Walkhoff	First prototype of a dental radiograph	1896
C. E. Kells	May have taken first dental radiograph in the United States Promoted the use of radiography in dentistry	1896
W. H. Rollins	An early advocate for radiation safety	1901
A. Cieszyński	Applied "rule of isometry" to bisecting technique	1907
W. D. Coolidge	Introduced the hot cathode tube	1913
H. R. Raper	Wrote first dental x-ray textbook Introduced bitewing radiographs	1913 1924
F. W. McCormack	Developed paralleling technique	1920
G. M. Fitzgerald	Designed a "long-cone" to use with the paralleling technique	1947
	Introduction of panoramic radiography	1948
	Introduction of "D" speed film	1955
	Introduction of "E" speed film	1981
Francis Mouyen	Developed the first digital imaging system called RadioVisioGraphy	1987
	CT imagery introduced for dentistry as CBCT	1997
	Introduction of "F" speed film	2000

As **digital imaging** continues to develop, exciting advances in the development of imaging systems that allow for enhanced two- and three-dimensional images are being used in the diagnosis and treatment of dental conditions, particularly implant evaluation and orthodontic interventions. Medical imaging modalities such as tomography and computed tomography (CT scans), methods of imaging a single selected plane of tissues, have been used to assist dentists with complex diagnosis and treatment planning since the early 1970s. Because these medical imaging modalities deliver high radiation doses, sometimes up to 600 times more than a panoramic radiograph, the 1997 development of cone beam volumetric imaging (CBVI) [now commonly referred to as **cone beam computed tomography (CBCT)**] with lower radiation doses (4 to 15 times that required for a panoramic radiograph) for dental application is purported to become the gold standard of diagnosis for certain dental applications in the very near future.

Dental X-ray Film

Although today it is increasingly common to see paperless dental practices equipped with computers and image receptors that allow for the digital capture of radiographic images, film has been the standard for producing dental radiographs since 1896. Early dental **x-ray film** packets consisted of glass photographic plates wrapped in black paper and rubber. In 1913, the Eastman Kodak Company marketed the first hand-wrapped, moisture-proof dental x-ray film packet. It was not until 1919 that the first machine-wrapped dental x-ray film packet became commercially available (also from Kodak).

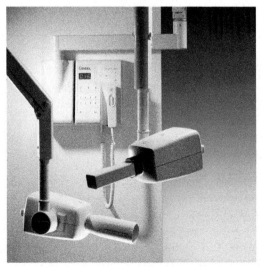

FIGURE 1–3 **Comparison of circular and rectangular PIDs.**
(Courtesy of Gendex Dental Corporation.)

Early film had emulsion on only one side and required long exposure times. Today, both sides of the dental x-ray film are coated with emulsion allowing for an exposure of only a fraction of the amount of radiation required to expose those early films. Film speeds continue to evolve, requiring less and less radiation.

Digital Image Receptors

Digital imaging systems (see Chapter 8) replace film as the image receptor with a **sensor**. In 1987, Francis Mouyen, a French dentist, introduced the use of a digital radiography system marketed for dental imaging, called RadioVisioGraphy. The first digital sensor was bulky and had limitations. Since that time image sensors have been improved and are now comparable to film in dimensions of the exposed field of view and approach film in overall radiographic quality. Their advantages include a reduction in radiation dosage, the elimination of film and processing chemistry, and the subsequent disposal of film packaging materials such as lead foils and spent processing chemicals, both potentially hazardous to the environment.

Dental X-ray Techniques

The two basic dental x-ray techniques still in use today were introduced early in the history of dental radiography. In 1907, A. Cieszyński, a Polish engineer, applied the *rule of isometry* to dental radiology, which was the basis for the **bisecting technique**. The bisecting technique was the only method used for many years. The search for a less-complicated technique that would produce better radiographic images more consistently resulted in the development of the **paralleling technique** by dentist Franklin McCormack in 1920. It was McCormack's dentist son-in-law G. M. Fitzgerald who, in 1947, designed a long "cone" PID that made the paralleling technique more practical.

Advances in Dental Radiographic Imaging

Radiography, aided by the introduction first of transistors and then computers, has allowed for significant radiation reduction in modern x-ray machines. Advances in two-dimensional and three-dimensional imaging systems are predicted to move radiography away from static interpretation of pictures of images and toward representations of real-life conditions. This introduction of a computed approach with its almost instantaneous images is sure to benefit the quality of oral health care.

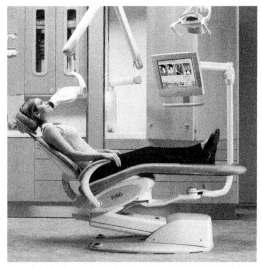

FIGURE 1–4 Radiography in a modern oral health care practice. (Courtesy of Gendex Dental Corporation.)

Today, an oral health care practice would find it impossible to provide patients with comprehensive dental care without dental radiographs (Figure 1–4 ■). Many practices have multiple intraoral dental x-ray machines (one in each operatory) and supplement these with a panoramic x-ray machine. Although no diagnosis can be based solely on radiographic evidence without a visual and physical examination, many conditions might go undetected if not for radiographic examinations (Box 1–1).

The discovery of x-radiation revolutionized the practice of preventive oral health care. Future technological advances undoubtedly will improve both the diagnostic use and the safety of radiography in the years ahead.

Box 1–1 Uses of Dental Radiographs

- Detect, confirm, and classify oral diseases and lesions
- Detect and evaluate trauma
- Evaluate growth and development
- Detect missing and supernumerary (extra) teeth
- Document the oral condition of a patient
- Educate patients about their oral health

REVIEW—Chapter summary

Wilhelm Conrad Roentgen's discovery of the x-ray on November 8, 1895, revolutionized the methods of practicing medicine and dentistry by making it possible to visualize internal body structures noninvasively. The usefulness of the x-ray as a diagnostic tool was recognized almost immediately as scientists and researchers contributed to its advancement. The use of radiographs in medical and dental diagnostic procedures is now essential.

In the early 1900s, scientists and researchers working in the field of radiography were not aware that radiation could be dangerous, resulting in exposure to unnecessary radiation. Early x-ray equipment was primitive and sometimes dangerous. Today improved equipment, advanced techniques, and educated personnel make it possible to obtain radiographs with high diagnostic value and minimal risk of unnecessary radiation to patient or operator.

Although film has been the standard image receptor since the discovery of the x-ray, dental practices continue to adopt the computer and digital sensor as the method of acquiring a dental radiographic image. Digital imaging reduces patient radiation dose, eliminates the need to maintain an inventory of film and processing chemistry, and avoids disposal of the potentially environmental hazards of lead foils and spent processing chemicals.

The two basic techniques for acquiring a dental radiographic image are the bisecting technique and the paralleling technique.

Cone beam computed tomography (CBCT) produces two- and three-dimensional images for dental diagnosis. This technology may become the gold standard for diagnosing certain dental conditions.

RECALL—Study questions

For questions 1–5, match each term with its definition.

a. Radiograph
b. Radiography
c. Radiology
d. Roentgen ray
e. X-ray

_____ 1. The study of x-radiation
_____ 2. Image or picture produced by x-rays
_____ 3. An older term given to x-radiation in honor of its discoverer
_____ 4. The original term Roentgen applied to the invisible ray he discovered
_____ 5. The making of radiographs by exposing and processing x-ray film

6. Who discovered the x-ray?
a. C. Edmund Kells
b. Howard Riley Raper
c. Franklin McCormack
d. Wilhelm Conrad Roentgen

7. When were x-rays discovered?
a. 1695
b. 1795
c. 1895
d. 1995

8. Who is believed to have exposed the prototype of the first dental x-ray film?
a. A. Cieszyński
b. Otto Walkhoff
c. G. M. Fitzgerald
d. Francis Mouyen

9. Who is considered by many to be an early advocate for the science of radiation protection?
a. Otto Walkhoff
b. A. Cieszyński
c. C. Edmund Kells
d. Franklin McCormack

10. Which of the following is credited with making early dental x-ray machines safer?
a. Replacing the open-ended PID with a pointed PID
b. Assisting the patient with holding the film in the mouth
c. Using the bisecting technique instead of the paralleling technique
d. Placing the x-ray tube in an oil-filled compartment

11. Replacing a pointed "cone" position indicating device (PID) with an open-cylinder PID reduces the radiation dose to a patient *because* open-cylinder PIDs eliminate scattered x-rays through contact with the cone material.
a. Both the statement and reason are correct and related.
b. Both the statement and reason are correct but NOT related.
c. The statement is correct, but the reason is NOT.
d. The statement is NOT correct, but the reason is correct.
e. NEITHER the statement NOR the reason is correct.

12. When was film speed "D" introduced?
a. 1919
b. 1955
c. 1981
d. 2000

13. Which imaging modality will most likely become the gold standard for imaging certain dental conditions in the near future?
a. RadioVisioGraphy
b. Crooke's tubes
c. Roentgenographs
d. Cone beam computed tomography

14. List five uses of dental radiographs.
a. _____
b. _____
c. _____
d. _____
e. _____

REFLECT—Case study

Your patient today tells you that she recently watched a television documentary on the dangers of excess radiation exposure. To put this patient at ease, develop a brief conversation between you and the patient based on your reading of this chapter, explaining how historical developments have increased dental radiation safety.

RELATE—Laboratory application

Perform an inventory of the x-ray machine used in your facility. Using the historical lessons learned in this chapter, identify the parts of the x-ray machine, type of film or digital sensor used, and the safety protocol and posted exposure factors in place. Specifically list the following:

a. Unit manufacturer

Using the Internet, research the manufacturer's website to determine the company origin. How old is the company? Are they a descendant of an original manufacturer? Who developed the design for the x-ray unit produced today? Do they offer different unit designs? What is the reason your facility chose this model?

b. Shape and length of the PID

Does the machine you are observing reduce radiation exposure? Why or why not? Why was the PID you are observing chosen over other shapes and lengths?

c. Names of the dials on the control panel.

How does this differ from the dental x-ray machines used in dental practices in the early 1900s? What exposure factors are inherent to the unit, and what factors may be varied by the radiographer? What are the advantages and disadvantages to using an x-ray machine where the exposure settings are fixed? Variable?

d. What are the recommended exposure settings for various types of radiographs? How do these differ from the settings used by the first dentists to use x-rays in practice in the early 1900s?

e. Describe the film or digital sensor used to produce a radiographic image.

What is the film size and speed, and how is it packaged? Does the film or sensor used in your facility allow you to produce a quality radiograph using the least amount of radiation possible? What is the rationale for using this film type in your facility?

f. Are the safety protocols regarding x-ray machine operation known to all operators? How is this made evident? List the safety protocols in place in your facility.

RESOURCES

American Dental Association Council on Scientific Affairs. (2012). The use of cone beam tomography in dentistry. An advisory statement from the American Dental Association Council on Scientific Affairs. *Journal of the American Dental Association*, 143, 899–902.

Bird, D. L., & Robinson, D. S. (2015). Radiographic imaging. *Modern dental assisting* (11th ed.). St. Louis, MO: Elsevier.

Horner, K., Drage, N., & Brettle, D. (2008). *21st century imaging.* London: Quintessence Publishing.

Thomson, E. M. (2012). Innovation improves safety. Dimensions in Brief. An educational supplement sponsored by Carestream Dental. *Dimensions of Dental Hygiene, 10*[supplement], 5–13.

Thunthy, K. H. (2013). Early pioneers of oral & maxillofacial radiology. American Academy of Oral and Maxillofacial Radiology. Retrieved from AAOMR website: www.aaomr.org.

Visit www.pearsonhighered.com/healthprofessionsresources to access the student resources that accompany this book. Simply select Dental Hygiene from the choice of disciplines. Find this book and you will find the complementary study tools created for this specific title.

Characteristics and Measurement of Radiation

CHAPTER OUTLINE

OBJECTIVES

Following successful completion of this chapter, you should be able to:

1. Define the key terms.
2. Draw and label a typical atom.
3. Describe the process of ionization.
4. Differentiate between radiation and radioactivity.
5. List the properties shared by all energies of the electromagnetic spectrum.
6. Explain the relationship between wavelength and frequency.
7. List the properties of x-rays.
8. Identify and describe the two processes by which kinetic energy is converted to electromagnetic energy within the dental x-ray tube.
9. Differentiate between primary, secondary, and scatter radiations.
10. List and describe the four possible interactions of dental x-rays with matter.
11. Define the terms used to measure x-radiation.
12. Match the *Système Internationale* (SI) units of x-radiation measurement to the corresponding traditional terms.
13. Identify three sources of naturally occurring background radiation.

KEY TERMS

Absorbed dose
Absorption
Atom
Binding energy
Coulombs per kilogram (C/kg)
Dose equivalent
Effective dose equivalent
Electromagnetic radiation
Electromagnetic spectrum
Electron
Energy
Energy levels

Exposure
Frequency
Gray (Gy)
Ion
Ion pair
Ionization
Ionizing radiation
Kinetic energy
Microsievert (μSv)
Molecule
Neutron
Particulate radiation
Photon
Primary radiation

Proton
Rad
Radiation
Radioactivity
Radiolucent
Radiopaque
Rem
Roentgen (R)
Scatter radiation
Secondary radiation
Sievert (Sv)
Useful beam
Velocity
Wavelength

Introduction

The word *radiation* is attention grabbing. When news headlines incorporate words such as *radiation, radioactivity,* and *exposure,* the reader often pays attention to what follows. Patients tend to link dental x-rays with other types of radiation exposure they read about or see on television and online. Patients assume that oral health care professionals who are responsible for taking dental x-rays are knowledgeable regarding all types of ionizing radiation exposures and can adequately answer their questions. Although the study of quantum physics is beyond the scope of this book, it is important that dental assistants and dental hygienists understand what dental radiation is, what it can do, and what it cannot do. This chapter explores the characteristics of x-radiation and looks at where dental x-rays fit in relation to other types and sources of radiations.

Prior to studying the production of x-rays, a radiographer should have a base knowledge of atomic structure. A scientist understands that the world consists of matter and energy. Matter is defined as anything that occupies space and has mass. Things that are seen and can be recognized are forms of matter. **Energy** is defined as the ability to do work and overcome resistance. Heat, light, electricity, and x-radiation are forms of energy. Matter and energy are closely related. Energy is produced whenever the state of matter is altered by natural or artificial means. The difference between water, steam, and ice is the amount of energy associated with molecules. Such an energy exchange is produced within the x-ray machine and will be discussed later.

Atomic Structure

To understand radiation, an understanding of atomic structure is required. Currently there are 118 known basic elements that occur either singly or in combination in natural forms. Each element is made up of atoms. An **atom** is the smallest particle of an element that still retains the properties of the element. If any given atom is split, the resulting components no longer retain the properties of the element. Atoms are generally combined with other atoms to form molecules. A **molecule** is the smallest particle of a substance that retains the properties of that substance. A simple molecule such as sodium chloride (table salt) contains only two atoms, whereas a complex molecule like deoxyribonucleic acid (DNA) may contain hundreds of atoms.

Atoms are extremely minute and are composed of three basic building blocks: electrons, protons, and neutrons.

- **Electrons** have a negative charge and are constantly in motion orbiting the nucleus.
- **Protons** have a positive charge; the number of protons in the nucleus of an element determines its atomic number.
- **Neutrons** have no charge.

The atom's arrangement in some ways resembles our solar system (Figure 2–1 ■). The atom has a nucleus as its center or sun, and the electrons revolve around it like planets. The protons and neutrons form the central core or nucleus of the atom. The electrons orbit around the nucleus in paths called shells or energy levels. Normally, the atom is electrically neutral, having equal numbers of protons in its nucleus and electrons in orbit.

The nucleus of all atoms, except hydrogen, contains at least one proton and one neutron (hydrogen in its simplest form has only a proton). Some atoms contain a very high number of each. The electrons and the nucleus normally remain in the same position relative to one another. To accommodate the electrons revolving about the nucleus, the larger atoms have several concentric orbits at various distances from the nucleus. These are referred to as electron shells, which some chemists call **energy levels**. The innermost level is referred to as the K shell, the next as the L shell, and so on, up to seven shells (see Figure 2–1).

Electrons are maintained in their orbits by the positive attraction of the protons, known as **binding energy**. The binding energy of an electron is strongest in the intermost K shell and becomes weaker in the outer shells.

Ionization

Atoms that have gained or lost electrons are electrically unstable and are called ions. An **ion** is a charged particle. It helps to understand the formation of ions by reviewing the

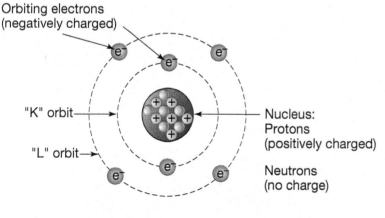

Orbiting electrons
(negatively charged)

"K" orbit

"L" orbit

Nucleus:
Protons
(positively charged)

Neutrons
(no charge)

⊕ Protons ◯ Neutrons e⁻ Electrons

FIGURE 2–1 Diagram of carbon atom. In the neutral atom, the number of positively charged protons in the nucleus is equal to the number of negatively charged orbiting electrons. The innermost orbit or energy level is the K shell, the next is the L shell, and so on.

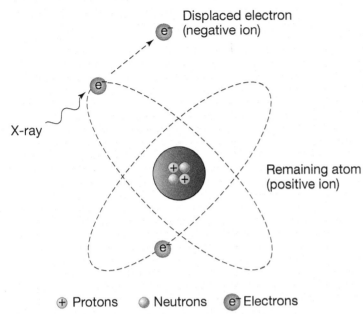

Displaced electron
(negative ion)

X-ray

Remaining atom
(positive ion)

⊕ Protons   ◯ Neutrons   ⓔ Electrons

FIGURE 2–2 Ionization is the formation of ion pairs. When an atom is struck by an x-ray, an electron may be dislodged, and an ion pair results.

normal structural arrangement of the atom. The atom normally has the same number of protons (positive charges) in the nucleus as it has electrons (negative charges) in the orbital levels. When one of these electrons is removed from its orbital level in a neutral atom, the remainder of the atom loses its electrical neutrality.

An atom from which an electron has been removed has more protons than electrons, is positively charged, and is called a positive ion. The negatively charged electron that has been separated from the atom is a negative ion. The positively charged atom ion and the negatively charged electron ion are called an **ion pair**. **Ionization** is the formation of ion pairs. When an atom is struck by an x-ray photon (a quantum or particular amount of electromagnetic radiation), an electron may be dislodged and an ion pair created (Figure 2–2 ▪). As high-energy electrons travel on, they push out electrons (like charges repel) from the orbits of other atoms, creating additional ion pairs. These unstable ions attempt to regain electrical stability by combining with another oppositely charged ion.

Ionizing Radiation

Radiation is defined as the emission and movement of energy through space in the form of **electromagnetic radiation** (x- and gamma rays) or **particulate radiation** (alpha and beta particles). Any radiation that produces ions is called **ionizing radiation**. Only a portion of the radiation portrayed on the electromagnetic spectrum, the x-rays and the gamma and cosmic rays, are of the ionizing type. In dental radiography, concern is limited to the changes that may occur in the cellular structures of the tissues as the ions are produced by the passage of x-rays through the cells. The mechanics of biologic tissue damage are explained in Chapter 5.

Radioactivity

Radioactivity is defined as the process whereby certain unstable elements undergo spontaneous disintegration (decay) in an effort to attain a stable nuclear state. Unstable isotopes are radioactive and attempt to regain stability through the release of energy, by a process known as decay. Dental x-rays do not involve radioactivity.

Electromagnetic Radiation

Electromagnetic radiation is the movement of wavelike energy through space as a combination of electric and magnetic fields. Electromagnetic radiations are arranged in an orderly fashion according to their energies in what is called the **electromagnetic spectrum** (Figure 2–3 ▪). The electromagnetic spectrum consists of an orderly arrangement of all known radiant energies. X-radiation is a part of the electromagnetic spectrum, which also includes gamma rays, ultraviolet rays, visible light, infrared, microwave, and radio waves. All energies of the electromagnetic spectrum share the following properties:

- Travel at the speed of light in a vacuum
- Have no electrical charge
- Have no mass
- Pass through space as particles and in a wavelike motion
- Give off an electrical field at right angles to their path of travel and a magnetic field at right angles to the electric field
- Have energies that are measurable and different

Electromagnetic radiations display two seemingly contradictory properties. They are believed to move through space as both a particle and a wave. Particle or quantum theory assumes the electromagnetic radiations are particles, or quanta. These particles are called photons. **Photons** are bundles of energy that travel through space at the speed of light. Wave theory assumes that electromagnetic radiation is propagated in the form of waves similar to waves resulting from a disturbance in water. Electromagnetic waves exhibit the properties of wavelength, frequency, and velocity.

- **Wavelength** is the distance between two similar points on two successive waves (Figure 2–4 ▪). Wavelength may be measured in the metric system or in angstrom (Å) units (1 Å is about 1/250,000,000 inch or 1/100,000,000 cm). The shorter the wavelength, the more penetrating the radiation.
- **Frequency** is a measure of the number of waves that pass a given point per unit of time. The special unit of frequency is the hertz (Hz). One hertz equals one cycle per second. The higher the frequency, the more penetrating the radiation.
- **Velocity** refers to the speed of the wave. In a vacuum, all electromagnetic radiations travel at the speed of light (186,000 miles/sec or 3×10^8 m/sec).

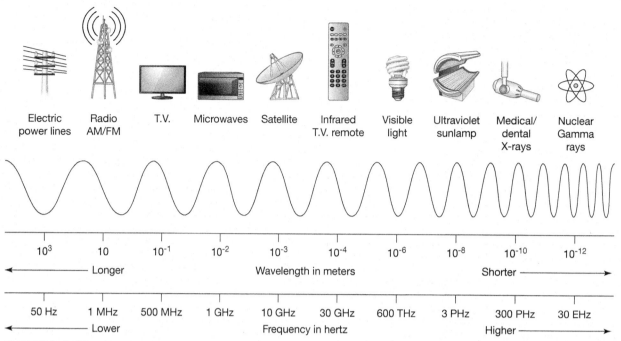

Electric power lines	Radio AM/FM	T.V.	Microwaves	Satellite	Infrared T.V. remote	Visible light	Ultraviolet sunlamp	Medical/ dental X-rays	Nuclear Gamma rays

10^3	10	10^{-1}	10^{-2}	10^{-3}	10^{-4}	10^{-6}	10^{-8}	10^{-10}	10^{-12}

← Longer   Wavelength in meters   Shorter →

50 Hz	1 MHz	500 MHz	1 GHz	10 GHz	30 GHz	600 THz	3 PHz	300 PHz	30 EHz

← Lower   Frequency in hertz   Higher →

FIGURE 2–3 The electromagnetic spectrum. Electromagnetic radiations are arranged in an orderly fashion according to their energies. (Cliparts from openclipart.org)

No clear-cut separation exists between the various radiations represented on the electromagnetic spectrum; consequently, overlapping of the wavelengths is common. Each form of radiation has a range of wavelengths. This accounts for some of the longer infrared waves being measured in meters, whereas the shorter infrared waves are measured in angstrom units. It therefore follows that all x-radiations are not the same wavelength. The longest of these are the Grenz rays, also called *soft radiation,* that have only limited penetrating power and are unsuitable for exposing dental radiographs. The wavelengths used in diagnostic dental radiography range from about 0.1 to 0.5 Å and are classified as *hard radiation,* a term meaning radiation with great penetrating power. Still shorter wavelengths are produced by supervoltage machines when greater penetration is required, as in some forms of medical therapy and industrial radiography.

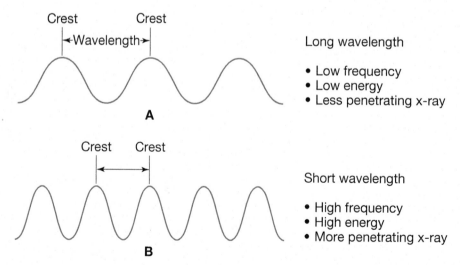

Crest   Crest
←Wavelength→

Long wavelength

- Low frequency
- Low energy
- Less penetrating x-ray

A

Crest   Crest

Short wavelength

- High frequency
- High energy
- More penetrating x-ray

B

FIGURE 2–4 Differences in wavelengths and frequencies. Only shortest wavelengths with extremely high frequency and energy are used to expose dental radiographs. Wavelength is determined by distances between crests. Observe that distance is shorter in (**B**) than in (**A**). Photons that comprise dental x-ray beam are estimated to have over 250 million such crests per inch. Frequency is number of crests of a wavelength passing a given point per second.

Properties of X-rays

X-rays are believed to consist of minute bundles (or quanta) of pure electromagnetic energy called photons. These have no mass, are invisible, and cannot be sensed. Because they travel at the speed of light (186,000 miles/sec or 3×10^8 meters/sec), these x-ray photons are often referred to as "bullets of energy." X-rays have the following properties; they:

- Are invisible
- Travel in straight lines
- Travel at the speed of light in a vacuum
- Have no mass
- Have no charge
- Interact with matter, causing ionization
- Can penetrate opaque tissues and structures
- Can affect photographic film emulsion (producing a latent image)
- Can affect biological tissue

X-ray photons have the ability to pass through gases, liquids, and solids. The ability to penetrate materials or tissues depends on the wavelength of the x-ray and the thickness and density of the object. The composition of the object or the tissues determines whether the x-rays will penetrate and pass through it or whether they will be absorbed in it. Materials that are extremely dense and have a high atomic weight will absorb more x-rays than thin materials with low atomic numbers. This partially explains why dense structures such as bone and enamel appear **radiopaque** (white or light gray) on a radiograph, whereas the less dense pulp chamber, muscles, and skin appear **radiolucent** (dark gray or black).

Production of X-rays

X-rays are generated inside an x-ray tube located in the tube head of a dental x-ray machine (see Chapter 3). X-rays are produced whenever high-speed electrons are abruptly stopped or slowed down. Bodies in motion have **kinetic energy** (from the Greek word *kineticos*, "pertaining to motion"). In a dental x-ray tube, the kinetic energy of electrons is converted to electromagnetic energy by the formation of general or *bremsstrahlung* radiation (German for "braking") and characteristic radiation.

- **General/bremsstrahlung radiation** is produced when high-speed electrons are stopped or slowed down by the tungsten atoms of the target located inside the dental x-ray tube. Referring to Figure 2–5 ▪, observe that

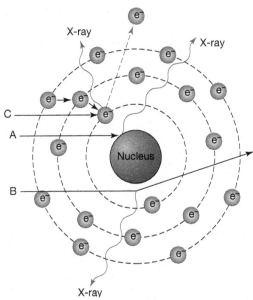

FIGURE 2–5 **General and characteristic radiation.** High-speed electron (**A**) collides with nucleus, and all its kinetic energy is converted into a single x-ray. High-speed electron (**B**) is slowed and bent off its course by positive pull of the nucleus. Kinetic energy lost is converted into an x-ray. Impact from both A and B electrons produce general radiation. High-speed electron (**C**) hits and dislodges a K-shell electron. Another electron in an outer shell quickly fills void, and x-ray energy is emitted. Impact from C electron produces characteristic radiation.

the impact from both (A) and (B) electrons produce general/bremsstrahlung. When a high-speed electron collides with the nucleus of an atom in the target metal, as in (A), all its kinetic energy is transferred into a single x-ray photon. In (B), a high-speed electron is slowed and bent off its course by the positive pull of the nucleus. The kinetic energy lost is converted into an x-ray. The majority of x-rays produced by dental x-ray machines are formed by general/bremsstrahlung radiation.

- **Characteristic radiation** is produced when the high-speed electrons collide with an orbiting K-shell electron of the tungsten target as shown in Figure 2–5 (C). The K-shell electron is dislodged from the atom. Another electron in an outer shell quickly fills the void, and x-ray energy is emitted as a result of this rearrangement. The x-rays produced in this manner are called characteristic x-rays. Characteristic radiation can only be produced when the x-ray machine is operated at or above 70 kilovolts (kV) because a minimum force of 69 kV is required to dislodge a K-shell electron from a tungsten atom. Characteristic radiation accounts for a small portion of the x-rays produced in a dental x-ray machine.

Description of X-ray Forms

It is important to understand that the terms *general radiation* and *characteristic radiation* describe the types of radiation generated inside the dental x-ray machine tube head. Once these x-rays leave the tube head this energy will have the opportunity to interact with the matter it comes in contact with, described in the next section. To better comprehend the interaction of x-rays with matter it is necessary to know these x-ray descriptions.

- **Primary radiation** refers to the general and/or characteristic radiation generated at the target (explained in detail in Chapter 3) inside the x-ray tube head. Primary radiation refers to the **useful beam**, or those x-rays generated for the purpose of making a radiographic image.
- **Secondary radiation** refers to radiation formed as a result of primary radiation striking and interacting with matter. In dental radiography matter consists of the patient's tissues, including soft tissues of the head and neck region and hard tissues of the teeth and facial bones. A description of this interaction follows in the next section. Secondary radiation is not as penetrating as primary radiation and is not only not useful in the production of a radiographic image but also can contribute to a lowered contrast, poor quality image.
- **Scatter radiation** is a form of secondary radiation and results when x-rays are deflected in all directions as a result of interaction with matter. Like secondary radiation, scatter radiation is not useful and can cause unnecessary additional exposure to patient tissues and to the careless operator who does not follow safety protocols to protect oneself during operation of the x-ray machine.

Interaction of X-rays with Matter

Once the primary radiation leaves the dental x-ray tubehead, the beam of x-rays passing through matter is weakened and gradually disappears. Such a disappearance is referred to as **absorption** of the x-rays. When so defined, absorption does not imply an occurrence such as a sponge soaking up water, but instead refers to the process of transferring the energy of the x-rays to the atoms of the material through which the x-ray beam passes. The basic method of absorption is ionization.

When a beam of x-rays passes through matter, four possibilities exist:

1. **No interaction.** The x-ray photon can pass through an atom unchanged and no interaction occurs (Figure 2–6 ■).
   - In dental radiography about 9 percent of the x-rays pass through the patient's tissues without interaction.
2. **Coherent scattering.** When a low-energy x-ray photon passes near an atom's outer electron, it may be scattered without loss of energy (see Figure 2–6). The incoming x-ray photon interacts with the electron by causing the electron to vibrate at the same frequency as the incoming x-ray photon. The incoming x-ray photon ceases to exist. The vibrating electron radiates another x-ray photon of the same frequency and energy as the original incoming x-ray photon, but in a different direction. Essentially, the new x-ray photon is scattered but unmodified.

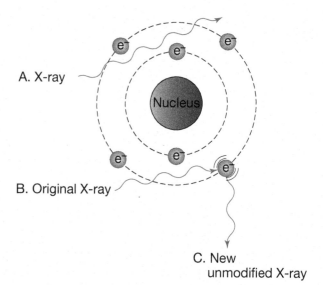

FIGURE 2–6 No interaction and coherent scattering. (**A**) X-ray photon passes through an atom unchanged. (**B**) Coherent scattering. Incoming x-ray photon causes an electron to vibrate at the same frequency as the incoming x-ray. Incoming x-ray photon ceases to exist. Vibrating electron radiates a new, unmodified x-ray photon that is scattered in a different direction (**C**).

- Coherent scattering accounts for about 8 percent of the interactions of matter with the dental x-ray beam.

3. **Photoelectric effect.** The photoelectric effect is an all-or-nothing energy loss. The x-ray photon imparts all its energy to an orbital electron of an atom. This x-ray photon, because it consisted only of energy in the first place, simply vanishes. The electromagnetic energy of the x-ray photon is imparted to the electron in the form of kinetic energy of motion and causes the electron to fly from its orbit with considerable speed. The result is the creation of an ion pair (Figure 2–7 ■). Remember, the basic method of the interaction of x-rays with matter is the formation of ion pairs. The high-speed electron (called a photoelectron) knocks other electrons from the orbits of other atoms (forming secondary ion pairs) until all its energy is used up.

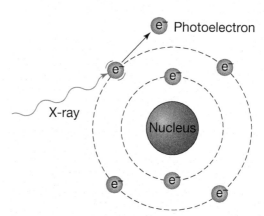

FIGURE 2–7 Photoelectric effect. Incoming x-ray photon collides with an orbital electron and imparts electromagnetic energy to the electron in the form of kinetic energy causing electron to fly from its orbit, creating an ion pair.

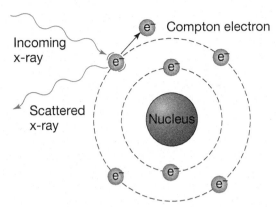

FIGURE 2–8 Compton scattering. Incoming x-ray photon collides with an orbital electron and ejects it. But, only a part of the x-ray energy is transferred to the electron, and a new, weaker x-ray photon is formed and scattered in a new direction.

The positive ion combines with a free electron, and the absorbing material is restored to its original condition.

- Photoelectric effect accounts for about 30 percent of the interactions of matter with the dental x-ray beam.

4. **Compton scattering** is similar to the photoelectric effect in that the x-ray photon interacts with an orbital electron and ejects it. But in the case of Compton scattering, only a part of the x-ray energy is transferred to the electron, and a new, weaker x-ray photon is formed and scattered in a new direction (Figure 2–8 ■). This secondary radiation may travel in a direction opposite that of the original x-ray photon. The new x-ray photon may undergo another Compton scattering or it may be absorbed by a photoelectric effect interaction. The positive ion combines with a free electron, and the absorbing material is restored to its original condition.

- Compton scattering accounts for about 60 percent of the interactions of matter with the dental x-ray beam.

A question often asked is, "Do x-rays make the material they pass through radioactive?" The answer is no. Dental x-rays have no effect on the nucleus of the atoms they interact with. Therefore, equipment, walls, and patients do not become radioactive after exposure to x-rays.

Units of Radiation

The terms used to measure x-radiation are based on the ability of the x-ray to deposit its energy in air, tissues of the body, or other substances. The International Commission on Radiation Units and Measurements (ICRU) has established standards that clearly define radiation units and radiation quantities (Table 2–1 ■). The most widely accepted terms used for radiation units of measurement come from the *Système Internationale* (SI), a modern version of the metric system. The SI units are

1. Coulombs per kilogram (C/kg)
2. Gray (Gy)
3. Sievert (Sv)

Older traditional units of radiation measurement are now considered obsolete, although they may be observed in some older documents, especially those dealing with health and safety. The traditional units are

1. Roentgen (R)
2. Rad (radiation absorbed dose)
3. Rem (roentgen equivalent [in] man)

The American Dental Association requires the use of SI terminology on national board examinations, and following the guidelines established by the National Institute of Standards and Technology, this book will use SI units first, followed by the traditional units in parentheses. It is important to note that numerical amounts of radiation expressed using SI terminology do not equal the numerical amounts of radiation expressed using the traditional terms. For example, consider the metric system of measurement adopted by most of the world with the traditional units of measurement used in the United States. Whereas the global community uses the term *kilometers* to measure distance,

Table 2–1 Radiation Measurement Terminology

Quantity	SI Unit	Traditional Unit
Exposure	coulombs per kilogram (C/kg)	roentgen (R)
Absorbed dose	gray (Gy)	rad
Dose equivalent	Sievert (Sv)	rem

in the United States distance is more commonly measured in *miles*. One kilometer does not equal 1 mile. Instead, 1 kilometer equals approximately 0.62 mile. When comparing measurements of radiation, it is important to remember that SI units and traditional units, although measuring the same thing, are not equal numerically.

An x-ray, or any form of radiation, has many properties such as wavelength, frequency, and energy. By using standardized units it is possible to obtain, or measure, the quantity (or value) of these properties.

For practical x-ray protection measurement the following are used:

1. Exposure
2. Absorbed dose
3. Dose equivalent
4. Effective dose equivalent

Exposure

Exposure can be defined as the measurement of ionization in air produced by x- or gamma rays. The unit for measuring exposure is **coulombs per kilogram (C/kg)** [**roentgen (R)**]. A coulomb is a unit of electrical charge. Therefore, the unit C/kg measures electrical charges (ion pairs) in a kilogram of air. Coulombs per kilogram (roentgen) only applies to x- or gamma radiation and only measures ion pairs in air. It does not measure the radiation absorbed by body tissues or other materials. Therefore, it is not a measurement of dose. An exposure does not become a dose until the radiation is absorbed in the tissues.

Absorbed Dose

Absorbed dose is defined as the amount of energy deposited in any form of matter, such as the tissues of the head and neck of a patient, by any type of radiation (alpha or beta particles, x- or gamma rays). The unit for measuring absorbed dose is the **gray (Gy)** (**rad**). One gray equals 100 rads.

Dose Equivalent

Dose equivalent is used to compare the biological effects of the various types of radiations. It is defined as the product of the absorbed dose times a biological-effect qualifying or weighting factor determined by quantum physicists. Because this weighting factor for x-rays is always "1", absorbed dose and dose equivalent are numerically equal. The unit for measuring dose equivalent is the **sievert (Sv)** (**rem**). One Sv equals 100 rem.

When pertaining to exposures from dental radiation, smaller multiples of these units are commonly used. For example, milligray (mGy) and millisievert (mSv), where the prefix *milli-* means "one-thousandth of," would more likely be used to express the smaller dose of radiation used in most dental applications.

Effective Dose Equivalent

To aid in making more accurate comparisons between different radiographic exposures, the **effective dose equivalent** is used to compare the risk of the radiation exposure producing a biological response. The effective dose equivalent is expressed using the term **microsievert (μSv)**, meaning 1/1,000,000 of a sievert. The effective dose equivalent compensates for the differences in area exposed and the tissues, critical or less critical, that may be in the path of the x-ray beam. For example, comparing the skin dose of a chest x-ray, which is approximately 0.2 mSv, to a single periapical dental radiograph, which is approximately 2.5 mSv, does not take into consideration that the chest x-ray delivers its dose to a larger area and to more tissues than the single periapical radiograph. Using the measurement for effective dose equivalent, the chest x-ray is approximately 80 μSv, and the effective dose equivalent for the single periapical using F-speed film and a round PID is approximately 1.3 μSv.

Background Radiation

Dental x-rays are considered man-made exposure, and when grouped with all other man-made medical applications of ionizing radiation including computed tomography (CT scans), nuclear medicine, and fluoroscopy, account for approximately 48 percent of the total radiation exposure to the U.S. population. Consumer products and activities such as building materials, cigarette smoking, and combustion of fossil fuels make up another approximately 2 percent of man-made exposure to the population. However, it is important to note that the remaining approximately 50 percent of total exposure to the population comes from naturally occurring background sources of radiation (Figure 2–9 ■). Background radiation is defined as ionizing radiation that is always present in our environment. The human race has always been subjected to exposure from natural background radiations originating from the following sources:

- Cosmic radiations from outer space
- Terrestrial radiations from the earth and its environments, including radon gas
- Background radiations from naturally occurring radionuclides (unstable atoms that emit radiations) that are deposited in our bodies by inhalation and ingestion

The average natural background radiation level for the U.S. population is estimated to be about 3.1 mSv or 310 mrem (millirem) per year or about 0.9 mSv per day. The exact amount varies according to locality, the amount of radioactive material present, and the intensity of the cosmic rays—this intensity varies according to altitude and latitude. For example, persons living on the Colorado plateau receive an increased dose of background radiation because of the increased cosmic radiation at the higher altitude and more terrestrial radiation from soils enriched in naturally occurring uranium that raise the levels of terrestrial radionuclides located there.

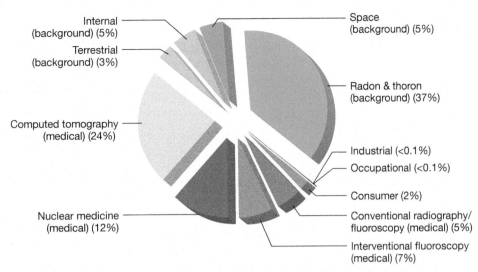

FIGURE 2–9 **Annual effective dose equivalent of ionizing radiations.** Approximate percentage of exposure of the U.S. population to background and man-made radiations. (Reprinted with permission of the National Council on Radiation Protection and Measurements, http://NCRPonline.org)

REVIEW—Chapter summary

The three basic building blocks of an atom are protons, neutrons, and electrons. Protons and neutrons make up the central nucleus, which is orbited by the electrons revolving in the energy levels. Binding energy between the positive protons and negative electrons maintains the electrons in their orbits.

Ionization is the formation of charged particles called ions. A positive ion and a negative ion are called an ion pair. Ionizing radiation is defined as any radiation that produces ions.

Electromagnetic radiation is the movement of wavelike energy through space. Electromagnetic radiation exhibits the properties of wavelength, frequency, and velocity. Short-wavelength x-rays, called hard radiation, are very penetrating. Long-wavelength x-rays, called soft radiation, have limited penetrating power. The electromagnetic spectrum consists of an orderly arrangement of all known radiant energies.

X-rays are invisible, travel in straight lines at the speed of light, interact with matter causing ionization, affect photographic film, and affect living tissue. An x-ray produced when high-speed electrons are abruptly stopped or slowed down is general radiation. An x-ray produced when high-speed electrons dislodge a K-shell electron in the tungsten target material within the x-ray tube is characteristic radiation. An x-ray generated for the purpose of exposing diagnostic radiographs is described as primary radiation. X-rays may pass through a patient with no interaction, or they may be absorbed by the photoelectric effect or scattered by either Compton scattering or coherent scattering. Following interaction with matter, radiation is described as secondary or scatter radiation.

Four x-ray measurement quantities are exposure (C/kg; roentgen), absorbed dose (gray/Gy; rad), dose equivalent (sievert/Sv; rem), and effective dose equivalent (microsievert/μSv).

All medical uses of ionizing radiations including dental and medical x-rays, CT scans, and nuclear medicine account for approximately 48 percent of the U.S. population's total ionizing radiation exposure. Background radiation consisting of cosmic radiation, terrestrial radiations and radon gas, and naturally occurring radionuclides accounts for 50 percent of the total radiation exposure. The average natural background radiation level for the U.S. population is estimated to be about 3.1 mSv or 310 mrem per year or 0.9 mSv per day.

RECALL—Study questions

1. What term describes the smallest particle of an element that retains the properties of that element?
   a. Atom
   b. Molecule
   c. Photon
   d. Isotope

2. Draw and label a typical atom.

3. Which of these subatomic particles carries a negative electric charge?
   a. Proton
   b. Neutron
   c. Nucleus
   d. Electron

4. Radiant energy sufficient to remove an electron from its energy level of an atom is called
   a. atomic.
   b. electronic.
   c. ionizing.
   d. ultrasonic.

5. What term describes the process by which unstable atoms undergo decay in an effort to obtain nuclear stability?
   a. Absorption
   b. Radioactivity
   c. Radiolucent
   d. Ionization

6. Which of the following is NOT a property shared by all energies of the electromagnetic spectrum?
   a. Have energy that is measurable and different
   b. Travel in a pulsating motion at the speed of sound
   c. Have no mass
   d. Emit an electrical field at right angles to the path of travel

7. What is the distance between two similar points on two successive waves called?
   a. Wavelength
   b. Frequency
   c. Velocity
   d. Energy level

8. Which of these electromagnetic radiations has the shortest wavelength?
   a. Radar
   b. Ultraviolet rays
   c. Infrared rays
   d. X-rays

9. Which of these forms of radiation has the greatest penetrating power?
   a. Visible light
   b. X-rays
   c. Sunlamp
   d. Radio waves

10. List five properties of x-rays.
    a. _____
    b. _____
    c. _____
    d. _____
    e. _____

11. Radiation produced when high-speed electrons are stopped or slowed down by the tungsten atoms of the target inside the dental x-ray tube is called
    a. general/bremsstrahlung.
    b. characteristic.
    c. coherent.
    d. Compton.

12. X-rays generated for the purpose of making a radiographic image are described as
    a. scatter radiation.
    b. tertiary radiation.
    c. primary radiation.
    d. secondary radiation.

13. What is the most likely result when dental x-rays interact with matter?
    a. No interaction
    b. Photoelectric effect
    c. Coherent scattering
    d. Compton scattering

14. Which of these terms is the unit used to measure radiation exposure?
    a. Angstrom (Å)
    b. Coulombs per kilogram (roentgen)
    c. Sievert (rem)
    d. Gray (rad)

15. The *Système Internationale* (SI) unit that has replaced the traditional unit rem is
    a. coulomb/kilogram.
    b. gray.
    c. rad.
    d. sievert.

16. Diagnostic tests used in medical and dental health care that employ ionizing radiations account for what approximate percentage of the overall total exposure to the U.S. population?
    a. 8 percent
    b. 28 percent
    c. 48 percent
    d. 88 percent

17. List three sources of background radiation.
    a. _____
    b. _____
    c. _____

18. What is the average annual amount of background radiation to which the U.S. population is exposed?
    a. 2.1 mSv (210 millirem)
    b. 3.1 mSv (310 millirem)
    c. 4.1 mSv (410 millirem)
    d. 6.1 mSv (610 millirem)

REFLECT—Case study

While taking a full mouth series of dental radiographs, your patient begins to consider the number of radiographs that are exposed in this operatory on a daily basis and decides to ask you questions such as, "How long do you have to wait after each exposure before you can reenter the room?" and "Are the walls and equipment in this room becoming radioactive from all the exposures taken in here?" Prepare a conversation with this patient addressing these two questions based on what you learned in this chapter on radiation physics.

RELATE—Laboratory application

Research recent media (magazine or journal articles, newspaper reports, or the Internet) for stories on radiation exposure. Select an article for review, and critique the article for clarity and readibility. Summarize how many different types of radiation are mentioned in the article. What units of radiation measurement does the author use? Does the article use these terms in a manner that is appropriate for what is being measured? Consider the type of radiation described in this article. Is it naturally occuring/background radiation or a radiation generated by an artificial or man-made source? How many key words from this chapter can you find in the article? Anticipate what questions a patient may have for you after reading this article.

RESOURCES

Bushberg, J. T., Seibert, J. A., Leidholdt, E. M., Jr., & Boone, J. M. (2012). *The essential physics of medical imaging*, 3rd ed. Philadelphia, PA: Lippincott Williams & Wilkins.

National Council on Radiation Protection and Measurements. (2009). *Report No 160: Ionizing radiation exposure of the population of the United States.* Bethesda, MD: Author.

Taylor, B. N., & Thompson, A. (Eds.). (2008). *The international system of units (SI)* [special publication 330]. Washington, DC: National Institute of Standards and Technology, U.S. Dept. of Commerce.

Thompson, A., & Taylor, B. N. (2016). *The NIST Guide for the use of the International System of Units (SI)* [special publication 811]. Gaithersburg, MD: National Institute of Standards and Technology.

United States Nuclear Regulatory Commission. (2015, September 30). Backgrounder on biological effects of radiation. Retrieved from the Nuclear Regulatory Commission website: http://www.nrc.gov/reading-rm/doc-collections/fact-sheets/bio-effects-radiation.html

United States Nuclear Regulatory Commission. (2015, December 2). Standards for protection against radiation, Title 10, Part 20, of the *Code of Federal Regulations.* Retrieved from the Nuclear Regulatory Commission website: http://www.nrc.gov/reading-rm/doc-collections/cfr/part020/part020-1201.html

United States Nuclear Regulatory Commission, Office of Public Affairs. (2003). *Fact sheet.* Washington, DC: Author.

White, S. C., & Pharoah, M. J. (2014). Physics. *Oral radiology. Principles and interpretation* (7th ed.). St. Louis, MO: Mosby Elsevier.

Visit www.pearsonhighered.com/healthprofessionsresources to access the student resources that accompany this book. Simply select Dental Hygiene from the choice of disciplines. Find this book and you will find the complementary study tools created for this specific title.

③

The Dental X-ray Machine: Components and Function

CHAPTER OUTLINE

OBJECTIVES

Following successful completion of this chapter, you should be able to:

1. Define the key terms.
2. Identify the three major components of a dental x-ray machine.
3. Identify and explain the function of the five controls on the control panel.
4. Differentiate between alternating and direct electrical currents.
5. Explain the relationships between AC and DC dental x-ray machines and their effects on film and digital image receptors.
6. State the three conditions necessary for the production of x-rays.
7. Draw and label the parts of a dental x-ray tube.
8. Trace the production of x-rays from the time the exposure button is activated until x-rays are released from the tube.
9. Demonstrate, in sequence, steps in operating a dental x-ray machine.

KEY TERMS

Alternating current (AC)
Anode
Cathode
Central ray
Collimator
Control panel
Direct current (DC)
Electron cloud
Exposure button

Extension arm
Filament
Filter
Focal spot
Focusing cup
Impulse
Kilovolt peak (kVp)
Milliampere (mA)
Polychromatic
Port

Primary beam
Radiator
Step-down transformer
Step-up transformer
Target
Thermionic emission
Tube head
Useful beam
X-ray tube
Yoke

Introduction

At the time of exposure, the radiographer who activates the exposure button is responsible for the radiation dose the patient incurs. The role of exposing dental radiographs is an important one for a dental assistant and dental hygienist, making it essential that these professionals understand how an x-ray machine works to produce ionizing radiation. To operate dental x-ray equipment safely and competently, a radiographer needs to develop a base knowledge of the components of the dental x-ray machine and possess an understanding of how these components work together to produce ionizing radiation. This chapter explains the dental x-ray machine, its components, and its function.

Dental X-ray Machine Components

Although dental x-ray machines vary in size and appearance, they have similar structural components (Figure 3–1 ■). A dental x-ray machine typically consists of three parts:

1. **Control panel,** which contains the master switch and other exposure buttons
2. **Extension arm** or bracket, which enables the tube head to be positioned
3. **Tube head,** which contains the x-ray tube from which x-rays are generated

Control Panel

Dental x-ray machines require an electrical source to produce x-rays. The electric current enters the control panel either through a cord plugged into a grounded outlet in the wall or through a direct connection to a power line in the wall. The control panel may be integrated with the extension arm and tube head for ease of access during exposures (Figure 3–2 ■), or it may be remote from the unit, mounted on a shelf or wall (Figure 3–3 ■). One control panel may serve two or more tube heads. In the past, dental x-ray machines were readily available with variable milliamperage and kilovoltage controls of the incoming electricity that an operator would adjust manually (Figure 3–4 ■). Increasingly more common are dental x-ray machines with these controls preset by the manufacturer (Figure 3–5 ■). If the milliamperage and the kilovoltage are preset by the manufacturer, the control panel will indicate at what variables these units are preset. Five major controls may be operated or will be preset on dental x-ray machines: (1) the line switch to an electrical outlet, (2) the milliampere selector, (3) the kilovoltage selector, (4) the timer, and (5) the exposure button. The function of each of these is discussed next.

LINE SWITCH The line switch on the control panel of a dental x-ray machine may be a toggle switch that can be flicked on or off with light finger pressure, or it may be an ON/OFF push button or a keypad (see Figure 3–5). When the line

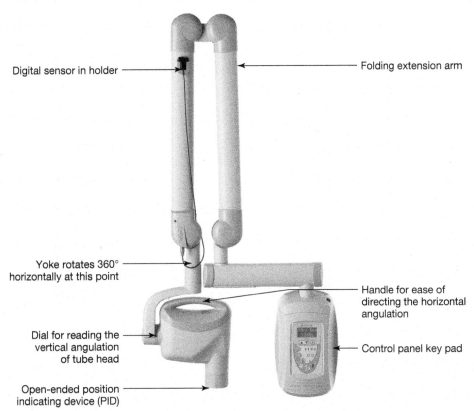

FIGURE 3–1 **Typical wall-mounted dental x-ray machine.** (Courtesy of Progeny, A Midmark Company.)

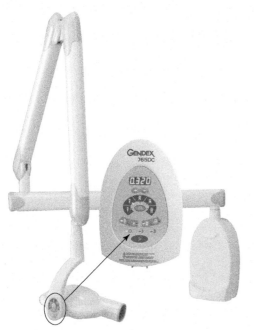

FIGURE 3–2 **Control panel integrated with tube head support.** (Courtesy of Gendex Dental Corporation.)

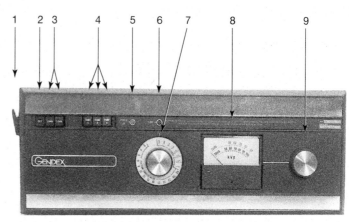

FIGURE 3–4 **Control panel of a dental x-ray machine that allows for manual adjustment of exposure variables.** (**1**) Exposure button holder, (**2**) main ON/OFF switch, (**3**) mA control, (**4**) x-ray tube selector (this master control accommodates three remote tube heads), (**5**) power ON light, (**6**) x-ray emission indicator light, (**7**) timer control, (**8**) kVp meter, (**9**) kVp control. This control panel allows settings of 50 kVp to 90 kVp at 15 mA, and 50 kVp to 100 kVp at 10 mA.

switch is in the ON position, an indicator light turns on, indicating the machine is operational.

MILLIAMPERE SELECTOR The **milliampere (mA)** measures the amount of current passing through the wires of the circuit. The mA is set by turning a selector knob, depressing the marked push button, or touching a keypad (see Figure 3–4). On a dental x-ray machine with the mA preset, its activation is connected directly to the ON/OFF switch (see Figure 3–5). The mA determines the available number of free electrons at the cathode filament and, therefore, the amount of x-rays that will be produced.

KILOVOLT PEAK SELECTOR The voltmeter measures the difference in current potential or voltage across an x-ray tube. A **kilovolt peak (kVp)** selector in the form of a dial, push button, knob, or keypad enables an operator to change the peak kilovoltage (see Figure 3–4). On a dental x-ray machine with the kVp preset, its activation is connected

directly to the ON/OFF switch (see Figure 3–5). The kVp determines the speed of electrons traveling toward the target on the anode and, therefore, the penetrating ability of the x-rays produced.

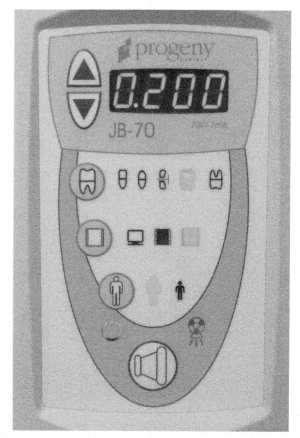

FIGURE 3–5 **Control panel with preset exposure variables.** Note the preset milliamperage and kilovoltage values and the preprogrammed settings for various teeth and patient types.

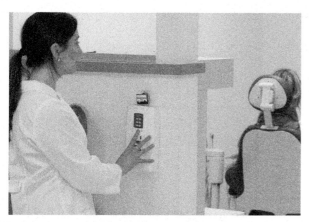

FIGURE 3–3 Control panel mounted in protected area.

TIMER The timer is set by turning the selector knob, depressing the marked push button, or touching a keypad (see Figure 3–5). The timer serves to regulate the duration of the interval that the current will pass through the x-ray tube. Dental x-ray machines are equipped with accurate electronic timers. Timer settings may be in fractions of a second or **impulses.** There are 60 impulses in a second. For example, a 1/10-second exposure lasts 6 impulses, a 1/5-second exposure lasts 12 impulses, and so forth. X-ray machines with electronic digital timers are accurate to 1/100-second intervals and work well with digital radiography systems. The time selected determines the duration of the exposure.

EXPOSURE BUTTON Depressing the **exposure button** activates the x-ray production process. The exposure button may be located on the handle of the timer cord (Figure 3–6 ■) or at a remote location in a protected area (see Figure 3–3). If the exposure button is located on the end of the timer cord, the cord must be sufficiently long to enable an operator to step into an area of protection from radiation, usually at least 6 ft (1.83 m) from the source of the x-ray beam. Because the possibility exists that an operator may not utilize the full length of a timer cord to be safely protected from the x-rays generated, an exposure switch permanently mounted to the control panel or wall in a protected area is preferred. In fact, many state regulations now require that the exposure button be permanently mounted in a protected area.

Dental x-ray machines use a "dead-man" exposure switch that automatically terminates the exposure when the operator's finger ceases to press on the timer button. This makes it necessary to maintain firm pressure on the button during the entire exposure. Failure to do so results in the formation of an insufficient number of x-rays to properly expose the image receptor. When the exposure button is activated, the operator will hear an audible beep (required by law) that indicates x-rays are being generated. Additionally, exposure buttons installed directly on the control panel allow an operator to observe an active light indicating that x-rays are being generated.

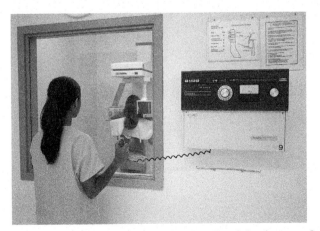

FIGURE 3–6 Exposure button on the handle of the timer cord. Operator is exposing a panoramic radiograph from behind a lead-lined glass window.

The manufacturing trend is toward simpler and automated controls. In addition to preset mA and kVp, many dental x-ray machines now have a default timer that automatically resets itself and does not have to be altered unless a change in the exposure time is desired. Also available are programmable preset exposure settings that an operator can select directly from the tube head for a quick change of settings chairside (see Figure 3–2).

Extension Arm

The folding extension arm is a support from which the tube housing is suspended (see Figure 3–1). The extension arm allows for moving and positioning the tube head. The extension arm is hollow to permit the passage of electrical wires from the control panel to the tube head from one or both sides at a point where the tube head attaches to a yoke. The tube head is attached to the extension arm by means of a **yoke** that can revolve 360 degrees horizontally where it is connected. In addition, the tube head can be rotated vertically within the yoke. All sections of the extension arm and yoke are heavily insulated to protect patient and operator from electrical shock.

Tube Head (Tube Housing)

The tube head (sometimes called tube housing) is a tightly sealed heavy metal (usually cast aluminum), lead-lined housing that contains the dental x-ray tube, insulating oil, and step-up and step-down transformers (Figures 3–7 ■ and 3–8 ■). The metal housing performs several important functions:

1. Protects the x-ray tube from accidental damage
2. Increases the safety of the x-ray machine by grounding its high-voltage components (the x-ray tube and the transformers) to prevent electrical shock
3. Prevents overheating of the x-ray tube by providing a space filled with oil, gas, or air to absorb the heat created during the production of x-rays
4. Lined with lead to absorb any x-rays produced that do not contribute to the primary beam that exits through the port in the direction of the position indicating device (PID)

Older dental x-ray machine tube heads were heavy and bulky. The trend now is toward using lighter weight materials and smaller digital components that reduce the size and

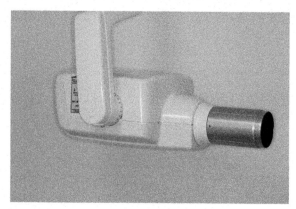

FIGURE 3–7 **Dental x-ray tube head.**

weight of the tube head making it easier for an operator to position (see Figure 3–7).

Electricity

Because electricity is needed to produce dental x-rays, an understanding of basic electrical concepts and terminology is necessary. Electricity can be defined as electrons in motion. Two electrical circuits are used in producing dental x-rays.

1. A filament circuit provides low voltage (3–8 V) to the filament of the x-ray tube to generate a source of electrons needed for the production of x-rays.
2. A high-voltage circuit provides the high voltage (50–100 kV) necessary to accelerate the electrons from the cathode filament to the anode target.

Transformers

A transformer is an electromagnetic device for changing the current coming into the dental x-ray machine. Transformers are required to decrease (step down) or increase (step up) ordinary 110-V or 220-V current that enters the x-ray machine. A **step-down** (low-voltage) **transformer** decreases the voltage from the wall outlet to approximately 5 V, just enough to heat the filament and form an electron cloud. A **step-up** (high-voltage) **transformer** increases the voltage from the wall outlet to approximately 50–100 kVp to propel the electrons toward the target.

Amperage

Amperage measures the number of electrons that move through a conductor. The ampere is the unit of quantity of electric current. An increase in amperage results in an increase

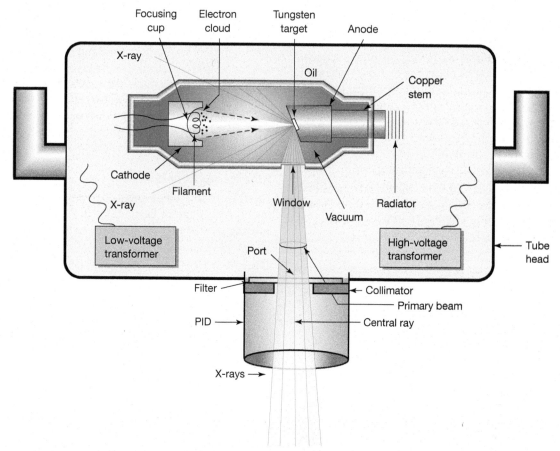

FIGURE 3–8 **Dental x-ray tube head, containing x-ray tube, transformers, and oil.** When an electric current is applied to the high-voltage circuit (between cathode and anode), boiled off electrons are propelled from the cathode to the target on the anode, producing heat and x-rays. The 20-degree angle of the anode target directs most of the x-rays through the window toward the port opening. These x-rays make up the primary x-ray beam. The central ray is the x-ray in the center of the primary beam.

in the number of electrons available to travel from the cathode to anode when the tube is activated. This results in a production of more x-rays. Only a small current is required to generate the number of electrons necessary to produce dental x-rays; therefore, the term *milliampere* (mA), denoting 1/1,000 ampere, is used. Dental x-ray machines typically operate in ranges from 4 to 15 mA. The setting will vary by manufacturer and is usually preset, although some x-ray machines allow an operator to choose the setting for different exposures.

Voltage

Voltage or volt (V) is the electrical pressure (sometimes called potential difference) between two electrical charges. In the production of x-rays the voltage determines the speed of the electrons when traveling from cathode to anode. This speed of electrons, in turn, determines the energy (penetrating power) of the x-rays produced. When the voltage is increased, the electrons travel faster and produce a harder type of radiation. Because dental x-ray machines operate at very high voltages, it is customary to express voltage in terms of kilovolts. A kilovolt equals 1,000 V and is abbreviated kV. The voltage varies during an exposure, producing a **polychromatic** beam (x-rays of many different energies) containing high-energy rays and also containing soft rays that have barely enough energy to escape from the tube. The highest voltage to which the current in the tube rises during an exposure is called the kilovolt peak (kVp), as mentioned. So if the x-ray machine controls are set at 70 kVp (70,000 V), the maximum x-ray energy that can be produced during this exposure is 70 kV. Dental x-ray machines may operate within a range of 50 kVp to 100 kVp. The setting will vary by manufacturer and is usually preset, although some x-ray machines allow an operator to choose the setting for different exposures.

Electrical Current

Dental x-ray machines are available that utilize either direct or indirect electrical current. Electrical current can flow steadily in one direction (direct current) or flow in pulses and change directions (alternating current). With the increase in the adoption of digital imaging, an understanding of the role these different electrical currents play in producing quality radiographs while reducing patient radiation exposure is important.

> **Alternating current (AC)** has two phases—one positive and the other negative—and alternates between these phases (Figure 3–9 ■). U.S. household electric current is called 60-cycle alternating current because the current changes its direction of flow 60 times a second. During the time that the x-ray tube is producing x-rays, the flow of current changes from negative to positive 60 times per second. The dental x-ray machine can produce x-rays only when the current is in the positive direction—or half of the 1/60-second cycle time frame—essentially 1/120 second. This alternation in current causes the dental x-ray machine to produce x-rays in a series of bursts, or pulses, rather than in a continuous flow.

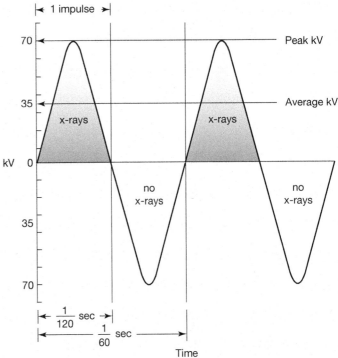

FIGURE 3–9 Illustration of alternating current (AC). Dental x-ray machines using AC are programmed to only produce x-rays when the current is flowing in the appropriate positive–negative direction resulting in bursts or pulses of x-ray output. Note that the kilovoltage fluctuates from 0 to a peak (kVp) of 70, but the actual output is closer to the average 35kV.

Direct current (DC) flows continuously in one direction eliminating the alternating cycles resulting in a more constant and even flow of x-rays (Figure 3–10 ■).

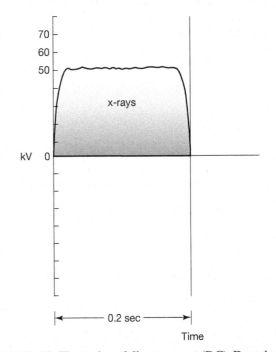

FIGURE 3–10 Illustration of direct current (DC). Dental x-ray machines using DC produce a more constant flow of x-rays and at a more consistent kilovoltage.

This unidirectional current is similar to that produced by battery power. This direct current flow causes a dental x-ray machine to produce x-rays at a more consistent wavelength.

Digital Trends

Historically dental x-ray machines have utilized alternating current. As dentistry moves away from film-based radiography and increasingly adopts digital imaging, manufacturers are marketing DC dental x-ray machines as better suited to exposing digital image receptors. Both AC and DC dental x-ray machines produce acceptable quality radiographic images when paired with film and when paired with digital image receptors, although there are differences. Specifically, DC dental x-ray machines may produce more consistent exposures at the very short exposure times associated with digital radiography and may slightly reduce patient radiation exposure.

The differences between AC and DC dental x-ray machines are explained here. An AC dental x-ray machine set at 70 kVp, for example, where the *p* indicates that the "peak" or most output the machine will have during the exposure is 70 kilovolts. However, because the dental x-ray machine cannot "know" at what point along this continuum of peak and trough of the alternating current wave that the exposure button will be activated, not all the x-ray energy generated will be of the same wavelength. Wavelength is determined by the kV setting. So if the wave of the alternating current rises and falls between 0 and 70 kV (in this example) it can be concluded that the actual kilovolts will more likely be an average between 0 and 70; in this case 35 kV (see Figure 3–9). This explains why the dial on an AC dental x-ray machine indicates a setting of kilovoltage "peak" because this setting does not represent a continuous output at the 70 kV level.

All this is important for three reasons:

1. Digital image receptors require a shorter radiation exposure time than do film receptors. Although the exposure timer on an AC dental x-ray machine currently set for exposure of film can be decreased to a lower setting to accommodate a digital image receptor, the results may be inconsistent. During the very short exposure time required for digital imaging, the exposure button may be initiated at any point along the peak and trough of the electric current wave. Depending on at what point in the wave the exposure is initiated, the amount of "usable" positive energy can vary due to the very short exposure time. As illustrated in Figure 3–11 ■, this can result in a one-third difference between the amount of radiation reaching the image receptor.
2. DC dental x-ray machines may in fact slightly reduce patient radiation exposure. Lower wavelength energy unneccesarily increases patient radiation exposure. All dental x-ray machines limit this long wavelength, low energy from exiting the tube head.

However, consider that in the example just presented, an AC dental x-ray machine set at 70 kVp actually exposes the patient to a low, average 35 kV energy. A direct current dental x-ray machine set at 70 kV would essentially expose the patient to a more homogeneous output of high energy. This fact influences the settings typically used by AC and DC machines. DC dental x-ray machines typically operate at 50 to 65 kV; AC machines typically operate at 70 kVp or higher.

3. Kilovoltage settings effect radiographic image contrast. A thorough discussion of image contrast follows in Chapter 4, but it can be noted here that AC dental x-ray machines generally produce images with higher contrast than those produced by DC machines; however, this difference is often negligible because DC machines typically operate at a lower kilovoltage setting than AC machines, which essentially can balance out and result in similar contrast levels.

The X-ray Tube

X-rays are produced when a stream of high-speed electrons is suddenly stopped or slowed down and diverted off course. Three conditions must exist for x-rays to be produced:

1. An available source of free electrons
2. High voltage to impart speed to the electrons
3. A target that is capable of stopping/slowing the electrons

The x-ray tube and the circuits within the machine are designed to create these conditions. The **x-ray tube,** located inside the tube head, is a glass bulb from which the air has been pumped to create a vacuum. A **cathode** (the negative electrode) and an **anode** (the positive electrode) are sealed within the vacuum tube, and the two protruding arms of the electrodes permit the passage of the current through the tube with minimum resistance. In most dental x-ray tubes, the space between the electrodes is less than 1 inch (25.4 mm; Figure 3–12 ■).

Cathode

The purpose of the cathode is to supply the electrons necessary to produce x-rays. The cathode, or negative electrode, consists of a thin, spiral filament of tungsten wire. This **filament** wire, when heated to incandescence (red hot and glowing), produces the electrons. This process is known as **thermionic emission.** Tungsten's high atomic number makes it possible to liberate electrons, through thermionic emission, from their orbital shells when the metal is heated. The released electrons form an **electron cloud** around the wire. The wire filament is recessed into a molybdenum **focusing cup,** which directs the electrons toward the target on the anode (Figure 3–13 ■). The mA setting accurately controls the thermionic emission and therefore controls the quantity of free electrons available.

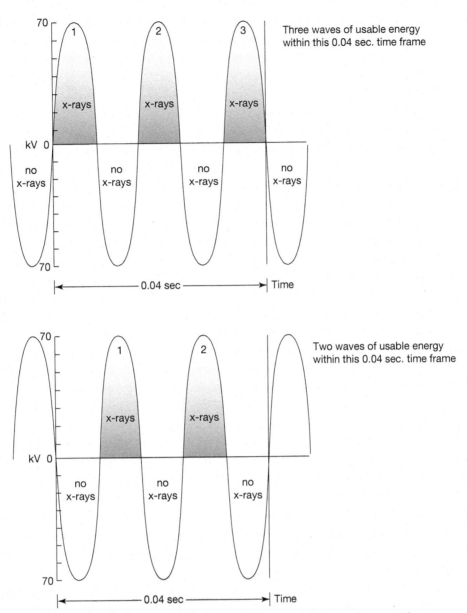

Three waves of usable energy within this 0.04 sec. time frame

Two waves of usable energy within this 0.04 sec. time frame

FIGURE 3–11 Illustration of difference in usable energy at low-exposure settings. Exposures can vary by one-third depending on when initiated during AC current.

Anode

The kilovoltage imparts speed to the electrons sending them flying across the tube from cathode to anode. The purpose of the anode is to provide a target to stop or significantly slow the high-velocity electrons, converting their kinetic energy into x-rays (electromagnetic energy). The anode, or positive electrode, consists of a copper bar with a tungsten plate imbedded in the end that faces the focusing cup of the cathode. This tungsten plate, called the **target,** is set into the copper at an angle of 20 degrees to the cathode. This angle directs most of the x-rays produced in one direction to become the **primary beam.** The **focal spot** is a small rectangular area on the target of the anode to which the focusing cup directs the electron beam. The focal spot size plays an important role in determining radiographic image sharpness (see Chapter 4).

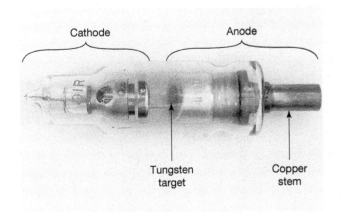

FIGURE 3–12 Dental x-ray tube.

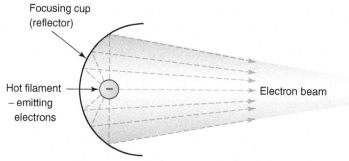

Focusing cup
(reflector)

Hot filament
– emitting
electrons

Electron beam

FIGURE 3–13 **Formation of electron beam by focusing cup.** A focusing cup, within the cathode structure into which the filament is placed, focuses the electron beam in a similar manner as light is focused by a flashlight reflector. When the high-voltage circuit is activated, the free electrons are accelerated toward the focal spot on the anode target.

A Summary of the Principles of X-ray Tube Operation

Before x-ray production can begin, the dental x-ray machine must be turned on. If not preset by the manufacturer, the radiographer must set the correct milliamperage and kilovoltage by adjusting the control panel dials. The radiographer will then set the correct exposure time. The process of x-ray production is initiated by firmly pressing the exposure button. This permits the current to enter the filament circuit of the x-ray machine. A step-down transformer reduces the voltage before it enters the filament circuit and heats the filament of the cathode to incandescence, separating electrons from their atoms. The degree to which the filament is heated depends on the milliamperage setting; the higher the milliamperes, the more electrons in the electron cloud. These electrons are now in a state of excitation as they hover around the tungsten filament recessed in the molybdenum focusing cup. After just a fraction of a second time delay, the line current enters the cathode–anode high-voltage circuit. A step-up transformer then increases the voltage to impart sufficient force to propel the free electrons toward the focal spot on the target at the anode. These high-velocity electrons are stopped or slowed when they collide with the tungsten atoms in the target resulting in the production of general radiation (also called bremsstrahlung radiation) and/or characteristic radiation. (See Chapter 2.) The kinetic energy (the high-velocity electrons) is converted into approximately 1 percent x-ray energy. The other 99 percent of the kinetic energy generated is lost as heat energy.

The metal tungsten (symbol W and atomic number 74; also known as wolfram) is ideally suited for use in the filament and target because it can withstand extremely high temperatures (melting point 3370°C). Because it is subjected to such extreme heat and has low thermal conductivity, the tungsten plate is imbedded in a core of copper. Copper is highly conductive and carries the heat generated off to the **radiator,** which is just outside the tube (see Figure 3–8). The large mass of copper conducts the heat out of the tube into a radiator that transfers the heat to the oil, gas, or air that surrounds the tube.

Although the target is set into the copper stem at an angle to direct most of the x-rays toward the window (a thin area in the glass tube) located at a point where the emission of x-rays is most intense, some x-rays are emitted out in all directions within the tube housing. These x-rays are absorbed by the glass tube, oil, air, wires, transformers, and the tube head lining. If the tube head is properly sealed, the **port** (an opening in the tube housing) is the only place through which the x-rays can escape the tube head (see Figure 3–8). This port is covered by a permanent seal of glass, beryllium, or aluminum. The PID fits over the port and can be positioned to aim the primary beam of x-rays in the desired direction. After completion of the predetermined exposure, the high-voltage current is automatically shut off, and x-ray production stops.

The X-ray Beam

X-rays are produced in 360-degree direction at the focal spot of the target; however, because of the angle of the anode, a high concentration of x-rays travels toward the port opening of the tube head. Only a beam of radiation the size of the port seal is allowed to exit the tube head. The other x-rays are stopped (absorbed) by the contents and walls of the tube head. After the x-ray beam exits through the port, the lead **collimator** (see Chapter 6) further restricts the x-ray beam to the desired size.

The x-ray beam is cone shaped because x-rays travel in diverging straight lines as they radiate from the focal spot. This beam of x-rays is called the primary beam or the **useful beam.** The primary beam is the original useful beam of x-rays that originates at the focal spot and emerges through the port of the tube head. The **central ray** consists of the x-rays in the center of the primary beam.

The x-ray beam formed at the focal spot is polychromatic, consisting of x-rays of various wavelengths. Only x-rays with sufficient energy to penetrate oral structures are useful for diagnostic dental radiographs. X-rays of low penetrating power (long wavelength) add to patient dose but not to the information recorded on the image receptor. To remove the soft x-rays, a thin sheet of aluminum called a **filter** is placed in the path of the x-ray beam (see Chapter 6).

Procedure 3–1

Operation of a dental x-ray machine

1. Turn power on. A light on the control panel will indicate that the machine is ready to operate.
2. Unless preset by the manufacturer, select mA and kV best suited for the exposure to be made.
3. Set timer for the desired exposure time.
4. Place the image receptor into the holding device and position in the patient's oral cavity.
5. Utilizing the extension arm and yoke, adjust the tube head by aligning the PID so that the central beam of radiation is directed toward the center of the image receptor at the appropriate horizontal and vertical angulations.
6. Move to the appropriate protected location away from the tube head.
7. Depress the exposure button and hold it down firmly until the exposure is completed. The audible signal and x-ray exposure indicator light will activate for the duration of the exposure.
8. Remove the image receptor and holder from the patient's oral cavity after the exposure.
9. When the procedure is complete, fold the tube head support extension arm into the closed, neutral position.
10. Turn off the power to the x-ray machine.

The intensity of the x-ray beam refers to the quantity and quality of the x-rays. Quantity refers to the number of x-rays in the beam. Quality refers to the energy strength or penetrating ability of the x-ray beam (see Chapter 4). Intensity is defined as the product of the number of x-rays (quantity) and the energy strength of the x-rays (quality) per unit of area per unit of time. Intensity of the x-ray beam is affected by milliamperage, kilovoltage, exposure time, and distance.

Operation of the Dental X-ray Machine

The specific steps to safe and effective use of a dental x-ray machine are outlined in the operating manual provided by the manufacturer. All persons operating an x-ray machine should study the manual until they are thoroughly familiar with the operational capability and maintenance requirements of the machine. To achieve consistent results, follow a systematic and orderly process (Procedure 3–1). Additionally, whenever x-ray exposures are made on patients, it is assumed here and in all subsequent instructions that:

- The radiographer is competent and can follow radiation safety protocol. (Some states require anyone

Practice Point

For maximum effectiveness in exposing dental radiographs, prepare the patient and the x-ray equipment and set the controls on the x-ray unit prior to positioning the image receptor in the oral cavity. Following an orderly sequence reduces the likelihood of errors and retakes.

placing and exposing dental radiographs to successfully complete a training course in radiation safety and protection protocols.)
- The radiographer performs all radiographic procedures in accordance with federal, state, and local regulations and recommendations.
- Infection control is maintained throughout the procedure (see Chapter 9).
- The procedure has been explained, and the patient has given consent.
- The patient has received instructions and is able to cooperate with the procedure.
- Image receptor holding devices are utilized for all intraoral radiographs.

REVIEW—Chapter summary

All x-ray machines, regardless of size and voltage range, operate similarly and have the same components (control panel, extension arm, and tube head) and electrical parts (x-ray tube, low- and high-voltage circuits, and a timing device).

The control panel may be integrated with the x-ray machine tube head support, or it may be remote from the unit, mounted on a shelf or wall. There are five major controls, some of which will be preset by a manufacturer or may be selected by an operator: (1) the line switch to the electrical outlet, (2) the milliampere selector, (3) the kilovoltage selector, (4) the timer, and (5) the exposure button. A folding extension arm is a support from which the tube housing is suspended. The tube head is a tightly sealed heavy metal housing that contains the dental x-ray tube, insulating oil, and step-up and step-down transformers.

Three conditions must exist to produce x-rays: (1) a source of free electrons, (2) high voltage to accelerate them, and (3) a target to stop them. The dental x-ray tube creates these conditions. X-rays are produced only when the unit is turned on and a firm pressure is maintained on the exposure button. Dental x-ray machines operate on alternating current (AC) or direct current (DC). DC dental x-ray machines are proving to be ideally matched to exposing digital image receptors. Electric current flows into the x-ray machine and proceeds either through the step-down transformer or the step-up transformer. The step-down transformer reduces the electric current from the wall outlet to heat the filament inside the focusing cup of the cathode (negative) side of the tube. Thermionic emission results in freed electrons available to make x-rays. The step-up transformer increases the electric current to impart kinetic energy to the freed electrons to cause them to propel across the tube to strike the target (at the focal spot) on the anode (positive) side of the tube.

The degree to which the filament is heated and, therefore, the quantity of electrons made available depends on the milliamperage setting. Quantity refers to the number of x-rays in the beam; the higher the milliamperage, the more electrons available. The penetrating ability or quality of the resultant x-rays is determined by the kilovoltage setting; the higher the kilovoltage, the more penetrating the x-rays. The beam of radiation that exits the port seal of the tube head is the primary or useful beam. The polychromatic beam must be filtered to allow only x-rays with sufficient energy to reach the oral structures.

A radiographer must be familiar with the operation of a dental x-ray machine, and a patient must understand the procedure and provide consent. To achieve consistent results, follow a systematic and orderly procedure.

RECALL—Study questions

1. The x-ray machine component that allows an operator to position the tube head is called the
   a. timer cord.
   b. control panel.
   c. dead-man switch.
   d. extension arm.
2. Each of the following EXCEPT one may be located on the control panel. Which one is the EXCEPTION?
   a. mA selector
   b. kV selector
   c. Focusing cup
   d. Line switch
3. To generate a larger quantity of electrons available to produce x-rays, increase the
   a. mA (milliamperage).
   b. kV (kilovoltage).
   c. PID (position indicating device).
   d. DC (direct current).
4. After depressing the exposure button the radiographer will hear an audible beep sound indicating that the
   a. kilovoltage has reached the peak.
   b. x-rays are being generated.
   c. cathode and anode are reversing polarity.
   d. alternating current has been transformed into direct current.
5. Which of the following will step up or step down the current coming into an x-ray machine?
   a. Radiator
   b. Collimator
   c. Transformer
   d. Filter
6. What term describes the electrical pressure (difference in potential) between two electrical charges?
   a. Amperage
   b. Voltage
   c. Ionization
   d. Incandescence

7. What term best describes an x-ray beam that is composed of a variety of energy wavelengths?
   a. Polychromatic
   b. Short scale
   c. Filtered
   d. Collimated
8. Alternating electrical current changes its direction of flow 60 times a second.
   AC dental x-ray machines are ideally suited for use with exposing digital image receptors.
   a. The first statement is true. The second statement is false.
   b. The first statement is false. The second statement is true.
   c. Both statements are true.
   d. Both statements are false.
9. A DC dental x-ray machine that is set at 60 kV would most likely have an x-ray output of
   a. 15 kV.
   b. 30 kV.
   c. 60 kV.
   d. 90 kV.
10. List the three conditions that must exist for x-rays to be produced.
    a. _____
    b. _____
    c. _____
11. Draw and label the parts of a dental x-ray tube.

12. The process of heating the cathode wire filament until red hot and electrons boil off is called
    a. autotransformation.
    b. focusing.
    c. thermionic emission.
    d. kilovoltage peak.

13. Which of these must be charged negatively during the time that the x-ray tube is operating to produce x-rays?
    a. Radiator
    b. Target
    c. Anode
    d. Cathode

14. What term describes the opening in the tube housing that allows the primary beam to exit?
    a. Yoke
    b. Port
    c. Filament
    d. Focusing cup

15. Which of the following removes the low-energy, long-wavelength energy from the beam?
    a. Filter
    b. Collimator
    c. Transformer
    d. Radiator

REFLECT—Case study

To help understand the practical use of altering exposure variables on a dental x-ray machine, consider the following patients with these characteristics:

- A 9-year-old female, height 4' 8" and weight 85 pounds, who has been assessed for bitewing radiographs to determine the evidence of caries
- A 21-year-old male college football player, height 6' 1" and weight 280 pounds, who has been assessed for periapical radiographs of suspected impacted third molars
- A 58-year-old female, with multiple edentulous regions (areas with no teeth present), who has been assessed for a full mouth series for the evaluation of periodontal disease

1. Would an increased or decreased amount of radiation produce diagnostic-quality radiographic images for each of these patients?

2. Which of these three exposure variables—milliamperage, kilovoltage, or time—control(s) the amount of radiation produced?

3. Which exposure variable would be the *best* choice to alter to increase or decrease the amount of radiation produced for each of these patients?

4. Would an increased or decreased penetrating ability of the x-ray beam produce diagnostic-quality radiographic images for each of these patients?

5. Which of the three exposure variables—milliamperage, kilovoltage, or time—control(s) the penetrating ability of the x-ray beam?

6. Which exposure variable would be the *best* choice to alter to increase or decrease the penetrating ability of the x-ray beam?

Think of other characteristics patients may present with that would require an adjustment to these x-ray machine variables. Keep in mind that increasing one factor may necessitate decreasing an opposing factor. Discuss the rationale for your choices.

RELATE—Laboratory application

For a comprehensive laboratory practice exercise on this topic, see Thomson, E. M., & Bruhn, A. M. (2018). *Exercises in oral radiography techniques: A laboratory manual* (4th ed.). Hoboken, NJ: Pearson. Chapter 1, "Introduction to Radiation Safety and Dental Radiographic Equipment."

RESOURCES

Bushberg, J. T., Seibert, J. A., Leidholdt, E. M., Jr., & Boone, J. M. (2011). *The essential physics of medical imaging* (3rd ed). Baltimore, MD: Lippincott Williams & Wilkins.

United States Air Force Dental Evaluation and Consultant Service. USAF synopsis of intra-oral x-ray units. Project 05-02. (2005). Retrieved from USAF website: http://airforcemedicine.afms.mil/idc/groups/public/documents/afms/ctb_108739.pdf

White, S. C., & Pharoah, M. J. (2014). Physics. *Oral radiology. Principles and interpretation* (7th ed). St. Louis, MO: Mosby Elsevier.

Factors Affecting Radiographic Quality

CHAPTER OUTLINE

OBJECTIVES

Following successful completion of this chapter, you should be able to:

1. Define the key terms.
2. Evaluate a radiographic image identifying the basic requirements of acceptability.
3. Differentiate between radiolucent and radiopaque areas on a dental radiograph.
4. Define radiographic density and contrast.
5. List the rules for casting a shadow image.
6. List the variables that affect film contrast.
7. Describe how geometric factors affect image sharpness.
8. Identify the causes of image magnification and distortion.
9. Explain the effect milliamperage, kilovoltage, and exposure time have on image density.
10. Explain the effect variations in target–surface, object–image receptor, and target–image receptor distances have on image quality.
11. Demonstrate practical use of the inverse square law.

KEY TERMS

Contrast
Density
Exposure factors

Geometric factors
Inverse square law
Long-scale contrast
Milliampere/second (mAs)

Penumbra
Radiolucent
Radiopaque
Short-scale contrast

Introduction

Each patient presents with a unique set of characteristics for which a customized approach to exposure settings is needed. A dental radiographer has an ethical responsibility to produce the highest diagnostic-quality radiographs for patients who have consented to be exposed to ionizing radiation. To consistently produce diagnostic-quality radiographs at the lowest possible radiation dose, a dental radiographer needs to understand the interrelationships of the components of the dental x-ray machine.

There are three basic requirements for an acceptable diagnostic radiograph (Figure 4–1 ■).

1. All parts of the structures recorded must be imaged as close to their natural shapes and sizes as a patient's oral anatomy will permit. Distortion and superimposition of structures should be kept to a minimum.
2. The area examined must be imaged completely, with enough surrounding tissue to distinguish between the structures.
3. The radiograph should be free of errors and show proper density, contrast, and definition.

The quality of a radiograph depends on both the physical factors and the subjective opinion of the individual who reads it. This chapter describes the physical attributes of a quality radiographic image and studies the factors that affect these attributes.

Terminology

The following terms should be used when describing radiographic images: *radiolucent, radiopaque, density, contrast,* and *sharpness.*

When a film-based dental radiograph is viewed on a light source and digital images are viewed on a computer monitor, the image appears black and white, with various shades of gray in between. The terms used to describe the black-and-white areas are *radiolucent* and *radiopaque,* respectively.

Radiolucent

Radiolucent refers to that portion of the image that is dark or black (see Figure 4–1). Structures that appear radiolucent permit the passage of x-rays with little or no resistance. The pulp chamber and periodontal ligament spaces are examples of structures that appear radiolucent on a radiograph.

Radiopaque

Radiopaque refers to that portion of the image that is light or white (see Figure 4–1). Structures that appear radiopaque are dense and absorb or resist the passage of x-rays. Enamel, dentin, and bone are examples of structures that appear radiopaque on a radiograph. Radiolucent and radiopaque are relative terms. For instance, even though both enamel and dentin are radiopaque, enamel is more radiopaque (appears lighter) than dentin.

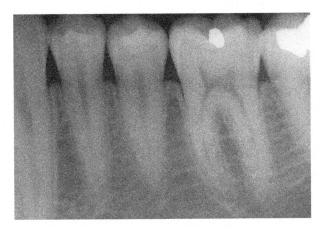

FIGURE 4–1 **A diagnostic-quality radiograph.**

Three visual image characteristics that directly influence the quality of a radiographic image are density, contrast, and sharpness.

Density

Density is the degree of darkness or image blackening (Figure 4–2 ■). A radiographic image that appears light is said to have little density. A radiographic image that appears dark is said to have more density. The blackness results when x-rays strike sensitive crystals in the film emulsion, and subsequent processing causes the crystals to darken. When using a digital sensor, sensitive pixels capture the radiation, and "processing" by computer software produces darker pixels. The degree of darkening of a radiograph is increased when the milliamperage or the exposure time is increased and more x-rays are produced to reach the film emulsion or digital sensor.

Radiographs need just the right amount of density to be viewed properly. If the density is too light or too dark, the images of the teeth and supporting tissues cannot be visually separated from each other. The ideal radiograph has the proper amount of density for an interpreter to view various radiolucencies and radiopacities.

Contrast

Contrast refers to the many shades of gray that separate the dark and light areas (Figure 4–3 ■). An image with good contrast will contain black, white, and enough shades of gray to differentiate between structures and their conditions.

High contrast (also called **short-scale contrast**) describes a radiograph in which the density differences

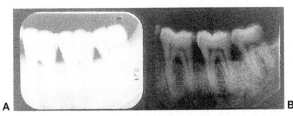

FIGURE 4–2 **Radiographic density.** Radiograph (**A**) is underexposed and appears too light (of decreased density). Radiograph (**B**) is overexposed and appears too dark (of increased density).

High contrast
Short scale

Low contrast
Long scale

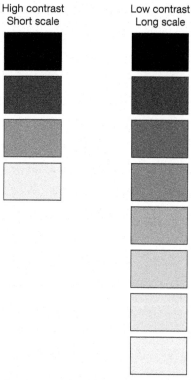

FIGURE 4–3 **Contrast.** A high-contrast image will have few shades of gray. A low-contrast image will have many shades of gray.

between adjacent areas are large (Figure 4–4 ■). The contrast is high because there are fewer shades of gray and more black against white. The gray tones indicate the differences in absorption of the x-ray photons by the various tissues of the oral cavity or the head and neck region. The radiograph is radiolucent where the tissues are soft or thin and radiopaque where the tissues are hard or thick. Such radiographs result when low kilovoltage is applied.

Low contrast (also called **long-scale contrast**) describes a radiograph in which the density differences between adjacent areas are small (see Figure 4–4). The contrast is low and very gradual because there are many shades of gray. Such radiographs result when high kilovoltage is applied.

Sharpness

Sharpness/definition is a geometric factor that refers to the detail and clarity of the outline of the structures shown on a radiograph. Unsharpness is generally caused by movement of the patient, image receptor, or tube head during

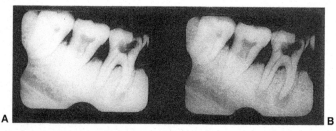

FIGURE 4–4 **Radiographic contrast.** Radiograph (**A**), exposed at 60 kVp, has higher contrast. Radiograph (**B**), exposed at 90 kVp, has lower contrast.

exposure. Digital imaging sharpness can be affected by pixel size and distribution (see Chapter 8).

Shadow Casting

A radiograph is a two-dimensional image of three-dimensional objects. Therefore, it is necessary to apply rules for creating a shadow image to produce a quality radiographic image. The following rules for casting a shadow image will help to reproduce the size and shape of the objects of the oral cavity accurately.

Rules for Casting a Shadow Image

1. Small focal spot: reduces size of **penumbra** (partial shadow around objects of interest) resulting in sharper image and slightly less magnification
2. Long target–object distance: reduces penumbra and magnification
3. Short object–image receptor distance: reduces penumbra and magnification
4. Parallel relationship between object and image receptor: prevents distortion of image
5. Perpendicular relationship between central rays of x-ray beam and both object and image receptor: prevents distortion of image

Because x-rays belong to the same electromagnetic spectrum as light (see Chapter 2), these two energies share many of the same characteristics. Therefore, when considering the application of shadow cast rules, it is helpful to compare the shadows cast by light with the shadows that x-rays will cast of the structures of the oral cavity. For example, if you were outside during the morning hours when the sun was low on the horizon, the sun's rays would be directed at your body at a low angle, casting a shadow that was elongated, or longer than your actual height. If you were outside at midday, when the sun was directly overhead, the sun's rays would be directed at your body at a steep angle, casting a shadow that was foreshortened, or shorter than your actual height. At some time during the day, the sun's light would be cast at the precise angle to your body that your shadow on the

Practice Point

Some clinicians prefer high-contrast radiographs that result from a low kV setting to diagnose caries and low-contrast radiographs that result from a high kV setting to diagnose periodontal disease. In theory, high-contrast images should be better at showing a radiolucency (such as decalcification indicating caries) against radiopaque tooth enamel, whereas low-contrast radiographs are purported to be better at showing subtle changes (gray areas) indicating alveolar bone changes. However, research indicates that both high- and low-contrast images perform equally well in providing a clinician with the necessary information for interpretation and diagnosis.

ground would be at the same length as your actual height. Directing a flashlight at an object, such as a child's game of producing hand puppet shadows, is another example of shadow casting. Depending on the direction of the flashlight beam alignment and the distance the light must travel to reach the object, accurate or distorted shadow images result.

Shadow cast rules are often referred to as **geometric factors** that contribute to the quality of a radiographic image. Geometric factors are those that relate to the relationships of angles, lines, points, or surfaces. Each of the shadow cast rules will be discussed in detail as to its role in producing quality radiographic images.

Factors Affecting a Radiographic Image

A dental radiographer must have a working knowledge of the factors that affect a radiographic image. Although density is important for producing the detail and visibility of a radiograph, the interpretation and diagnosis of oral conditions depend on radiographic contrast and sharpness/definition (Table 4–1 ■).

Radiographic Contrast

Radiographic contrast defined as the visible difference between densities depends on the following variables.

1. **Subject (types of tissues being imaged).** Subject contrast is the result of differences in absorption of

x-rays by the tissues under examination. The subject to be imaged must have contrast. A radiograph of a 1-inch-thick sheet of plastic would show no contrast because the plastic is of uniform thickness and composition. Patients have contrast because human tissues vary in size, thickness, and density.

2. **Kilovoltage (kV).** There is an inverse relationship between kV and contrast. In relative terms, higher kilovoltages produce lower contrast. The blacks are grayer, the whites are grayer, and there are many shades (or steps) of gray in between. Lower kilovoltages produce higher contrast. The blacks are blacker, the whites are whiter, and there are fewer shades (or steps) of gray in between (see Figure 4–4).

3. **Scatter radiation.** Chapter 2 discussed that Compton scattering occurs whenever dental x-rays interact with matter such as the tissues of a patient's head. These scattered x-rays add a uniform exposure to a radiograph that adversely decreases contrast. To assist with minimizing scatter when exposing intraoral radiographs (inside the mouth), a collimator (lead diaphragm) is used to restrict the size of the x-ray beam. A grid composed of thin alternating strips of lead and plastic is placed between a patient and image receptor to absorb scatter when exposing extraoral radiographs (outside the mouth). Use of a collimator and grid plays a role in radiographic contrast.

Table 4–1 Summary of Factors Influencing Radiographic Image Contrast

Factors	Variables	Image Contrast
Subject thickness (different tissues of the body)	Region with tissues of different densities (enamel, dentin, pulp) Region with tissues of similar densities (supporting alveolar bone)	Higher contrast between these different tissues Lower contrast between different areas of bone
kV (kilovoltage)	High kV Low kV	Lower contrast Higher contrast
Scatter radiation	Increased scatter radiation (large beam diameter used for intraoral radiographs/ no grid used for extraoral radiographs) Decreased scatter radiation (beam diameter narrowed with collimation for intraoral radiographs/grid used for extraoral radiographs)	Lower contrast Higher contrast
Image receptor type	Different manufacturers	Higher or lower contrast is inherent and depends on manufacturer
Exposure	Under- or overexposure and film fog	All will lower contrast
Processing	Accurate time-temperature processing followed Inaccurate time-temperature processing followed	Adequate contrast Lower or poor contrast

4. **Film/digital sensor type.** Each film has its own inherent (built-in) contrast that may vary by manufacturer. The effects of digital sensor pixel size on image contrast and density will be discussed in detail in Chapter 8.

5. **Exposure.** An underexposed or an overexposed radiograph will result in diminished or poor contrast. Accidental exposure of film to stray radiation or other conditions such as heat and humidity will create film fog (see Chapter 7). Fog is the formation of a thin, cloudy appearance that reduces image contrast. A radiograph that is too light, too dark, or fogged will not have significantly different shades of gray to provide optimal contrast.

6. **Processing.** Maximum film contrast can only be obtained through meticulous film processing procedures (see Chapter 7). A radiograph will not have the ideal contrast the manufacturer built into it if improper development time or temperature is used.

Sharpness/Definition

Sharpness, also known as definition, refers to the clarity of the outline of the structures on a radiograph. Radiographic image sharpness depends on the following variables (Table 4–2 ■).

1. **Focal spot size.** As explained in Chapter 3, the focal spot is the small area on the target where bombarding electrons are converted into x-rays. The smaller the focal spot area, the sharper the image appears (Figure 4–5 ■). A large focal spot creates more penumbra and therefore loss of image sharpness (Figure 4–6 ■). Ideally, the focal spot should be a point source, then no penumbra would be present. However, a single point source would

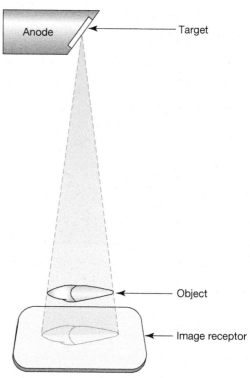

FIGURE 4–5 Using a small focal spot on the target, a long target–image receptor distance, and a short object–image receptor distance will result in a sharp image.

create extreme heat and burn out the x-ray tube. An x-ray machine manufacturer determines focal spot size. To ensure that the focal spot remains small, the tube head must remain perfectly still during exposure; even slight vibration of the tube head increases the size of the focal spot (Figure 4–7 ■).

Table 4–2 Summary of Factors Influencing Radiographic Image Sharpness

Factors	Variables	Image Sharpness
Focal spot size	Small focal spot Large focal spot	Increase sharpness Decrease sharpness
Target–image receptor distance	Long target–image receptor distance Short target–image receptor distance	Increase sharpness Decrease sharpness
Object–image receptor distance	Short object–image receptor distance Long object–image receptor distance	Increase sharpness Decrease sharpness
Motion	No movement Movement	Increase sharpness Decrease sharpness
Screen thickness	Thin screen Thick screen	Increase sharpness Decrease sharpness
Screen–film contact	Close contact Poor contact	Increase sharpness Decrease sharpness
Film crystal/pixel size	Small crystals/pixels Large crystals/pixels	Increase sharpness Decrease sharpness

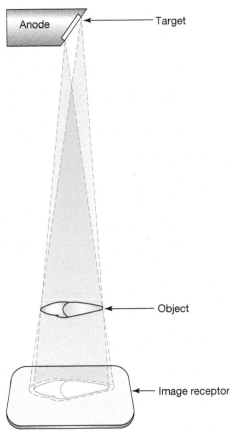

FIGURE 4–6 Large focal spot on the target and long object–image receptor distance results in more penumbra and loss of image sharpness.

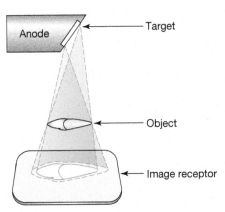

FIGURE 4–8 Large focal spot on the target and short target–image receptor distance results in more penumbra and loss of image sharpness.

2. **Target–image receptor distance.** The target–image receptor distance is the distance between the source of x-ray production (which is at the target on the anode inside the tube head) and the image receptor. PIDs are used to establish the target–image receptor distance. PIDs are classified as being short or long and come in standard lengths of 8 inches (20.5 cm), 12 inches (30 cm), and 16 inches (41 cm) for intraoral projections. The shorter the target–image receptor distance, the more divergent the x-ray beam (Figure 4–8 ■). A long target–image receptor distance has x-rays in the center of the beam that are nearly parallel. Therefore, the image on the radiograph will be sharper. Additionally, a longer target–image receptor distance will result in less image magnification (explained later in this chapter).

3. **Object–image receptor distance.** The object–image receptor distance is the distance between the object being radiographed (the teeth) and the dental x-ray

image receptor. The image receptor should always be placed as close to the teeth as possible. The closer the proximity of the image receptor to the teeth, the sharper the image and the less magnification (image enlargement). The image will become fuzzy (more penumbra) and magnified as the object–image receptor distance is increased (see Figure 4–6).

4. **Motion.** Movement of the patient and/or the image receptor in addition to the tube head results in a loss of image sharpness (Figure 4–9 ■).

5. **Screen thickness.** Intensifying screens (often referred to as screens), used in extraoral radiography, are made of crystals that emit light when struck by x-rays (see Chapter 17). The light, in turn, exposes the film and helps to produce an image. Intensifying screens

Practice Point

The tube head must remain perfectly still during exposure. Even slight vibration of the tube head increases the size of the focal spot, which in turn produces an unsharp image.

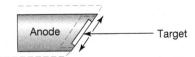

FIGURE 4–7 **Movement of the tube head.** Motion, even slight, of the tube head will effectively create a larger surface area of the focal spot, resulting in penumbra.

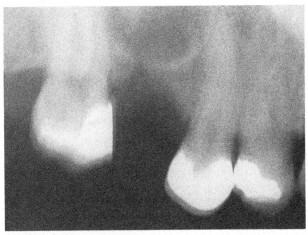

FIGURE 4–9 **Blurry, unsharp image** caused by movement of the patient, the image receptor, or the tube head.

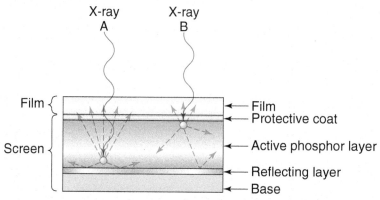

FIGURE 4–10 **Screen thickness.** X-ray A strikes a crystal far from the film and the divergent light exposes a wide area of the film, resulting in unsharpness. X-ray B strikes a crystal close to the film, resulting in less divergence of the light that exposes the film and therefore a sharper image. The thicker the screen, the less sharp the image.

require less radiation to produce a radiographic image than direct exposure film, resulting in less radiation exposure to a patient. However, the use of intensifying screens decreases the sharpness of a radiographic image (Figure 4–10 ■). The thicker the screen, the less radiation required to expose a film. However, these thicker screens produce a less sharp radiographic image. In general, use the highest speed screen and film combination, determined by the thickness of the phosphor layer that is consistent with good diagnostic results.

6. **Screen–film contact.** Film should be in close physical contact with the intensifying screen. Poor screen- film contact results in a wider spread of emitted light that increases penumbra. Intensifying screens should be examined periodically for proper functioning. Additionally, only one film should be placed in contact with the screen. Attempting to make a duplicate image by placing two films into one cassette is not acceptable practice unless using a film type made especially for this purpose.

7. **Crystal/pixel size of intraoral image receptors.** X-ray film emulsion contains crystals that receive x-ray exposure and in turn produce a radiographic image (see Chapter 7). Digital sensors use pixels that capture x-ray exposure as discrete units of information that computer software combines into a radiographic image (see Chapter 8). Image sharpness is influenced by the size of these crystals/pixels. Similar to the crystal size of intensifying screens, the smaller the size of the crystals within the film emulsion, and the pixels within a digital sensor, the sharper the radiographic image. However, small crystal/pixel size contributes to a slower speed image receptor, requiring a patient to receive a larger dose of radiation in order to obtain an image of appropriate density. Manufacturers strive to produce image receptors with the smallest sized crystals/pixels possible to avoid loss of image sharpness and yet maintain image density with a maximum reduction in radiation exposure.

Magnification/Enlargement

Magnification or enlargement is an increase in size of the image on a radiograph compared to the actual size of an object. Chapter 3 explained that x-rays travel in diverging straight lines as they radiate from the focal spot of the target. Because of these diverging x-rays, there is some magnification present in every radiographic image.

Magnification is most influenced by the target–object distance and the object–image receptor distance. The target–object distance is determined by the length of the PID. When a long PID is used, the x-rays in the center of the beam are more parallel, resulting in less image magnification (Figure 4–11 ■). The object–image receptor distance should be kept to a minimum. Always place an image receptor as close to the teeth as possible, while maintaining a parallel relationship between the long axes of the teeth and the plane of the image receptor, to decrease magnification.

Increasing the target–object distance and decreasing the object–image receptor distance will minimize image magnification. Note that these two shadow cast rules for reducing magnification also increase image sharpness.

Practice Point

When positioning an x-ray tubehead for intraoral exposures, it is important to place the open end of the PID as close as possible to (without touching) the skin surface of a patient's face. Image quality is improved when the target–surface distance is increased. However, it should be noted that increasing the distance between the target and the skin surface is determined by the length of the PID and not by positioning the PID a greater distance away from the patient (Figure 4–12 ■). Positioning the open end of the PID away from the skin surface of the patient's face will result in a larger diameter of radiation exposure and an underexposed image.

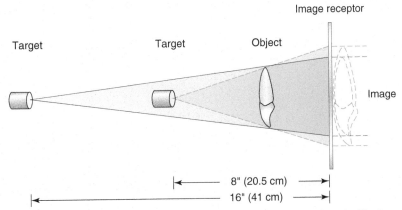

FIGURE 4–11 Magnification. Comparison of 8 inch (20.5 cm) and 16 inch (41 cm) target–object distances. Image magnification is reduced at the increased target–object distance.

Distortion

Distortion is the result of unequal magnification of different parts of the same object and results when an image receptor is not parallel to the object and/or when the central rays of the x-ray beam are not perpendicular to the object and the plane of the image receptor (Figures 4–13 ■ and 4-14 ■). To minimize image distortion, follow the two shadow cast rules for placement of the image receptor and x-ray beam positioning. Rules four and five state that the plane of the image receptor must be positioned parallel to the long axes of the teeth, and the central rays of the x-ray beam must be aligned perpendicular to both the image receptor and the teeth.

Effects of Varying Exposure Factors

Density and contrast have a tremendous influence on the diagnostic quality of a radiograph. X-ray machine exposure settings can affect both density and contrast (Table 4–3 ■).

Milliamperage, exposure time, and kilovoltage are known as **exposure factors.** Whenever one exposure factor is altered, one or a combination of the other factors must be altered proportionally to maintain radiographic density and contrast. For example, exposure time will need to be decreased when milliamperage or kilovoltage is increased to maintain optimal image density.

Variations in Milliamperage

The amount of electric current used in an x-ray machine is expressed in milliamperes (mA). The mA selected by an operator, or preset by a unit manufacturer, determines the quantity or number of x-rays that are generated within the tube. The density of a radiograph is affected whenever the mA is changed. Increasing mA increases the density of a radiograph, whereas decreasing mA decreases the density of the radiograph.

Variations in Exposure Time

Exposure time is the interval that an x-ray machine is fully activated and x-rays are produced. The principal effect of changes in exposure time is on density of a radiograph. Increasing exposure time darkens a radiograph, whereas it will lighten with decreasing exposure time. Opinions differ on optimum density and contrast because visual perception varies from person to person; some practitioners may prefer lighter radiographs, wherease others may prefer darker

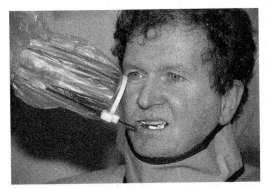 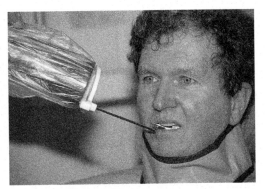

FIGURE 4–12 Correct and incorrect PID positioning. Left image illustrates the correct position of the open end of the PID as close to the patient's skin as possible. Right image illustrates an incorrect position of the PID. This PID position will result in a greater beam diameter of exposure to the patient and will produce an underexposed image.

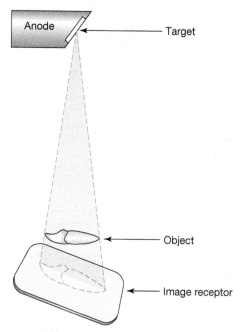

FIGURE 4–13 Object and image receptor are not parallel, resulting in distortion.

Table 4–3 **Effect of Varying Exposure Factors on Image Density**

Exposure Adjustment[a]	Image Density
Increase mA	Darker
Decrease mA	Lighter
Increase time	Darker
Decrease time	Lighter
Increase kV	Darker[b]
Decrease kV	Lighter[b]

[a]When any exposure factor is increased, or decreased, one or more of the other exposure factors must be adjusted to maintain optimum image density.
[b]Varying kV primarily affects image contrast, but it will also (secondarily) affect image density. Increase kV for less contrast and decrease kV for more contrast.

radiographs. Of the three controls, exposure time is easiest to change. In fact, many x-ray machines today have preset fixed milliamperage and kilovoltage, so that time is the only exposure factor that can be changed by an operator.

Milliampere/seconds

Because both milliamperage and exposure time are used to regulate the number of x-rays generated and have the same effect on radiographic density, they are often combined into a common factor called **milliampere/seconds (mAs)**. Combining the milliamperage with exposure time is an effective way to determine total radiation generated.

A simple formula for determining this total is: mA multiplied by exposure time (in seconds) equals mAs.

$$mA \times s = mAs$$

PROBLEM. Consider a practical problem using this formula. Assume the following exposure factors are in use: 10 mA, 0.6 sec, 50 kV, and 12 inch (30 cm) target–image receptor distance. If mA is increased to 15, but kV and target–image receptor distance remain constant, what should the new exposure time be to maintain image density?

SOLUTION. The only exposure factor that was changed is mA, which was increased from 10 mA to 15 mA. To compensate for the increase in mA, exposure time needs to be decreased.

$$mA \times s = mAs$$

$$10\,mA \times 0.6\,sec. = 6\,mAs$$

$$15\,mA \times ?\,sec. = 6\,mAs$$

$$?\,sec. = \frac{6\,mAs}{15\,mAs}$$

$$?\,sec. = 0.4\,sec$$

ANSWER. The new exposure time is 0.4 sec.

When mA is increased, exposure time must be decreased to produce identical radiographic image density between the first and second radiographs. A practical use for applying this formula would be when patient movement is anticipated—in this case, increasing the amount of radiation produced, so that the duration of exposure can be shortened.

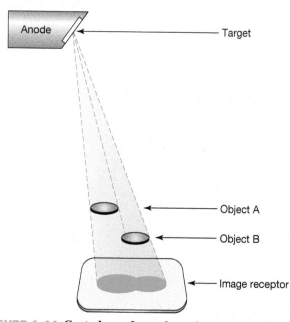

FIGURE 4–14 **Central ray of x-ray beam is not perpendicular to the objects and image receptor.** This results in distortion and overlapping of object A and object B. Note that object A is magnified larger than object B because object A is a greater distance from the image receptor than object B.

Variations in Kilovoltage

The quality of the radiation (wavelength or energy of the x-ray photons) generated by an x-ray machine is determined by kilovoltage (kV). The more the kV is increased, the shorter the wavelength and the higher the energy and penetrating power of the x-rays produced. Kilovoltage is the only exposure factor that directly influences contrast of a dental radiograph; however, increasing kV will also increase the number (quantity) of x-rays reaching the image receptor and, therefore, increase the density of a radiograph. As kV of an x-ray beam is increased for the purpose of producing a lower contrast image, the density of the radiograph is held constant by reducing the milliampere-seconds (mAs) or exposure time. Because exposure time is usually the easiest exposure factor to change, the following rule applies: When increasing kV by 15, for example from 50 kV to 65 kV, decrease exposure time by dividing by two; when decreasing kV by 15, increase exposure time by multiplying by two. One exposure factor balances the other to produce a radiographic image of acceptable density.

Effects of Variations in Distances

A radiographer must take into account several distances to produce an ideal diagnostic quality image—that is, the distances between the:

- x-ray source (at the focal spot on the target) and the surface of the patient's skin.
- object to be x-rayed (usually the teeth) and the image receptor.
- x-ray source and the recording plane of the image receptor.

Various terminology is used to describe these distances. In this text, *target–surface distance, object–image receptor distance, target–object distance,* and *target–image receptor distance* will be used (Figure 4–15 ■).

Target–Surface Distance

Generally, whenever an image receptor is positioned intraorally, the length of the target–surface distance is determined by the length of the PID. All intraoral techniques require that the open end of a PID be positioned to almost touch a patient's skin to standardize the distance in order to produce consistent image density.

Object–Image Receptor Distance

The object–image receptor distance depends largely on the method employed to hold a receptor in position next to the teeth. When the bisecting technique is used, an image receptor is placed against the palatal or lingual tissues as close as the oral anatomy will permit (see Chapter 14). This results in the object–image receptor distance being shorter in the area of the crown where the tooth and image receptor touch, than in the area of the root where the thickness of the bone and gingiva may cause a divergence between the long axis of the tooth and the image receptor (Figure 4–16 ■). The least divergence occurs naturally in the mandibular molar areas. The greatest divergence is in the maxillary anterior areas, where the palatal structures may curve sharply.

With the paralleling technique, most image receptor holders are designed so that a receptor is held parallel to the long axis of the tooth of interest. This necessitates positioning a receptor sufficiently into the middle of the oral cavity, away from the teeth, to avoid impinging on the supporting bone and gingival structures. This technique results in object–image receptor distances that are often more than 1 inch (25 mm). The paralleling technique compensates for this increased object–image receptor distance

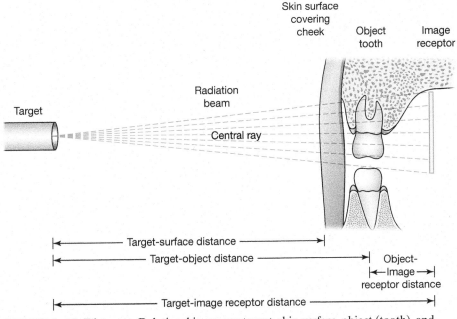

FIGURE 4–15 **Distances.** Relationship among target, skin surface, object (tooth), and image receptor distance.

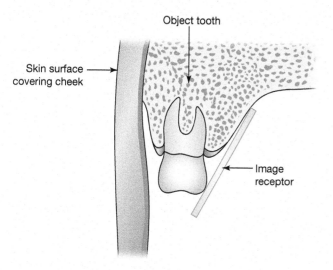

FIGURE 4-16 Object–image receptor distance. This placement of the image receptor places the crown of the tooth closer to the receptor than the root.

by recommending an increase in the target–image receptor distance (use a longer PID) to help offset the distortion, as explained next.

Target–Image Receptor Distance

The target–image receptor distance is the sum of the target–object and the object–image receptor distance (see Figure 4–15). The quality of a radiographic image improves whenever the target–image receptor distance is increased. Magnification and penumbra are reduced, and image definition is increased. Therefore, positioning an image receptor far enough from the teeth to enable it to be held parallel and using a longer, 12 inch (30 cm) or 16 inch (41 cm) PID will increase image definition quality. These techniques are described in detail in Chapter 12.

The location of the x-ray tube within the tube housing can affect the target–image receptor distance. In some dental x-ray machines, the target is situated in the tube head in front of the transformers. The attached PID length can be visibly determined. When the tube is recessed within the tube head, located behind the transformers, enough space is gained within the tube head so that a long target–image receptor distance is achieved even though a short PID is in place (Figure 4–17 ∎).

Inverse Square Law

X-ray photons, traveling in straight lines, spread out (diverge) as they radiate away from the source (target). As an x-ray beam spreads out, the intensity of the radiation decreases (Figure 4–18 ∎). How much the beam intensity decreases is based on the **inverse square law**, which states that the intensity of radiation varies inversely as the square of the distance from its source. The inverse square law formula may be written as:

$$\frac{\text{Original Intensity}}{\text{New Intensity}} = \frac{\text{New Distance}^2}{\text{Original Distance}^2}$$

Using this formula will show that if the distance is increased by two, the intensity will be decreased by four.

PROBLEM. A dental radiographer removes an 8 inch PID and replaces it with a 16 inch PID. What is the effect on the intensity of the radiation at this new distance?

SOLUTION. Let's assume that the original intensity is known as "1" at the original distance of 8 inches. To identify the new intensity at the new distance of 16 inches, use x for this unknown new intensity. Use the inverse square law formula to find the answer.

Original Intensity is 1 at an Original Distance of 8 inches
New Intensity is x at a New Distance of 16 inches

Place this data into the inverse square law formula:

$$\frac{1}{x} = \frac{16^2}{8^2}$$

Prior to squaring 16/8, reduce the fraction to 2/1 to make the arithmetic manageable. So after calculations, the formula now looks like this:

$$\frac{1}{x} = \frac{2^2}{1^2}$$

Perform the remainder of the calculations.

$$\frac{1}{x} = \frac{4}{1}$$

ANSWER.

$$x = \frac{1}{4}$$

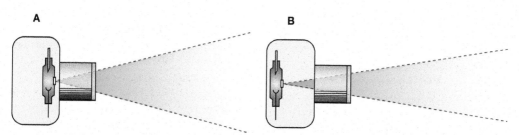

FIGURE 4-17 Comparison of conventional and recessed tube position within the tube head. (**A**) Conventional position with tube in front of the tube head. Note how quickly the x-ray beam pattern flares out. (**B**) With a recessed tube, a relatively more parallel x-ray beam is produced, resulting in a sharper radiographic image.

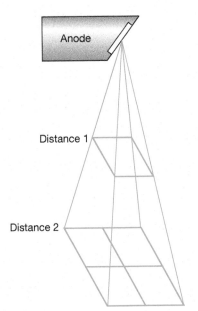

FIGURE 4–18 Inverse square law. When the target–image receptor distance is doubled the radiation spreads out and the intensity decreases by four.

Because the radiation intensity is now one-fourth what it was, a corresponding change must be made to the exposure time to make up for this decrease. Since the intensity decreased by four, the exposure time must now be increased by four to maintain image density.

This modified inverse square law formula can be applied to confirm this need for an increase in exposure time:

$$\frac{\text{Original Exposure Time}}{\text{New Exposure Time}} = \frac{\text{Original Distance}^2}{\text{New Distance}^2}$$

PROBLEM. Going back to the previous problem, if the exposure time with the 8 inch PID was 3 impulses, then what should the new exposure time be with the 16 inch PID?

SOLUTION. The original exposure time was 3 impulses at the original distance of 8 inches. To identify what the appropriate

new exposure time should be set to at the new distance of 16 inches, use x for this unknown new exposure time. Use the modified inverse square law formula to find the answer.

Original Exposure Time was 3 impulses at an Original Distance of 8 inches

New Exposure Time is x at a New Distance of 16 inches

Place this data into the modified inverse square law formula:

$$\frac{3}{x} = \frac{8^2}{16^2}$$

Prior to squaring 8/16, reduce the fraction to 1/2 to make the arithmetic manageable. So after calculations, the formula now looks like this:

$$\frac{3}{x} = \frac{1^2}{2^2}$$

Perform the remainder of the calculations.

$$\frac{3}{x} = \frac{1}{4}$$

ANSWER.

$$x = 12$$

Exposure Charts

Radiographers may memorize exposure factors needed for a particular technique; however, safety protocol dictates that exposure charts, available commercially or custom made by an oral healthcare practice, be posted at an x-ray machine control panel for easy reference. In fact, in some locations regulations require that exposure charts be posted.

Some dental x-ray machine manufacturers have incorporated commonly used exposure factors into the dial of the control panel. With these units, a radiographer only has to set the pointer to the desired region to be examined, and the unit automatically sets the required exposure factors (see Figure 3–5).

REVIEW—Chapter summary

An acceptable diagnostic radiograph must show the areas of interest—the designated teeth and surrounding bone structures—completely and with minimum distortion and maximum sharpness. When evaluating a radiographic image, utilize appropriate scientific terminology such as density, contrast, sharpness, magnification, and distortion. The term *radiolucent* refers to the dark or black portion of an image, whereas the term *radiopaque* refers to the light or white portion of an image. High-contrast images, those with black and white and few shades of gray, are called short scale, whereas low-contrast images, those with grayer whites and grayer blacks with many shades of gray, are called long scale.

Radiographic contrast depends on the subject (types of tissues being imaged), kilovoltage (kV) setting, scatter

radiation, film/digital sensor type, exposure, and processing. Sharpness is determined by geometric factors including focal spot size, target–image receptor distance, object–image receptor distance, motion, screen thickness, and screen–film contact, and by crystal/pixel size within an image receptor.

To create a sharp image, follow the rules for casting a shadow image: small focal spot, long target–image receptor distance, short object–image receptor distance, parallel relationship between object and image receptor, and perpendicular relationship between central rays of the x-ray beam and the object and image receptor. Image magnification and loss of sharpness is further reduced by limiting movement of the tube head and PID, the patient, and the image receptor during exposure.

Although not all dental x-ray machines allow a radiographer to manually alter all exposure factors, when available, take advantage of the ability to vary exposure factors to produce radiographs that have the desired image qualities. When altering one exposure factor, a corresponding change must be made to another factor to produce identical radiographic image density. The formula for altering exposure time and milliamperage is mA × s = mAs, where the mA is multiplied by the exposure time to determine the milliamperage seconds. The formula for altering kilovoltage is, if increasing kV by 15, then decrease the exposure time by dividing by two; if decreasing kV by 15, then increase the exposure time by multiplying by two.

When changing PID length, the inverse square law is used to adjust the exposure time to produce identical radiographic image density. The inverse square law states that the intensity of radiation varies inversely as the square of the distance from its source.

RECALL—Study questions

1. List the three criteria for acceptable radiographs.
   a. _____
   b. _____
   c. _____

2. Dense objects appear radiolucent *because* dense objects absorb the passage of x-rays.
   a. Both the statement and reason are correct and related.
   b. Both the statement and reason are correct but NOT related.
   c. The statement is correct, but the reason is NOT.
   d. The statement is NOT correct, but the reason is correct.
   e. NEITHER the statement NOR the reason is correct.

3. The degree of darkening of a radiographic image is referred to as
   a. contrast.
   b. definition.
   c. density.
   d. penumbra.

4. Which of the following describes the radiographic image produced with a kVp exposure setting of 90?
   a. Short scale
   b. Long scale
   c. High contrast
   d. Low density

5. Image contrast is NOT likely to be affected by
   a. processing procedures.
   b. type of film.
   c. scatter radiation.
   d. milliamperage.

6. Which of these factors has the greatest effect on image sharpness?
   a. Movement
   b. Filtration
   c. Kilovoltage
   d. Amperage

7. Film emulsion with large crystals produces increased radiographic image sharpness *because* a decreased amount of radiation is required to expose a film with large size crystals.
   a. Both the statement and reason are correct and related.
   b. Both the statement and reason are correct but NOT related.
   c. The statement is correct, but the reason is NOT.
   d. The statement is NOT correct, but the reason is correct.
   e. NEITHER the statement NOR the reason is correct.

8. What term best describes a fuzzy shadow that outlines anatomy recorded on a radiographic image?
   a. Magnification
   b. Distortion
   c. Penumbra
   d. Detail

9. Distortion results when
   a. an object and image receptor are not parallel.
   b. an x-ray beam is perpendicular to an object and image receptor.
   c. using a short object–image receptor distance.
   d. using a small focal spot.

10. A dental radiograph will appear less dense (lighter) if which of the following is increased?
    a. mA
    b. kVp
    c. Exposure time
    d. Target–image receptor distance

11. The exposure factors used at an oral health care facility are 10 mA, 0.9 sec, 70 kV, and 16 inch (41 cm) target–image receptor distance. A radiographer increases the mA to 15, but leaves the kV and target–image receptor distance constant. To maintain identical image density, what should be the new exposure time?
    a. 0.3
    b. 0.6
    c. 1.2
    d. 1.8

12. Which of the following is appropriate to increase radiographic contrast while maintaining image density?
    a. Increase kV and increase exposure time.
    b. Increase kV and decrease exposure time.
    c. Decrease kV and increase exposure time.
    d. Decrease kV and decrease exposure time.

13. Based on the inverse square law, what happens to the intensity of an x-ray beam when the target–image receptor distance is doubled?
    a. Intensity is doubled.
    b. Intensity is not affected.
    c. Intensity is one-half as great.
    d. Intensity is one-fourth as great.

14. A patient presents whose radiographs must be taken utilizing the bisecting technique. The radiographer decides to replace the 16 inch (41 cm) PID with an 8 inch (20.5 cm) PID to better accommodate this technique. Currently the impulse setting, with the 16 inch (41 cm) PID, is 12. To maintain image density, what will the new impulse setting be with the 8 inch (20.5 cm) PID?
    a. 3
    b. 6
    c. 24
    d. 48

REFLECT—Case study

You have just been hired to work in a new oral health care facility. Prior to providing patient services, you are asked to help develop exposure settings and equipment recommendations for the practice. The equipment and image receptor manufacturers' suggestions are as follows:

F Speed Film	8 in. (20.5 cm) PID	65 kVp
	Impulses	
Bitewings	Adult	Child
Posterior	10	8
Anterior	6	4
Periapicals		
Maxillary anterior	8	6
Maxillary premolar	12	8
Maxillary molar	14	10
Mandibular anterior	6	4
Mandibular premolar	8	6
Mandibular molar	10	8

1. You recommend that the facility replace the 8 inch (20.5 cm) PID with a 16 inch (41 cm) PID. Develop a new exposure chart for using the new 16 inch (41 cm) PID.

2. You recommend using a kVp setting of 50 to produce high-contrast images. Develop a new exposure chart for 50 kVp.

3. You recommend using a kVp setting of 80 to produce low-contrast images. Develop a new exposure chart for 80 kVp.

RELATE—Laboratory application

Obtain an inanimate object with varying densities that can be exposed at different exposure variables and compare the results. For example, expose a seashell placed on a size 2 intraoral film at the following exposure settings: 7 mA, 70 kVp, 10 impulses. Expose subsequent films varying one or more of the exposure settings and process normally. Using a view box, analyze the resultant radiographic images. Identify which settings produced darker or lighter images, and which settings produced low- or high-contrast images.

RESOURCES

Carestream Health Inc. (2007). *Exposure and processing for dental film radiography.* Rochester, NY: Author.

Thomson, E. M. (2012). Innovation improves safety. Dimensions in brief. An educational supplement sponsored by Carestream Dental. *Dimensions of Dental Hygiene, 10*[supplement], 5–13.

U.S. Air Force Dental Evaluation and Consultant Service. USAF synopsis of intra-oral x-ray units. Project 05-02. (2005).

Retrieved from USAF website: http://airforcemedicine.afms .mil/idc/groups/public/documents/afms/ctb_108739.pdf

White, S. C., & Pharoah, M. J. (2014). Physics. *Oral radiology: Principles and interpretation* (7th ed.). St. Louis, MO: Mosby Elsevier.

Visit www.pearsonhighered.com/healthprofessionsresources to access the student resources that accompany this book. Simply select Dental Hygiene from the choice of disciplines. Find this book and you will find the complementary study tools created for this specific title.

PART

II

Radiation Biology and Radiation Safety

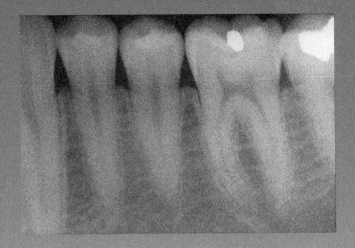

OUTLINE

(5) Effects of Radiation Exposure

OBJECTIVES

Following successful completion of this chapter, you should be able to:

1. Define the key terms.
2. Differentiate between the direct and indirect theories of biological damage.
3. Differentiate between a threshold dose–response curve and a nonthreshold dose–response curve.
4. List the sequence of events that may follow exposure to radiation.
5. Identify factors that determine whether radiation injuries are likely.
6. List three conditions that influence the radiosensitivity of a cell.
7. Determine the relative radiosensitivity or radioresistance of various kinds of cells in the body.
8. Explain the difference between deterministic and stochastic effects.
9. Explain the difference between somatic and genetic effects.
10. Explain the difference between short- and long-term effects of irradiation.
11. Identify critical tissues for dental radiography.
12. Discuss the risks versus benefits of dental radiographs.
13. Utilize effective dose equivalent to make radiation exposure comparisons.

KEY TERMS

Acute radiation syndrome (ARS)
Cumulative effect
Deterministic effect
Genetic effect
Latent period
Lethal dose (LD)
Mitosis
Radiolysis of water
Radioresistant
Radiosensitive
Somatic effect
Stochastic effect

Introduction

Patients are often concerned with the safety of dental x-ray procedures. Oral health care professionals also share such concerns. The fact that ionizing radiation produces biological damage has been known for many years. The first x-ray burn was reported just a few months following Roentgen's discovery of x-rays in 1895. As early as 1902, the first case of x-ray-induced skin cancer was reported in the literature (Figure 5–1 ■). Events such as the 1945 bombing of Hiroshima and the 2011 Fukushima nuclear power plant accident continue to generate unfavorable attitudes toward ionizing radiation and concern over the use of x-rays in health care, including dentistry. Although public concern is warranted, there are also some sensational and unsubstantiated articles appearing in newspapers and magazines, on television, and on the Internet. Much of what is known about the effects of radiation exposure comes from data extrapolated from high doses and high dose rates. Studies of occupational workers exposed to chronic low levels of radiation have shown no adverse biological effect. However, even the radiation experts have not been able to determine whether a threshold level exists below which radiation effects would not be a risk. Because even the experts cannot always predict a specific outcome from an amount of radiation exposure, the radiation protection community conservatively assumes that any amount of radiation may pose a risk. This chapter explains the theories of radiation injury and identifies factors that increase the risk of producing a biological response.

Theories of Biological Effect Mechanisms

As discussed in Chapter 2, x-rays belong to the ionizing portion of the electromagnetic spectrum. X-rays have the ability to detach and remove electric charges from the complex atoms that make up the molecules of body tissues. This process, known as ionization, creates an electrical imbalance within normally stable cells. Because disturbed cellular atoms or molecules generally attempt to regain electrical stability, they often accept the first available opposite electrical charge. In such cases, undesirable chemical changes become incompatible with surrounding body tissues. During ionization, the delicate balance of cell structure is altered, and a cell may be damaged or destroyed.

There are two generally accepted theories on how radiation damages biological tissues: (1) the direct theory and (2) the indirect (radiolysis of water) theory.

- **Direct theory:** X-ray photons collide with important cell chemicals and break them apart by ionization, causing critical damage to large molecules. One-third of biological alterations from x-radiation exposure result from a direct effect; however, most dental x-ray photons probably pass through a cell with little or no damage. A healthy cell can repair any minor damage that might occur. Moreover, the body contains

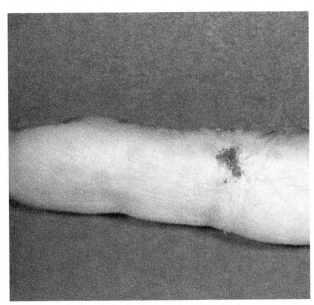

FIGURE 5–1 **Early carcinoma.** Found on the finger of a dentist who admitted to regularly holding films in the patient's oral cavity during exposures. This occurred many years ago, prior to the profession embracing ALARA.

so many cells that the destruction of a single cell or a small group of cells will have no observable effect.
- **Indirect theory** (**radiolysis of water**): is based on the assumption that radiation can cause chemical damage to a cell by ionizing the water within it (Figure 5–2 ■). Because about 80 percent of body weight is water and ionization can dissociate water into hydrogen and hydroxyl radicals, this theory proposes that new chemicals such as hydrogen peroxide could be formed under certain conditions. These chemicals act as toxins (poisons) to the body, causing cellular dysfunction. Two-thirds of biological alterations from x-radiation exposure result from indirect effects. Fortunately, when a water molecule is ionized, the ions have a strong tendency to recombine immediately to form water again instead of seeking out new combinations, keeping cellular damage to a minimum. Under ordinary circumstances, even when a new chemical such as hydrogen peroxide is formed, other cells that are not affected can take over the functions of the damaged cells until recovery takes place. Only in extreme instances, where massive irradiation has taken place, will entire body tissues be destroyed or death result. However, it should be remembered that cellular destruction is not the only biological effect; the potential exists for a cell to become malignant.

Dose–Response Curves

Radiation doses, like those of drugs or other biologically harmful agents, can be plotted onto a graph to illustrate the probability of a tissue response or damage. Plotting the two variables, the amount of radiation and the anticipated response of the biological tissues, creates a dose–response curve. A threshold dose–response curve indicates that there

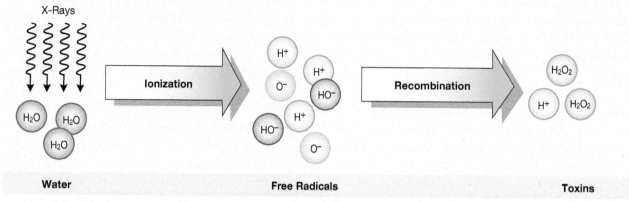

FIGURE 5–2 **Indirect theory.** X-rays ionize water, resulting in the formation of free radicals, which can recombine to form toxins such as hydrogen peroxide.

is a "threshold" amount of radiation, below which no biological response would be expected. A nonthreshold dose–response curve indicates that any amount of radiation, no matter how small, has the potential to cause a biological response (Figure 5–3 ■).

Radiobiologists have been unable to determine radiation effects at very low levels of exposure (for example, doses below 100 mSv) and cannot be certain whether a threshold dose exists. (To help put 100 mSv into perspective, a full mouth series of 18 F-speed films, at 90 kVp with 16 inch [41 cm] length PID is approximately 30 mSv skin exposure.) Therefore, the radiation protection community takes a conservative approach and considers any amount of ionizing radiation exposure as being nonthreshold. This assumption is the basis for radiation protection guidelines and radiation control activities. The concept that every dose of radiation may produce damage and should be kept to the minimum necessary to meet diagnostic requirements is known as the ALARA concept, where ALARA stands for "as low as reasonably achievable" (see Chapter 6).

Sequence of Events Following Radiation Exposure

The sequence of events following radiation exposure are latent period, period of injury, and recovery period, assuming, of course, that the dose received was nonlethal.

- **Latent period:** Following initial radiation exposure, and before the first detectable effect occurs, a time lag called the latent period occurs. The **latent period** may be very short or extremely long, depending on the initial dose and other factors described next. Effects that appear within a matter of minutes, days, or weeks are called short-term effects, and those that appear years, decades, and even generations later are called long-term effects.
- **Period of injury:** Following the latent period, certain effects can be observed. One of the effects seen most frequently in growing tissues exposed to radiation is the stoppage of mitosis (cell division). This may be temporary or permanent, depending on the radiation dose. Other effects include breaking or clumping of chromosomes, abnormal mitosis, and formation of giant cells (multinucleated cells) associated with cancer.
- **Recovery period:** Following exposure to radiation, recovery can take place. This is particularly apparent in the case of short-term effects. Nevertheless, there may be a certain amount of damage from which no recovery occurs, and it is this irreparable injury that can give rise to later long-term effects.

Factors that Determine Radiation Injury

Biological responses to low doses of radiation exposure are often too small to be detected. The body's defense mechanisms and ability to repair molecular damage often result in

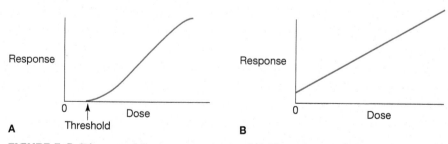

FIGURE 5–3 **Diagram of dose–response curve.** (**A**) The point at which the curve intersects the base line (horizontal line) is the threshold dose—that is, the dose below which there is no response. If an easily observable radiation effect, such as erythema (reddening of the skin) is taken as "response," then this type of curve is applicable. (**B**) A linear "nonthreshold" curve, in which the curve does not intersect the base line. Here it is assumed that any dose, no matter how small, has potential to cause a response.

no residual effects. In fact, the following five outcomes are possible: (1) nothing—the cell is unaffected by the exposure; (2) the cell is injured or damaged but repairs itself and functions at preexposure levels; (3) the cell dies, but is replaced through normal biological processes; (4) the cell is injured or damaged, repairs itself, but now functions at a reduced level; or (5) the cell is injured or damaged and repairs itself incorrectly or abnormally, resulting in a biophysical change (tumor or malignancy). Determining which of these five outcomes might occur depends on each of the following:

- **Total dose:** This dose refers to the type, energy, and duration of the radiation; the greater the dose, the more severe the probable biological effect.
- **Dose rate:** The rate at which the radiation is administered or absorbed is very important in the determination of what effects will occur. Because a considerable degree of recovery occurs from radiation damage, a given dose will produce less effect if it is divided (allowing time for recovery between dose increments) than if it is given in a single exposure. For instance, an exposure of 1 R/week for 100 weeks would result in less injury than a single exposure of 100 R. (R = Roentgen, a unit of measurement; see Chapter 2.)
- **Area exposed:** The larger the exposure area, other factors being equal, the greater the injury to an organism. Intraoral dental radiographic exposures use a very small (2.75 inch or 7 cm) beam diameter (or less if using rectangular collimation, see Figure 6–4) to limit the area of radiation exposure to the area of diagnostic concern.
- **Variation in species:** Various species have a wide range of sensitivity to radiation. Lethal doses for plants and microorganisms are usually hundreds of times higher than those for mammals.
- **Individual sensitivity:** Individuals vary in sensitivity within the same species. The genetic makeup of some individuals may predispose them to ionizing radiation damage. For this reason the **lethal dose (LD)** for each species is expressed in statistical terms, usually as the LD 50/30 for that species, or the dose required to kill 50 percent of the individuals in a large population in a 30-day period. For humans, the LD 50/30 is estimated to be 4.5 gray (Gy) or 450 rad (gray and rad are units of absorbed dose; see Chapter 2).
- **Variation in cell and tissue sensitivity:** All cells and tissues are not equally sensitive to radiation (Table 5–1 ■). The terms **radiosensitive** and **radioresistant** are used to describe the degree of susceptibility of various cells and body tissues to radiation. The relative sensitivity of cells to radiation is influenced by the following:

Mitotic activity. Cells are more susceptible to radiation injury during mitosis. Cells that undergo frequent mitosis are said to be more radiosensitive.

Table 5–1 Cell and Tissue Sensitivity to Radiation*

Most sensitive	Lymphocytes and blood-forming cells Reproductive cells
Moderately sensitive	Gastrointestinal (GI) cells Skin cells and lens of the eye
Least sensitive	Mature bone and cartilage Nerve, brain, and muscle cells

*Because research data may be interpreted differently, the listing order presented here is for general comparison along a continuum of relative radiosensitivities.

Metabolism. Cells with a high activity (metabolism) are more susceptible to radiation injury.

Differentiation. Immature cells and cells that are not highly specialized as to their function are more susceptible to radiation.

- **Age:** Within the same cell families, the immature forms, which are generally primitive and rapidly dividing, are more sensitive to radiation than the older, mature cells, which have specialized function and have ceased to divide. It follows that children will be more susceptible to injury than adults from an equal dose of radiation. Additionally, an increase in radiation sensitivity is observed again in old age. As the body ages, the cells may begin to lose the ability to repair damage.

Radiation Effects on Tissues of the Body

Low levels of radiation exposure do not usually produce an observable adverse biological effect. As a dose of radiation increases and enough cells are destroyed, the affected tissue will begin to exhibit clinical signs of damage. For example, erythema (redness of the skin) would not be expected to result from exposing the skin to the ionizing radiation of the sun's rays for a few seconds. However, as the time of exposure to the sun's rays is increased, the erythema would be expected to increase proportionally. When the severity of the tissue change is dependent on the dose, the effect is called a **deterministic effect** (or nonstochastic effect). In addition to erythema, cataract formation (affecting the lens of the eye), hair loss (depilation), and infertility are also examples of deterministic effects.

When a biological response is based on the probability of occurrence rather than the severity of the change, it is called a **stochastic effect**. The occurrence of cancer is an example of a stochastic effect of radiation exposure. The risk of developing cancer increases as the radiation dose increases; the severity of the cancer does not depend on the dose. When the dose of radiation is increased, the "probability" of the stochastic effect (cancer) occurring increases, but not its severity.

Somatic and Genetic Effects

All of the cells making up body tissues can be classified as somatic cells or genetic cells. Somatic cells are all the cells of the body, except the reproductive cells. A **somatic effect** occurs when a biological change or damage occurs in the irradiated individual, but is not passed along to offspring. A **genetic effect** describes changes in hereditary tissues that do not manifest in the irradiated individual, but show up in the individual's offspring.

Experts do not fully understand all these effects or their future consequences. Scientists believe that some of these effects are **cumulative**, especially if exposure is too great and the intervals between exposures too frequent for body cells to repair or replace themselves. Unless the damage is too severe or the subject is in extremely poor health, many body (somatic) cells have a recovery rate of almost 75 percent during the first 24 hours following exposure.

In determining whether an exposure is potentially harmful, consider the quantity and the duration of an exposure and which body area is to be irradiated. Continued exposure over prolonged periods alters the ability of the genetic cells (eggs and sperm) to reproduce normally. Current evidence indicates that chromosome damage is cumulative, increasing in effect by each successive additional radiation exposure, and genetic cells cannot repair themselves. Radiation may alter the genetic material in the reproductive cells so that mutations (abnormalities) may be produced in future generations.

Short- and Long-Term Effects of Radiation

The effects of radiation are classified as either short term or long term. Short-term effects of radiation are those seen minutes, days, or months after exposure. When a very large dose of radiation is delivered in a very short period of time, the latent period is short. If a dose of radiation is large enough (generally over 1.0 Gy or 100 rads, whole body), the resultant signs and symptoms that comprise these short-term effects are collectively known as **acute radiation syndrome (ARS)**. ARS symptoms include erythema, nausea, vomiting, diarrhea, hemorrhage, and depilation. ARS is not a concern in dentistry because dental x-ray machines cannot produce the very large exposures necessary to cause it.

Long-term effects of radiation are those that are seen well beyond the original exposure. The latent period is much longer (years) than that associated with ARS. Delayed radiation effects may result from a previous acute, high exposure that the individual has survived or from chronic low-level exposures delivered over many years.

No unique disease associated with the long-term effects of radiation has been established. Instead, there can be a statistical increase in the incidence of certain conditions that can have causes other than radiation exposure such as cancer, embryological defects, and genetic mutations. Because of the low natural incidence of these conditions in the population, large numbers of exposed persons must be observed to evaluate whether the increases can be linked to long-term radiation exposure.

Critical Tissues and Radiation Risks

A risk may be defined as the likelihood of injury or death from any given hazard. Since exposure of dental radiographs uses a small radiation dose, deterministic effects are not a concern. The primary risk from dental radiography is a stochastic effect: radiation-induced cancer. However, it is important to note that the facial and oral structures are fairly radioresistant, being composed largely of bone, nerve, and muscle tissue. The potential risk of a full mouth series of dental radiographs inducing cancer in a patient has been estimated to be approximately 3 in 1 million radiographic examinations. To put this into perspective, the risk that a fatal cancer will develop spontaneously is 3,300 per 1 million people. It is equally important to consider the risk of NOT exposing necessary dental radiographs, and the potential to miss pathology and other problems that can lead to diminished oral and general health.

While the risk of dental radiographs inducing cancer is low, the following are identified as critical tissues for dental radiography because of their relative radiosensitivity and their location in the path of the primary beam: skin of the head and neck regions, bone marrow of the mandible, and the thyroid gland (Table 5–2 ■). Because the lens of the eye is made up of radiosensitive cells it used to be considered a critical tissue even though dental x-rays have never been reported to cause cataracts. It takes at least

Practice Point

To assist patients in understanding potential risks, it may be tempting to compare dental radiation with unrelated activities, such as comparing risks of dental x-ray exposure with risks associated with riding in an automobile or traveling in an airplane. Merely looking at the number of fatalities that occur from accidents involving these other activities does not take into consideration a multitude of other variables. Patients are familiar with using statistics in this manner to nullify and justify a multitude of other occurrences in daily living, and a comparison between the risk of a dental radiograph compared to an accidental death may appear as if the radiation exposure is being trivialized. Instead, risk management experts recommend comparing risks between the same type of occurrence. In this case a more realistic conversation would compare dental radiation exposure with other types of ionizing radiation exposures.

Table 5–2 **Select Tissues and Doses for Dental Radiography***

Tissue	Effect	Minimum Estimated Acute Dose Required to Produce Effect	Approximate Dental Dose from a FMS
Skin	Erythema Cell death	3,000–6,000 mSv 5,000–10,000 mSv	12.6 mSv
Bone marrow	Reduction of blood cell production	500 mSv	8 mSv
Thyroid gland	Cancer	65 mSv	0.4 mSv
Lens of eye	Detectable opacities Cataracts	500–2,000 mSv 5,000 mSv	0.4 mSv
Gonads	Temporary sterility Permanent sterility	150 mSv 2,500–6,000 mSv	0.005 mSv (*no lead apron*) to 0.0003 mSv (*with lead apron*)

*Because research data may be interpreted differently, the amounts presented here are estimates for general comparisons only.

5,000 milliseiverts (mSv) of x-radiation to cause cataract formation. The potential radiation dose to the eyes from a full mouth series of radiographs is less than 1 mSv. Most experts no longer consider the lens of the eye a critical tissue for dental radiography.

Additionally, the highly radiosensitive gonadal tissues are not likely to be impacted by dental radiographic exposures. Because scatter radiation reaching the gonads from a dental radiographic examination is less than 0.0001 that of the exposure to the surface of the face, the risk of genetic mutations or sterility is negligible. Using a lead or lead-equivalent barrier apron substantially reduces the radiation reaching these tissues to zero.

While the potential risks associated with low doses of radiation are not well understood, there have been no reports of radiation injuries caused by normal dental radiographic procedures since safety protocols were adopted. Dental radiographs are prescribed and exposed when the benefit of a diagnosis outweighs the risk of biologic injury to a patient. It is important to understand that when determining the need for a radiographic examination, a risk assessment must include consideration of the potential risks to a patient's oral and overall health with not performing a selection criteria-based radiographic examination (see Chapter 6).

Radiation Exposure Comparisons

Patients often have questions regarding the amount of radiation dental radiographs are adding to their accumulated lifetime exposure. The exact amount of radiation exposure produced when taking dental radiographs varies, depending on many factors, such as film speed or use of a digital imaging receptor, technique used, and collimation (circular or rectangular). Additionally, dental exposures are often

quoted as skin surface amounts rather than amounts to deeper bone marrow and other critical tissues.

Effective dose equivalent can be used to compare dental radiation exposures with days of natural background ionizing radiation exposure (see Chapter 2). The average effective dose equivalent from naturally occurring background ionizing radiation to the U.S. population is approximately 8 μSv (microseiverts) per day. A full mouth series of radiographs using F-speed film and a round collimator has an effective dose equivalent of approximately 23.4 μSv. Therefore, a full mouth series is equal to approximately 2.9 days of naturally occurring background ionizing radiation exposure (Table 5–3 ■).

Much about radiation effects remains to be discovered. Future research may demonstrate that human beings are not as sensitive to radiation damage as we now believe. But until we have such evidence, common sense dictates improving radiographic safety techniques in every way possible.

Practice Point

Be careful not to tell a patient that a full mouth series is equal to 2.9 days "in the sun." Naturally occurring background radiation includes not only the sun, or cosmic energy, but also terrestrial and internal sources of ionizing radiation (see Chapter 2). Additionally, most patients are aware that exposure to the sun's rays is harmful and many people take precautions against putting themselves at risk for skin damage. To compare dental x-rays to sun exposure may provoke a response from a patient to avoid dental x-rays as well.

Table 5–3 Effective Dose Equivalent

Examination	Effective Dose	Days of Natural Exposure[a]
Single intraoral exposure[b]	1.3 μSv	0.2
Bitewing radiographs[b] (4 films)	5.2 μSv	0.7
Full mouth series[b] (18 films)	23.4 μSv	2.9
Panoramic radiograph	7 μSv	0.9
CT scan of the maxilla	240–1200 μSv	40–200
CT scan of the mandible	480–3324 μSv	80–547.5
Cone beam CT mandible	75 μSv	12.5
Cone beam CT maxilla	42 μSv	7
Chest x-ray	80 μSv	10
Upper GI	2440 μSv	305
Lower GI	4060 μSv	507.5

[a]Fractions rounded up.
[b]F-speed, round PID.

REVIEW—Chapter summary

Ionizing radiation has the potential to produce biological damage because x-rays can detach subatomic particles from larger molecules and create an imbalance within a normally stable cell. The two generally accepted theories on how radiation may cause damage to cellular tissues are (1) the direct theory, and (2) the indirect theory or the radiolysis of water. Whether cell damage from radiation is physical or chemical, it has been established that a healthy body soon repairs minor damage.

Dose–response curves are used to plot the dosage of radiation administered with the response produced to establish responsible levels of radiation exposure. The non-threshold dose–response curve illustrates the conservative view that every dose of radiation potentially produces damage and should be kept to a minimum. Assuming that a radiation dose is not lethal, the sequence of events following radiation exposure are (1) a latent period, (2) a period of injury, and (3) a recovery period.

Factors that influence a biological response to irradiation include dose amount, dose rate, area exposed, species exposed, individual sensitivity, cell sensitivity, tissue sensitivity, and age. The terms *radiosensitive* and *radioresistant* are used to describe the degree of susceptibility of various cells and body tissues to radiation. The susceptibility of cells is influenced by mitotic activity, metabolism, and differentiation.

The term *deterministic effect* is used when referring to a tissue response, such as erythema, whose severity is directly

related to the radiation dose. The term *stochastic effect* is used when referring to a tissue response, such as cancer, that is based on the probability of occurrence rather than the severity of the response. Biological changes or damage from radiation exposure that occur in somatic cells will affect the irradiated individual but will not be passed along to offspring. Biological changes or damage that do not affect the irradiated individual but are passed to offspring are called genetic effects. The cumulative effect of irradiation is defined as an amount of radiation damage from which no recovery occurs, giving rise to later long-term effects.

The effects of radiation exposure may be short term (occurring within hours, days, or weeks after exposure) or long term (occurring years after exposure). Acute radiation syndrome (ARS) is a short-term, extremely high-dose exposure outcome. No unique disease associated with the long-term effects of radiation has been established. Cancer, cataracts, embryological defects, and genetic abnormalities may result from radiation exposure and from exposure to other agents and conditions. The risk of dental radiographic examinations causing a fatal cancer is estimated to be 3 per 1 million examinations. The potential benefits of dental radiographs outweigh the risk. Because of their relative sensitivity and their location in the path of the primary beam of radiation, the critical tissues for dental radiography include skin, bone marrow in the mandible, and thyroid gland. With proper radiation safety protocol, there is minimal risk of injury caused by necessary dental radiographic procedures. The effective dose equivalent can be used to compare risks of different radiation exposures and to compare dental radiation exposure with days of exposure to natural background ionizing radiation.

RECALL—Study questions

1. The primary cause of biological damage from radiation is
   a. ionization.
   b. direct effect.
   c. indirect effect.
   d. genetic effect.

2. Indirect injury from radiation occurs when x-ray photons
   a. strike critical cell molecules.
   b. pass through the skin into deeper tissues.
   c. ionize water and form toxins.
   d. break DNA bonds in the cell nucleus.

3. A dose–response curve indicating that any amount of radiation, no matter how small, has the potential to cause a biological response is called
   a. stochastic.
   b. nonstochastic.
   c. threshold.
   d. nonthreshold.

4. Which of the following is the correct sequence of events following radiation exposure?
   a. Period of injury, latent period, recovery period
   b. Latent period, period of injury, recovery period
   c. Latent period, recovery period, period of injury
   d. Recovery period, latent period, period of injury

5. List the five possible biological responses of an irradiated cell.
   a. _____
   b. _____
   c. _____
   d. _____
   e. _____

6. Each of the following is a factor in determining the occurrence of tissue injury from radiation EXCEPT one. Which one is the EXCEPTION?
   a. Size of the irradiated area
   b. Amount of radiation dose
   c. Gender of the patient
   d. Rate at which the dose is delivered

7. According to the factors that determine radiation injury, based on age, which of the following patients would potentially be the most radiosensitive?
   a. 6-year-old
   b. 16-year-old
   c. 26-year-old
   d. 46-year-old

8. An increase in each of the following puts a cell in a radiosensitive state EXCEPT one. Which one is the EXCEPTION?
   a. Mitotic activity
   b. Presence of immature cells
   c. Metabolic rate
   d. Specialization

9. When a biological response is based on the probability of occurrence rather than the severity of the change, it is called what kind of effect?
   a. Short term
   b. Long term
   c. Stochastic
   d. Deterministic

10. When an effect of a radiation exposure is observed in the offspring of an irradiated person, but not in the irradiated person, this is called what kind of effect?
    a. Somatic
    b. Genetic
    c. Direct
    d. Indirect

11. Which of these are considered short-term outcomes following radiation exposure?
    a. Embryological defects
    b. Cataracts
    c. Acute radiation syndrome
    d. Cancer

12. Each of the following may be in the region of the x-ray beam during exposure of an intraoral dental radiograph on an adult patient. Which one, because of its relative radioresistancy, is NOT considered critical for dental radiography?
    a. Spinal cord
    b. Lens of the eye
    c. Mandible
    d. Thyroid gland

13. Which of these cells/tissues is most radiosensitive?
    a. Mature bone
    b. Lymphocyte
    c. Nerve cell
    d. Brain cell

14. Which of these cells/tissues is most radioresistant?
    a. Blood-forming cell
    b. Lens of the eye
    c. Skin cell
    d. Mature cartilage

15. The potential risk of a full mouth dental x-ray examination inducing cancer in a patient has been estimated to be
    a. 3 per 1,000 examinations.
    b. 3 per 10,000 examinations.
    c. 3 per 100,000 examinations.
    d. 3 per 1,000,000 examinations.

16. What term best expresses comparisons between dental radiation exposures and natural background exposure?
    a. Absorbed dose
    b. Accumulated dose
    c. Effective dose equivalent
    d. Lethal dose

REFLECT—Case study

Retaking a radiograph because of a technique or processing error causes an increase in radiation exposure for a patient.

Discuss ways a retake radiograph affects the factors that determine radiation injury.

RELATE—Laboratory application

Calculate your radiation dose. Visit the American Nuclear Society at http://www.ans.org/pi/resources/dosechart/msv.php, where you can estimate your average annual radiation dose. Based on the questions posed by this calculator, what conclusions can you draw about (1) the source of radiation exposure, (2) the region in which people live, (3) sources of internal radiation exposure, and (4) situations and/or products with the ability to increase your dose of radiation exposure?

RESOURCES

American Dental Association Council on Scientific Affairs. (2006). The use of dental radiographs: Update and recommendations. *Journal of the American Dental Association, 137*(9), 1304–1312.

American Dental Association Council on Scientific Affairs. U.S. Department of Health and Human Services: Public Health Service. Food and Drug Administration. (2012). *Dental radiographic examinations: Recommendations for patient selection and limiting radiation exposure.* Washington, DC: Author.

Bird, D. L., & Robinson, D. S. (2015). Radiographic imaging. *Modern dental assisting* (11th ed.). St. Louis, MO: Elsevier.

Carestream Health Inc. (2007). *Kodak Dental Systems. Radiation safety in dental radiography.* Rochester, NY: Author.

Iannucci, J. M., & Howerton, L. J. (2014). Radiation biology. *Dental radiography. Principles and techniques* (4th ed.). St. Louis, MO: Elsevier Saunders.

Ludlow, J. B. (2012). The risks of radiographic imaging. *Dimensions of Dental Hygiene, 10*(6), 56–61.

National Council on Radiation Protection and Measurements. (2009). *Ionizing radiation exposure of the population of the United States.* Report No 160. Bethesda, MD: Author.

Peck, D. J., & Samei, E. (2010). *How to understand and communicate radiation risk.* Retrieved from American College of Radiology website: http://www.imagewisely.org/imaging-modalities/computed-tomography/medical-physicists/articles/how-to-understand-and-communicate-radiation-risk

U.S. Nuclear Regulatory Commission. (2015). *Biological effects of radiation.* Retrieved from Nuclear Regulatory Commission website: http://www.nrc.gov/reading-rm/doc-collections/fact-sheets/bio-effects-radiation.pdf

U.S. Nuclear Regulatory Commission. (2016, February 2). *Standards for protection against radiation,* Title 10, Part 20, of the Code of Federal Regulations. Retrieved from Nuclear Regulatory Commission website: http://www.nrc.gov/reading-rm/doc-collections/cfr/part020/

White, S. C., & Pharoah, M. J. (2014). Biology. *Oral radiology: Principles and interpretation* (7th ed.). St. Louis, MO: Mosby Elsevier.

Visit www.pearsonhighered.com/healthprofessionsresources to access the student resources that accompany this book. Simply select Dental Hygiene from the choice of disciplines. Find this book and you will find the complementary study tools created for this specific title.

Radiation Protection

OBJECTIVES

Following successful completion of this chapter, you should be able to:

1. Define the key terms.
2. Adopt the ALARA concept.
3. Use the selection criteria guidelines to explain the need for prescribed radiographs.
4. Explain the roles communication, working knowledge of quality radiographs, and education play in preventing unnecessary radiation exposure.
5. Explain the roles technique and exposure choices play in preventing unnecessary radiation exposure.
6. Compare inherent, added, and total filtration.
7. State the federally mandated limited diameter of the intraoral dental x-ray.
8. List two functions of a collimator.
9. Explain how PID shape and length contribute to reducing patient radiation exposure.
10. Identify film speeds currently available for use in dental radiography.
11. Explain the role image receptor holders play in reducing patient radiation exposure.
12. Advocate the use of a lead/lead equivalent thyroid collar and apron.
13. Explain the role darkroom protocol and film handling play in reducing patient radiation exposure.
14. Summarize radiation protection methods for a patient.
15. Explain the roles time, shielding, and distance play in protecting a radiographer from unnecessary radiation exposure.
16. Utilize distance and location to take a position an appropriate distance and angle from the x-ray source during an exposure.
17. Describe radiation safety protocol for use with portable, handheld x-ray devices.
18. Describe radiation monitoring devices.
19. Summarize radiation protection methods for a radiographer.
20. List organizations responsible for recommending and setting exposure limits.
21. State the maximum permissible dose (MPD) for radiation workers and for the general public.

KEY TERMS

Added filtration

ALARA (as low as reasonably achievable)

Aluminum equivalent

Backscatter ring shield

Collimation

Direct ion storage (DIS) dosimeter

Filtration

Half-value layer (HVL)

Handheld x-ray device

Inherent filtration

Lead/lead-equivalent apron

Maximum permissible dose (MPD)

Optically stimulated luminescence (OSL) dosimeter

Personnel monitoring

Radiation worker

Retake radiograph

Selection criteria

Thermoluminescent dosimeter (TLD)

Thyroid collar

Total filtration

Introduction

Radiation exposure in sufficient doses may produce harmful biological changes in humans. Although it is the consensus of radiobiologists that the dose received from a dental x-ray exposure is not likely to be harmful, even the experts do not know what risk a small dose carries. Therefore, it must be assumed that any dose carries a potential risk. The patient has given consent to the radiation exposure because of the benefits he or she expects to receive. An oral health care practitioner is obligated to follow safety protocols that minimize the patient's risk.

This chapter discusses radiation safety protocols, including selection criteria used in prescribing dental radiographs and methods to minimize x-ray exposure to both dental patient and radiographer.

ALARA

Radiation from dental imaging has attracted more attention as the use of computed tomography (CT) scans has become more common in oral health care. The oral health care team has an ethical responsibility to embrace the **ALARA (as low as reasonably achievable)** concept, recommended by the International Commission on Radiological Protection to minimize radiation risks. The ALARA concept implies that "any radiation dose that can be reduced without major difficulty, great expense, or inconvenience should be reduced or eliminated." ALARA is not simply a phrase, but a culture of professional excellence; it should guide practice principles. In an ideal world, an oral health care team would like to get the diagnostic benefits of dental radiographs with a zero dose radiation exposure to a patient. In reality, this is not possible; all dental radiographs will result in a small but acceptable level of risk. The best way to prevent this risk from increasing is to keep the exposure ALARA.

Protection Measures for the Patient

Patient protection measures should be used at all times to keep radiation exposures as low as possible (Box 6–1). The benefits of radiographs in dentistry outweigh the risks when proper safety procedures are followed. Patient protection measures begin with a professional assessment of need for a radiographic examination and are implemented by a skilled radiographer following recommended technique standards using safe equipment.

Professional Judgment

The most important way to ensure that a patient receives a reasonably low dose of radiation is to use evidence-based **selection criteria** when determining which patients need radiographs. Guidelines developed by an expert panel of health care professionals convened by the Public Health Service and adopted by the American Dental Association have been published, and are periodically updated, to assist in deciding when, what type, and how many radiographs should be taken (Table 6–1 ■). These guidelines allow a dentist to base the decision regarding x-rays for a patient on

Box 6–1: Summary of Protection Methods for the Patient

- Evidence-based prescribing
- Good communication between radiographer and patient
- Radiographer's working knowledge of quality radiographs
- Education and skills of the radiographer
- Selection of technique used for the examination.
- Posted exposure factors to avoid mistakes
- Filtration of the x-ray machine
- Collimation of the x-ray machine
- Open-ended, 16 inch (41 cm) rectangular PID
- Digital image receptors or F-speed film
- Image receptor holders for the examination
- Lead/lead-equivalent thyroid collar/apron
- Darkroom protocol to avoid retake radiographs

Practice Point

Completing an accurate dental history may reveal that a new patient has recently had radiographs taken at another oral health care practice. Every effort should be made to secure a copy of these radiographs to avoid additional radiation exposure for the patient.

expert recommendations. Although a dentist prescribes a radiographic exam for a patient based on these guidelines, the recommendations are subject to clinical judgment and may not apply to every patient.

Evidence-based selection criteria guidelines are applied only after reviewing a patient's health history and completing a clinical examination. The time frames suggested in the guidelines are used in the absence of positive historical findings and signs and symptoms presented by a patient. For example, a patient who presents with a toothache would most likely be assessed for a radiographic exam of this symptom even if the patient had radiographs within the suggested time frame for this patient's category. Additionally, a radiographic examination should not wait until a patient presents with pain or other symptom of pathology. The time frames suggested by the selection criteria guidelines are preventive measures that are evidence-based effective. A dentist uses these guidelines to prescribe a radiographic exam for a patient, and a dental hygienist may use the guidelines during initial examination of a patient to make a preliminary assessment for the recommendation of radiographic need. Both the dental hygienist and the dental assistant rely on the selection criteria guidelines to assist with explaining radiographic need to a patient. Once the decision to expose radiographs is made, every reasonable effort must be made to minimize exposure to the patient and to the operator and to those who may be in the area of the x-ray machine.

Technical Ability of the Operator

- **Communication.** Reduction of radiation exposure begins with communication skills. A patient's cooperation must be secured to perform radiographic examinations accurately and safely. Patient protection during a radiographic procedure should begin with clear, concise instructions. When responsibilities are adequately defined through effective communication, a patient understands what must be done and can more fully cooperate with a radiographer and avoid retake mistakes.

- **Working knowledge of quality radiographs.** A radiographer should understand what a quality dental radiograph should image. Based on this knowledge, a radiographer needs to take every precaution against retaking radiographs. **Retake radiographs** are necessary when the first exposure results in errors that compromise image quality. When a radiograph is retaken, the second exposure doubles the dose and dose rate of radiation for the patient. The best way to avoid retake radiographs is to develop an understanding of common technique and processing errors (see Chapter 18). Armed with this knowledge, a radiographer can better avoid mistakes that lead to an increase in patient radiation exposure.

- **Education.** Continuing education is the cornerstone of all health care professions. Rapidly advancing technology is constantly changing the scope of oral health care practice. Some of the methods and procedures learned for the practice of oral health care just a few years ago may be obsolete in today's world. For example, we are currently witnessing the possible elimination of film-based dental radiography. With the increasing use of computers and the advancement of digital imaging, new technology will surely contribute more to the reduction of dental radiation exposure. The radiographer who continues to learn about and adopt these new practices will further help decrease radiation exposure for the patient and the radiographer.

Technique Standards

- **Intraoral technique choice.** The paralleling technique should be the operator's first choice when exposing periapical radiographs, as this technique yields more accurate and precisely sized radiographic images (see Chapter 13). However, consideration should also be given to which technique, paralleling or bisecting, will produce the best results for the patient. The more efficient and convenient the technique, the less likely there will be retake radiographs. A radiographer

Practice Point

Not every undiagnostic radiograph must be retaken. If multiple radiographs are taken at the same time, for example, when exposing a full mouth series or set of bitewings, check to see if the area of interest is imaged on an adjacent radiograph. Sometimes a retake radiograph may be avoided if the area of interest is imaged diagnostically on an adjacent radiograph.

Practice Point

The ease with which retakes can be taken quickly, often without removing a digital image sensor from a patient's mouth, can lead to a higher retake rate than when using film-based radiography resulting in additional radiation exposure for a patient. Practitioners should be cognizant of assuming that the real or the perceived radiation dose reduction expected with digital imaging will make retakes easily justifiable.

Table 6–1 Guidelines for Prescribing Dental Radiographs

Type of Encounter	Children		Adolescent	Adult	
	Primary dentition (prior to eruption of first permanent tooth)	Transitional dentition (after eruption of first permanent tooth)	Permanent dentition (prior to eruption of third molars)	Dentate or partially edentulous	Edentulous
New Patient					
Being evaluated for dental disease and dental development	Individualized radiographic exam consisting of selected periapical/occlusal views and/or posterior bitewings if proximal surfaces cannot be visualized or probed; patients without evidence of disease and with open proximal contacts may not require radiographic exam	Individualized radiographic exam consisting of posterior bitewings with panoramic exam or posterior bitewings and selected periapical images	Individualized radiographic exam consisting of posterior bitewings with panoramic exam or posterior bitewings and selected periapical images: full mouth intraoral radiographic exam is preferred when patient has clinical evidence of generalized dental disease or history of extensive dental treatment		Individualized radiographic exam, based on clinical signs and symptoms
Recall Patient*					
With clinical caries or at increased risk for caries**	Posterior bitewing exam at 6- to 12-month intervals if proximal surfaces cannot be examined visually or with probe			Posterior bitewing exam at 6- to 18-month intervals.	Not applicable
Recall Patient*					
With no clinical caries and not at risk for caries**	Posterior bitewing exam at 12- to 24-month intervals if proximal surfaces cannot be examined visually or with probe		Posterior bitewing exam at 18- to 36-month intervals	Posterior bitewing exam at 24- to 36-month intervals	Not applicable
Recall Patient*					
With periodontal disease	Clinical judgment as to need for and type of radiographic images for evaluation of periodontal disease; imaging may consist of, but not limited to, selected bitewing and/or periapical images of areas where periodontal disease (other than nonspecific gingivitis) can be identified clinically				Not applicable

Patient*

		Not usually indicated
For monitoring of growth and development	Clinical judgment as to need for and type of radiographic images for evaluation and/or monitoring of dentofacial growth and development	Clinical judgment as to need for and type of radiographic images for evaluation and/or monitoring of dentofacial growth and development; panoramic or periapical exam to assess developing third molars

Patient*

With other circumstances including, but not limited to, proposed or existing implants, pathology, restorative/endodontic needs, treated periodontal disease and caries remineralization	Clinical judgment as to need for and type of radiographic images for evaluation and/or monitoring in these circumstances

*Clinical situations for which radiographs may be indicated include but are not limited to:

A. Positive historical findings
1. Previous periodontal or endodontic treatment
2. History of pain or trauma
3. Familial history of dental anomalies
4. Postoperative evaluation of healing
5. Remineralization monitoring
6. Presence of implants or evaluation for implant placement

B. Positive clinical signs/symptoms
1. Clinical evidence of periodontal disease
2. Large or deep restorations
3. Deep carious lesions
4. Malposed or clinically impacted teeth
5. Swelling
6. Evidence of dental/facial trauma
7. Mobility of teeth
8. Sinus tract ("fistula")
9. Clinically suspected sinus pathology
10. Growth abnormalities
11. Oral involvement in known or suspected systemic disease
12. Positive neurologic findings in the head and neck
13. Evidence of foreign objects
14. Pain and/or dysfunction of the temporomandibular joint
15. Facial asymmetry
16. Abutment teeth for fixed or removable partial prosthesis
17. Unexplained bleeding
18. Unexplained sensitivity of teeth
19. Unusual eruption, spacing, or migration of teeth
20. Unusual tooth morphology, calcification, or color
21. Unexplained absence of teeth
22. Clinical erosion

**Factors increasing risk for caries may include but are not limited to:
1. High level of caries experience or demineralization
2. History of recurrent caries
3. High titers of cariogenic bacteria
4. Existing restoration(s) of poor quality
5. Poor oral hygiene
6. Inadequate fluoride exposure
7. Prolonged nursing (bottle or breast)
8. High-sucrose frequency diet
9. Poor family oral health
10. Developmental or acquired enamel defects
11. Developmental or acquired disability
12. Xerostomia (dry mouth)
13. Genetic abnormality of teeth
14. Many multisurface restorations
15. Chemo/radiation therapy
16. Eating disorders
17. Drug/alcohol abuse
18. Irregular dental care

Data from American Dental Association: Council on Scientific Affairs. U.S. Dept. of Health and Human Services: Public Health Service. Food and Drug Administration. (2012). *Dental radiographic examinations: Recommendations for Patient Selection and Limiting Radiation Exposure.*

should be skilled at both techniques and should possess the knowledge on which to base the decision regarding which one to use.

- **Exposure factors.** Operating a dental x-ray machine includes selecting the appropriate exposure factors—kilovoltage (kV), milliamperage (mA), and time—for the size of a patient and for the specific area of the oral cavity to be imaged. Additionally, experts agree that a kilovoltage setting between 60 and 70 kVp produces quality radiographs while maintaining low radiation dosage; and a kilovoltage setting above 90 kVp will unnecessarily increase patient dose and should not be used. Although a radiographer should possess a working knowledge of appropriate exposure factors, to assist in radiation safety for all patient sizes and all regions of the oral cavity, exposure charts should be posted near the control panel for easy reference. These size-based exposure charts must be periodically evaluated and updated, especially if a change occurs in film speed or digital sensor types.

Equipment Standards

All dental x-ray machines in the United States are safe from a radiological health point of view. The Federal Performance Standard for Diagnostic X-Ray Equipment became effective on August 1, 1974. The provisions of this standard require that all x-ray equipment manufactured after that date meet certain radiation safety requirements including filtration, collimation, and position indicating device (PID).

- **Filtration** is the absorption of the long wavelength, less penetrating x-rays of the polychromatic x-ray beam by passage of the beam through a sheet of material called a filter (Figure 6–1 ■). A filter is an absorbing material (usually aluminum) placed in the path of the x-ray beam to remove a high percentage of the soft x-rays (the longer wavelengths) and to reduce patient radiation dose.

  In a dental x-ray machine, these aluminum filter disks vary in thickness. The **half-value layer**

(HVL) of an x-ray beam is the thickness (measured in millimeters) of aluminum that will reduce the intensity of the beam by one-half. Measuring the HVL determines the penetrating quality of the x-ray beam. The HVL is more accurate than kilovoltage to describe the x-ray beam quality and penetration. Two similar x-ray machines operating at the same kilovoltage may not produce x-rays of the same quality and penetration. The half-value layer is used by radiological health personnel when determining filtration requirements.

Filters may be sealed into the tube head or inserted into the port where the PID attaches. Pure aluminum or its equivalent will not hinder the passage of high-energy x-rays, but will absorb a high percentage of the low-energy x-rays. The latter do not contribute to the radiographic image. Low-energy x-rays are harmful to a patient because they are absorbed by the skin, increasing a patient's dose (Figure 6–2 ■).

Any material an x-ray beam passes through filters the beam. Filtration may be built into the tube head (inherent), or it may be added.

Inherent filtration is built into the machine by the manufacturer, and includes the glass of the x-ray tube, the insulating oil, and the material that seals the port. All x-ray machines have some built-in filtration; usually the inherent filtration is not sufficient to meet state and federal standards, requiring that additional filtration be added.

Added filtration is the placement of aluminum discs in the path of the x-ray beam between the port seal of the tube head and the PID. When the inherent filtration is not sufficient to meet safety standards, a disk of aluminum of the appropriate thickness (usually 0.5 mm) is inserted between the port of the tube head and the PID. Several manufacturers have introduced x-ray units in which the traditional aluminum filter is replaced with samarium, a rare-earth metal that performs the same function as aluminum.

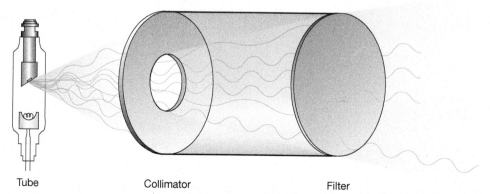

Tube   Collimator   Filter

FIGURE 6–1 **Collimator and filter.** The collimator is a lead washer that restricts the size of the x-ray beam. The filter is an aluminum disc that filters (removes) the long wavelength x-rays.

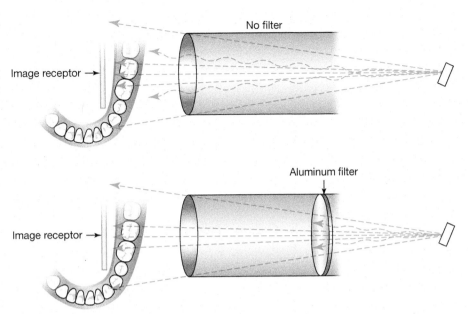

FIGURE 6–2 **Effect of filtration on skin exposure.** Aluminum filters selectively absorb the long wavelength x-rays.

Total filtration is the sum of the inherent and added filtration expressed in millimeters of **aluminum equivalent**. Beam filtration must comply with state and federal laws. Present safety standards require an equivalent of 1.5 mm aluminum for x-ray machines operating in ranges below 70 kVp and a minimum of 2.5 mm aluminum for machines operating at or above 70 kVp.

- **Collimation** controls the size and shape of the useful beam. While filtration reduces patient radiation exposure by filtering out the longer wavelengths of the x-ray beam, collimation restricts the x-ray beam to reduce scatter radiation. Scatter radiation leads to an increase in patient exposure as the radiation is deflected in all directions during its passage through matter. A lead diaphragm collimator is placed in the path of the primary beam as it exits the tube housing at the port (Figure 6–3 ■). The opening in the lead diaphragm collimator allows only a precise, narrow beam to reach a patient's tissues. Collimators may have either a round or a rectangular opening. Federal regulations require that round collimators restrict the

x-ray beam to 2.75 inches (7 cm) at the patient end of the PID. Rectangular collimators restrict the beam to an even smaller area of exposure, the approximate size of the image receptor (Figure 6–4 ■). In addition to decreasing patient radiation dose, collimation (and especially rectangular collimation) reduces scatter radiation that causes poor contrast of the radiograph (see Chapter 4).

A PID is an extension of the tube housing and is used to direct the primary x-ray beam. The shape (round or rectangular) of a PID plays a corresponding role with the collimator (Figures 6–5 ■ and 6–6 ■). Although rectangular collimation, which is strongly recommended by the American Dental Association (ADA) and U.S. Food and Drug Administration (FDA) guidelines on radiography, reduces patient radiation exposure by up to 70 percent over a round-collimated beam, many dental x-ray machines have round PIDs

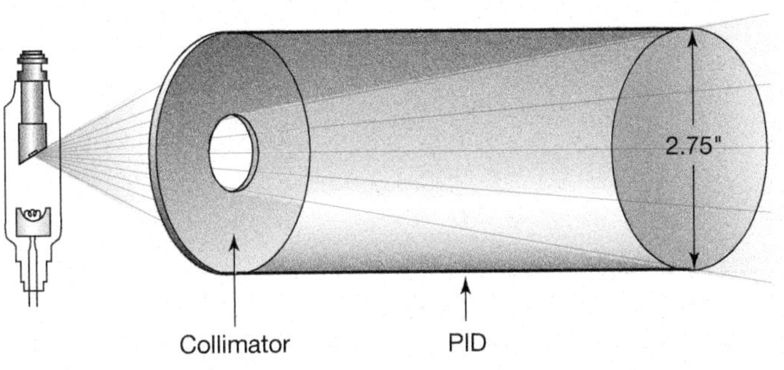

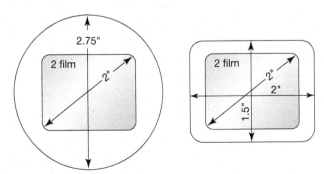

FIGURE 6–4 **Exposure comparison.** (**A**) Round collimation provides a large area of exposure to adequately cover a size 2 image receptor; patient receives excess radiation not needed for exposure. (**B**) Rectangular collimation reduces excess exposure to approximate size of the image receptor; precise alignment of the x-ray beam is required to avoid conecut error.

Collimator   PID

FIGURE 6–3 The collimator restricts the size of the primary beam to 2.75 inches (7 cm) at the end of the PID.

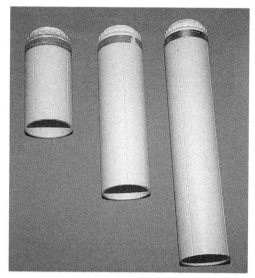

FIGURE 6–5 **Round PIDs** are available in 8, 12, and 16 inches (20.5, 30, and 41 cm).

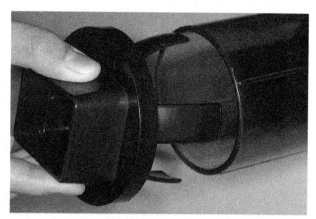

FIGURE 6–7 **External collimator** attaches to the PID to reduce the area of radiation exposure.

attached. Practitioners may be reluctant to make the change to a rectangular PID, citing a perception of increased conecut errors with a smaller x-ray beam, and the expense of upgrading equipment to meet this recent emphasis on using a rectangular PID to reduce radiation exposure. To help overcome these barriers, image receptor positioners are available with external aiming devices to assist with proper alignment of the x-ray beam; and rectangular PID attachments can be purchased, avoiding the expense associated with buying a new x-ray machine (see Figure 13–11; Figures 6–7 ■ and 6–8 ■).

- **PID length** also has an effect on the radiation dose a patient receives. The length of a PID helps to establish the desired target-surface distance (see Chapter 4). Both round and rectangular PIDs are available in different lengths, usually 8 inch (20.5 cm), 12 inch (30 cm),

and 16 inch (41 cm), as shown in Figures 6–5 and 6–6. The 16 inch PID can reduce patient radiation exposure by 10 to 25 percent because of its length, and results in better quality radiographic images. With a longer PID, there is less divergence of the x-ray beam, creating a smaller diameter of exposure (Figure 6–9 ■).

It is important to note that a dental x-ray machine may appear to have a short PID while still achieving long target–surface distance. Some dental x-ray machines feature a recessed PID, where the x-ray tube is recessed back in the tube head behind the transformers, thereby creating a longer target–surface distance (see Figure 4–17).

- **Fast film and digital image sensors** require less radiation for exposure and are essential for dose reduction. Currently, intraoral dental x-ray film is available in three speed groups: D, E, and F. F-speed film reduces radiation exposure approximately 25 percent as compared to E-speed film, and approximately 60 percent as compared to D-speed film. The American Dental Association and the American Academy of Oral and Maxillofacial Radiology recommend the use of the fastest

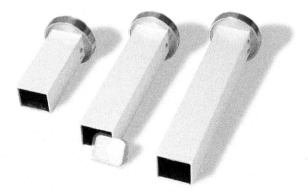

FIGURE 6–6 **Rectangular PIDs** restrict the x-ray beam to the approximate size of a 2 intraoral image receptor. Rectangular PIDs are available in 8, 12, and 16 inches (20.5, 30, and 41 cm). (Courtesy of Margraf Dental Manufacturing Inc.)

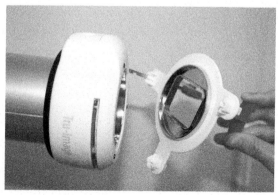

FIGURE 6–8 **External collimator** attaches to the PID to reduce the area of radiation exposure.

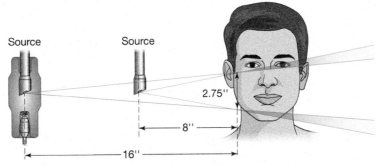

FIGURE 6–9 **Target-surface distance.** The longer the target–surface distance, the more parallel the x-rays and the less tissue exposed. Note that the beam size at the patient's skin entrance is 2.75 inches (7 cm) for both target–surface distances. It is the exit beam size on the other side of the patient's head that increases to expose a larger area when using the shorter target–surface distance.

Practice Point

Pointed, closed-end cones, originally designed to aid in aiming an x-ray beam at the center of a film packet, are no longer used (Figure 6–10 ▪). Pointed cones cause the deflection or scattering of x-rays through contact with the material of the cones. Because these pointed cones were used for so many years, some still refer to the PID as a "cone." The term *position indicating device (PID)* is more descriptive of its function of directing the x-rays, rather than of its shape.

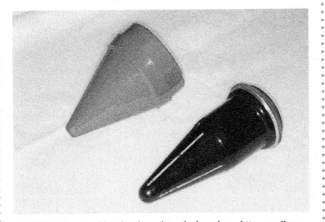

FIGURE 6–10 Plastic closed-ended, pointed "cones" are no longer used.

speed film currently available. Digital image sensors can further reduce the amount of radiation required to produce a diagnostic image (see Chapter 8).

- **Image receptor holding devices** that position a film packet or digital sensor intraorally are recommended to avoid having a patient hold the receptor in the oral cavity with his or her fingers (Figure 6–11 ▪). Unnecessarily exposing a patient's fingers is not ethical practice in keeping with ALARA. The use of image receptor holders with external aiming devices will assist in aligning the x-ray beam, which may afford a patient additional protection by reducing the number of retakes that may result from alignment errors. These devices also stabilize an image receptor in the mouth and reduce the possibility of movement and of film bending that can result when a patient uses a finger to hold the receptor in position.

- **A lead or lead equivalent apron** placed over a patient's abdomen to protect the reproductive organs and other radiosensitive tissues from potential scatter radiation during exposure of dental radiographs was first recommended many years ago when dental x-ray machine output was less reliable and film speeds were slower than today's standards. Use of fast-speed film or digital image sensors and dental x-ray machines that are appropriately collimated and filtered essentially eliminate the need for covering the patient's abdomen with a lead apron. The National Council on Radiation Protection and Measurements has determined that

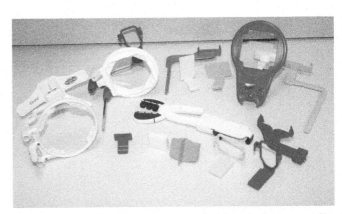

FIGURE 6–11 Many image receptor holding devices are available to fit most situations. The use of a holder prevents asking patients to put their fingers in the path of the primary beam.

lead aprons do not significantly reduce doses from intraoral dental exposures. Nevertheless some states still have laws requiring the use of a lead apron over the abdominal area, and patients have come to expect it. Additionally, the use of a lead or lead-equivalent apron is in keeping with ALARA and remains a prudent if not essential practice (Figure 6–12 ■). To offer maximum protection, lead aprons must be made of at least 0.25 mm lead. Protective aprons made of lead-equivalent materials provide a comparable, lightweight alternative to leaded aprons. However, it is important to determine with the manufacturer that a lead-equivalent apron is constructed to provide protection from the radiation generated at the level set by the x-ray machine kilovoltage.

Lead and lead-equivalent aprons should be stored flat or hung unbent. Folding the apron may cause the material inside to crack. This is most likely to occur when aprons are repeatedly folded in the same place day after day. Cracks in the material allow radiation to penetrate and render the apron less effective.

A lead or lead-equivalent **thyroid collar** when in place around a patient's neck, protects the thyroid gland and other radiosensitive tissues in the neck region during exposure of intraoral radiographs (Figure 6–13 ■). Because of the direction of the dental

Practice Point

The use of a thyroid collar is contraindicated when exposing panoramic radiographs using rotational panoramic equipment because the collar or upper part of the apron to which it is attached may obscure diagnostic information or interfere with the rotation of the panoramic unit. This is one of the reasons lead aprons are available without thyroid collars.

x-ray beam in this region, lead or lead-equivalent thyroid collars are recommended for all patients. Lead and lead-equivalent aprons are available with or without an attached thyroid collar.

Optimum Film Processing

Film-based radiographs require meticulous processing procedures to avoid errors that can result in undiagnostic images. Poor-quality radiographic images that have to be retaken increase patient radiation exposure. Careful attention to chemical replenishment and the following of time–temperature method processing produces radiographs of ideal quality and avoids retakes (see Chapter 7).

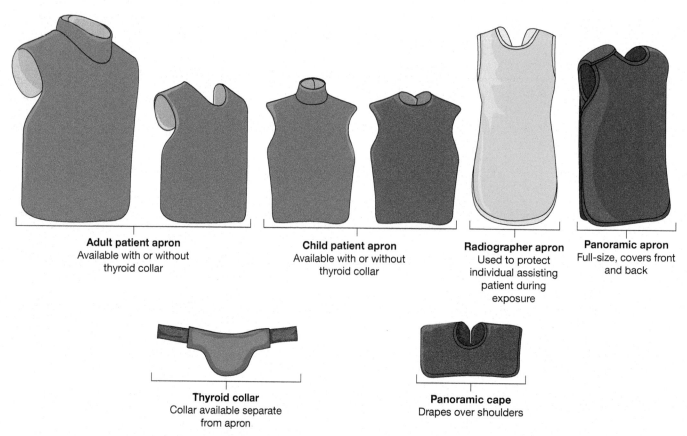

Adult patient apron
Available with or without thyroid collar

Child patient apron
Available with or without thyroid collar

Radiographer apron
Used to protect individual assisting patient during exposure

Panoramic apron
Full-size, covers front and back

Thyroid collar
Collar available separate from apron

Panoramic cape
Drapes over shoulders

FIGURE 6–12 **Lead aprons and thyroid collars** are available in a wide range of sizes. Aprons are available with an attached thyroid collar, or the thyroid collar may be a separate part.

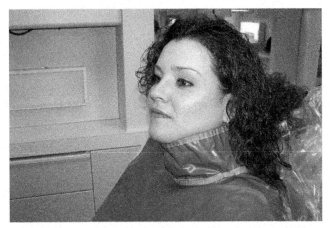

FIGURE 6–13 Patient protected with lead apron with thyroid collar in place.

Protection Measures for the Radiographer

All measures taken to protect a patient from radiation also benefit a radiographer (Box 6–2). Specific radiation protection methods for a radiographer include time, shielding, and distance. A radiographer should spend a minimal amount of time, protected by shielding, at the greatest distance from the source of radiation to avoid unnecessary exposure.

Time

When careful attention is focused on producing the highest quality radiographs, the need for retake radiographs is decreased, which in turn decreases the time a radiographer spends near an x-ray machine. Additionally, avoid the pitfalls that may lure movement into the path of the primary beam. For example, a drifting tube head should never be held during an exposure. Radiation leakage from the tube head can expose an operator to radiation. If the tube head drifts, it should be serviced for stabilization.

If a patient must be stabilized during a procedure, as is sometimes the case with a child, a parent or guardian may have to be asked to assist with the procedure. The parent or guardian should be protected with lead/lead-equivalent barriers such as an apron or gloves, when in the path of the x-ray beam. The radiographer must never be positioned in the primary beam.

Image receptor holding devices should be used to stabilize the receptor in a patient's oral cavity. If placement with an image receptor holding device is difficult to achieve, as is the case with a patient with a small mouth, low and/or sensitive palatal vault, or an exaggerated gag reflex, experiment with other holders, smaller image receptors, or the bisecting technique. A radiographer must not hold an image receptor in a patient's mouth. Additionally, another member of the oral health care team must not be allowed to place themselves in the path of the primary beam while the radiographer presses the exposure button.

Shielding

Structural shielding provides protection from potential scattered radiation. Safe installation of dental x-ray machines requires that an exposure button be permanently mounted behind a protective barrier, providing protection for an operator (see Figure 3–3). Most oral health care practices are located in buildings that have incorporated adequate shielding in walls such as these regularly used construction materials: plaster, cinderblock, 3 inches of drywall, 3/16 inch steel, or 1 millimeter of lead. Additionally, lead-lined walls or windows, thick or specially constructed partitions between rooms, or specially constructed lead screens offer excellent protection during exposure (see Figure 3–6).

Distance

If a protective barrier is not present, as may be the case in an open-bay designed practice setting, distance plays an important role in safeguarding a radiographer during patient exposures. Always stand as far away as practical—at least 6 ft (1.8 m)—from the head of a patient (the source of scatter radiation) while making an exposure. The intensity of the x-radiation diminishes the farther the x-rays travel. In addition to distance, it is important to remain in a position 45 degrees to the primary x-ray beam as it exits the patient, as this is the area of minimum scatter when the patient is seated upright. Maximum scatter is most likely to occur back in the direction of the tube head (Figure 6–14 ■). If exposing radiographs while a patient is in a supine position (lying prone in the examination chair), take a position at an angle of 135 to 180 degrees behind the patient's head where the least scatter radiation occurs. All persons, whether other oral health care team members or other patients not directly involved with the x-ray exposure, must be protected by shielding and/or distance.

Handheld X-ray Devices

Portable, battery-operated handheld x-ray generating equipment is increasingly being marketed for use in dental applications. **Handheld x-ray devices**, commonly referred to as

---

Box 6–2: Summary of Methods to Protect the Radiographer

- Follow all patient protection measures.
- Avoid contact with the tube head during exposure.
- Avoid retakes.
- Do not hold the image receptor for a patient.
- Use a protective barrier/shield.
- Use lead/lead-equivalent protective clothing when necessary.
- Remain 6 ft (1.82 m) away and at a 45-degree angle from the exiting primary beam.
- Use radiation monitoring.

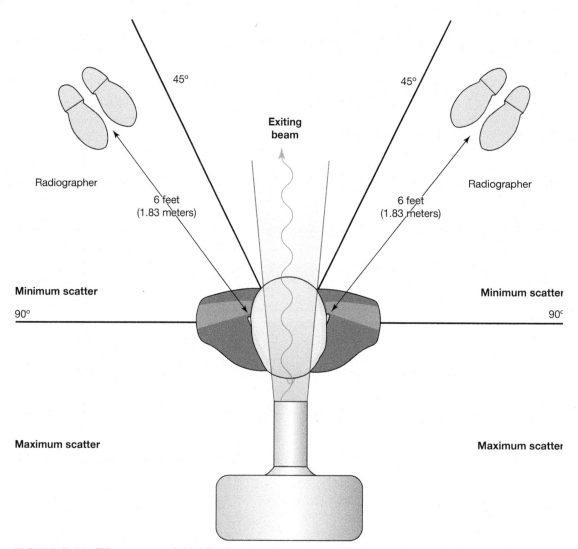

FIGURE 6–14 When structural shielding is not available, the radiographer should stand in a position at least 6 ft (1.83 m) from the head of the patient at an angle of 45 degrees to the exiting primary beam.

handhelds, provide a convenient way to bring beneficial radiographic diagnostic examinations into situations where a traditional x-ray machine would not be available, such as outreach health care screenings and onsite clinics in temporary, emergency settings (see Chapter 30). Handhelds should only be used when a conventional wall-mounted x-ray machine is not available, or when it is not practical to move a patient to where a conventional x-ray machine is located.

Only those brands of handheld devices that have been certified safe by the Federal Food and Drug Administration (FDA) should be used. Handhelds that are deemed safe are those that are manufactured with, and tested for, increased inherent tube head shielding; additional shielding around the PID; and a leaded acrylic external **backscatter ring shield** (Figure 6–15 ■). This shielding needs to be in place to protect against radiation leakage because an operator must hold the device during exposure. The 2.4 inch (6 cm) diameter round PID further helps limit scatter radiation by reducing the area exposed, compared with the 2.75 inch (7 cm) diameter of round PIDs fitted to stationary dental x-ray machines.

Research indicates that FDA-approved handheld devices present no greater radiation risk to a patient or to an operator than a conventional dental x-ray machine when safety protocols are followed. Prior to use, a radiographer

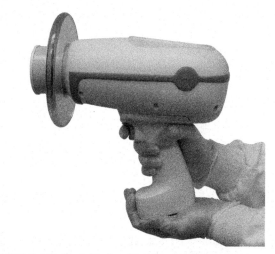

FIGURE 6–15 Portable handheld x-ray device.

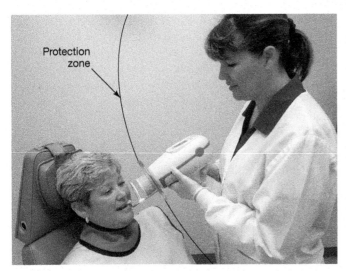

FIGURE 6–16 **Portable handheld x-ray device.** Note the protection zone provided by the backscatter ring shield.

must be familiar with the operating instructions supplied by the manufacturer. Safety protocol for the use of these portable devices differs from that used for traditional wall-mounted dental x-ray machines. For maximum radiation protection during exposure an operator must support the device with both hands, in front of the body at mid-torso height; remain within the backscatter ring shield protection zone; and position the PID as close to the patient's face as possible (Figure 6–16 ■). The backscatter ring shield only provides protection when the radiographer is holding the handheld upright with the PID parallel to the floor. Excessive vertical angulation of the PID or less than ideal patient positioning leads to increased angulation, which can alter the effectiveness of the backscatter ring shield and result in scatter radiation exposure to the radiographer. Handheld devices must not be used if the backscatter shield is not affixed to the unit or is damaged or broken. While some operators may choose to wear a lead/lead-equivalent apron while operating a handheld, studies continue to show that this is not necessary if recommended safety protocol is followed. Some state and local regulations require persons using portable x-ray devices to wear a radiation monitoring dosimeter. To prevent misuse or theft, the handheld device must be securely stored, preferably in a locked cabinet when not in use. The battery should be removed and, ideally, stored separately from the device.

Radiation Monitoring

The only way to determine what amount of radiation is emitting from dental x-ray equipment and that operators are not receiving more than the maximum permissible dose, is to use radiation measuring devices to monitor equipment and personnel. Because dental radiography equipment produces a very small amount of radiation, only that necessary to travel a short distance, radiation monitoring is not considered a requirement by many regulatory agencies unless employing a handheld, portable dental x-ray device.

Radiation monitoring is defined as periodic or continuing measurement to determine the exposure rate in a given area or the dose received by an operator.

Area Monitoring

Area monitoring involves making an onsite survey to measure the output of a dental x-ray machine, to check for possible high-level radiation areas in the operatory, and to determine if any radiation is passing through walls. Special equipment is needed to detect the exact amount of ionizing radiation at any given area. Numerous companies specialize in area monitoring. In some regions qualified state inspectors must perform this service.

Personnel Monitoring

Personnel monitoring requires oral health care professionals to wear a radiation monitoring device or dosimeter (Figures 6–17 ■ and 6–18 ■). For a fee, radiation monitoring companies provide the dosimeters, such as traditional **thermoluminescent (TLD) dosimeter**, **optically stimulated luminescence (OSL) dosimeter**, or an instant-dose monitor called a **direct ion storage (DIS) dosimeter**. The dosimeter is made to clip on or otherwise attach to the outside front of a radiographer's apparel and is to be worn throughout the day when exposing radiographs or when in the vicinity of radiographic equipment. After use, the dosimeter is returned to the company or the information recorded by the device is transmitted to the company via the Internet. The company evaluates the information captured by the dosimeter and provides the oral health care practice with a report regarding exposure. This report compares an operator's exposure reading with the maximum allowable level, and the monitoring company updates the subscriber's records to keep the wearer informed regarding compliance with federal and state safety regulations. The reports from a radiation monitoring service provide a reliable permanent record of accumulated doses of occupational radiation exposure. There are several different types of personnel monitoring devices currently on the market (Table 6–2 ■).

The likelihood of dental radiation exposing an oral health care professional who is following ALARA is so

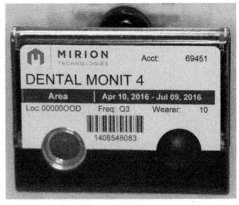

FIGURE 6–17 **Thermoluminescent dosimeter (TLD)** worn by a radiographer to monitor radiation exposure.

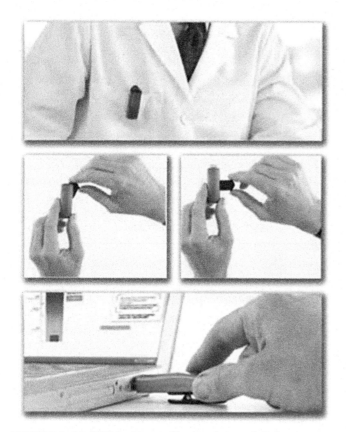

FIGURE 6–18 DIS dosimeter. Sized and shaped similar to a thumb drive. Clip allows a radiographer to wear the dosimeter while working with ionizing radiation. Dosimeter uses a USB connector to plug into a computer with Internet access. When logged on to the manufacturer's Web site, real-time radiation exposure readings may be downloaded from the device. (Courtesy of Mirion Technologies.)

small that only a few states consider dental radiation monitoring mandatory, unless operating a mobile or handheld x-ray device. Even so, more oral health care professionals are deciding to secure monitoring devices and services for themselves and their employees, even when not mandated by law. As a risk management tool, monitoring radiation exposure—or more likely, documenting the lack of exposure—helps to determine whether the operator is maintaining radiation safety protocols; aids in providing the radiographer with peace of mind; and assists with risk management by providing a health record of exposure, or more likely, the lack of exposure, for personnel.

Although personnel monitoring dosimeters play a valuable role, it should be noted that they are limited in their ability to be precise at estimating very low levels of exposure. Advancing technology in this area continues to improve the ability of dosimeters to estimate low-dose exposures. Monitors that have been approved by the National Voluntary Laboratory Accreditation Program (NVLAP) can be expected to be accurate. However, personnel monitoring dosimeters do not "protect" the wearer from radiation.

Organizations Responsible for Recommending/Setting Exposure Limits

As early as 1902, studies were undertaken to determine the effect of radiation exposure on the body and to consider setting limits on radiation exposure. The International Commission on Radiological Protection (ICRP) was formed in 1928, and in 1929 the National Council on Radiation Protection and Measurements (NCRP) was created in the United States. The ICRP and the NCRP do not actually set laws governing the use of ionizing radiation, but their suggestions and recommendations are so highly regarded that most all regulatory bodies use recommendations from these organizations to formulate legislation controlling the use of radiation. The American Dental Association (ADA) and its various committees and affiliated organizations, such as the American Academy of Oral and Maxillofacial Radiology (AAOMR), work closely with all organizations to ensure

Table 6–2 Types of Personnel Monitoring Dosimeters

Type	How It Works	Advantages	Limitations
Thermoluminescent dosimeter (TLD)	Contains crystals, usually lithium fluoride, that absorb radiation; crystals are heated after being exposed, and energy emitted, in the form of visible light, is proportional to the amount of radiation absorbed	Reliably used for many years	Badge must be returned to the monitoring company at specific intervals for reading
Optically stimulated luminescence (OSL) dosimeter	Absorbs radiation similar to TLD, but crystals release energy during optical stimulation instead of heat	Allows multiple readouts for reanalysis	Badge can only be used once
Direct ion storage (DIS) dosimeter	Uses miniature ion chamber to absorb radiation; exposure is determined through digital processing	Instant real-time unlimited readouts	Requires onsite reader or connection to the Internet

Table 6–3 Radiation Protection Organizations

Organization	Web Site
International Commission on Radiological Units and Measurements (ICRU)	www.icru.org
International Commission on Radiological Protection (ICRP)	www.icrp.org
National Council on Radiation Protection and Measurements (NCRP)	www.ncrponline.org
U.S. Nuclear Regulatory Commission (NRC)	www.nrc.gov
U.S. Environmental Protection Agency (EPA)	www.epa.gov
U.S. Food and Drug Administration (FDA)	www.fda.gov
U.S. Occupational Safety and Health Administration (OSHA)	www.osha.gov
American Academy of Oral and Maxillofacial Radiology (AAOMR)	www.aaomr.org
American Dental Association (ADA)	www.ada.org

that oral health care patients receive state-of-the-art treatment in radiation safety (Table 6–3 ■).

Maximum Permissible Dose

The United States Nuclear Regulatory Commission has developed radiation protection guidelines referred to as the **maximum permissible dose (MPD)** for the protection of radiation workers and the general public (Table 6–4 ■). MPD is defined as the dose equivalent of ionizing radiation that, in the light of present knowledge, is not expected to cause detectable body damage to average persons at any point during their lifetime. These limits do not apply to medical or dental radiation used for diagnostic or therapeutic purposes. Maximum limits are set higher for workers than for the general population, but the suggested limits of the MPD for both groups are purposely set far lower than it is believed the human body can safely accept.

- **Radiation workers.** The MPD for oral health care professionals is the same as for other **radiation workers**. According to these guidelines, the whole-body dose may not exceed 50 mSv (5 rem) per year. There is no established weekly limit, but state public health personnel often use a weekly dose upper limit of 1.0 mSv (0.1 rem) when inspecting oral healthcare facilities that employ dental x-ray equipment.

The 50 mSv (5 rem) yearly limit for radiation workers has two very important exceptions. It does not apply to persons under 18 years of age or to any pregnant member of the oral health care team. Persons under age 18 are classified as part of the general public and can accumulate only 5 mSv (0.5 rem) per year. In the case of pregnancy, it is recommended that exposure to the fetus be limited to 5 mSv (0.5 rem), not to be received at a rate greater than 0.5 mSv (0.05 rem) per month.

Table 6–4 U.S. Nuclear Regulatory Commission Occupational Dose Limits

Tissue	Annual Dose Limit
Whole body	50 mSv (5 rem)
Any organ	500 mSv (50 rem)
Skin	500 mSv (50 rem)
Extremity	500 mSv (50 rem)
Lens of eye	150 mSv (15 rem)

U.S. Nuclear Regulatory Commission. (2015, December 2). *Standards for protection against radiation*, Title 10, Part 20, of the Code of Federal Regulations. Retrieved from the Nuclear Regulatory Commission website: http://www.nrc.gov/reading-rm/doc-collections/cfr/part020/part020-1201.html

- **General public.** The general public is permitted 5 mSv (0.5 rem) per year, or one-tenth the dose permitted radiation workers. It should be noted that the MPD has been established for incidental or accidental exposures and does not include doses from medical and dental diagnostic or therapeutic radiation. Necessary medical and dental diagnostic or therapeutic radiation is not counted in the permissible dose limits. If a patient is prescribed a radiographic examination, that amount of radiation does not contribute to the patient's MPD. An oral health care team member who requires medical, dental diagnostic, or therapeutic radiation would become a "patient," again, without having an effect on the MPD.

Guidelines for Maintaining Safe Radiation Levels

Radiation Safety Legislation

The U.S. Tenth Amendment gives states the constitutional authority to regulate health, but because many federal agencies are involved in the development and use of atomic energy, the federal government has preempted the control of radiation. Certain provisions of the Constitution and Public Law 86-373 have enabled states to assume this preempted power and pass laws that spell out radiation safety measures to protect patient, radiographer, or anyone (general public) near a source of radiation. Some counties and cities have passed ordinances to protect their citizens from radiation hazards.

The entry of the federal government into the regulation of x-ray machines began in 1968 with the enactment of the Radiation Control for Health and Safety Act, which standardized the performance of x-ray equipment. Subsequently, the Consumer-Patient Radiation Health and Safety Act of 1981 was passed, requiring states to develop minimum standards for operators of dental x-ray equipment. Several states responded to this by enacting educational requirements for the certification of individuals who place and expose dental radiographs.

Because laws concerning radiation control vary from state to state, individuals working with x-rays must be familiar with regulations governing the use of ionizing radiation in their locale. Regardless of laws, failure to observe safety protocol cannot be justified ethically.

REVIEW—Chapter summary

Oral health care professionals have an ethical responsibility to adopt the "as low as reasonably achievable" (ALARA) concept—which implies that any dose that can be reduced without major difficulty, great expense, or inconvenience should be reduced or eliminated. The most important step in keeping a patient's exposure to a minimum is the use of evidence-based selection criteria to assess patients for radiographic need.

The technical ability (communication, working knowledge of quality radiographs, and education) of a radiographer aids in preventing unnecessary radiation exposure to a patient. Technique standards, including the radiographic technique, and the selection of exposure factors also aid in preventing unnecessary radiation exposure. A kilovoltage setting between 60 and 70 kVp is recommended; settings above 90 kVp should not be used. Size- and density-based exposure charts should be posted near the dental x-ray control panel for easy reference. Equipment standards that play important roles in reducing patient radiation dose include filtration, collimation, and PID length. Filtration is the absorption of long wavelength, less penetrating x-rays from the x-ray beam by passage through a sheet of material called a filter. The half-value layer (HVL) of an x-ray beam is the thickness (measured in millimeters) of aluminum that will reduce the intensity of the beam by one-half. Present safety standards require an equivalent of 1.5 mm aluminum filtration for dental x-ray machines operating in ranges below 70 kVp and a minimum of 2.5 mm aluminum for machines operating at or above 70 kVp. Total filtration is the sum of inherent and added filtration.

Collimation is the control of the size and shape of the useful beam. Federal regulations require that round opening collimators restrict the x-ray beam to 2.75 inches (7 cm) at the patient end of the PID. Rectangular collimation reduces patient radiation dose by up to 70 percent over round collimation. Collimation reduces scattered radiation that contributes to poor contrast of radiographic images.

A PID is an extension of the tube housing and is used to direct the primary x-ray beam. The length of a PID helps to establish the desired target–surface distance. PIDs have either a round or rectangular shape and are available in 8 inch (20.5 cm), 12 inch (30 cm), and 16 inch (41 cm) lengths. There is less radiation dose to the patient when using a long, 16 inch rectangular PID.

Fast film requires less radiation for exposure. Film speed groups D, E, or F are currently available for use in dental radiography. F-speed film reduces radiation exposure approximately 25 percent compared to E-speed film and approximately 60 percent compared to D-speed film. The use of digital image receptors can further reduce the radiation dose to a patient. The use of image receptor holders eliminates using the patient's fingers to stabilize the receptor intraorally, avoiding unnecessary radiation exposure to the patient's fingers; and assists the radiographer in obtaining quality radiographic images.

A lead or lead-equivalent thyroid collar with apron should be placed on all patients during intraoral x-ray exposures. Optimum film processing using time-temperature techniques in an adequately equipped darkroom will help avoid retakes that lead to an increase in patient radiation exposure. To reduce the chance of operator exposure, time spent near the source of radiation should be reduced; structural shielding employed; or the operator should be in a position at least 6 feet away from the source of radiation at a 45-degree angle to the exiting primary beam.

Handheld portable x-ray devices are advantageous for use in situations where wall-mounted units are unavailable or impractical. The tube head and PID of handhelds must have increased shielding and a backscatter ring shield must be affixed to the device to provide a protection zone for an operator during exposure. For maximum radiation protection during exposure, an operator must support the device with both hands, in front of the body at mid-torso height; remain within the backscatter ring shield protection zone; and position the PID as close to the patient's face as possible.

Thermoluminescent (TLD), optically stimulated luminescence (OSL), and direct ion storage (DIS) dosimeters that have been approved by the National Voluntary Laboratory Accreditation Program (NVLAP) can be used to monitor area and personnel exposure to radiation. The International Commission on Radiological Protection (ICRP) and the National Council on Radiation Protection and Measurements (NCRP) recommend dose limits. Federal, state, and local agencies set regulations governing exposure. The American Dental Association and the American Academy of Oral and Maxillofacial Radiology work closely with all agencies responsible for radiation safety. The maximum permissible dose (MPD) is 50 mSv (5 rem) per year for radiation workers and 5 mSv (0.5 rem) for the general public, radiation workers who are pregnant, and children under 18 years of age.

RECALL—Study questions

1. Who has an ethical responsibility to adopt ALARA?
   a. Dental assistants
   b. Dental hygienists
   c. Dentists
   d. All of the above

2. Based on the selection criteria guidelines, what is the radiographic recommendation for bitewing radiographs on an adult recall patient with no clinical caries and no high-risk factors for caries?
   a. Every 6–12 months
   b. Every 12–18 months
   c. Every 18–24 months
   d. Every 24–36 months

3. Communication, working knowledge of a quality radiographic image, and education all aid in protecting a patient against unnecessary radiation exposure by
   a. using lower exposure factors.
   b. reducing the risk of retake radiographs.
   c. collimating and filtering the primary beam.
   d. creating a longer target–surface distance.

4. What is the minimum total filtration required by a dental x-ray machine that can operate in ranges above 70 kVp?
   a. 1.5 mm of aluminum equivalent
   b. 1.5 mm of lead equivalent
   c. 2.5 mm of aluminum equivalent
   d. 2.5 mm of lead equivalent

5. What is the federally mandated maximum diameter size of the primary beam at the end of a round PID (at the skin of a patient's face)?
   a. 1.75 inches (4.5 cm)
   b. 2.75 inches (7 cm)
   c. 3.75 inches (10 cm)
   d. 4.75 inches (12 cm)

6. Radiation protection from secondary radiation may be increased by the use of an aluminum filter and a lead collimator *because* the filter regulates the size of the tissue area that is exposed and the collimator prevents low-energy radiation from reaching the tissue.
   a. Both the statement and reason are correct and related.
   b. Both the statement and reason are correct but NOT related.
   c. The statement is correct, but the reason is NOT.
   d. The statement is NOT correct, but the reason is correct.
   e. NEITHER the statement NOR the reason is correct.

7. Which of the following exposes a patient to less radiation?
   a. 8 inch (20.5 cm) round PID
   b. 12 inch (30 cm) round PID
   c. 16 inch (41 cm) round PID
   d. 16 inch (41 cm) rectangular PID

8. Which of the following contributes the most to reducing patient radiation exposure?
   a. D-speed film
   b. E-speed film
   c. F-speed film

9. During dental x-ray exposure, the lead/lead-equivalent thyroid collar with apron should be placed on
   a. children.
   b. females.
   c. males.
   d. all patients.

10. Each of the following aids in reducing patient radiation exposure EXCEPT one. Which one is the EXCEPTION?
    a. Slow-speed film
    b. Careful film handling
    c. Darkroom protocol
    d. Image receptor holders

11. If a protective barrier is not present, what is the recommended minimum distance that the operator should stand from the source of the radiation?
    a. 3 ft (0.91 m)
    b. 6 ft (1.83 m)
    c. 9 ft (2.74 m)
    d. 12 ft (3.66 m)

12. Which of the following is NOT a radiation safety feature of an FDA-approved handheld dental x-ray device?
    a. Increased inherent tube head shielding
    b. Additional shielding around the PID
    c. A leaded acrylic external backscatter ring shield
    d. A removable battery

13. TLD, OSL, and DIS dosimeters are used to
    a. protect an operator from unnecessary radiation exposure.
    b. reduce the radiation exposure received by a patient.
    c. monitor radiation exposure a dental radiographer may incur.
    d. record an onsite survey of the radiation output of the x-ray unit.

14. The annual maximum permissible whole-body dose for oral health care personnel is
    a. 0.5 mSv.
    b. 5.0 mSv.
    c. 50 mSv.
    d. 500 mSv.

15. The annual maximum permissible whole-body dose for the general public is
    a. 0.5 mSv.
    b. 5.0 mSv.
    c. 50 mSv.
    d. 500 mSv.

16. List three radiation protection organizations.
    a. _____
    b. _____
    c. _____

REFLECT—Case study

Use the selection criteria guidelines to make a preliminary recommendation and/or to explain to a patient why a dentist has prescribed or has not prescribed radiographs. Consider the following three cases:

1. A 17-year-old patient presents with a healthy oral assessment. No active caries clinically detected. No periodontal pockets noted. Record indicates last radiographs were bitewings taken 6 months ago. Based on the evidence-based selection criteria guidelines, what would be the most likely recommendation for radiographs for this patient?

2. A 25-year-old recall patient presents for a 6-month checkup. Although good home care is noted, Class II (multisurface) restorations are present on several molars and premolars. Last radiographs were bitewings taken 3 years ago. Based on the evidence-based selection criteria guidelines, what would be the most likely recommendation for radiographs for this patient?

3. A 45-year-old patient, new to the practice, presents with a moderate periodontal condition and evidence of generalized dental disease. No professional oral care in several years. Based on the evidence-based selection criteria guidelines, what would be the most likely recommendation for radiographs for this patient?

RELATE—Laboratory application

Using Box 6-1, Summary of Protection Methods for the Patient, and Box 6-2, Summary of Methods to Protect the Radiographer, as guides, perform an inventory of your facility, including a list of all used radiation protection methods. Compare and contrast these with the safety protocols learned in this chapter.

Begin with the first patient radiation protection method listed in Box 6-1, evidence-based prescribing. Investigate how the dentist at your facility determines who will need radiographs. What guidelines do the dental hygienist and the dental assistant use to help in explaining the need for necessary radiographs to a patient? Does your facility use guidelines similar to the evidence-based guidelines you learned about in this chapter? Describe them. Compare and contrast the methods your facility uses to determine radiographic need to the guidelines you learned about in this chapter. Is your facility meeting or exceeeding this safety method for reducing patient radiation dose? If not, what is the rationale for not meeting this standard?

Proceed to the next item on the list in Box 6-1, communication. Observe the communication between oral health care professionals at your facility prior to, during, and following patient x-ray exposure. What are some examples of dialogue that contributed to aiding in the protection of patients from unnecessary radiation exposure? Was there any communication that you think could have been added? Again, compare and contrast the communication standards the professionals at your facility use to decrease the likelihood of unnecessary radiation exposure using the guidelines you learned about in this chapter. Is your facility meeting or exceeeding this safety method for reducing patient radiation dose? If not, what is the rationale for not meeting this standard?

Proceed through the list of items in Box 6-1 and Box 6-2. Use observation and interviewing techniques to thoroughly investigate how each of these items is applied at your facility. Based on what you learned in this chapter, determine whether your facility is adequately applying all possible methods of reducing radiation exposure to patients and radiographers.

RESOURCES

American Dental Association: Council on Scientific Affairs. U.S. Dept. of Health and Human Services: Public Health Service. Food and Drug Administration. (2012). *Dental radiographic examinations: Recommendations for patient selection and limiting radiation exposure.* Washington, DC: Author.

Bruhn, A. M., Newcomb, T. L., & Tolle, S. L. (2015). Ensuring safe practice in dental radiology. *Dimensions of Dental Hygiene, 13*(12), 30–33.

Carestream Health, Inc. (2007). *Kodak Dental Systems: Radiation safety in dental radiography.* Pub. N-414. Rochester, NY: Author.

Castellanos, S., & Jain, R. K. (2013). Reduce radiation with rectangular collimation. *Dimensions of Dental Hygiene, 11*(2), 46, 48–50.

Christodoulou, E. G., Goodsitt, M. M., et al. (2003). Evaluation of the transmitted exposure through lead equivalent aprons used in a radiology department, including the contribution from backscatter. *Medical Physics, 30,* 1033–1038.

Danforth, R. A., Herschaft, E. E., & Leonowich, J. A. (2009). Operator exposure to scatter radiation from a portable hand-held dental radiation emitting device (Aribex™NOMAD™) while making intraoral dental radiographs. *Journal of Forensic Science, 54*(2), 415–421.

Harrison, L. (2013, February 11). New dental x-ray guidelines spell out radiation reduction. Retrieved from Medscape Today News website: http://www.medscape.com /viewarticle/779091

Kuroyanagi, K., Yoshihiko, H., Hisao, F., & Tadashi, S. (1998). Distribution of scattered radiation during intraoral radiography with the patient in supine position. *Oral Surgery Oral Medicine, Oral Pathology, Oral Radiology 85*(6), 736–741.

National Council on Radiation Protection and Measurements. (1991). *Implementation of the principle of as low as reasonably achievable (ALARA) for medical and dental personnel.* NCRP Report No. 107. Washington, DC: NCRP.

National Council on Radiation Protection and Measurements. (2003). *Radiation protection in dentistry.* NCRP Report No. 145. Washington, DC: NCRP.

Thomson, E. M. (2012). Putting ALARA into practice. Dimensions in Brief, an educational supplement sponsored by Carestream Dental. *Dimensions of Dental Hygiene, 10*[supplement], 14–15.

U.S. Food and Drug Administration Center for Devices and Radiological Health. (2014, July 30). *Dental radiography: Doses and film speed.* Retrieved from FDA website: http:// www.fda.gov/Radiation-EmittingProducts/RadiationSafety /NationwideEvaluationofX-RayTrendsNEXT/ucm116524.htm.

Zuguchi, M., Chida, K., Taura, M., et al. (2008). Usefulness of non-lead aprons in radiation protection for physicians performing interventional procedures. *Radiation Protection Dosimetry, 131,* 531–434.

Visit www.pearsonhighered.com/healthprofessionsresources to access the student resources that accompany this book. Simply select Dental Hygiene from the choice of disciplines. Find this book and you will find the complementary study tools created for this specific title.

Dental X-ray Image Receptors and Image Production

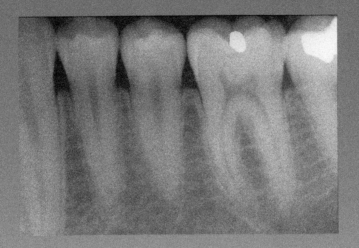

OUTLINE

Dental X-ray Film and Processing Methods

CHAPTER OUTLINE

OBJECTIVES

Following successful completion of this chapter, you should be able to:

1. Define the key terms.
2. List and describe the four parts of an intraoral film.
3. Describe latent image formation and explain how it becomes a visible radiographic image.
4. List and describe the four parts of an intraoral film packet.
5. Identify the intraoral film speeds currently available for dental radiographs.
6. Explain how duplicating film is different than radiographic film.
7. List in sequence the steps in processing dental films.
8. Identify and explain the role developer plays in processing a radiographic image.
9. Identify and explain the role fixer plays in processing a radiographic image.
10. List requirements for safelighting a darkroom.
11. Identify equipment needed for manual film processing.
12. Identify equipment needed for automatic film processing.
13. Compare manual and automatic processing methods, stating advantages and disadvantages of each.
14. Explain the role chemical replenishment and solution changes play in maintaining optimal processing chemistry.
15. List conditions that will diminish the quality of stored dental x-ray film.

KEY TERMS

Antihalation coating
Automatic processor
Darkroom
Daylight loader
Developer

Duplicating film
Elon
Emulsion
Extraoral film
Film feed slot
Film hanger
Film packet

Film recovery slot
Film speed
Fixer
Gelatin
Hydroquinone
Identification dot
Intraoral film

Introduction

Technological advances in digital imaging may one day render film-based radiography obsolete. Until that day, film remains a reliable method for acquiring diagnostic images to assess oral health and plan treatment for oral disease. Dental assistants and dental hygienists should possess a working knowledge of how radiographic film records an image, because radiation's interaction with film is what allows for the use of x-rays in preventive oral health care. Determining how film can best be used to provide the greatest amount of diagnostic information while exposing a patient to the least amount of radiation possible is key to radiation safety. This chapter explains film composition and types, outlines the fundamentals of film processing, and discusses film protection and storage to aid dental assistants and dental hygienists in making appropriate decisions regarding film use and handling.

Composition of Dental X-ray Film

The film used in dental radiography is photographic film that has been especially adapted in size, emulsion, speed, and packaging for dental uses. Figure 7–1 ■ illustrates the composition of dental x-ray film.

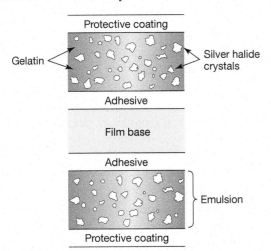

FIGURE 7–1 Schematic cross-section drawing of dental x-ray film. The rigid but flexible film base is coated on both sides with an emulsion consisting of silver halide (bromide and iodide) crystals embedded in gelatin. Each emulsion layer is attached to the base by a thin layer of adhesive. The emulsion layers are covered by a supercoating of gelatin to protect the emulsion from scratching and handling.

Film Base

Film base provides support for the fragile emulsion and strength for handling. Films used in dental radiography have a thin, flexible, clear, or blue-tinted polyester base. The blue tint enhances contrast and image quality. The base is covered with a photographic emulsion on both sides. Each emulsion layer is attached to the base by a thin layer of adhesive.

Emulsion

Emulsion is composed of **gelatin** in which crystals of silver halide salts are suspended. The main function of the gelatin is to keep the silver halide crystals evenly suspended over the base. The gelatin swells when placed in liquid, exposing the silver halide crystals to the chemicals in the developing solution. A supercoat layer of gelatin shrinks as it dries to protect the emulsion from handling, leaving a smooth surface that becomes the radiograph.

Silver halide crystals are compounds of a halogen (either bromine or iodine) with another element. In radiography, as well as in film photography, that element is silver. Dental film emulsion is about 90 to 99 percent silver bromide and 1 to 10 percent silver iodide. Silver halide crystals are sensitive to radiation; it is these crystals that, when exposed to x-rays, retain the latent image.

Latent Image Formation

During radiation exposure x-rays strike and ionize some, but not all, of the silver halide crystals resulting in the formation of a **latent (invisible) image** (Figure 7–2A ■). Not all the radiation penetrating the patient's tissues will reach the film emulsion. As discussed in Chapter 4, the varying thicknesses of the objects in the path of the beam will allow more or less radiation to pass through and reach the film emulsion. For example, enamel and bone will absorb, or stop, more x-rays

Practice Point

Patients have the right to access their dental records, including radiographs. The use of double film packets produces two original radiographs, allowing the practice to keep one as part of the patient's permanent record and to provide a ready copy for the patient when requested.

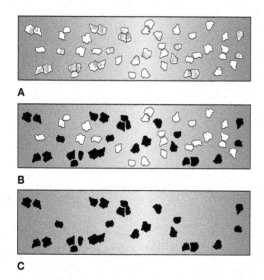

FIGURE 7–2 Cross section of dental x-ray film emulsion.
(**A**) X-rays strike silver halide crystals, forming latent image sites (shown in gray). (**B**) After development, crystals struck by x-rays (latent image sites) reduced to black metallic silver. (**C**) Fixer removes unexposed, undeveloped crystals, leaving the black metallic silver.

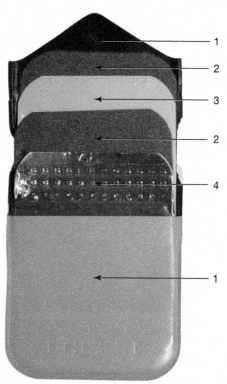

FIGURE 7–3 Open film packet as viewed from the back.
(**1**) Moisture-resistant outer wrap. (**2**) Black paper. (**3**) Film. (**4**) Lead foil backing.

from reaching the film than the less dense structures such as the dentin or pulp chambers of the teeth. When radiation does reach the emulsion, the silver halide crystals are ionized, or separated into silver and bromide and iodide ions that store this energy as a latent image. These energy centers store the invisible image pattern until the processing procedure produces a visual image, as discussed later.

Types of Dental X-ray Film

Intraoral Film

Intraoral film is designed for use inside the oral cavity. The use of an intraoral film outside the oral cavity is contraindicated because of the increased dose of radiation needed to produce an acceptable radiographic density.

FILM PACKET Film manufacturers cut films to the sizes required for dentistry. Small films suitable for intraoral radiography are made into what are called **film packets.** The terms *film packet* and *film* are often used interchangeably. All intraoral film packets (Figure 7–3 ■) are assembled similarly, and consist of:

1. **Film.** Film packets contain one or two films. When a packet containing two radiographic films is exposed, a duplicate radiograph results at no additional radiation exposure to the patient. A small raised **identification dot** is located in one corner of the film. The raised dot is used to determine film orientation and to distinguish between radiographs of the patient's right and left sides (see Chapter 20).
2. **Black paper wrapping.** The film is wrapped in black paper that adds additional protection from light exposure.

3. **Lead foil.** A sheet of lead foil is located in the back of the film packet, behind the film. The lead foil backing absorbs scattered radiation that strikes the film emulsion from the back side of the film (the side away from the tube), fogging or reducing the clarity of the image. The lead foil is embossed with a pattern that becomes visible on the developed radiograph in the event that the packet is accidentally positioned backward during the exposure.
4. **Moisture-resistant outer wrapping.** Consists of paper or soft vinyl plastic and holds the packet contents and protects the film from light and moisture. This wrapping is either smooth or slightly pebbly to prevent slippage. Each film packet has two sides, a front side or tube side that faces the tube (radiation source) and a back side that faces away from the source of radiation (Figure 7–4 ■). The tube side is usually solid white. The tab for opening the film packet is on the back side and may be white or a color depending on the manufacturer.

To aid in determining which is the front and the back side of the film packet, the following information is usually printed on the back side:

- Manufacturer's name
- Film speed
- Number of films in the packet (one or two)
- Circle or mark indicating the location of the identifying dot
- The statement "Opposite side toward tube"

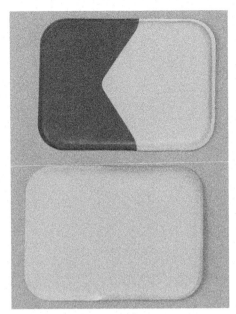

FIGURE 7–4 **Intraoral film packets**. Color-coded back side (*top*) and white, front or tube side (*bottom*).

FILM EMULSION SPEEDS (SENSITIVITY) Speed refers to the amount of radiation required to produce a radiograph of acceptable density. The faster the **film speed,** the less radiation required. Factors that determine film speed include size of the silver halide crystals, thickness of the emulsion, and the addition of special radiosensitive dyes.

Although a thick emulsion and the addition of radiosensitive dyes aid in increasing film speed (film sensitivity), the most important factor in increasing film speed is the size of the silver halide crystals in the emulsion. The larger the crystals, the faster the film speed, resulting in less radiation exposure to produce an acceptable image. However, image sharpness is more distinct when the crystals are small. The larger crystals used in high-speed (fast) film result in a certain amount of graininess that reduces the sharpness of the radiographic image. It has been determined that this slight loss of image sharpness does not interfere with diagnosis and is tolerated because of the reduction in patient radiation exposure.

SPEED GROUPS Trademark names like *Ultra*-speed or *Insight* are names assigned by the manufacturer and do not indicate the actual film speed. The American National Standards Institute (ANSI) groups film speed using letters of the alphabet: speed group A for the slowest through F, which is presently the fastest film available. In addition to labeling the film packages, film speed is printed on the back side of each individual film packet.

Currently only D-speed, E-speed, and F-speed films are available. Film speeds slower than D are no longer used, and some manufacturers have stopped producing E-speed film. Both the American Dental Association and the American Association of Oral and Maxillofacial Radiology recommend using the fastest speed film currently available to aid in reducing unnecessary radiation to patients. Although F-speed film requires less radiation to produce an acceptable image, some practitioners have not stopped using the slower D-speed film. Faster speed films contain a larger crystal size that may contribute to a slight decrease in image resolution. Some practitioners who are accustomed to viewing D-speed images resist the change. However, it should be noted that changes in the visual acuity of today's films have improved the image of the faster speed films, and studies of film speed comparisons have failed to indicate that faster speed films are less diagnostic. The use of high-speed film has made it possible to reduce patient exposure to radiation to a fraction of the time formerly deemed necessary.

FILM SIZE There are five sizes of intraoral film: 0, 1, 2, 3, and 4. The larger the number, the larger the size of the film (Figure 7–5 ■). These five film sizes are used to expose three

Practice Point

During intraoral film packet placement, the embossed dot should be positioned away from the area of interest. Usually, when taking periapical radiographs, the area of interest is the apices of the teeth. Therefore, the embossed dot should be positioned toward the occlusal. To assist with positioning the embossed dot out of the way, intraoral film manufacturers have packaged film so that the embossed dot can be observed on the outer moisture-resistant wrapping.

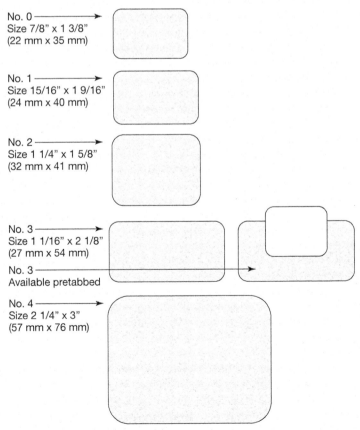

No. 0 ——→
Size 7/8" x 1 3/8"
(22 mm x 35 mm)

No. 1 ——→
Size 15/16" x 1 9/16"
(24 mm x 40 mm)

No. 2 ——→
Size 1 1/4" x 1 5/8"
(32 mm x 41 mm)

No. 3 ——→
Size 1 1/16" x 2 1/8"
(27 mm x 54 mm)

No. 3 ——→
Available pretabbed

No. 4 ——→
Size 2 1/4" x 3"
(57 mm x 76 mm)

FIGURE 7–5 **Intraoral film sizes.**

types of intraoral film projections: bitewing, periapical, and occlusal, which are described in detail in Chapter 12.

- **Size 0** film is especially designed for small children and is often called pedo (from the Greek word *paidos*, child) or pedodontic film.
- **Size 1** film may also be used for children. In adults, the use of the narrow 1 film is normally limited to exposing radiographs of the anterior teeth. Although it images only two or three teeth, this film is ideal for areas where the oral cavity is narrow.
- **Size 2** film is generally referred to as the standard film, or periapical film (PA). This film size is used to take both periapical and bitewing radiographs in adults and children whose oral cavities are large enough to tolerate its placement, making size 2 film the most selected size used in all intraoral radiography.
- **Size 3** film comes with a preattached bite tab and is used exclusively to take bitewing radiographs. Its longer horizontal dimension will record more teeth than size 2 film, allowing for the exposure of two size 3 films compared to four size 2 films in a set of bitewing radiographs (see Chapter 15).
- **Size 4** film is the largest of the intraoral films. Size 4 films are generally referred to as occlusal films, used exclusively for taking occlusal radiographs (see Chapter 16).

Extraoral Film

Extraoral film, classified as screen film, is larger in size and designed for use outside the mouth. **Screen film** (indirect-exposure film) is exposed primarily by a fluorescent type of light given off by special emulsion-coated intensifying screens that are positioned between the film and the x-ray source. The intensity of the fluorescent light emitted by the intensifying screens permits a significant reduction in the amount of radiation required to produce an image. The image produced on an extraoral film results from exposure to this fluorescent light, instead of directly from the x-rays (see Chapter 17).

PACKAGING Larger extraoral films are generally packaged 25, 50, or 100 to a box (Figure 7–6 ■). The films are sometimes sandwiched between two pieces of protective paper, and the entire group is wrapped in protective foil. Because these films are designed for extraoral use with a cassette, they require neither individual lead backing nor moisture-resistant wrappings.

FILM SIZE Extraoral films vary in size. The two most common sizes used to record the oral cavity and various regions of the head and neck are:

- 8 × 10 inch (20 × 26 cm), used for lateral views of the jaw, cephalometric profiles, and posteroanterior views of the skull
- 5 or 6 inch × 12 inch (13 or 15 cm × 30 cm), used for panoramic radiographs of the entire dentition

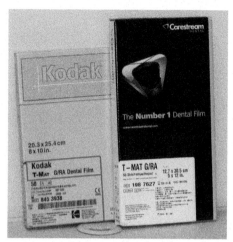

FIGURE 7–6 **Extraoral film packages** in sizes 8 × 10 inch (20.3 × 25.4 cm) and 5 × 12 inch (12.7 × 30.5 cm).

Duplicating Film

When a duplicate radiograph, a copy identical to an original, is needed, oral health care practices often use two- or double-film intraoral packets. However, if an additional copy is needed or a two-film packet was not used when the original radiograph was exposed, a duplicating machine with special duplicating film can be used.

Duplicating film is different than x-ray film and is exposed by the action of infrared and ultraviolet light rather than by x-rays. Only one side of the duplicating film is coated with emulsion. The emulsion side appears dull and lighter when observed under safe light conditions in the darkroom. The nonemulsion side is shiny and appears darker under safe light conditions. To make a copy of a radiograph, the emulsion side of the film is placed against the original radiograph with the nonemulsion side up (see Chapter 30). When duplicating film is exposed to ultraviolet light from a duplicating machine, the **solarized emulsion** records the copy. Solarized emulsion is different than x-ray film emulsion in that the image produced in response to light exposure gets darker with less light exposure and lighter with more light exposure. The nonemulsion side contains an **antihalation coating.** The dye in the antihalation coating absorbs the ultraviolet light coming through the film to prevent back-scattered light from reexposing the film and creating an unsharp image.

Dental X-ray Film Processing

Processing transforms the latent image, which is produced when the x-ray photons are absorbed by the silver halide crystals in the emulsion, into a visible, stable image by means of chemicals. The basic steps of processing dental x-ray film are:

1. Developing
2. Rinsing (automatic processors often omit this step)
3. Fixing
4. Washing
5. Drying

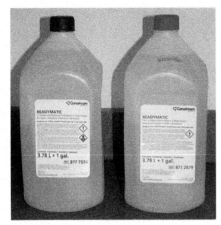

FIGURE 7–7 **Processing chemicals.** Ready to use developer and fixer.

Developing

The role of the **developer** solution is to reduce the exposed silver halide crystals within the film emulsion to black metallic silver (Figure 7–7 ■). Basically, the developer is responsible for creating the film's radiolucent appearance. The chemical ingredients in the developer solution are developing agents (also called reducing agents), a preservative, an activator (also called alkalizer), and a restrainer (Table 7–1 ■). The developing agents reduce the exposed silver halide crystals to metallic silver but have no effect on the unexposed crystals at recommended **time–temperatures.**

This is called **selective reduction,** meaning that only the nonmetallic elements, the halides, are removed, and the exposed silver remains (see Figure 7–2).

Developer contains two reducing agents, **hydroquinone** and **elon.** The hydroquinone works slowly but steadily to build up density and contrast in the image. The elon works fast to bring out the gray shades (contrast) of the image. Both chemicals are affected by extreme temperatures; therefore, regulating the temperature of the developer solution is critical.

Rinsing

The purpose of the rinsing step is to remove as much of the alkaline developer as possible before placing the film in the fixer solution. Rinsing preserves the acidity of the fixer and prolongs its useful life.

Fixing

After brief rinsing, the film is immersed in the **fixer** solution (see Figure 7–7). The fixing step (1) stops further film development—thereby establishing the image permanently on the film; (2) removes (dissolves) the unexposed/undeveloped silver halide crystals (those that were not exposed to x-rays); and (3) hardens (fixes) the emulsion. The chemical ingredients in the fixer solution are a fixing agent (also called a clearing agent), a preservative, a hardening agent, and an acidifier (Table 7–2 ■).

Table 7–1 Composition of Developer

Ingredient	Chemical	Action
Developing agent (reducing agent)	Hydroquinone	Reduces (converts) exposed silver halide crystals to black metallic silver; slowly builds up black tones and contrast
	Elon	Reduces (converts) exposed silver halide crystals to black metallic silver; quickly builds up gray tones
Preservative	Sodium sulfite	Prevents rapid oxidation of developing agents
Activator	Sodium carbonate	Activates developing agents by providing required alkalinity
Restrainer	Potassium bromide	Restrains developing agents from developing unexposed silver halide crystals, which produce film fog

Table 7–2 Composition of Fixer

Ingredient	Chemical	Action
Fixing agent (clearing agent)	Ammonium thiosulfate or sodium thiosulfate	Removes unexposed and any remaining undeveloped silver halide crystals
Preservative	Sodium sulfite	Slows rate of oxidation and prevents deterioration of fixing agent
Hardening agent	Potassium alum	Shrinks and hardens gelatin emulsion
Acidifier	Acetic acid	Stops further development by neutralizing alkali of developer

The fixing (clearing) agent, ammonium thiosulfate or **sodium thiosulfate,** also known as "hypo" or hyposulfate of sodium, removes all unexposed and any remaining undeveloped silver halide crystals from the emulsion. Basically, the fixer is responsible for creating the film's radiopaque appearance.

Washing

After the film is completely fixed, it is washed in running water to remove any remaining traces of the chemicals. If not thoroughly washed, chemicals will continue to react within the dried emulsion and degrade the image over time.

Drying

The final step is drying the film for storage as a part of the patient's permanent record. Films may be air-dried at room temperature or they may be dried in a heated cabinet especially made for this purpose.

Darkroom

The **darkroom** provides an area where x-ray films can be safely handled and processed. A well-equipped room with adequate safelighting aids in producing high-quality radiographic images. Films can be processed outside the darkroom with chairside manual processing mini-darkrooms or with a **daylight loader**–equipped automatic processor (Figures 7–8 ■ and 7–9 ■). A darkroom remains the standard in most film-based practices, especially because safelight conditions are required to handle larger tasks associated with extraoral film. The darkroom should be located near the area where radiographs will be exposed for convenient access and should be large enough to meet the requirements of the practice. The darkroom should be equipped with correct lighting and be plumbed for a water supply.

Lighting

X-ray film is sensitive to white light. Any white light in the darkroom can blacken the film or cause film fog. Therefore, the darkroom must be **light-tight.** A light-tight room is one that is completely dark and excludes all light. Felt strips may have to be installed around the door(s) to the darkroom or any other area such as around water pipes where a light leak is discovered. Although darkroom walls are sometimes painted black, this is not necessary if the room is completely sealed to white light. The following forms of illumination are desirable in the well-equipped darkroom.

1. **White ceiling light.** An overhead white ceiling light that provides adequate illumination for the size of the room will allow the clinician to perform equipment maintenance and other tasks requiring visibility.
2. **Safelight.** Safelighting is achieved through the use of a filtered white lightbulb or a special light-emitting diode (LED) bulb that provides enough light in the darkroom to allow the clinician to perform activities without exposing or fogging the film (Figure 7–10 ■). Older style **safelights** consist of a 7.5 or 15 watt white incandescent lightbulb with a **safelight filter** placed over it (Figure 7–11 ■). The safelight filter removes the short wavelengths in the blue-green region of the visible light spectrum. The longer wavelength red-orange light is allowed to pass through the filter to illuminate the darkroom. A variety of filters are available. Orange or yellow filters allow for safe handling of D-speed film, but E- and F-speed film and most extraoral films require a red filter. The type of safelight required for film processing can usually be found on the film package. LED safelights emit pure red light and are safe for all film speeds and types.

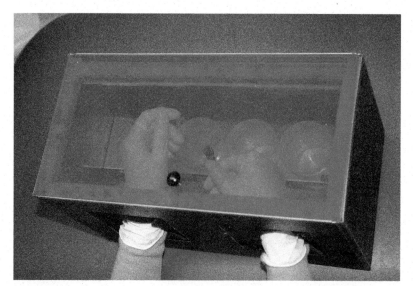

FIGURE 7–8 Chairside mini darkroom box with view-through plastic safelight filtered top. First cup is filled with developer, second cup with rinse water, third cup with fixer, and fourth cup with wash water.

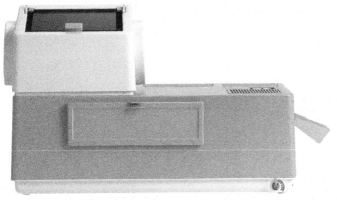

FIGURE 7–9 **Automatic processor with daylight loader attachment for use outside the darkroom.** (Courtesy of Air Techniques, Inc.)

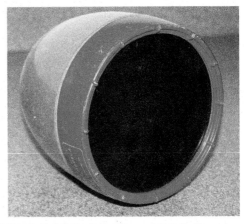

FIGURE 7–11 **Safelight.** Incandescent lightbulb enclosed inside a bracket-style lamp with red safelight filter shield.

The term "safe" light is relative. Film emulsion can be damaged by prolonged exposure even to filtered safelight. Film handling should be limited to 2.5 minutes under safelight conditions or fogging may occur. The distance between the lamp and the film is critical. The rule is 2.25 watts per foot (0.3 m) and a 4 ft (1.2 m) minimum distance between the source of light and the counter space where the film will be handled.

3. **Viewbox.** A **viewbox** or illuminator is a light source (generally a lamp behind an opaque glass) used for viewing radiographs. A darkroom equipped with a wall-mounted or countertop viewbox or illuminator will allow a clinician the opportunity for a quick reading, viewing the radiograph without leaving the darkroom. A viewbox emits considerable white light, and care must be taken not to turn it on when film packets are unwrapped. Additionally, if films are undergoing the developing process in a manual processor, the manual processor tank cover must remain on during the use of a viewbox.

4. **In-use light.** The darkroom door should be locked when processing films to prevent someone from entering and inadvertently allowing white light into the darkroom. Some darkrooms are equipped with a

warning light outside the darkroom, which indicates that it is not safe to open the door.

Maintenance

Cleanliness and orderliness are essential for the production of quality radiographs and the safety and health of the clinician using the area. Infection control protocol for opening film packets (see Chapter 9) must be strictly adhered to, and chemicals and other radiographic wastes must be properly handled and disposed (see Chapter 19). Because safelight conditions reduce visibility, a clinician must be skilled in the procedures to be performed. Needed materials should be within easy reach, and the person doing the processing should be familiar with where each item is located. The workspace counter must be free of substances that can contaminate films such as water, chemicals, and dust.

A utility sink large enough to accommodate cleaning the processing equipment should be available in the darkroom. A wastebasket should be placed in the darkroom for the disposal of general waste items. Lead foil is separated from other film wrappings and must be placed in an appropriate container for safe disposal, and the remainder of the film packet must be placed in a biohazard container for disposal (see Chapter 19).

Manual Film Processing

Manual processing is a method used to process films by hand in a series of steps (Procedure Box 7–1). Although no longer in widespread use, advantages of manual film processing are that it is reliable and not subject to equipment malfunction. A clinician has more control over the processing procedure, including the ability to adjust the time–temperature and the ability to read the radiographs prior to the end of the processing procedure (wet reading). Clinicians often make use of the manual processing procedure to "rapid" or "hot" process working films discussed at the end of this section. The biggest disadvantage of manual processing is the time required to produce a finished radiograph.

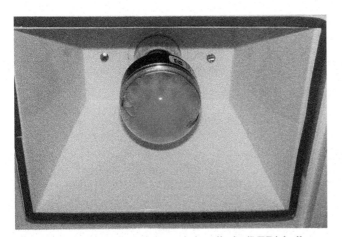

FIGURE 7–10 **Safelight.** Light-emitting diode (LED) bulb.

Procedure 7–1

Manual film processing

1. Maintain infection control (see Chapter 9).
2. Select a film hanger and label with patient information.
3. Open the light-tight cover of the manual processing tank to check solution levels to ensure adequate coverage of films when submerged. Add replenisher chemicals if necessary.
4. Stir the developer and fixer solutions to ensure even concentration throughout the tank. Use a different stirring paddle for each, developer and fixer, to prevent contamination of solutions.
5. Check the developer temperature and bring in line with manufacturer's recommendations. Chemical reaction is sluggish at low temperature, and high temperature increases film fog.
6. Refer to the time–temperature recommendations of the solution manufacturer and set timer. Optimal time–temperature for manually processed radiographs is 68°F for 5 minutes. Slight temperature variations from the ideal may be acceptable as long as the developing time is correspondingly adjusted (Table 7–3 ■).
7. Lock the darkroom door, turn off the white light, and turn on the safelight.
8. Open the film packets (see Figure 9-15) and place films on hanger.
9. Immerse the films into the developer solution and agitate film hanger for 5 seconds to release trapped air bubbles.
10. Set the timer. (Time is dependent on temperature of the developer solution.)
11. Close the light-tight cover while the film is developing.
12. When the developing time is complete, under safelight conditions, open the light-tight cover and remove film hanger with films attached from developer solution.
13. Pause a few seconds over the developer tank to allow the excess solution to drain from the films.
14. Immerse the film hanger into the water rinse and agitate for 30 seconds.
15. Pause a few seconds over the water tank to allow the excess water to drain from the films.
16. Immerse the film hanger into the fixer solution and agitate for 5 seconds to release trapped air bubbles.
17. Activate the timer for double the time in the developer or 10 minutes. Fixing time need not be as precisely controlled as developing time. However, excessively short fixing time results in slow drying and poor hardening of the emulsion, and loss of detail and darkening of the radiographic image over time. Excessively long fixing time will adversely lighten the image.
18. Close the light-tight cover for the first 2 to 3 minutes of fixation. (It is safe to view the films under white light after 2 or 3 minutes of fixation for a wet reading, following which the films must be returned to the fixer solution for completion of the fixation time for archival quality.)
19. Remove the film hanger from the fixer solution when the time is up.
20. Pause a few seconds over the fixer tank to allow the excess solution to drain from the films.
21. Immerse the films into the water wash for 20 minutes.
22. Remove the film hanger from the water wash when the time is up.
23. Place the film hanger in a commercially made film dryer or hang to air dry when the wash is complete.
24. Mount and label the dried radiographs.
25. Turn on white overhead light and clean up as needed. At end of workday, turn off water and drain water compartment. Leave cover in place over developer and fixer tanks to prevent oxidation and to contain chemical fumes.

Equipment

Manual processing requires the use of:

1. **A processing tank.** The **processing tank** has two insert tanks placed inside the master tank (Figure 7–12 ■). The insert tanks hold the developer and fixer solutions and should be labeled to prevent confusion as to which tank contains which chemical. Usually, the left insert tank holds the developer solution, and the right insert tank contains the fixer solution. The master tank holds water between the insert tanks for rinsing and washing the films. The master tank is usually equipped with a water-mixing valve that mixes the hot and cold water to any desired temperature. A close-fitting lightproof cover completes the tank assembly.

2. **A thermometer and timer.** To achieve selective reduction at recommended time–temperatures and eliminate guesswork, a thermometer and timer are necessary. The timer should have an audible alarm. Timers with a digital readout should emit red safelight only so as not to fog the film.

3. **Film hangers.** A **film hanger**, sometimes called a film rack, is a stainless steel frame to which the films can

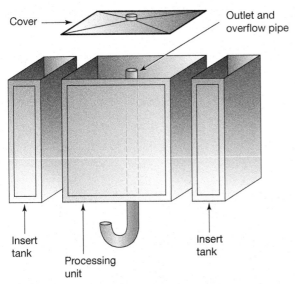

FIGURE 7–12 **Processing tank with removable inserts.** The central compartment holds the rinse/wash water and the inserts hold the developer and fixer solutions.

Cover
Outlet and overflow pipe
Insert tank
Processing unit
Insert tank

be attached (Figure 7–13 ■). A film hanger allows the radiographer to transport the films between each of the processing solutions. Various film hanger sizes are available that accommodate from 1 to 20 films.

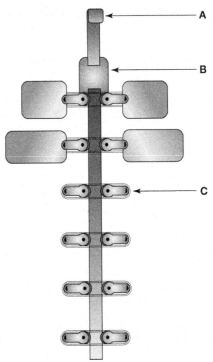

FIGURE 7–13 **Intraoral film hanger with 12 clips. (A)** Curved portion at the top allows the hanger to rest on the rim of the tank insert for the duration of the time required. **(B)** Identification tag on which the patient's name can be written. **(C)** Clamps hold the film securely in place.

Practice Point

If the radiograph is needed immediately for a quick reading of the image, the film may be read under white light conditions after 2 or 3 minutes of fixing. This is called a **wet reading.** The film can be rinsed in water for a short interval and viewed at a viewbox. The film must be returned to the fixer as soon as possible to complete fixation and permit further shrinking of the emulsion. If this is not done, some of the unexposed silver halide grains may be left on the film, giving it a fogged and discolored appearance after it dries.

Rapid (Chairside) Film Processing

Manual processing can be used to produce a **working radiograph** without a darkroom in about 30 seconds. Rapid or chairside processing with the use of special, faster-acting chemicals and a compact light-tight box that acts as a miniature darkroom can be valuable in endodontic practices, oral surgery practices, and at remote sites such as community outreach oral health projects where a darkroom is not available (see Figure 7–8). Rapid processing has limitations and is not intended to replace conventional processing. Short developing and fixing times, combined with minimal washing, result in a substandard radiograph. Rapid processing chemistry does not produce archival

Table 7–3 Time–Temperature Chart

Temperature		Development Time (min)
60°F (15.5°C)		9
65°F (18.3°C)		7
68°F (20°C)	optimum	5
70°F (21.1°C)		4.5
75°F (23.9°C)		4
80°F (26.7°C)		3

(permanent) results, and the films will eventually discolor. In the event that the film is to be retained with a patient's permanent record, it should be placed into the fixer solution for 4 minutes and washed for 20 minutes at normal conventional darkroom temperatures and conditions. Although rapid processing fulfills a need to view a radiograph quickly, it is at the expense of image quality and longevity.

Equipment

Rapid processing requires the use of a light-tight countertop box that has two light-tight openings, or baffles, through which a radiographer's hands can be passed into the working compartment when the lid is closed (see Figure 7–8). A transparent plastic top functions to filter out unsafe light while permitting the operator to see into the box to unwrap the film packet and manually proceed through the processing steps. Four cups are set up inside the box containing developer, rinse water, fixer, and wash water. A small film hanger with a single clip is used to manually transfer the film from solution to solution. Developing and fixing solutions made especially for rapid processing can be heated to 85°F (29.4°C) by a calibrated heater in the unit. Chemicals used for chairside processing are used for processing a limited number of films and then discarded appropriately (see Chapter 19).

Automatic Film Processing

Automatic processing has largely replaced manual processing for acquiring film-based radiographs because of its ability to produce a large volume of radiographs in less time (usually 5 minutes from developer to dried finished radiograph) (Procedure Box 7–2). Another advantage of an **automatic processor** is the machine's ability to regulate automatically the temperature of the processing solutions and the time of the development process. Disadvantages of automatic processing include possible equipment malfunction, increased

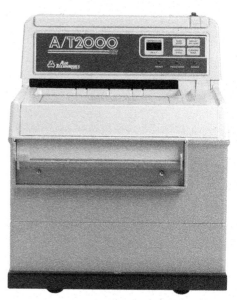

FIGURE 7–14 Automatic processor. (Courtesy of Air Techniques, Inc.)

maintenance required for optimal output, and more rapid chemical depletion than with manual processing chemistry.

Equipment

Automatic processing equipment varies in size and complexity (see Figure 7–9; Figure 7–14 ■). Some processors have a limited capacity and process only intraoral or certain sizes of extraoral films; others can handle any dental film regardless of size. Most are intended for use in the darkroom under safelight conditions. Automatic processors equipped with daylight loaders have a light-tight baffle for inserting the hands while unwrapping the film and can be used under normal white light conditions with a filter that acts as a safelight over the film entry slots.

Most automatic processors consist of three tanks or compartments, one each for the developer, fixer, and water, and a drying chamber (Figure 7–15 ■). All automatic processors require water. Some machines are connected to

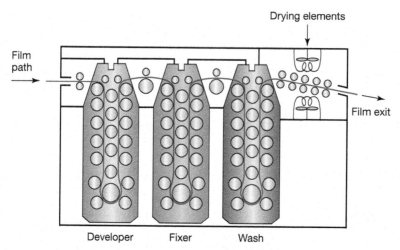

FIGURE 7–15 Schematic illustration of automatic film processor. Film is transported by roller assemblies through each of the processing steps.

Practice Point

In addition to being less effective, a breakdown in the integrity of the processing chemicals will occur if chemicals are not replenished or changed at the recommended intervals. This breakdown causes the solutions to become slick. Slick solutions cause the films to slide or slip through the roller transport system of the automatic processor, making it difficult for the rollers to advance the film and resulting in films that get stuck inside the machine.

existing plumbing, whereas others have a self-contained water supply. A heating unit warms the processing chemicals to the required temperature so there may be a warming-up period before the unit is operational.

The automatic film processing sequence usually consists of four steps: developing, fixing, washing, and drying. The use of a **roller transport system** helps "squeeze" excess solution from the film surface, allowing the automatic processor to omit the rinsing step between developing and fixing.

Unwrapped film is fed into the **film feed slot** on the outside of the processor. The roller transport system moves the film through the developer, fixer, water, and drying compartments. Motor-driven gears or belts propel the roller transport system. The film emerges from the processor through an opening on the outside of the processor called the **film recovery slot.** Most machines process a film in approximately

5 minutes. Some automatic processors have a 2-minute setting for producing working radiographs for a quick reading, similar to the wet reading produced with manual processing.

Processing Chemistry Maintenance

Both manual and automatic processing methods require chemical maintenance and solution replenishing and changing. Protective eyewear, mask, utility gloves, and a plastic or rubber apron should be worn when cleaning the processing tanks or changing the solutions.

Processing chemistry becomes weakened or lost in several ways. A small amount of developer and fixer is lost when chemicals adhere to the film surfaces during transfer from solution to solution. During manual processing stirring paddles, the thermometer, and film hangers all contribute to the loss of solution. Additionally, transfer of films between solutions will slowly contaminate the chemicals and weaken them.

Weakened chemistry also occurs through **oxidation**, the union of a substance—in this case, the developer and fixer—with the oxygen in the air. The developer is especially subject to oxidation in the presence of air and loses its effectiveness very quickly. Whenever possible, the processing tank covers should remain in place to slow oxidation and evaporation. The cover should be removed only when adding solutions to the proper level; when checking the temperature of the developer; and when inserting, removing, or changing the film hangers from one compartment or insert to another (manual processing). Care must be taken not to rotate the processor cover when it is removed. Causing only

Procedure 7–2

Automatic film processing

1. Maintain infection control (see Chapter 9).
2. Turn on water supply or fill water tanks of self-contained models.
3. Check solution levels to ensure adequate coverage of roller transports. Add replenisher chemicals if necessary.
4. Turn on the automatic processor and allow machine to warm to optimum temperature as determined by manufacturer.
5. Employ a method for labeling the feed slots used for retrieval and identification of films.
6. If it is the beginning of the day, or after several hours of inactivity, run a specially manufactured cleaning sheet through the processor and discard.
7. Unless the automatic processor is equipped with daylight loader baffles, lock the darkroom door, turn off the white light, and turn on the safelight.
8. Open the film packets (see Figure 9-15) and place films into the automatic processor feed slot.
9. Allow the rollers to grasp the film before releasing. Multiple films should be placed, one at a time, into alternating feed slots with 5 to 10 seconds wait between to prevent films from overlapping and getting stuck in the machine.
10. Ten seconds after feeding the last film into slot, turn on overhead white light and clean up the area as needed.
11. Retrieve the processed films when the cycle is complete, usually about 5 minutes.
12. Unless equipped with an automatic shutoff, turn off or place machine in standby mode to conserve water that would continue to run after the films have finished processing
13. Mount and label the radiographs.
14. At the end of the workday, turn off main power and water supply. Leave cover in place over developer and fixer tanks to prevent oxidation and to contain chemical fumes.

a few drops of condensed developer to fall into the fixer or vice versa will contaminate and weaken the solutions. All chemistry must be changed periodically to avoid diminishing quality. The useful life of the solutions depends on:

- The original quality or concentration of the solution
- The original freshness of the solution used
- The number of films that are processed
- Contamination, oxidation, and evaporation of the chemicals

Many chemical manufacturers recommend that processing solutions be changed at least every 4 weeks under "normal" use. Because normal use may be defined differently among different practices, refer to the manufacturer recommendations to determine reasonable intervals to change solutions. One way to maintain solution strength in between changes is through replenishment.

Replenishment consists of removing a small amount of developer and fixer and replacing with fresh chemistry or chemical replenisher specifically made for this purpose. For every 30 intraoral films processed, it is recommended that 6 to 8 ounces of developer and fixer be removed and discarded. (See Chapter 19 for safe and environmentally sound protocols for discarding radiographic wastes.) Fresh chemicals should be added to raise the solution levels in the tanks to the full level. Some processors automatically replenish the solutions; others depend on the operator to keep them at the correct level.

Automatic processors require strict adherence to manufacturers' instructions for chemical replenishment and changes and for cleaning the unit to maintain optimal performance. Few pieces of equipment in the oral health care practice require such diligence and regular care. Depending on the workload, automatic processors require daily, weekly, or monthly cleaning. A specially designed cleaning sheet may be run through the processor to remove debris and residual gelatin from the rollers daily or more often if the processor sits idle for several hours (Figure 7–16 ■). However, complete cleaning and maintenance of the roller transports and solution-holding

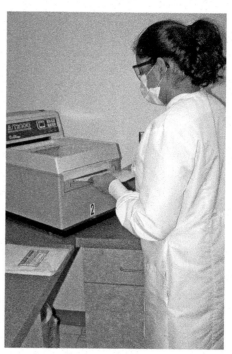

FIGURE 7–16 Specially prepared cleaning sheet run through the processor to remove any residual debris from the rollers.

tanks is also required. If the rollers are not kept free of debris, radiographs emerge streaked, stained, or worse, with scratched emulsion. Most manufacturers recommend that the roller assembly be removed and cleaned weekly, in warm running water and special cleansers. It is important to follow manufacturer's instructions concerning care and maintenance.

Film Storage and Protection

All radiographic film is extremely sensitive to radiation, light, heat, humidity, chemical fumes, and physical pressure. Additionally, film is sensitive to aging, having a shelf life determined by the manufacturer. Precautions for safely storing and protecting films from these conditions must be followed. Film fogging is the darkening of the finished radiograph caused by one or more of these factors.

Radiation

Stray radiation, not intended for primary exposure, can fog film. Film should be stored in its original packaging in an area shielded from radiation. Individual film packets should also be kept in a shielded area. This is especially important while in the process of exposing several radiographs at one time, as is the case when exposing a set of bitewings or full mouth series. Once a film has been exposed to radiation, the crystals within the emulsion increase in their sensitivity. The exposed film should be placed in a shielded area while the next film is exposed. All exposed films should be kept safe from radiation until processing.

Practice Point

It is important to note that the processing chemicals used in automatic processors differ from those used in manual procedures. Solutions for use in automatic processors are supersaturated, and the developer contains more hardening agents. The chemical solutions in automatic processors are heated to temperatures much higher than those used in manual processing—as high as 125°F (52°C) in some units. Advanced film technology has produced film emulsions that can withstand these temperatures for the short times required in automated processing without excessive softening or melting.

Light

Care should be taken when handling intraoral film packets so as not to tear the outer light-tight wrap. Extraoral cassettes must be closed tightly to prevent light leaks. Safe lighting in the darkroom must be periodically examined to ensure safe light conditions (see Chapter 19).

Heat and Humidity

To prevent fogging, film should be stored in a cool, dry place. Ideally, all unexposed film should be stored at 50°F to 70°F (10°C–21°C) and 30 to 50 percent relative humidity.

Chemical Fumes

Film should be stored away from the possibility of contamination by chemical fumes. Film should not be stored in the darkroom near processing chemicals.

Physical Pressure

Physical pressure and bending can fog film. When storing, boxes of film must not be stacked so high as to increase the pressure on the packets. Heavy objects should not be placed or stored on top of film.

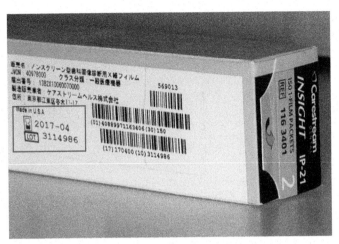

FIGURE 7–17 **Film package showing expiration date.**

Shelf Life

Dental x-ray film has a limited shelf life. The expiration date is printed on the film packaging (Figure 7–17 ■). All intraoral film should be stored so that the expiration date can be readily seen and the appropriate films used first. Expired film compromises the diagnostic quality of the image and should not be used.

REVIEW—Chapter summary

X-ray film serves as a radiographic image receptor. The film used in dental radiography is photographic film that has been especially adapted in size, emulsion, film speed, and packaging for dental uses. All x-ray film has a polyester base that is coated with a gelatin emulsion containing silver halide (bromide and iodide) crystals. During radiation exposure, the x-rays strike and ionize some of the silver halide crystals, forming a latent image. The image does not become visible until the film is processed.

An intraoral film packet consists of film, light-protective, black paper wrapping, lead foil, and a moisture-resistant outer wrapping. Intraoral film packets have a white, unprinted front or tube side. The lead foil and the tab for opening the film packet are on the back side. Film speed (sensitivity) refers to the amount of radiation required to produce a radiograph of acceptable density. Currently only D-, E-, and F-speed films are available for dental radiographs. The five intraoral film sizes are 0, 1, 2, 3, and 4.

Larger extraoral films designed for use outside the mouth are classified as screen films because fluorescent light from intensifying screens is used to help the x-rays produce the image. Duplicating film is used in conjunction with a duplicating machine that emits light to make copies of radiographs. Duplicating film differs from radiographic film in that the solarized emulsion gets darker with less light exposure and lighter with more light exposure.

Film processing is a series of steps that converts the invisible latent image on the dental x-ray film into a visible permanent image called a radiograph. The sequence of processing steps is developing, rinsing, fixing, washing, and drying. Developing reduces the exposed silver halide crystals within the film emulsion to black metallic silver. Rinsing removes the alkaline developer before the film enters the fixer solution. Fixing removes the unexposed and/or undeveloped silver halide crystals from the film emulsion. Washing removes any remaining traces of the chemicals. Drying preserves the film and allows for storage as a part of the patient's permanent record.

With the exception of automatic processors equipped with daylight loaders and chairside rapid processing miniature darkroom boxes, all processing must be done in the darkroom under safelight conditions. Safelighting is achieved with a red light-emitting diode (LED) or a white incandescent lightbulb with a filter that eliminates short wavelength, blue-green light.

Manual processing requires a processing tank, thermometer, timer, and film hangers. The ideal time–temperature for manual processing is 68°F (20°C) for 5 minutes. Colder developer solution requires a longer developing time; warmer developer solution requires a shorter developing time. With specially adapted chemistry, the rapid processing method can produce a radiographic image in less than 1 minute. Automatic processors use a roller transport assembly to advance the films automatically from solution to solution, producing a finished radiograph in 5 minutes.

Oxidation over time and chemical contamination through normal use prompt solution changes and regularly scheduled equipment maintenance and cleaning. The useful life of the solutions is determined by the original quality or concentration of the solution, the freshness of the solution, the number of films that have been processed, and the contamination of the chemicals. Replenishment helps prolong the life of the processing solutions.

X-ray film is sensitive to radiation, light, heat, humidity, chemical fumes, physical pressure, and aging. Care must be exercised in storing and in handling film before, during, and after exposure.

RECALL—Study questions

1. Which of the following provides support for the fragile film emulsion?
   a. Base
   b. Adhesive
   c. Silver halide crystals
   d. Protective coating

2. Which of the following is light and x-ray sensitive?
   a. Lead foil
   b. Adhesive
   c. Gelatin
   d. Silver halide crystals

3. During x-ray exposure, crystals within the film emulsion become energized with a(n)
   a. visible image.
   b. slow image.
   c. latent image.
   d. intensified image.

4. What is the function of the lead foil in the film packet?
   a. Protect against moisture
   b. Absorb backscatter radiation
   c. Give rigidity to the packet
   d. Protect against fluorescence

5. Each of the following can be found on the back side of an intraoral film packet EXCEPT one. Which one is the EXCEPTION?
   a. Film speed
   b. Film size
   c. Embossed dot location
   d. Number of films in packet

6. Which of the following film speeds has the greatest sensitivity to radiation?
   a. D
   b. E
   c. F

7. Which of the following is FALSE regarding duplicating film?
   a. Emulsion is solarized.
   b. Emulsion is on one side only.
   c. Requires more radiation exposure than radiographic film.
   d. Requires exposure to infrared and ultraviolet light to produce an image.

8. Which of the following is the correct processing sequence?
   a. Rinse, fix, wash, develop
   b. Fix, rinse, develop, wash
   c. Rinse, develop, wash, fix
   d. Develop, rinse, fix, wash

9. During which step of the processing procedure are the exposed silver halide crystals reduced to metallic silver?
   a. Developing
   b. Fixing
   c. Rinsing
   d. Washing

10. Which ingredient removes the unexposed/undeveloped silver halide crystals from the film emulsion?
    a. Acetic acid
    b. Potassium bromide
    c. Sodium thiosulfate
    d. Hydroquinone

11. Which of the following colors of safelight filters is safe for processing all film speeds?
    a. Yellow
    b. Green
    c. Red
    d. Blue

12. A thermometer is used for manual processing to determine the temperature of the
    a. developer solution.
    b. water.
    c. fixer solution.
    d. Both a and c are correct.

13. Each of the following is an advantage of automatic processing over manual processing EXCEPT one. Which one is the EXCEPTION?
    a. Decreased processing time
    b. Less maintenance
    c. Increased capacity for processing
    d. Self-regulation of time and temperature

14. Replenisher is added when necessary to the developing solution to compensate for
    a. oxidation.
    b. loss of volume.
    c. loss of solution strength.
    d. all of the above.

15. X-ray films should be stored
    a. away from heat and humidity.
    b. near the source of radiation.
    c. in the darkroom.
    d. stacked in columns.

REFLECT—Case study

You work for a temporary agency that provides staffing for oral health care practices in your area. Today your employer has sent you to a practice organized and set up for a left-handed practitioner. Your first patient requires a bitewing series of radiographs. You expose the films and proceed to the darkroom for processing. Unknown to you, this practice has set up the manual processing tanks with the developing solution tank on the right and the fixer tank on the left. You are used to working with processing tanks set up with the developing solution on the left and the fixer on the right, and you proceed to process your films in this manner. What effect will this have on the resultant radiographs? Why will they look this way? Explain why the processing solutions will produce this result. What can you do to avoid this mistake in the future? What can this practice do to prevent this mistake from happening again?

RELATE—Laboratory application

Obtain one each of a size 0, size 1, size 2, size 3, and size 4 intraoral film packet. Beginning with the size 0 film packet, consider the following. Repeat with each of the film sizes. Write out your observations.

1. What is the film speed? How did you get the answer to this question?

2. What information is written on the outside of the film packet? Where is this information written: on the front or back of the film packet?

3. How many films do you expect to find inside this packet? How did you get the answer to this question?

4. Where is the embossed dot located? How did you find it? What is this used for?

5. What about this film packet's size makes it ideal; less than ideal; or not suited for an adult patient? A child patient?

6. Now open the film packet. List the four parts of the packet and explain the purpose of each.

7. Next, hold the film up horizontally (parallel to the floor) at eye level and observe it from the edge. Can you see the film base with the emulsion coating on the top and the bottom?

8. Next, observe the metal foil. What is the reason for the embossed imprint?

9. When you opened the film packet, did you utilize the inner black paper's tab? This tab plays an important role in opening a contaminated film packet aseptically. This is discussed in detail in Chapter 9.

RESOURCES

Carestream Health, Inc. (2015). *Exposure and processing for dental film radiography.* Pub. N-414. Rochester, NY: Author.

Visit www.pearsonhighered.com/healthprofessionsresources to access the student resources that accompany this book. Simply select Dental Hygiene from the choice of disciplines. Find this book and you will find the complementary study tools created for this specific title.

8

Digital Radiography and Image Acquisition

CHAPTER OUTLINE

OBJECTIVES

Following successful completion of this chapter, you should be able to:

1. Define the key terms.
2. Explain the fundamental concepts of digital radiography and image acquisition.
3. Describe the characteristics of a digital image.
4. List equipment needed to acquire a digital image.
5. Explain the use of software in digital image interpretation.
6. Differentiate between direct and indirect digital imaging.
7. Describe the difference between narrow and wide dynamic range.
8. Describe and compare three types of digital image receptors.
9. Discuss digital imaging's effect on radiation dose to a patient.
10. Identify benefits and limitations of digital radiographic imaging.

KEY TERMS

Analog
Artificial intelligence
Charge-coupled device (CCD)
Complementary metal oxide
    semiconductor active pixel
    sensor (CMOS-APS)

Digital subtraction
Dynamic range
Gray scale
Gray value
Line pair (lp/mm)
Noise
Photostimulable phosphor (PSP)

Pixel
Sensor
Solid state
Spatial resolution
Storage phosphor
Transfer box

Introduction

Digital imaging is an integral part of the paperless oral health care practice. The introduction of digital image receptors, which function as radiographic film, and a computer that functions as a darkroom processor has the potential to improve the quality of oral health care while possibly reducing radiation exposure for a patient (Table 8–1 ■). Dental assistants and dental hygienists must possess an understanding of the concepts of digital radiography and develop the skills necessary to safely use digital technology. This chapter presents the fundamental concepts of digital radiography, introduces the types of digital imaging systems currently available, and discusses the benefits and limitations of digital radiography.

Fundamental Concepts

The term *digital imaging* has come to replace the term *radiography*. Using film to "take a radiograph" is being replaced with digital terminology to "acquire an image." The difference between a digital image and a film-based radiograph is that a digital image has no physical form. Digital images

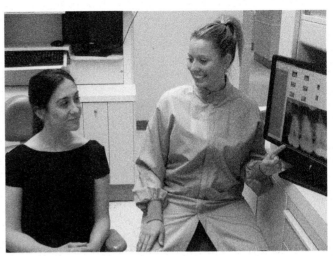

FIGURE 8–1 **Effective viewing of radiographic images.**

exist as bits of information in a computer file that special software constructs into an image on a monitor or other viewing device (Figure 8–2 ■). Digital radiography systems are not limited to intraoral images; panoramic and other extraoral radiographic digital imaging systems are also available. The techniques and methods learned for exposing intra- and extraoral radiographs are the same whether using traditional film or a digital sensor. The significant difference between film-based radiography and digital imaging is that the film is replaced with a digital image receptor and there is no longer a need for processing chemistry and darkroom equipment.

Table 8–1 Benefits and Challenges of Digital Imaging over Film

Benefits	Challenges
• Almost instantaneous viewing of image • Elimination of darkroom: processing time; potential processing errors; generation of hazardous wastes (processing chemistry and lead foils) • Images can be manipulated to improve visual acuity avoiding retakes; software enhances interpretation and diagnosis • Remote electronic consultation and sending of images • Easy-to-understand viewing that enhances discussion of treatment plan and oral hygiene education (Figure 8–1 ■) • Possibly less radiation exposure • Long-term costs may be less when compared to costs associated with purchasing film and processing chemicals	• Ease of retakes may result in excess radiation exposure • Smaller recording dimensions; additional exposures may be required to image an area entirely • Thick sensor size (CCD and CMOS-APS) and attached wire may be less tolerated by patient • Concerns with reliability and security: system malfunction, computer crash, or temporary inability to access images delaying treatment; computer viruses; secure space for image storage; changes in technology requiring expensive equipment updates • Environmentally friendly in short term, but disposal of broken, obsolete digital equipment must be considered

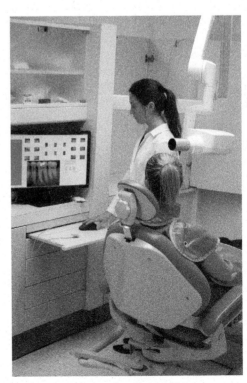

FIGURE 8–2 **Digital intraoral radiographic system.**

Characteristics of a Digital Image

Digital imaging systems produce a radiographic image on a computer monitor. The term *digital image* is used to distinguish this radiographic image from a film-based analog image. An **analog** image can be compared to a painting that has a continuous smooth blend from one color to another. A digital image is like a mosaic, made up of many small pieces put together to make a whole. A digital image is composed of structurally ordered **pixels**. Pixels (*pix,* plural of *pic*ture and *el,* short for *el*ement) are tiny dots representing discrete units of information that together constitute an image. Each pixel is a single dot in a digital image. The more pixels in an image, the higher the resolution and the sharper the image.

Spatial Resolution

The number and size of pixels determines **spatial resolution**, the discernible separation of closely adjacent details of an image. When the number of pixels is low, the image appears to have jagged edges and is difficult to see (Figure 8–3 ■). Spatial resolution is measured in line pairs. A **line pair (lp/mm)** refers to the greatest number of paired lines visible in 1 millimeter (mm) of an image. For example, a resolution of 10 line pairs/mm would mean that when 10 ruled lines are squeezed into 1 mm of an image, the individual lines can still be distinguished from each other. The greater the spatial resolution in an image, the sharper it looks.

Gray Scale

Gray scale refers to the number of shades of gray visible in an image. The gray scale of a radiographic image is probably its most important characteristic. Detection and diagnosis of oral conditions depend on gray scale to provide the appropriate image contrast. A practitioner most often relies on the radiograph's contrast, its radiolucency, and radiopacity to determine the presence or absence of disease. The ability to record subtle changes in the gray areas of images improves diagnosis. Digital radiographic systems claim the ability to produce up to 65,500 gray levels. However, computer monitors can display only 256 gray levels. A number stored for each pixel determines the number of shades of gray visible (Figure 8–4 ■). Each pixel has a number from 0 to 255, representing pure black at 0 to pure white at 255

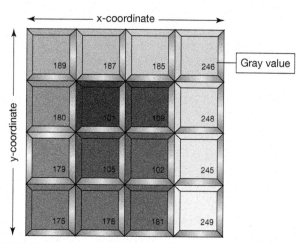

FIGURE 8–4 **Diagram of sensor grid.** Each square represents a pixel "well," which stores an exposure. Numbers correspond to gray values that a computer will reconstruct into an image.

for a total of 256 gray levels in an image. The human eye can distinguish only about 32 shades of gray unaided. However, this does not necessarily mean that the large range of gray scale captured by digital imaging systems is wasted. When aided by computer software features, which can be used to enhance the gray levels, it may be possible to detect changes that might be overlooked in film-based images.

The goal of digital imaging systems is to produce high-quality diagnostic images. It is the combination of pixels, spatial resolution, and gray scale that determines the quality of the final image. Manufacturers are continuing to improve the capability of digital equipment and software to aid in the early detection of oral diseases.

Acquiring a Digital Image

Digital imaging systems use a dental x-ray machine, a computer, and specialized software to acquire radiographic images.

Dental X-ray Machine

Both alternating current (AC) and direct current (DC) dental x-ray machines produce acceptable quality radiographic images when paired with digital image receptors. However, as explained in Chapter 3, DC dental x-ray machines may produce more consistent exposures at the very short exposure times associated with digital radiography (see Figure 3–11). If pairing digital imaging receptors with an AC dental x-ray machine, the impulse timer should be evaluated and possibly updated to ensure that it is capable of producing the low exposure output required to produce quality digital images. Generally speaking, a DC dental x-ray machine with settings at 60 kV or lower and a low 5 mA is ideally suited to digital radiography.

Computer

Digital radiography requires a computer to capture, and a monitor to view, the image. The type and size of computer required depends on several variables, such as the

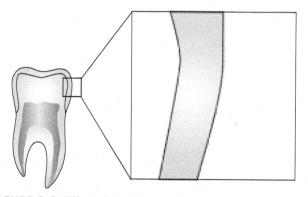

FIGURE 8–3 **Effect of pixel size on image.**

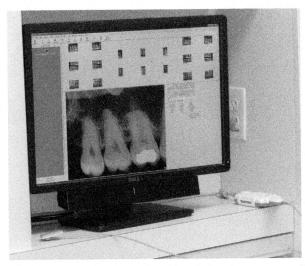

FIGURE 8–5 **Radiographic image displayed on computer monitor.**

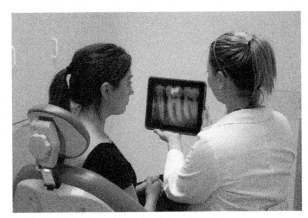

FIGURE 8–6 **Tablet device.** Viewing radiographic images via network.

speed of the operating system, the amount of storage space required, whether an Internet connection will be used, and the requirements of the digital imaging software. Digital imaging software allows a computer to digitize, process, and store information received from a digital image receptor.

The computer must be equipped to support visual image displays on a high-resolution monitor for accurate diagnoses (Figure 8–5 ■). There are different types of monitors available, all of which are capable of displaying digital images within 0.5 to 120 seconds after the image receptor is exposed to radiation. Plasma and liquid crystal display (LCD) monitors are increasingly being marketed to replace traditional cathode ray tube (CRT) monitors. Current research indicates that these monitor technologies perform equally well; however, digital imaging system manufacturer guidelines should be consulted to best match computer and monitor for optimal compatibility.

The ability to wirelessly network a computer used to capture digital radiographs has several advantages. Digital radiographs obtained in one location may be viewed over a networked system by other oral health care specialists for the purpose of consultation, or by a practice manager for the purpose of obtaining third-party payment for dental treatment (see Chapter 10). Access to a networked service within the practice allows for viewing radiographs between operatories. Handheld devices such as a tablet computer can serve as a convenient chairside viewing opportunity for patient education (Figure 8–6 ■). When needed, a photocopy or plain-paper copy of digital radiographs may be obtained by connecting the computer to a printer.

Software

Manufacturers of digital radiographic systems provide software programs that when loaded onto a computer will allow an operator to manipulate the images (Figure 8–7 ■). These programs offer a variety of features to aid in viewing and interpreting the images. For example, images can be enlarged for viewing on the computer monitor to assist with evaluating subtle changes not easily detected by the

unaided eye; image density and contrast can be increased or decreased to improve visual acuity; and measurement tools can be useful to assess the length of root canals in endodontic therapy and for estimating periodontal bone levels.

A software tool that fully utilizes computing capabilities is **digital subtraction**. This feature allows for comparison of digitally stored images to detect changes over time or prior to and after treatment interventions. Digital subtraction merges two radiographic images of the same area, taken at different times and matches gray values between the two images to eliminate data that is similar and highlight changes (differences in the images). Merged together electronically, those portions of the images that are alike (i.e., did not change over time) will cancel each other out as data are matched and then subtracted from each image. The portions of the images where change occurred will stand out conspicuously. Digital subtraction is an effective method of measuring periodontal changes such as bone loss or regeneration, assessment of implants, and healing of periapical pathosis.

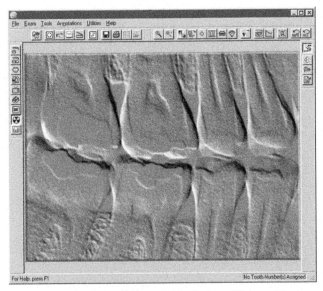

FIGURE 8–7 **Digital software manipulation of image.** (Courtesy of Dentrix Dental Systems.)

Practice Point

The ability to increase or decrease digital image density will not compensate for a severely under- or overexposed image. For example, if the exposure setting is too low, the resultant image will be too light. Often a light image will not reveal such subtle changes as an early or incipient carious lesion. If the original image does not detect the radiolucency of the caries because it was underexposed (too light), then merely darkening the image with the digital software density control tool will not "put" the caries into the picture. If it was not detected to begin with, the software will not reveal it.

Table 8–2 Comparison of Direct and Indirect Digital Imaging

Direct Digital Sensors	Indirect Phosphor Plates
• Narrow dynamic range • Almost instantaneous image viewing • Thick, rigid sensor may be less tolerated by patient • Relatively durable; less likely to be damaged by normal use of disinfecting chemicals; sensor cord susceptible to damage from crimping and careless handling • Increased spatial resolution	• Wide dynamic range • Scanning "processing" step required to transfer latent image into computer system • Similar to film size and flexibility may improve patient tolerance • Easily damaged or scratched during handling; sensitive to disinfectant chemicals • Require additional time to prepare and package for intraoral placement • Decreased spatial resolution

Software technology continues to find ways to improve the diagnostic yields from digital imaging. Predictions have been made that **artificial intelligence**, programming a computer to make decisions regarding the diagnosis of the images acquired, will one day be used to assist a practitioner with reading and interpreting digital images. Possible uses for artificial intelligence would be to develop computer software to analyze bone around a dental implant to determine if osseointegration (anchoring in bone) has occurred or to analyze bone densities of the jaws to screen for osteoporosis with a dental radiograph. Although certainly very beneficial ideas, these uses of artificial intelligence have not yet been realized.

Types of Digital Image Receptors

There are two types of dental radiographic digital imaging systems: direct and indirect. The difference between the two imaging systems is based on the type of image receptor used, and how this image receptor captures and produces a radiographic image on a computer monitor. The adoption of one system over the other depends on practitioner preference, and is often influenced by manufacturers' marketing in different locations of the country and globally. Studies continue to compare different digital imaging systems and find that all systems currently on the market produce acceptable images in terms of spatial resolution and gray scale when compared to intraoral film. Each has benefits and limitations (Table 8–2 ■).

Direct Digital Imaging

Direct digital imaging uses an electronic sensor to produce a radiographic image *directly* on a computer screen, with the computer almost instantly transforming exposure to x-rays to produce an image. A **solid-state sensor**, containing an electronic chip replaces film. Sensors are based on **charge-coupled device (CCD)** technology or **complementary metal oxide semiconductor active pixel sensor (CMOS-APS)**. These two technologies differ in their electronic framework, but work equally well at converting x-rays into an electronic

signal that is sent to a computer. While CCD and CMOS-APS sensors use slightly different components, each capture x-ray energy to produce a radiographic image in a similar manner.

Direct digital sensors are made up of a grid of x-ray or light-sensitive cells (see Figure 8–4). Each cell represents one pixel in the final image. A pixel serves as a small box or "well" into which the electrons produced by the x-ray exposure are deposited. A pixel is the digital equivalent of a silver halide crystal used in film-based radiography (see Chapter 7). As opposed to film emulsion that contains a random arrangement of silver halide crystals, pixels are arranged in a structured order of rows and columns. Each pixel has an x-coordinate, a y-coordinate, and a gray value. The x- and y-coordinates are numbers that represent where the pixel is located; the row and column, respectively, in the grid. The **gray value** is a number that corresponds to the amount of radiation received by a pixel. When x-rays strike the sensor, the pixels are excited in such a way that an electronic charge is produced on the surface of the sensor. The number that represents the gray value increases or decreases inversely proportional to the number of x-rays striking each pixel. A value of zero represents a maximum exposure; a value of 255 represents no exposure. The sensor then transmits the x- and y-coordinates and the gray value, through a wire or wirelessly via radio frequency to a circuit board inside the computer. The computer software processes the x- and y-coordinates and a gray value number to reconstruct an image to display on the monitor.

The newer CMOS-APS with its less expensive technology is becoming increasingly more common. Additionally, CMOS-APS may provide increased abilities compared to older CCD sensor technology. Unlike CCD technology, CMOS-APS has an active component built into each pixel, allowing digital data to be transferred together as an entire row reducing the need for computer system power requirements and possibly increasing longevity of the sensor.

CMOS-APS and CCD technologies differ in their respective **dynamic range**, the range of radiation exposure able to produce a diagnostic image. Dynamic range is expressed as being wide or narrow. A wide dynamic range means that a wide range of exposure settings will produce an image of acceptable density and contrast. A narrow dynamic range means that the exposure settings must be relatively precise, not slightly high and not slightly low in order to capture an image at an acceptable density and contrast. In general, digital sensors and PSP plates exhibit a wider dynamic range than radiographic film. Exposure settings used with radiographic film that are slightly high or slightly low, will readily produce an image that exhibits characteristics of over- or underexposure respectively; which may prompt a need for a retake. An image receptor with a wide dynamic range is capable of capturing an image using a wide variation of exposures, without any, or with barely noticeable changes in density and contrast; avoiding over- and underexposure errors that result in retakes.

A comparison of CMOS-APS and CCD technologies has demonstrated that CMOS-APS sensors, while maintaining a wider dynamic range than radiographic film, have a narrower dynamic range than CCD sensors. Additionally, some CMOS-APS sensors cannot process extremely high or extremely low radiation exposure settings—that is, settings that fall outside their programmed range will not produce an image. Consider that a very high exposure setting will result in a very dark, or black, film radiograph. This might not be the result with some CMOS-APS sensors. An exposure setting outside the dynamic range might not capture an image. When this occurs, a warning message may be displayed on the computer monitor indicating the sensor's inability to capture data.

The ability of an image receptor with a wide dynamic range to produce a radiograph with acceptable density and contrast with a wide range of exposure settings may assist in avoiding over- and underexposure errors. However, when a small to moderate increase in the exposure setting does not produce a noticeable difference in density and contrast, there is no indicator to alert a radiographer that more radiation is being used than is required. This phenomenon may possibly lead to an unnecessary increased radiation dose.

Another problem that occurs with a wide dynamic range is electronic noise. If exposure time is set too low, an increase in **noise**, an electrical disturbance, will "fog" or clutter a digital image. The practitioner will often increase the exposure time to eliminate noise. While it is acceptable to change exposure settings to achieve desired results, it is important to be aware of these phenomena of sensors with wide dynamic range to avoid unnecessary radiation exposure to a patient.

Digital image receptors may be wired or wireless. Wired sensors use a universal serial bus (USB) cable to connect either directly to a computer or to a USB interface module or box that has been attached to the computer via a USB port (Figure 8–8 ■). The USB interface module assists in obtaining radiographic images and troubleshooting problems. Light emitting diode (LED) indicator lights let the radiographer know when the sensor is connected and ready

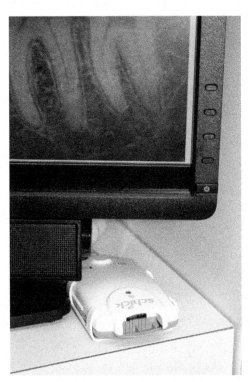

FIGURE 8–8 **USB interface module for connecting a direct digital sensor to the computer.**

for exposure. Wired sensor cables vary in length, with popular lengths from 3 to 9 ft (1 to 3 m). The shorter the cable, the more limited the range of motion. Intraoral dental x-ray machines are available that allow for convenient attachment of a wired sensor (Figure 8–9 ■).

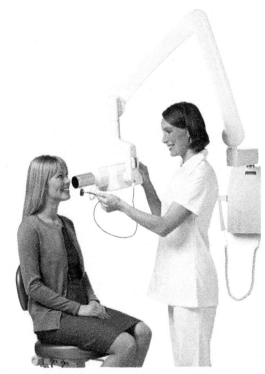

FIGURE 8–9 **Digital radiography system** with conveniently attached sensor. (Courtesy of Planmeca.)

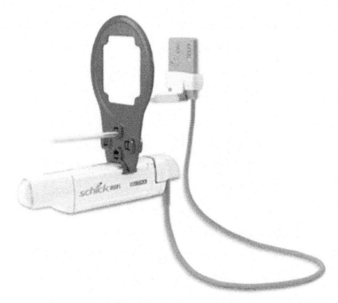

FIGURE 8–10 **Wireless digital sensor.** (Courtesy of Sirona Dental, Inc., Long Island City, NY.)

While CCD technology utilizes wired sensors exclusively, CMOS-APS technology allows for the use of either wired or wireless technology. Wireless CMOS-APS sensors incorporate a battery attachment that supplies power to the sensor allowing it to communicate with a computer via a radio frequency eliminating the need for a direct cable connection (Figure 8–10 ■). Eliminating long wires between a sensor and a computer provides freedom of movement, and ease of sensor placement. Wireless technology may be sensitive to signals or noise from other electronic devices being used in the vicinity, preventing the sensor from capturing and the computer from displaying the radiographic image. Wireless technology is more expensive than the comparable wired technology, due in part to the additional cost of the disposable batteries.

While design is unique to the manufacturer, sensors are readily available in the equivalent of intraoral film sizes 0, 1, and 2 (Figure 8–11 ■). It is important to note that the active recording dimensions of a digital sensor may be slightly smaller than the film size the sensor represents. Sensors are available with contoured edges and angled wire attachments (Figure 8–12 ■), and some have been reduced to just over 3 mm in thickness—all characteristics designed to enhance patient acceptance of intraoral image receptor positioning.

Indirect Digital Imaging

Indirect digital imaging replaces film with a **photostimulable phosphor (PSP)** plate that captures x-ray energy as analog data and *indirectly* produces a digital radiographic image on a computer screen. PSP uses different technology than direct digital imaging sensors in that there is no wire connection to a computer (Figure 8–13 ■). PSP technology requires a processing step in between exposure to x-rays and viewing the radiographic image on a computer monitor. PSP sensors, often referred to as storage phosphor *plates*, very closely parallel film in the way they capture an invisible image that is made visible through a "processing" step.

PSP technology uses polyester plates coated with a **storage phosphor** (europium activated barium fluorohalide). When exposed to x-rays this storage phosphor captures and stores x-ray energy as a latent image similar to the way silver halide crystals within film emulsion store a latent image. Each PSP plate can be exposed only one time until the scanning step reads the latent image. If exposing a series of radiographic images, several individual PSP plates will be required. After exposure, a PSP plate must be kept protected from bright light, which can adversely affect image quality and erase the data. Placing an exposed PSP plate into a light-tight **transfer box** until ready for the scanning step will assist with protecting it from prolonged light exposure, especially if exposing a series of multiple PSP plates Figure 8–14 ■).

Following exposure, the transfer box with the exposed PSP plates inside is taken to the location of the PSP system's

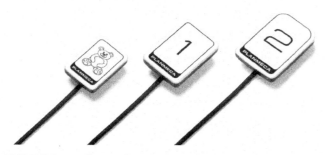

FIGURE 8–11 **Sensor sizes similar to film.** (Courtesy of Planmeca.)

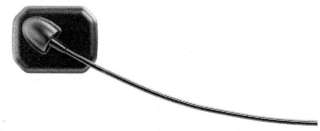

FIGURE 8–12 **Sensor with contoured edges and angled wire attachment.** (Courtesy of DEXIS, LLC.)

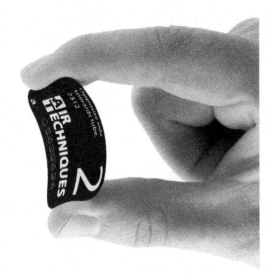

FIGURE 8–13 **PSP plate.** (Courtesy of Air Techniques, Inc.)

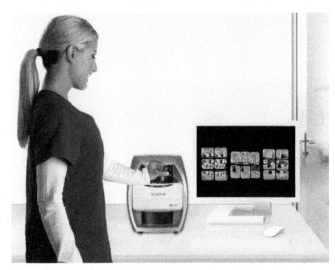

FIGURE 8–15 **PSP digital imaging system.** Operator placing exposed PSP sensor plates into the laser scanning device. (Courtesy of Air Techniques, Inc.)

laser scanning device. It is recommended that the laser scanner be located in an area or room with subdued lighting to further protect the exposed plates from white light. The exposed PSP sensors are placed into the laser scanning device, which is connected to a computer and monitor (Figure 8–15 ■). The laser scanner provides mounts into which the plates are positioned for scanning (Figure 8–16 ■). It is important that the plates be fed into the mounts in the correct position to avoid displaying images upside down, or in the wrong place on the computer monitor template.

The scanner directs a helium-neon laser beam to pass over the PSP plate causing the stored latent image to be released in the form of light. The light intensity released is directly related to the x-ray energy absorbed by the storage phosphor. This released energy is converted to an electrical signal that is then converted into digital values. The computer uses these digital values to reconstruct an image on a monitor. Scanning time can take between 10 seconds to produce an image for a single periapical radiograph and

5 minutes to produce an extraoral panoramic image. The laser scanner processing step makes PSP technology seem similar to film-based radiography in that an image receptor is exposed and then "developed" later. Because of this additional laser scanning step, this method of acquiring a digital image is referred to as indirect digital imaging. In general, PSP technology produces images with less spatial resolution compared to solid-state sensors, which is related to the time necessary for scanning the images. After processing with the laser scanner, PSP plates must be erased by exposing them to bright light before using again.

PSP plates have a wider dynamic range and are less sensitive to variations in radiation exposure than both CCD and CMOS-APS technology. As with CCD sensors, it is possible to overexpose PSP plates, with more radiation than is necessary, without the image appearing darker. Essentially overexposed PSP plates will not alert a radiographer that too much radiation is being used to produce the image. Intraoral PSP plates very closely resemble intraoral film sizes 0, 1, 2, 3, and 4

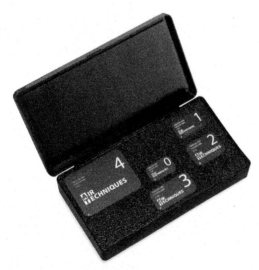

FIGURE 8–14 **PSP transfer box.** (Courtesy of Air Techniques, Inc.)

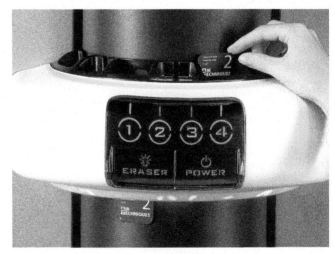

FIGURE 8–16 **PSP scanner.** (Courtesy of Air Techniques, Inc.)

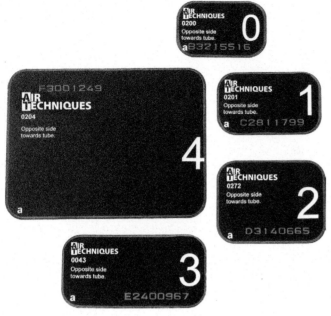

FIGURE 8–17 PSP plates in sizes comparable to film. (Courtesy of Air Techniques, Inc.)

and extraoral PSP plates are placed into a cassette (without intensifying screens) in the same manner as extraoral film (Figure 8–17 ■; see Chapter 17). Intraoral PSP plates are thin and slightly flexible making them susceptible to damage from bending or scratching (see Figure 18–18).

Practice Point

Because the computer can record more data than the human eye can detect, software is being studied that might be able to "learn" oral disease. Consider this future possible use of artificial intelligence. Through the input of data, a computer can develop "neural networks" that could potentially aid a practitioner in detecting subtle dental disease. For example, a computer could be directed to color healthy enamel, with a certain level of density, yellow. Enamel density that falls below this established healthy level could be colored purple. Essentially, the computer would be identifying caries with the color purple.

REVIEW—Chapter summary

Digital imaging systems replace film with a sensor that captures radiation exposure and uses a computer to display a radiographic image on a monitor. A digital image is composed of pixels, short for picture elements. The number and size of pixels, arranged in columns, and rows, determines the spatial resolution, sharpness, and gray scale of an image. Spatial resolution is measured as line pairs (lp/mm). Gray scale is represented digitally by a number from 0 (pure

Radiation Exposure

When digital imaging first became available, one of the advantages most often cited was a reduction in radiation exposure compared to radiographic film in use at that time. Claims for up to 50% radiation reduction were reasonably accurate when comparing digital exposures with slower film speeds (D-speed) commonly in use at that time. While digital image receptors are more sensitive to radiation than film, capturing x-rays more efficiently, the radiation reduction realized is smaller when compared with faster speed film in use today (E- and F-speed). It should be noted that CCD sensors are slightly less sensitive to radiation, and may require an approximate 25 percent increase in radiation exposure over CMOS-APS sensors. PSP plates are less sensitive to radiation than both CCD and CMOS-APS direct sensors. Radiation reduction over film may not be realized in practice with PSP technology. There may be no radiation reduction realized when comparing extraoral CCD, CMOS-APS, or PSP technology to extraoral film-screen combinations. In fact, some extraoral systems using PSP technology actually require an increase in radiation exposure over film-screen radiographs. As with all types and makes of digital imaging systems, evaluate results in practice and adjust the exposure time as necessary to produce a diagnostically acceptable image.

Another important consideration when discussing radiation exposure is the possibility of a higher retake rate and more exposures being taken with direct digital imaging when compared with indirect digital imaging and film-based radiographs. Possible explanations for this higher incidence of exposure with direct digital imaging include the:

- Ease with which retakes can be immediately taken without removing the sensor from the patient's mouth.
- Real and the perceived radiation dose reduction expected by digital imaging which makes retakes seem easily justifiable.
- Recording dimensions of the sensors which are smaller than film and PSP plates, requiring multiple exposures to adequately record all areas of interest.
- Size and rigidity of the sensor and the wire and plastic infection-control barrier protruding from the oral cavity which can compromise placement, leading to increased chance of errors.

black) to 255 (pure white). Digital imaging works best with a direct-current dental x-ray machine set at a low kV and low mA. A computer and specialized software produce a visible image on a monitor. Digital subtraction software allows for comparison of digitally stored images to detect changes over time.

Direct digital imaging uses a solid-state sensor, containing an electronic chip based on either charge-coupled device (CCD) technology or complementary metal oxide semiconductor active pixel sensor (CMOS-APS) technology. CMOS-APS may be wired or wireless. CCD sensors and CMOS-APS transmit x- and y-coordinates of pixels and gray value to a circuit board inside a computer. Computer software processes the information to reconstruct a radiographic image to display on a monitor. CMOS-APS may provide increased abilities compared to older CCD sensor technology.

Indirect digital imaging uses a photostimulable phosphor (PSP) plate covered with a storage phosphor that captures analog data similar to the action of radiographic film. PSP plates are not attached to the computer with a wire. A transfer box protects exposed PSP plates from bright light until the scanning step is performed. After exposure to x-rays, PSP plates are placed into a laser scanner that converts the digital signal to an image on a computer monitor. PSP plates must be erased by exposing to bright light before reusing.

Dynamic range, the range of radiation exposure that can produce images of acceptable quality, varies among digital image receptor types. The wider the dynamic range, the wider the range of exposure that will produce an acceptable image. PSP plates have the widest dynamic range, followed by CCD sensor technology, followed by CMOS-APS technology, which has the narrowest range. The ability to produce an image with acceptable density and contrast with a range of exposure settings may assist in avoiding over- and under-exposure errors. However, slight to moderate increases in exposure settings that do not produce increased image density will not alert a radiographer that more radiation is being used than necessary.

Benefits of digital radiographic imaging include almost instantaneous viewing of images; possible radiation dose reduction over film-based radiography; elimination of darkroom, including need for chemical handling and disposal of potentially hazardous wastes; potential for improved interpretation through image manipulation; and ability to transmit images electronically. Challenges include possible increased radiation exposure as a result of increased number of retakes; smaller recording dimensions than film; thick size and wire attachment may be less tolerated by patient; and possible reliability and security issues with electronic data.

RECALL—Study questions

For questions 1 to 5, match each term with its definition.

   a. Analog
   b. Dynamic range
   c. Gray scale
   d. Pixels
   e. Spatial resolution

_____ 1. Discrete units of information that together constitute an image

_____ 2. Discernable separation of closely adjacent image details

_____ 3. Allowable radiation exposure able to produce a diagnostic image

_____ 4. Data represented by continuously variable physical quantities

_____ 5. Shade levels from pure black to pure white visible in an image

6. A digital radiographic image exists as bits of information in a computer file.
   A computer converts this information into an image that appears on a monitor.
   a. The first statement is true. The second statement is false.
   b. The first statement is false. The second statement is true.
   c. Both statements are true.
   d. Both statements are false.

7. The larger the number of pixels in an image the sharper the spatial resolution, *because* each pixel stores a number representing a different shade of gray.
   a. Both the statement and reason are correct and related.
   b. Both the statement and reason are correct but NOT related.
   c. The statement is correct, but the reason is NOT.
   d. The statement is NOT correct, but the reason is correct.
   e. NEITHER the statement NOR the reason is correct.

8. Each of the following is needed to produce digital radiographic images EXCEPT one. Which one is the EXCEPTION?
   a. Dental x-ray machine
   b. Solid-state sensor or phosphor coated plate
   c. Computer and monitor
   d. Special software
   e. Darkroom

9. Each of the following dental x-ray machine parameters is considered ideally suited to producing quality digital radiographic images EXCEPT one. Which one is the EXCEPTION?
   a. Direct current
   b. 60 kV or lower
   c. Low 5 mA
   d. Round PID

10. Which of the following is NOT true regarding digital subtraction?
    a. Merges two radiographic images of the same region.
    b. Matches gray values between two image files.
    c. Eliminates a need for a second radiograph after treatment intervention.
    d. Allows digital images to detect changes over time.

11. Digital sensors are made up of _____ that are arranged _____.
    a. pixels; randomly
    b. pixels; in a structured order of rows and columns
    c. silver halide crystals; randomly
    d. silver halide crystals; in a structured order of row and columns

12. The dynamic range of a digital image receptor is wider than the dynamic range of radiographic film.
    A digital image receptor with a wide dynamic range requires precise exposure settings to produce acceptable image density and contrast.
    a. The first statement is true. The second statement is false.
    b. The first statement is false. The second statement is true.
    c. Both statements are true.
    d. Both statements are false.

13. Which digital image receptor has the widest dynamic range?
    a. Charge-coupled device (CCD)
    b. Complementary metal oxide semiconductor active pixel sensor (CMOS-APS)
    c. Photostimulable phosphor (PSP)

14. Which digital image receptor captures and stores x-ray energy until stimulation by a laser beam converts it into a digital image?
    a. Charge-coupled device (CCD)
    b. Complementary metal oxide semiconductor active pixel sensor (CMOS-APS)
    c. Photostimulable phosphor (PSP)

15. Digital radiography requires less radiation exposure to produce an image than film-based radiography because the
    a. chemical processing steps are eliminated.
    b. radiation used for digital imaging is different than radiation used for film-based imaging.
    c. computer can control the amount of radiation output better than a radiographer.
    d. image receptor (CCD or CMOS-APS) is more sensitive to x-rays than film.

16. Each of the following describes PSP plates EXCEPT one. Which one is the EXCEPTION?
    a. Almost instantaneous viewing of the image.
    b. Easily damaged or scratched during handling.
    c. Must be exposed to white light to erase previous image before reusing.
    d. Similar to intraoral film in size and flexibility.

17. Each of the following is a possible limitation of CMOS-APS technology over film-based imaging EXCEPT one. Which one is the EXCEPTION?
    a. Requires an increased radiation setting.
    b. Ease of retakes may result in excess radiation exposure.
    c. Thick, rigid sensor size.
    d. Smaller recording dimensions.

REFLECT—Case study

Using the Internet, search for a digital imaging system marketed for oral health care practice. Evaluate the system based on the information presented in this chapter. Consider the following.

a. Does the system use direct or indirect technology? What is the difference?

b. What image receptor sizes are available? Why are different sizes important?

c. What is the dynamic range of the image receptor? What does a narrow or wide range mean?

d. Does the manufacture list the values for pixel size, spatial resolution, gray scale, or line pair? What do these

mean? What other terminology does the manufacturer use to describe the system?

e. What are the software features for viewing the images? Why are these important?

f. Does the manufacturer make recommendations for dental x-ray machines or computer systems and monitors to pair with their system? Why are these considerations important?

g. Does the manufacturer state radiation exposure reductions over film-based exposures? What are these?

h. Are there advantages and limitations of this system? What are they?

RELATE—Laboratory application

For a comprehensive laboratory practice exercise on this topic, see Thomson, E. M., & Bruhn, A. M. (2018). *Exercises in oral radiography techniques: A laboratory manual* (4th ed.). Hoboken, NJ: Pearson. Chapter 3, "Introduction to digital radiographic imaging."

RESOURCES

Brullmann, D. D., Kempkes, B., d'Hoedt, B., & Schulze, R. S. (2013). Contrast curves of five different intraoral x-ray sensors: A technical note. *Oral Surgery, Oral Medicine, Oral Pathology, Oral Radiology 115*, 55–61.

Farman, A. G., Levato, C., Gane, D., & Scarfe W. (2008). In practice: How going digital will affect the dental office. *Journal of the American Dental Association, 139*, S14–S19.

Francisco, E. F., Horlak, D., & Azevedo, S. (2010). The balance between safety and efficacy: Understanding the technology available that will produce high quality radiographs while reducing patient risk to ionizing radiation. *Dimensions of Dental Hygiene, 8*, 26–30.

Kitagawa, H., Scheetz, J. P., & Farman, A. G. (2003). Comparison of complementary metal oxide semiconductor and charge-coupled device intraoral x-ray detectors using subjective image quality. *Dentomaxillofacial Radiology, 32*, 408–411.

Paurazas, S. B., Geist, J., Pink, F. E., Hoen, M. M., & Steiman, H. R. (2000). Comparison of diagnostic accuracy of digital imaging by using CCD and CMOS-APS sensors with E-speed film in the detection of periapical bony lesions. *Oral Surgery, Oral Medicine, Oral Pathology, Oral Radiology, 89*, 356–362.

Wenzel, A., & Moystad, A. (2010). Work flow with digital intra-oral radiography: A systematic review. *Acta Odontologica Scandinavica, 68*(2), 106–114.

White, S. C., & Pharoah, M. J. (2014). Digital imaging. *Oral radiology: Principles and interpretation* (7th ed.). St. Louis, MO: Elsevier.

Visit www.pearsonhighered.com/healthprofessionsresources to access the student resources that accompany this book. Simply select Dental Hygiene from the choice of disciplines. Find this book and you will find the complementary study tools created for this specific title.

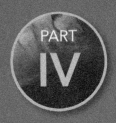

Dental Radiographer Fundamentals

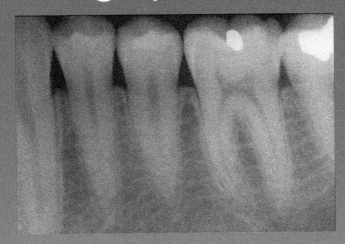

9

Infection Control

CHAPTER OUTLINE

OBJECTIVES

Following successful completion of this chapter, you should be able to:

1. Define the key terms.
2. List the conditions that make up the chain of infection.
3. State the purpose of infection control.
4. Identify methods of breaking the chain of infection.
5. State the roles the Centers for Disease Control and Prevention (CDC) and the Occupational Safety and Health Administration (OSHA) play in providing guidelines for infection control.
6. List personal protective equipment (PPE) recommended for dental radiographers.
7. Explain how to maintain hand and respiratory hygiene.
8. Compare the different levels of Environmental Protection Agency (EPA)-regulated disinfectants.
9. Explain the role of surface barriers in infection control.
10. Differentiate between semicritical and noncritical objects used during radiographic procedures.
11. Demonstrate competency in following infection control protocol prior to, during, and after radiographic procedures.
12. Demonstrate competency in following infection control protocol for handling and processing intraoral image receptors.
13. Demonstrate competency in following infection control protocol when using an automatic processor with a daylight loader attachment.

KEY TERMS

Aseptic
Barrier envelope
Chain of infection
Cough etiquette
Disinfection
Hand hygiene

Microbial aerosol
Overgloves
Pathogen
Personal protective equipment (PPE)
Portal of entry/exit
Reservoir
Respiratory hygiene

Spatter
Standard precautions
Sterilization
Susceptible host
Surface barriers
Transmission
Universal precautions

Introduction

The purpose of infection control procedures used in oral health care is to prevent the transmission of disease among patients and between patients and oral health care practitioners. Maintaining infection control throughout the radiographic procedure can be challenging. Radiographers need a thorough understanding of recommended infection control protocols that must be followed before, during, and after radiographic exposures. Specific steps required to skillfully and aseptically handle radiographic equipment and supplies require practice to achieve competency. This chapter provides step-by-step guidelines for infection control throughout all aspects of a dental radiographic examination.

Fundamentals of Infection Control

Chain of Infection

Human beings have always lived with the possibility of infection occurring through invasion of the body by pathogens. A **pathogen** is a microorganism capable of causing disease. Bacteria and viruses are examples of pathogens. Because of the special risk diseases carry, of particular concern to oral health care professionals are the human immunodeficiency virus (HIV), hepatitis B virus (HBV), hepatitis C virus (HCV), tuberculosis (TB), and herpes virus diseases. For infection to occur, the following must be present (Figure 9–1 ■):

- A **susceptible host** (not immune)
- Disease-causing microorganisms (pathogens)
- Sufficient numbers of pathogens to initiate infection (**reservoir**)
- Appropriate routes (portals) for a pathogen to exit a reservoir and enter a host
- A mode of **transmission**

Infectious diseases may be transmitted from patient to oral health care personnel, from oral health care personnel to patient, and from patient to patient. Routes of transmission include direct contact with pathogens in open lesions, blood, saliva, or respiratory secretions; and with airborne contaminants present in aerosols of oral and respiratory fluids; or by indirect contact with contaminated objects such as

radiographic equipment. The purpose of infection control is to alter one of these conditions to prevent the transmission of disease. To break the **chain of infection** consider each of the following:

- Improve health and immunize a susceptible host. A weakened immune system is more susceptible to infection. Maintaining a condition of health will help to resist infection. Follow the Centers for Disease Control and Prevention (CDC) vaccination recommendations for oral health care personnel and keep immunizations up to date with current guidelines.
- Remove the pathogen. Use sterilization and high-level disinfection techniques.
- Reduce the numbers of pathogens. Thoroughly clean and disinfect surfaces and equipment. Sterilize instruments; use protective barriers on devices that cannot be sterilized.
- Block the **entrance/exit portals** of transmission. Use personal protective equipment (PPE) barriers including protective clothes, masks, eyewear, and gloves to avoid contact with pathogens. Avoid contact with contaminated objects or instruments. Maintain healthy, intact skin especially on hands and fingers.
- Block the routes of transmission. Avoid direct contact with pathogens in open lesions, blood, saliva, or respiratory secretions. Minimize airborne contaminants present in aerosols of oral and respiratory fluids. Practice good **hand hygiene** by frequent and effective handwashing. Aid patients and those accompanying patients with measures for cough etiquette. Disinfect and use protective barriers on surfaces and equipment.

Infection Control Guidelines

Two government agencies that play major roles in developing, recommending, and/or regulating infection control for oral health care practice are the Occupational Safety and Health Administration (OHSA) and the CDC.

OHSA'S BLOOD-BORNE PATHOGENS STANDARD. OHSA's role in developing standards to protect oral health care personnel is regulatory, meaning that the standards set forth form the basis of laws that govern the conduct and practice of oral health care. Regulations require that an oral health care practice comply with OHSA's Blood-Borne Pathogens Standard, which mandates that employers of oral health care personnel establish a written exposure control plan for following universal precautions. The infection control concept of **universal precautions** states that human blood and all other body fluids, including saliva, are potentially infectious for blood-borne diseases such as HIV and HBV. Some patients may be reluctant to admit to having an infectious condition. Taking a thorough medical history and performing an oral examination will not always identify potential infected patients. The concept of universal precautions uses a single standard that takes into consideration the potential for all patients to be a risk for transmitting blood-borne infection.

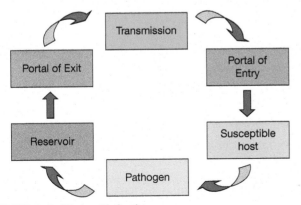

FIGURE 9–1 Chain of infection.

CDC STANDARD PRECAUTIONS. The CDC's role in providing guidelines for infection control is advisory. Recommendations provided by the CDC have assisted OSHA with developing regulatory standards. In 2003 the CDC issued *Guidelines for Infection Control in Dental Healthcare Settings*. Earlier guidelines focused on universal precautions for blood-borne infections. The CDC guidelines introduced the use of **standard precautions**, expanding the potential for transmission of not only blood-borne pathogens, but now to include all body fluids (except sweat), of all patients, whether known to be infected or not. Since saliva was categorized as a potentially infectious material under both universal and standard precautions, there is no operational difference for infection control protocol for clinical practice of oral health care, including those used for safe radiographic procedures. The CDC's infection control guidelines that directly relate to dental radiography are listed in Box 9–1.

Personal Protective Equipment (PPE)

Clothing, masks, eyewear, and gloves worn by oral health care personnel act as a protective infection control barrier (Figure 9–2 ■). **Personal protective equipment (PPE)** prevents the transmission of infective microorganisms between oral health care practitioners and patients.

PROTECTIVE CLOTHING. Scrubs, laboratory coats, gowns, and uniforms must be made from materials that provide protection from exposure to body fluids. Change protective clothing daily, or more frequently if soiled or wet; remove it before leaving the treatment facility; and launder it separately to prevent contamination of other items. Ideally, protective clothing should be laundered by a commercial biohazard service that can remove and isolate the items for safe laundering.

PROTECTIVE MASKS. Although radiographic procedures are much less likely than other dental procedures to produce aerosols and **spatter** (a heavier concentration of microbial aerosols), protection from **microbial aerosols** may

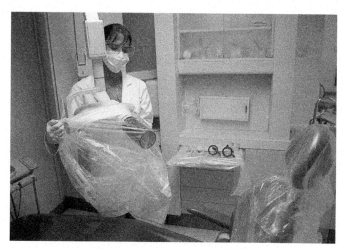

FIGURE 9–2 Infection control and PPE. Radiographer wearing PPE to place barriers to cover the x-ray tube head and PID. Note assembled image receptor holders on a plastic barrier on countertop.

be achieved through the use of a mask. Masks should be changed when soiled or wet and between patients.

PROTECTIVE EYEWEAR. Although radiographic procedures are much less likely than other types of dental procedures to cause physical eye accidents, the use of protective eyewear will protect against microbial aerosols and spatter. Types of protective eyewear include glasses with side shields, goggles, and full-face shields. Protective eyewear must be washed with appropriate cleaning agents following patient treatment procedures and as needed.

GLOVES. Gloves must be worn at all times throughout a radiographic procedure. A variety of gloves are available for specialized uses. Use sterile gloves for surgical procedures; use medical examination (nonsterile) gloves for most dental procedures, including radiographic examinations; plastic overgloves have temporary applications as a protectant cover of patient treatment gloves; and utility gloves are appropriate for cleaning and disinfecting of equipment. Medical examination gloves are made of latex or a nonlatex material such as vinyl or nitrile. Avoid powdered gloves as the powder residue can cause radiographic artifacts (see Chapter 18). Do not wash gloves with soap or disinfect for reuse. Soap may damage gloves in a way that would allow the flow of liquid through undetected holes. Change punctured, torn, or cut gloves immediately. Change and discard gloves between patients. Do not touch unprotected surfaces not directly associated with the procedure, such as doorknobs to access a darkroom or patient records with contaminated gloves.

Hand and Respiratory (Cough Etiquette) Hygiene

HANDWASHING. Protective clothing, mask, and eyewear should be in place to prepare for handwashing prior to putting on examination gloves. Clean hands thoroughly before putting on, and after removing gloves (Procedure 9–1). It is important to remove potentially infectious pathogens from the hands that can grow rapidly inside a warm, moist glove. Completely dry hands prior to putting on gloves.

Box 9–1: CDC-Recommended Infection Control Practices for Oral Radiography

- Wear patient treatment gloves when exposing radiographs and handling contaminated image receptors.

- Use protective eyewear, mask, and gown if spattering of blood or other body fluids is likely.

- Use heat-tolerant or disposable image receptor holding devices whenever possible; at a minimum, disinfect semicritical heat-sensitive devices such as digital radiographic sensors, according to the manufacturer's instructions.

- Transport and handle exposed image receptors in an **aseptic** manner to prevent contamination of processing equipment.

- Use Food and Drug Administration (FDA)-cleared protective barriers on digital radiographic image receptors.

Procedure 9–1

Handwashing for radiographic procedures

1. Put on protective clothing, mask, and eyewear.
2. Remove rings, wristwatch,* and other jewelry.
3. Wet hands with cool/tepid water and apply liquid antimicrobial soap.
4. Vigorously lather for 15 seconds; interlace fingers and thumbs, and move hands back and forth; work lather under nails.
5. Rinse well, allowing water to run from fingertips.
6. Dry each hand thoroughly with a separate paper towel.
7. Unless equipped with a foot pedal or hands-free activator, turn off the water by placing a clean paper towel between clean, dry hand and the faucet.

*Wristwatch may be replaced after handwashing as long as it will remain protected under the gown or covered with the glove during the procedure.

Wash visibly dirty hands with an antimicrobial liquid soap and water. If hands are not visibly soiled, an alcohol-containing preparation designed for reducing the number of viable microorganisms on the hands may be used. Remove all jewelry, including watches and rings, prior to handwashing. Avoid long fingernails, false fingernails, and nail polish, as these may harbor pathogens and have the potential to puncture treatment gloves. Handwashing is most effective when nails are cut short and well manicured.

RESPIRATORY HYGIENE/COUGH ETIQUETTE. The CDC's *Summary of Infection Prevention Practices in Dental Settings*, published in 2016, recommends that oral health care practices take steps to prevent transmission of respiratory pathogens from patients, those who may accompany patients, and from oral health care professionals who show signs of illness by coughing, sneezing, runny nose, and other symptoms indicating a respiratory illness (Figure 9–3 ■).

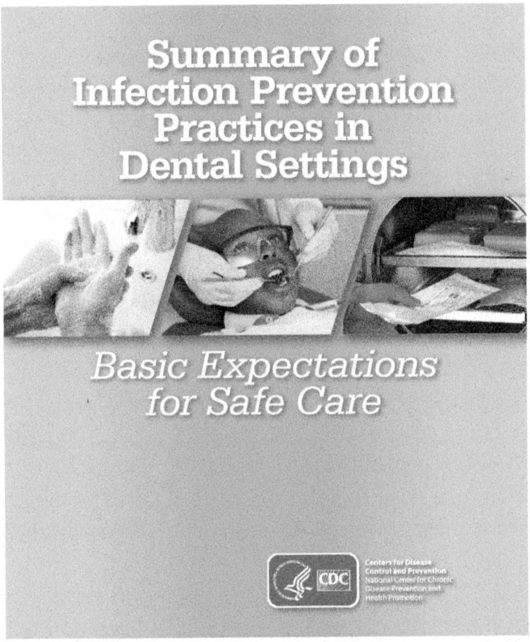

FIGURE 9–3 CDC Guidelines Summary. (Centers for Disease Control and Prevention. Summary of Infection Prevention Practices in Dental Settings: Basic Expectations for Safe Care. Atlanta, GA: U.S. Department of Health and Human Services; March 2016.)

Post a sign outlining **respiratory hygiene** or **cough etiquette**, including instructions to appropriately cover mouth and nose when coughing and sneezing, at the entrance to the oral health care facility. Provide a ready supply of tissues, an appropriate disposal, and no-touch hand sanitizer for patient access. Be cognizant of the need for hand hygiene when in contact with respiratory secretions. While not feasible during a radiographic examination procedure, offer a patient with symptoms a mask to wear while in the vicintiy of other patients and personnel.

Disinfection, Surface Barriers, and Sterilization

Cleaning, disinfection, and sterilization break the chain of infection, preventing transmission of infective microorganisms. Prior to and following radiographic procedures, clean and disinfect equipment and surfaces in the treatment area and/or protect with a barrier. Preclean radiographic equipment and surfaces that will come in contact, directly or indirectly, with potential contaminates. Clean all surfaces prior to disinfecting. Disinfectant is not effective on a surface that has not been precleaned, unless using a disinfectant product specifically designed to both clean and disinfect simultaneously.

Disinfection

Disinfection is the use of a chemical or physical procedure to reduce, destroy, or inactivate pathogens to an acceptable level on inanimate objects. Disinfectants do not inactivate all pathogens and cannot destroy particularly resistant bacterial spores. Disinfecting agents are too toxic for use on living tissue, so use only on clinical surfaces and on some instruments that cannot be heat sterilized. Because of their corrosive and toxic properties, carefully and selectively use disinfectants that have been registered as effective by the Environmental Protection Agency (EPA). The EPA regulates and classifies chemical disinfectants as follows:

- **High-level disinfectant** requires a relatively short contact time and may be considered a sterilant, capable of inactivating spores, with a longer contact time. Can be used to disinfect heat-sensitive semicritical equipment, such as digital sensors.

- **Intermediate-level disinfectant** is labeled as hospital-grade disinfectant with tuberculocidal properties. *Mycobacterium tuberculosis* is highly resistant to chemical disinfectant. A product with the ability to inactivate *M. tuberculosis* is considered especially effective against all less-resistant bacteria and viruses. Hospital-grade disinfectant with tuberculocidal properties can be used to disinfect noncritical equipment, such as the x-ray tube head and position indicating device (PID).
- **Low-level disinfectant** is non-tuberculocidal, but is effective against certain other pathogens and can be used to clean and disinfect housekeeping surfaces, such as the handwashing sink.

Surface Barriers

Some clinical surfaces may be difficult to clean, preventing effective disinfection. Disinfectants have the potential to affect electrical connections, so directly spraying or saturating an x-ray control panel, dials, or exposure button may damage an x-ray machine. Therefore, protective **surface barriers** should be used whenever practical. Plastic wrap or barriers are commonly used to cover those surfaces most likely to be contaminated during the radiographic procedure, such as the x-ray tube head and PID, control panel and dials, exposure switch, and counter surfaces (Figures 9–2 and 9–4 ■). At the beginning of the day, preclean and disinfect surfaces prior to applying a barrier. Carefully remove

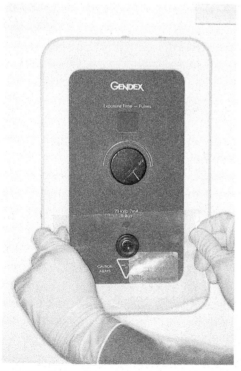

FIGURE 9–4 **Plastic barrier wrap covering x-ray control panel.**

and discard barriers after the procedure. A new barrier may be placed in between patients without cleaning and disinfecting the surface under the barrier again, provided that the surface was not touched or contaminated during the removal of the barrier. Disinfectants have residual activity, the ability to remain effective at neutralizing pathogens for a considerable time after application. Remove the barrier and perform cleaning and disinfecting again at the end of the day.

Sterilization

Sterilization is the total destruction of all pathogens and spores and is usually accomplished by steam autoclave or dry heat processes. Only when a device cannot withstand the autoclave or dry heat processes should sterilization be achieved through a prolonged exposure to an EPA-registered high-level disinfectant. Ideally, all critical and semicritical equipment and instruments should be sterilized.

Classification of an Object's Risk of Transmitting Infection

The CDC classifies instruments and devices used in oral health care according to risk of transmitting infection (Table 9–1 ■). Disinfect or sterilize instruments and devices according to the object's classification as critical, semicritical, or noncritical.

Critical instruments are those used to penetrate soft tissue or bone. Examples include needles, forceps, and scalers. Critical objects must be discarded or sterilized after each use. No critical instruments or equipment are used in radiographic procedures.

Semicritical instruments are those that contact oral mucosa without penetrating soft tissue or bone, such as intraoral dental mirrors. Image receptor holding devices and digital sensors fall into this category. Semicritical instruments must be discarded or sterilized after use. Only disposable image receptor holders, or ones that the manufacturer states can be sterilized, are recommended for use. Digital sensors and photostimulable phosphor (PSP) plates are semicritical instruments, but are heat sensitive, and usually cannot be submerged in liquid chemical disinfectant to achieve sterilization, presenting a challenge to maintaining infection control. Prior to use, a digital sensor and PSP plate must be protected with a plastic barrier that has been approved as minimally effective by the FDA. FDA-cleared plastic barriers do not completely protect a sensor from contamination, prompting a need for disinfection after removal of the barrier. Consult the digital sensor manufacturer's recommendations for which EPA-registered intermediate- or high-level disinfectant chemical to use.

Noncritical instruments are those devices that may contact intact skin or may become contaminated by microbial aerosols or spatter, but do not come into contact with mucous membranes. Examples include an intraoral x-ray tube head and PID, and the chin rest and head positioner

Table 9–1 Classification of Equipment Used in Radiographic Procedures

Category	Radiographic Equipment	Risk of Disease Transmission	Sterilize, Disinfect, or Discard
Critical	None	High	N/A
Semicritical	Image receptor positioner Digital sensor/PSP plate* Panoramic biteblock	Moderate	Sterilize or use disposable devices; clean/disinfect/cover heat-sensitive digital sensors
Noncritical	X-ray tube head, PID, support arm Extraoral radiographic machine positioner guides Lead/lead equivalent apron/thyroid collar	Low or none	Clean/disinfect with appropriate level EPA-registered disinfectant
Clinical contact surfaces	Exposure controls** Treatment chair controls** Countertop used to transfer devices/supplies needed to complete examination Countertop in darkroom	Low or none	Clean/disinfect with appropriate level EPA-registered disinfectant
Housekeeping surfaces	Countertop in vicinity not used to transfer devices/supplies Handwashing sink Floors/walls	Low or none	Clean/disinfect with appropriate level EPA-registered disinfectant

*Consult manufacturer's recommendations.
**Liquid disinfectants can damage electrical components. Consult manufacturer's recommendations.

guides of an extraoral panoramic machine (see Chapter 17). Noncritical instruments can be disinfected using EPA-registered intermediate- or low-level disinfectants; or thoroughly cleaned.

CLINICAL CONTACT AND HOUSEKEEPING SURFACES. Environmental infection control refers to procedures used to protect, clean, and disinfect equipment used as clinical contact surfaces and housekeeping surfaces that do not directly come in contact with patients.

Clinical contact surfaces may be contaminated directly by touching the surface, or indirectly as when an instrument is placed on the surface. Examples of clinical contact surfaces include an x-ray control panel and the treatment room counter being used to transfer image receptors and holders. Thoroughly clean clinical contact surfaces and protect with a barrier prior to the procedure; and disinfect using EPA-registered intermediate- or low-level disinfectants after the procedure.

Housekeeping surfaces are those not directly involved in the radiographic procedure that may be contaminated by indirect aerosol or spatter. Examples of housekeeping surfaces include the handwashing sink and countertops not directly involved with the radiographic procedure. Thoroughly clean housekeeping surfaces and depending on the level of contamination disinfect using EPA-registered intermediate- or low-level disinfectants.

Infection Control Protocol for the Radiographic Procedure

Infection control for the radiographic procedure can be divided into three categories: prior to, during, and after the exposure examination.

Protocol Prior to the Radiographic Procedure

Clean, disinfect, and/or cover with a protective barrier all treatment area surfaces likely to come in contact with potential contaminants either directly or indirectly. Obtain image receptors, holding devices, and other needed supplies and place for easy access during the procedure to avoid having to open drawers or leave the treatment area during the examination — actions that can complicate infection control.

INTRAORAL DENTAL FILM. Intraoral film packets inside original packaging are not sterile, but are considered "industrially clean," which means they are not expected to be contaminated with pathogens. To avoid contamination, dispense intraoral film packets just prior to use in a disposable container such as a paper cup. Because they are heat sensitive, film packets cannot be sterilized, and liquid saturation with disinfectant is not recommended.

To prevent transmission of microorganisms to an intraorally placed film packet use a **barrier envelope** (Figure 9–5 ■). Plastic barrier envelopes are specifically designed to create a

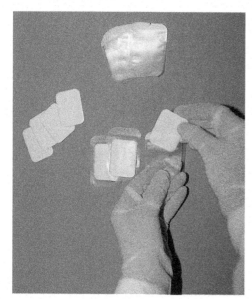

FIGURE 9–5 **Barrier envelopes** being placed on intraoral film packets.

moisture-proof seal that prevents microorganisms from coming into contact with a film packet when placed in the oral cavity for exposure. Film packets are available presealed inside barrier envelopes, or envelopes may be obtained separately. Following removal from the oral cavity, open the barrier envelope and discard appropriately (Figure 9–6 ■). The sealed film packet in the barrier envelope may now be handled with clean hands (or new gloves) to complete the processing procedure.

DIGITAL IMAGE RECEPTORS. PSP plates used in indirect digital imaging systems and direct imaging digital sensors cannot withstand sterilization procedures, so clean, disinfect, and cover with a plastic barrier prior to placing intraorally. Consult the image receptor manufacturer's recommendations for maintaining infection control which will usually include wiping with an appropriate level disinfectant prior to and after placement of a plastic barrier (Figure 9–7 ■). PSP plates must be sealed in plastic barrier envelopes in a similar manner as used for intraoral film packets (Figure 9–8 ■). Follow the same careful handling recommended for film packets to avoid contamination of a PSP plate when removing the barrier following exposure. Direct imaging digital sensors require the use of

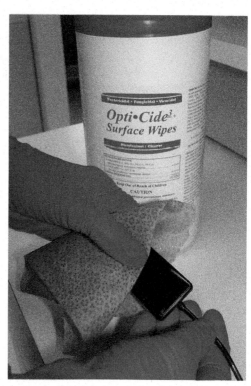

FIGURE 9–7 Disinfectant wipe for digital sensor infection control.

open-ended plastic sheath barriers that adapt to the universal serial bus (USB) cord that attaches the sensor to a computer. There are many sizes and styles of barrier envelopes and sheaths to accommodate various sizes of digital image receptors (Figure 9–9 ■). It is important to note that barriers are subject to tearing and are not always totally protective, making the proper use of disinfectants all the more important.

Prepare the digital imaging system computer keyboard and mouse that will be contacted during the radiographic exposure sequence (Figure 9–10 ■). Advances in digital technology have made available computer keyboards that can be cleaned and disinfected, and then covered with a plastic surface barrier. Because of its close proximity to patient treatment, take care to protect the computer monitor from possible contact with potential contaminants. Computer monitors

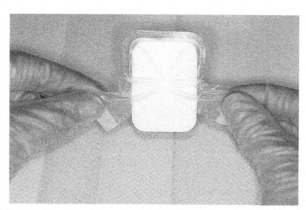

FIGURE 9–6 Aseptic opening of barrier envelope allows film packet to drop onto a paper towel.

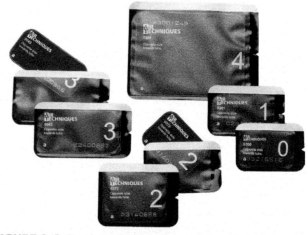

FIGURE 9–8 **Barrier envelopes for phosphor plates.** Note notched edge to facilitate opening. (Courtesy of Air Techniques, Inc.)

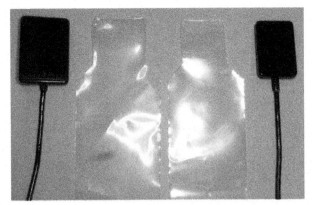

FIGURE 9–9 Barrier sheaths to fit different size digital sensors.

are available with glass fronts that can be cleaned and disinfected. Infection control products and techniques that ensure the safety of digital radiographic imaging are continuing to evolve. Always consult a product manufacturer's recommendations for appropriate infection control (Procedure 9–2).

Protocol During the Radiographic Procedure

PATIENT PREPARATION. Prepare the treatment area and ready the supplies prior to seating the patient. Take care when making adjustments to the treatment chair and headrest so as not to compromise the infection control process; or cover with a plastic barrier. Provide the patient with an optional antimicrobial mouth rinse to reduce oral microorganisms that contribute to infectious aerosols. Have the patient remove any items that may interfere with the procedure, such as eyeglasses and dentures, and place them in a remote area protected from contamination and where they will not contaminate other objects. Drape the patient with a lead/lead equivalent apron and thyroid collar. Have available tissues or other disposable paper products for appropriate cough etiquette or other need the patient may have to contain respiratory and oral secretions during the procedure (Figure 9–11 ■).

DURING EXPOSURES. Once the procedure has begun, take care to touch only covered surfaces. The best way to minimize contamination is to touch as few surfaces as possible.

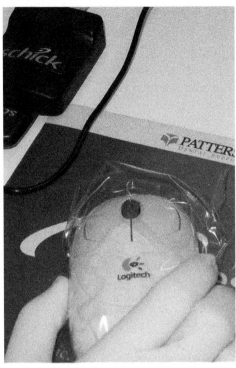

FIGURE 9–10 Disposable plastic barrier placed to protect mouse during digital radiographic procedure.

If drawers or cabinets must be opened to retrieve additional supplies, or a need to leave the treatment area arises, remove treatment gloves and perform hand hygiene. Perform hand hygiene again prior to putting on a new pair of treatment gloves when restarting the procedure. Plastic barrier **overgloves** provide another option if treatment must be interrupted. Rinse patient treatment gloves briefly with water only if necessary (do not use soap, as it will compromise the integrity of the protection), dry, and cover with overgloves. Remove overgloves and discard when restarting the procedure.

IMAGE RECEPTOR MANAGEMENT. Immediately after removing an image receptor from the oral cavity wipe dry with gauze or a paper towel to remove excess saliva (Figure 9–12 ■).

Procedure 9–2

Infection control prior to the radiographic procedure

1. Perform handwashing (Procedure 9–1) or apply an alcohol-based hand rub.*
2. Put on utility gloves.
3. Clean and disinfect with appropriate disinfectant all surfaces that will come in contact either directly or indirectly with potential contaminants:
   a. X-ray tube head, PID, extension arm
   b. Exposure control panel**
   c. Treatment chair, including headrest, back support, arm rests, body and back of chair
   d. Bracket table, countertop, or other clinical contact surfaces used during the procedure
   e. Lead/lead equivalent apron/thyroid collar
   f. Digital sensor/PSP plates
   g. Computer keyboard and mouse**

(continued)

Procedure 9–2 *(continued)*

4. Wash and remove utility gloves. Disinfect, dry, and store gloves.
5. Perform hand hygiene.
6. Put on clean overgloves.
7. Obtain plastic barriers and cover all surfaces that will come in contact either directly or indirectly with the patient:
   a. X-ray tube head, PID, extension arm
   b. Exposure control panel
   c. Treatment chair, including headrest, back support, arm rests, body and back of chair
   d. Bracket table, countertop, or other clinical contact surfaces that will be used during the procedure
   e. Digital sensor/PSP plates/film packets
   f. Computer keyboard and mouse
8. Obtain radiographic supplies:
   a. Image receptors (film packets/digital sensors/PSP plates)
   b. Disposable/sterile image receptor holding devices
   c. Film mount (film-based imaging)
   d. Disposable paper/plastic cup/bag or transfer box
   e. Gauze/paper towels
   f. Miscellaneous supplies (e.g., cotton rolls, extra disposable image receptor holders)
9. Place film mount under plastic barrier on countertop workspace.
10. Place intraoral film packets on top of plastic barrier; position within windows of film mount.
11. Place paper/plastic cup, gauze/paper towel next to film mount on top of the plastic barrier.
12. Prepare antimicrobial mouth rinse for patient use prior to procedure.***

*Alcohol-based hand rub can be used when hands are not visibly soiled. Refer to manufacturer's recommendations for use.

**Electronic equipment can be damaged by disinfectants. Consult manufacturer's recommendations. Protect with a plastic barrier.

***Scientific evidence has not demonstrated that preprocedural mouth rinsing prevents the spread of infections; however, the number of microorganisms that may be released in the form of aerosols/spatter may be reduced.

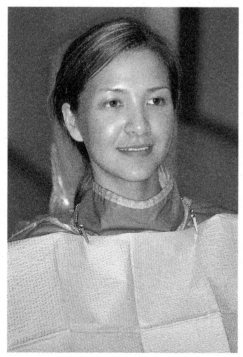

FIGURE 9–11 Respiratory hygiene/cough etiquette. Patient napkin over lead apron provides disposable paper product for containment of potential infective microorganisms.

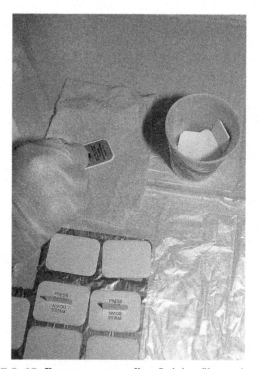

FIGURE 9–12 Remove excess saliva. Swiping film packet across paper towel after removal from oral cavity prior to dropping into containment cup.

If using a digital sensor, wipe the plastic sheath barrier dry prior to placing it for the next exposure. After drying a film packet drop into a containment paper/plastic cup/bag without touching the outside edges of the cup/bag. The cup/bag will contain the contaminated film packet and serves as the transport method of getting the image receptor safely to the darkroom for processing.

Management of PSP plates during a radiographic procedure varies regarding when to remove the barrier envelope. If exposing only one or a small number of PSP plates, it may not be necessary to use a light-tight containment box because scanning will take place almost immediately following exposure. If this is the case, then follow protocol used for film packets, and wipe the plate dry and drop into a containment cup/bag. If the time between exposure and scanning is longer, PSP plates must be protected from light exposure by placing in a light-tight box specifically designed for this purpose (see Figure 8–14). To avoid contamination of the transfer box, remove the barrier envelope. Holding the PSP plate directly over the transfer box, carefully tear the plastic by gripping the corners on either side of the notched edge and allow the plate to drop into the box (Figure 9–13 ■). Do not touch the plate with gloved hands.

IMAGE RECEPTOR HOLDER MANAGEMENT. Transfer image receptor holding devices from a barrier-protected surface to the oral cavity and then back to the same covered surface. Do not place contaminated instruments on an uncovered surface (Procedure 9–3).

Protocol After the Radiographic Procedure

When the examination is complete, do not immediately remove the lead/lead equivalent apron and thyroid collar

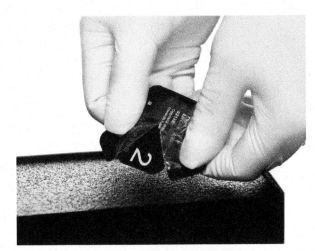

FIGURE 9–13 Aseptic opening of barrier envelope allows PSP plate to drop into containment box. (Courtesy of Air Techniques, Inc.)

from the patient while still wearing treatment gloves. The apron and collar can be difficult to clean and disinfect so do not touch it with contaminated gloves. Request that the patient remain seated to allow time to remove treatment gloves and perform hand hygiene, then remove the apron and collar with clean, dry hands. Clean and prepare reusable image receptor holders for sterilization according to manufacturer's recommendations. Usually holders can be washed with soap and water or ultrasonic cleaned in detergent and dried and packaged in an autoclave bag for sterilization. If using a digital sensor, carefully remove the barrier sheath to avoid tearing the plastic and contaminating the sensor (Figure 9–14 ■). Clean and disinfect digital sensors and PSP plates according to manufacturer's recommendations (Procedure 9–4).

Procedure 9–3

Infection control during the radiographic procedure

1. Perform handwashing (Procedure 9–1) or apply an alcohol-based hand rub.*

2. Put on patient treatment gloves.

3. Place overgloves over patient treatment gloves to place lead/lead equivalent apron and thyroid collar on the patient.

4. Remove overgloves and place on countertop for possible use later.

5. With patient treatment gloves in place, assemble image receptor into disposable or sterile holding device, place intraorally, position the x-ray tube head and PID, depress exposure button.

6. Remove image receptor and holding device from oral cavity and remove excess saliva by wiping with gauze or paper towel. Drop film or PSP plate into containment cup/bag.

7. If additional supplies are needed that require contact with uncovered surfaces or an interruption requires leaving the treatment area:

   a. Rinse treatment gloves with plain water if necessary (no soap) and dry. Place overgloves over treatment gloves. Remove overgloves when restarting the procedure.

   OR

   b. Remove and discard treatment gloves and perform hand hygiene. Prior to restarting the procedure, perform hand hygiene and put on a new pair of treatment gloves.

*Alcohol-based hand rub can be used when hands are not visibly soiled. Refer to manufacturer's recommendations for use.

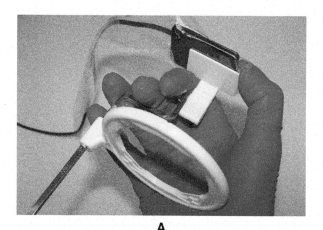
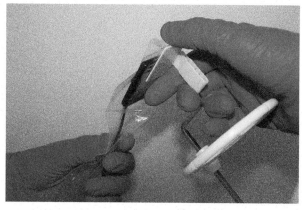

A   **B**

FIGURE 9–14 **Removal of plastic barrier from a digital sensor.** Remove sticky-backed biteblocks carefully to avoid tearing sheath. **(A)** Grasp holder in the palm of one hand, press on the sensor with thumb. **(B)** As the sensor begins to move, guide it out of the plastic sheath with the other hand.

Procedure 9–4

Infection control after the radiographic procedure

1. Remove and discard patient treatment gloves. Perform handwashing (Procedure 9–1) or apply an alcohol-based hand rub.*
2. Remove lead/lead equivalent apron with thyroid collar and dismiss patient.
3. Put on utility gloves.
4. Prepare and package image receptor holders for sterilization.
5. Clean, disinfect, dry, and store digital image receptors.
6. Discard disposable contaminated items. Remove and discard plastic surface barriers.
7. Clean and disinfect surfaces that were not protected with a barrier.
8. Wash, dry, and remove utility gloves. Disinfect, dry, and store gloves.
9. Perform hand hygiene.

*Alcohol-based hand rub can be used when hands are not visibly soiled. Refer to manufacturer's recommendations for use.

Infection Control Protocol for Radiographic Processing

The use of digital sensors eliminates the need for challenging infection control protocol during image processing; and the use of barrier envelopes for protecting indirect digital PSP plates has already been discussed. Intraoral film processing requires special consideration to maintain infection control. Use a containment cup/bag to transport film packets to the darkroom. Once the darkroom countertop space has been cleaned, disinfected, and covered with an appropriate barrier, put on treatment gloves to separate film packets from a protective barrier envelope; or when not using a barrier envelope, to separate films from the outer plastic packet wrap. Place the containment cup with the contaminated film packets next to an empty cup or a clean paper towel placed on the countertop.

Protocol for Film with Barrier Envelopes

If using a film packet covered with a plastic barrier, infection control protocol is the same as that used for PSP plates. Remove a film packet from the containment cup, and holding it over the empty cup or paper towel tear open the plastic barrier allowing the film packet to drop into the cup or onto the paper towel (see Figure 9–6). Be careful to not touch the film packet. Repeat until all film packets are separated from the barrier envelopes. Remove treatment gloves and perform hand hygiene. Using clean, dry hands or new treatment gloves, open film packets and place the films into the automatic processor or prepare to process manually.

Protocol for Film Without Barrier Envelopes

Remove a film packet from the containment cup, and holding it over the empty cup or paper towel locate the plastic/paper tab and pull to open the packet's outer wrapping. Locate the folded black paper tab, grasp it to unfold and gently pull straight out while holding the packet directly over the empty cup or paper towel. Continue to slowly pull the tab allowing the film inside to drop out into the cup or onto the paper towel (Figure 9–15 ■). Be careful to not touch the film. Repeat until all films have been separated from the packets. Remove treatment gloves and perform hand hygiene. Using clean, dry hands or new treatment gloves, place films into

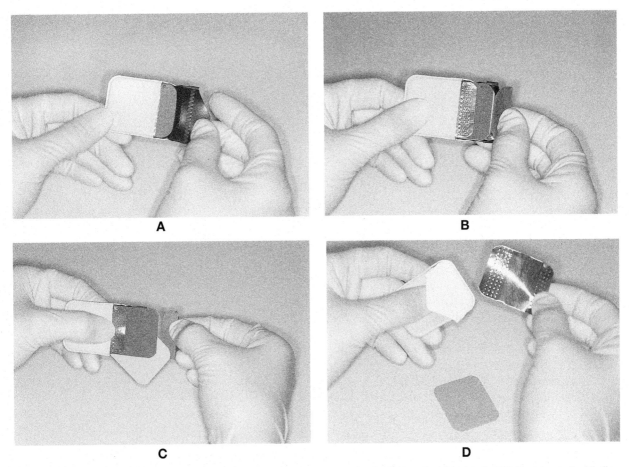

FIGURE 9–15 **Steps for removing film from contaminated packet. (A)** Open by lifting the plastic tab. **(B)** Locate, and with finger and thumb grasp the black paper folded tab. **(C)** Gently pull on tab, sliding film out of the packet. **(D)** Allow film to drop out onto a surface barrier. Separate lead foil for appropriate disposal.

the automatic processor or prepare to process manually. To avoid damage, handle films by the edges.

After processing, put on utility gloves to separate lead foils from the film packet outer wrap for disposal according to local and state regulations for handling this type of waste (see Chapter 19); and dispose of cups, paper towels, and other supplies used during the procedure. Clean and disinfect surfaces as needed. Aseptically opening film packets in a timely manner under safelight conditions requires practice. Be careful to avoid dropping and potentially losing films in the dim lighting. Film is sensitive to prolonged safelight exposure, requiring that packets be opened and films placed into the processor within two to three minutes (Procedure 9–5).

Procedure 9–5

Infection control for processing radiographic films without barrier envelopes

1. Transport contaminated film packets to darkroom in containment cup/bag.
2. Place two paper towels on the counter workspace in front of the automatic processor.
   a. Place containment cup with contaminated films on one paper towel; designate this paper towel as *contaminated*.
   b. Place new, clean treatment gloves on the other paper towel; designate this paper towel as *uncontaminated*.
3. Secure darkroom door. Turn off white overhead light and turn on safelight.
4. Put on clean treatment gloves.
5. Select a film packet from the containment cup; hold just above the *uncontaminated* paper towel and aseptically open, allowing the film to drop out onto the *uncontaminated* paper towel. Be careful to not touch the film.
6. Deposit the empty film packet onto the *contaminated* paper towel.
7. Repeat until all films have been separated from the packets.

(continued)

Procedure 9–5 *(continued)*

8. Remove and discard patient treatment gloves. Perform hand hygiene.

9. With clean, dry hands, grasp films by the edges and place into the automatic processor film feed slot or load onto manual processing film racks for processing.

10. Turn on the overhead white light. Put on utility gloves

11. Separate lead foil from film packets and dispose of according to local and state regulations for handling this type of waste; appropriately discard film packets, paper towel, cup/bag, and other supplies used for the procedure.

12. Clean and disinfect surfaces that were not protected with a barrier.

13. Wash, dry, and remove utility gloves. Disinfect, dry, and store gloves.

14. Perform hand hygiene.

Protocol for Daylight Loader Processors

Daylight loader attachments on automatic processors have light-tight flaps or sleeves that allow a radiographer's hands to slide through to access the intake slots on the front of a processor. Although film packets with and without plastic barrier envelopes can be processed in an automatic processor with a daylight loader attachment, because of the complexity of infection control protocol for its use, using film packets that were protected with barriers is recommended. Separate the films from the barriers prior to placing into the daylight loader compartment and then continue the process with clean, dry hands.

The key to infection control using a daylight loader to process films that were not secured in barrier envelopes is to open the light-filter cover when placing and removing items (Figure 9–16 ■). Never slide gloved hands or push items through the light-tight baffles. After placing items into the compartment, close the light-filter cover and insert clean, dry hands through the baffles. Looking through the light-filter cover, put on treatment gloves once hands are inside the unit and proceed to aseptically open the film packets, separate the lead foil, and contain all contaminated items

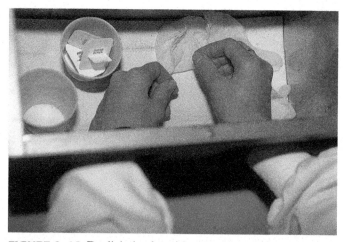

FIGURE 9–16 Daylight loader with cover opened illustrating operator has placed clean, dry hands through the baffles. Note that gloves will be put on once the hands are inside the compartment.

in the same manner as darkroom processing. When all films have been loaded into the processor, remove the contaminated treatment gloves before sliding ungloved hands out through the light-tight baffles (Procedure 9–6).

Procedure 9–6

Infection control for an automatic processor with a daylight loader attachment

1. Transport contaminated film packets to the processor in the containment cup/bag.

2. Open the light-filter cover and line the floor of the compartment with paper towels. Designate one side of the space as *contaminated* and the other side as *uncontaminated*.

3. Place the containment cup on the *contaminated* side; place new, clean treatment gloves on the *uncontaminated* side.

4. Close the light-filter cover and insert clean, dry hands through the light-tight baffles.

5. Once inside, put on the treatment gloves.

6. Aseptically open each film packet allowing film to drop onto the *uncontaminated* side of the compartment floor.

7. Drop the contaminated film packet onto the paper towel on the *contaminated* side of the compartment floor.

8. Repeat until all films have been separated from the packets.

9. Remove patient treatment gloves and place on the *contaminated* side of the compartment floor.

10. With clean, dry hands, grasp film by the edges and place into the automatic processor film feed slot.

11. When all films have completely entered the processor, remove ungloved hands through the light-tight baffles.

Procedure 9–6

12. Perform hand hygiene and put on utility gloves.

13. Open the light-filter cover and remove the cups, contaminated film packets, and paper towels and discard appropriately; separate lead foils and dispose of according to local and state regulations for handling this type of waste.

14. Clean and disinfect surfaces that were not protected with a barrier.

15. Wash, dry, and remove utility gloves. Disinfect, dry, and store gloves.

16. Perform hand hygiene.

REVIEW—Chapter summary

Infectious diseases may be transmitted from patient to oral health care personnel, from oral health care personnel to patient, and from patient to patient. Routes of transmission include direct and indirect contact with pathogens. The conditions for the chain of infection are a susceptible host, pathogens in sufficient numbers to initiate infection, portals of exit and entry, and an appropriate route for the pathogen to be transmitted. The purpose of infection control is to prevent the transmission of disease between patients and operators and between patients by breaking the chain of infection.

The Centers for Disease Control and Prevention (CDC) and the Occupational Safety and Health Administration (OHSA) play a role in developing, recommending, and/or enforcing guidelines for infection control. The CDC expanded on OSHA's blood-borne pathogen standard of universal precautions and introduced standard precautions, which expands the potential for transmission of pathogens to all body fluids (except sweat), of all patients whether known to be infected or not.

Personal protective equipment (PPE) includes protective clothing, masks, eyewear, and gloves that act as barriers to prevent the transmission of infective microorganisms. Following protocols for hand and respiratory hygiene can break the chain of infection. Use the appropriate Environmental Protection Agency (EPA)-regulated high-, intermediate-, or low-level disinfectant to reduce, destroy, or inactivate pathogens to an acceptable level on inanimate objects. Sterilization is required to inactivate resistant bacterial spores. Equipment used in the radiographic procedure is classified as semi- or noncritical for infection

control. Environmental infection control consideration must include clinical contact and housekeeping surfaces that should be cleaned, disinfected as needed, and/or covered with a surface barrier.

Plastic barrier envelopes and sheaths are available to protect intraoral dental film packets, PSP plates, and digital sensors from contact with microorganisms when placed in the oral cavity. Film packets obtained directly from a manufacturer's packaging are considered industrially clean and may be placed intraorally without barrier envelope protection. Perform step-by-step infection control methods prior to, during, and after the radiographic procedures. Key points of infection control for radiographic procedures include clean, disinfect as needed, and/or cover all surfaces that may come in contact either directly or indirectly with potential contaminants; use disposable or autoclavable image receptor holders; use overgloves to cover treatment gloves when needed; use gauze or paper towel to remove excess saliva from an image receptor upon removal from the oral cavity; utilize a containment cup/bag/box to hold contaminated image receptors; aseptically remove PSP plates from barrier envelopes prior to dropping into the light-tight transfer box; use aseptic technique to remove a digital sensor from a barrier sheath without tearing.

Perform specific step-by-step infection control procedures when opening contaminated barrier envelopes and film packets. Aseptically open film packets in a timely manner under safelight conditions. Follow strict infection control protocol when using an automatic processor with a daylight loader.

RECALL—Study questions

1. Each of the following is a condition of the chain of infection EXCEPT one. Which one is the EXCEPTION?
   a. Susceptible host
   b. Reservoir of pathogens
   c. Portals of exit and entry
   d. Critical instruments

2. The purpose of infection control is to prevent the transmission of disease between
   a. patients.
   b. patient and operator.
   c. operator and patient.
   d. all of the above.

3. Each of the following will break the chain of infection EXCEPT one. Which one is the EXCEPTION?
   a. Use of a digital sensor
   b. Use of personal protective equipment
   c. Sterilization of radiographic equipment
   d. Immunization of oral health care practitioners

4. Which of these agencies develops and provides recommendations for adoption of infection control guidelines, but does not act as an enforcer of these guidelines?
   a. Centers for Disease Control and Prevention (CDC)
   b. Occupational Safety and Health Administration (OHSA)
   c. U.S. Food and Drug Administration (FDA)
   d. U.S. Environmental Protection Agency (EPA)

5. List four items of PPE recommended for a dental radiographer.
   a. _____
   b. _____
   c. _____
   d. _____

6. The use of a chemical or physical procedure to reduce disease-producing microorganisms to an acceptable level on inanimate objects is the definition of
   a. asepsis.
   b. antiseptic.
   c. disinfection.
   d. sterilization.

7. Radiographic image receptor holders are classified for infection control as
   a. critical instruments.
   b. semicritical instruments.
   c. noncritical instruments.
   d. clinical contact surfaces.

8. A dental x-ray tube head and PID are classified for infection control as
   a. semicritical objects.
   b. noncritical objects.
   c. clinical contact surfaces.
   d. housekeeping surfaces.

9. Spraying disinfectant directly on which of these should be avoided?
   a. Digital sensor
   b. Treatment chair head rest
   c. X-ray machine exposure switch
   d. Bracket table or countertop

10. Each of the following may be protected with a plastic barrier to maintain infection control during the radiographic procedure EXCEPT one. Which one is the EXCEPTION?
    a. PSP plate
    b. Image receptor holder
    c. Exposure button
    d. Tube head and PID

11. Which of the following is more likely to be heat-sterilized following use?
    a. Digital sensor
    b. PSP plate
    c. Film packet
    d. Image receptor holder

12. What should be done with an image receptor immediately after removing it from the oral cavity?
    a. Remove and reapply a clean plastic barrier.
    b. Wipe off excess saliva with gauze or paper towel.
    c. Drop into a containment cup/bag without touching the sides.
    d. Rinse briefly with plain water, do not use soap.

13. Following a radiographic procedure, clean and disinfect clinical contact surfaces using
    a. utility gloves.
    b. patient treatment gloves.
    c. plastic overgloves.
    d. clean, dry hands.

14. The purpose of the black paper tab inside an intraoral film packet is to
    a. protect the film from bright light exposure.
    b. prevent glove print artifacts from appearing on the film.
    c. provide a way to aseptically slide the film out of the packet.
    d. facilitate removal of the lead foil.

15. Each of the following will assist in maintaining ideal infection control conditions when using an automatic processor with a daylight loader attachment EXCEPT one. Which one is the EXCEPTION?
    a. Open light-filter cover to place and remove items.
    b. Slide gloved hands through the baffles prior to and after processing.
    c. Use film packets that have been removed from barrier envelopes.
    d. Line the compartment floor with paper towels.

REFLECT—Case study

While exposing a full mouth series of radiographs, you accidentally drop the image receptor holding device with one of the unexposed films on the floor. Explain in detail what infection control protocol you would follow to respond to this situation to be able to complete the examination.

RELATE—Laboratory application

For a comprehensive laboratory practice exercise on this topic, see Thomson, E. M., & Bruhn, A. M. (2018). *Exercises in oral radiography techniques: A laboratory manual* (4th ed.). Hoboken, NJ: Pearson. Chapter 9, "Infection control for the Radiographic Procedure."

RESOURCES

Bird, D. L., & Robinson, D. S. (2015). Disease transmission and infection prevention. Principles and techniques of disinfection. Principles and techniques of instrument processing and sterilization. *Modern dental assisting* (11th ed.). St. Louis, MO: Elsevier.

Centers for Disease Control and Prevention. (2016, March). *Summary of infection prevention practices in dental settings: Basic expectations for safe care.* Atlanta, GA: U.S. Department of Health and Human Services, Centers for Disease Control and Prevention, National Center for Chronic Disease Prevention and Health Promotion, Division of Oral Health.

Hokett, S. D., Honey, J. R., Ruiz, F., Baisden, M. K., & Hoen, M. M. (2000). Assessing the effectiveness of direct digital radiography barrier sheaths and finger cots. *Journal of the American Dental Association, 131,* 463–467.

Kalathingal, S. M., Moore, S., Kwon, S., Schuster, G. S., Shrout, M. K., & Plummer, K. (2009). An evaluation of microbiologic contamination on phosphor plates in a dental school. *Oral Surgery, Oral Medicine, Oral Pathology, Oral Radiology, 107,* 279–282.

Kuperstein, A. S. (2012). Defective plastic infection-control barriers and faulty technique may cause PSP plate contamination used in digital intraoral radiography. *Journal of Evidence Based Dental Practice, 12,* 46–47.

Organization for Safety, Asepsis and Prevention. (2004, January). *Infection Control in Practice, 3*(1), entire issue. Retrieved from http://www.osap.org

OSHA Fact Sheet. (2011, January 28). OSHA's bloodborne pathogen standard. Retrieved from OSHA website: https://www.osha.gov/OshDoc/data_BloodborneFacts/bbfact01.pdf

U.S. Department of Health and Human Services for Disease Control and Prevention, Centers for Disease Control and Prevention. (2003, December 19). Guidelines for infection control in dental health-care settings. *MMWR, 52*(RR17), 1–61.

Visit www.pearsonhighered.com/healthprofessionsresources to access the student resources that accompany this book. Simply select Dental Hygiene from the choice of disciplines. Find this book and you will find the complementary study tools created for this specific title.

10

Legal and Ethical Responsibilities

OBJECTIVES

Following successful completion of this chapter, you should be able to:

1. Define the key terms.
2. Discuss federal and state regulations concerning the use of dental x-ray equipment.
3. Describe licensure requirements for individuals who expose dental radiographs.
4. Identify specific risk management strategies pertaining to dental radiography.
5. Respond to a patient exercising self-determination in refusing a radiographic examination.
6. List criteria for informed consent.
7. List the details that must be documented in a patient's record regarding a radiographic examination.
8. Describe elements required before releasing a copy of a patient's radiographic images.
9. State how long radiographic images should be maintained and available.
10. Describe the role of DICOM.
11. List the advantages of cloud sharing over other methods of storing and sharing digital radiographic images.
12. Identify a cloud sharing system that is HIPAA compliant.
13. Explain Joint Photographers' Expert Group (JPEG) impact on digital radiographic images.
14. Identify the role professional ethics play in guiding a radiographer's behavior.

KEY TERMS

Cloud file sharing systems
Code of Ethics
Confidentiality
Digital Imaging and Communications in Medicine (DICOM)
Direct supervision
Disclosure
Encryption
Ethics
Health Insurance Portability and Accountability Act (HIPAA)
Informed consent
Liable
Malpractice
Negligence
Protected health-related information (PHI)
Self-determination
Statute of limitations

Introduction

To perform radiographic services for patients safely and legally, a dental radiographer needs to be aware of laws and regulations pertaining to dental radiography, and the dental profession's codes of ethics that guide decisions regarding the use of ionizing radiation and protection of digital health records. This chapter discusses regulations that apply to dental radiography and presents the ethical use and protection of dental radiographic images.

Regulations and Licensure

The Federal Performance Act of 1974 requires that all dental x-ray equipment manufactured or sold in the United States meet federal performance standards. These standards include safety requirements for filtration, collimation, and other x-ray machine characteristics. Additionally, federal regulations, state, county, and city laws may also apply to the use of dental x-ray equipment. State laws often require that registration and inspection of dental x-ray machines be conducted every two to four years. Because laws and regulations vary by location, and are subject to change, contact individual state bureaus of radiological health for specific information.

Of particular interest to operators of dental x-ray machines are laws that establish guidelines for who can place and expose radiographs. In 1981, then updated in 1991, the federal Consumer-Patient Radiation Health and Safety Act was passed to protect patients from unnecessary radiation. This act established minimum standards for state certification and licensure of personnel who administer radiation in medical and dental radiographic procedures. Adoption of the act's standards was made discretionary with each state. Although a few states have not voluntarily established licensure laws for personnel who place and expose dental radiographs, a majority of states require that operators of x-ray equipment be trained and certified or licensed to take dental radiographs. Many states consider dental hygienists and dental assistants who have passed the National Board Dental Hygiene Examine (NBDHE) and the Dental Assisting National Board Examination (DANB), respectively, and hold a license to practice in the state as a Registered Dental Hygienist or Certified Dental Assistant, respectively, to meet this requirement. However, some states require dental hygienists and dental assistants to take an additional examination or to fulfill continuing education requirements annually to be certified specifically in radiation safety or radiographic technique competency.

State laws regulating personnel who expose dental radiographs vary considerably for "on-the-job" trained dental assistants. Whereas many states have a mandatory state examination or a continuing education requirement, a few states allow uncertified dental assistants with "on-the-job" training to take radiographs under the direct supervision of a dentist. **Direct supervision** means that the dentist is present in the office when the radiographs are taken. Each state's Dental Commission controls the scope of practice for oral health care professionals. Because laws and regulations vary and are subject to change, contact individual state Dental

Box 10–1: Web Sites for Professional Dental Organizations

American Dental Assistant Association (ADAA)	www.adaausa.org
American Dental Hygienists' Association (ADHA)	www.adha.org
American Dental Association (ADA)	www.ada.org
Hispanic Dental Association (HDA)	www.hdassoc.org
National Dental Association (NDA)	www.ndaonline.org
National Dental Assistants Association (NDAA)	Link from www .ndaonline.org
National Dental Hygienists Association (NDHA)	www.ndhaonline .org

Commissions directly to learn about legal requirements for placing and exposing dental radiographs in that state. A complete list of state Dental Commissions can be viewed on the American Dental Association's Web site (www.ada.org) (Box 10–1).

Legal Considerations

Malpractice actions against health care providers have increased in number and amount of awards in recent years. Risk management includes policies and procedures that reduce the chance that a patient will file legal action against a dentist and the oral health care team. In addition to developing good patient relations with clear communication, following standard protocols and performing procedures correctly will help reach the goals of providing quality care and minimizing risk. See Procedure 10–1 for a radiography safety audit for avoiding risk.

Specific risk management procedures that can be a good defense when performed correctly or a liability if performed poorly include obtaining a duplicate copy of a new patient's radiographs rather than reexposing the patient to ionizing radiation; using the best equipment currently available, including fast-speed film or digital imaging, rectangular collimation, lead/lead-equivalent thyroid collar barriers, and film-holding devices; and establishing a quality assurance plan and conducting quality control tests for all radiographic procedures (see Chapter 19). Personnel radiation monitoring, whether required by law or not, can be a good risk management tool. Monitoring radiation exposure, or more precisely the lack of exposure, will provide personnel and the oral health care practice with documentation of safe work habits.

Good patient relations can reduce the risk of possible legal action. It is important to make a patient feel comfortable by establishing a relaxing and confident chairside manner (see Chapter 11). Always explain to the patient what and how procedures are to be performed. Answer all questions the patient may have concerning the procedures.

Procedure 10–1

Safety Audit for Radiography Risk Management

- **Do radiographers:**

  Possess legal credentials, and are they properly trained to work with the x-ray equipment?

  Wear a radiation dosimeter to monitor work habits (Figure 10–1 ■)?

  Wear personal protective equipment (PPE) when working with processing chemistry?

  Know the location of the Safety Data Sheets (SDS) for potentially hazardous radiographic materials (see Chapter 19)?

- **Does dental x-ray equipment:**

  Have current license and inspection certificates?

  Have inspection certificates posted as may be required by law?

  Undergo quality control testing at regular intervals (see Chapter 19)?

- **Is signage posted:**

  To confirm credentials and continuing education achievements of radiographers?

  To announce the use of ionizing radiation in the area (Figure 10–2 ■)?

  That lists radiation safety protocols for use of the dental x-ray machine?

  For ease of reference to recommended exposure settings?

  To warn of accident prevention (i.e., "Watch head when pulling x-ray tube head away from the wall.")?

- **Is documentation kept for:**

  Informed patient consent prior to radiographic procedures?

  Patient assessment of need, number and type of exposures, retakes, name of radiographer who took the radiographs?

  Radiographic interpretation findings and how these are communicated to a patient following the appointment?

  How patient radiographs, film and digital images, are kept confidential?

  Updating digital software for accessing radiographs currently and in the future?

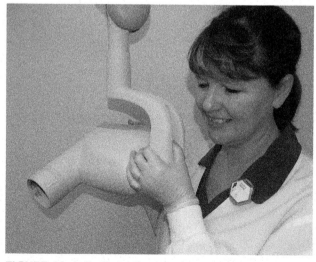

FIGURE 10–1 **Radiographer wearing a radiation monitoring badge.**

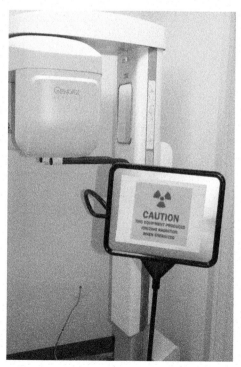

FIGURE 10–2 **Ionizing radiation in-use sign.**

Avoid negative remarks about procedures, equipment, and the dental staff. Statements like, "The digital image software is not working again" or "This tube head always drifts" should never be made to a patient or in front of a patient. These statements imply that you have chosen to use known defective equipment on a patient. This is not the same as saying, "The digital image software is not working. The radiographs must be retaken. However, we will not retake any more images until a thorough investigation is made to correct the problem with the software." or "This tube head is drifting. Because this is a problem, we cannot use it to take your x-rays until it is repaired. Let's move to another room for your procedure." If equipment is not working properly, it should be repaired or serviced.

Patients have a legal right to make choices about the health care they receive. This is called **self-determination**, and includes the right to refuse treatment. Occasionally, a patient may express opposition to recommended radiographs. The patient may believe that such radiographs are unnecessary or that the x-ray exposure risks are not warranted. The best response is to explain in clear terms the benefits to the patient to be realized from the radiographs, including the ability to determine a diagnosis, evaluate prognosis, and recommend treatment options. If a patient continues to refuse required radiographs, a dentist must carefully decide whether treatment can be provided. In rare situations, a patient may offer to sign a document to release the dentist from the responsibilities of going ahead with treatment without the required radiographs. Legally, such a document will not release a dentist from liability and is not valid because a patient cannot legally consent to negligent care. **Negligence** in this case might manifest as the failure to use a reasonable amount of care (obtaining a radiograph to determine diagnosis) that results in injury or damage (inappropriate treatment).

To be able to provide **informed consent** prior to undergoing radiographic examinations, a dentist must explain the nature and purpose of the examination to a patient. While state laws vary regarding the elements of informed consent, the following are general guidelines that must be presented to a patient with regard to radiographic procedures:

- Purpose of taking radiographs
- Benefits radiographs will supply
- Possible risks of radiation exposure
- Possible risks of refusing radiographs
- Identification of person who will perform procedure

This informing process is called **disclosure**. A patient should be given an opportunity to ask questions prior to radiographic procedures. Answer all questions completely in terms the patient understands.

A dentist is responsible for discussing all aspects of treatment to assist a patient with making an informed decision. It is important to understand that even though radiographers work under the supervision of a dentist, they are legally liable for their own actions. **Liable** means to be legally obligated to make good any loss or damage that may occur. Both dentists and dental radiographers are liable for procedures performed by a dental radiographer. In malpractice cases, legal action can be brought against both a supervising dentist and a dental radiographer.

Confidentiality of Dental Radiographs

Document all exposures of dental radiographs in a patient's dental record. Entries in the record should be made by a dentist or under a dentist's supervision, and must include:

- Patient's informed consent to the radiographic examination
- Number and type of radiographs exposed, including retakes
- Date radiographs are taken and name of radiographer who took them
- Reason for taking radiographs
- Interpretive and diagnostic results

Radiographs are considered part of a patient's dental record and are the property of a dentist. Patients have a right to reasonable access of their records and may request a copy of their radiographs; or that their radiographs be made available to another professional, such as when changing dentists or for the purpose of obtaining a consultation with a specialist (Procedure 10–2). A copy of the radiographs can be made available to the patient, but the original radiographs should be retained by the practice.

Dental records, including dental radiographic images, are part of a patient's confidential medical record and considered

Procedure 10–2

Procedure for releasing a copy of a patient's radiographs

1. Patient requests copy of radiographs in writing.
2. Keep the letter requesting radiographs in the patient's record.
3. Duplicate film-based radiographs, print out a paper copy of digital images or use cloud file sharing systems that allow patient access to electronic health records and digital radiographs.
4. Send duplicate radiographs or paper copy of digital images by the U.S. Postal Service's Certified Mail™ or use HIPAA-certified cloud file sharing systems.
5. Keep the postal receipt or electronic email confirmation in the patient's record.
6. Document the date and where and to whom the copies were sent in the patient's record.

Box 10–2: Elements of a Radiographic Release

- Name and address of dentist or practice facility
- Patient's name and identifying information
- Description of radiographs (type, number of images, etc.) to be released
- Name and address of individual or facility to which radiographs are to be sent
- Statement authorizing release of radiographs
- Patient acknowledgment of acceptance of potential risks associated with sending digital images if via unsecured email
- Signature of patient or authorized individual
- Time period for which release remains valid

American Dental Association. (2007). *Dental Records*. Council on Dental Practice Division of Legal Affairs. Chicago: Author.

to be **protected health-related information (PHI)**. The federal government signed into law privacy standards to protect patients' medical records and other health information, including radiographs. Developed by the Department of Health and Human Services (DHHS) as part of the **Health Insurance Portability and Accountability Act (HIPAA)**, this federal law is designed to provide patients with control over how their personal health information is used and disclosed. **Confidentiality** laws designed to protect a patient's privacy state that radiographs must not be viewed or discussed with anyone outside the oral health care practice without first obtaining a current, signed release from a patient (Box 10–2). More discussion on this topic follows in the next section on securing digital radiographic images.

How long an oral health care practice is required to keep dental radiographs depends on various factors. Legal action that can be brought against a dentist depends on malpractice and limitation statues that vary from state to state. For adult patients, the **statute of limitations**, the time period during which a patient may bring a malpractice action against a dentist or radiographer, generally begins at the time of an injury that results from negligent dental treatment, or when an injury should have reasonably been discovered. For children, the statute of limitations does not begin until a child reaches the age of majority (18 to 21 years old, depending on the state). Because these time periods vary, it is recommended that radiographs be retained indefinitely.

Securely Storing and Sharing Digital Radiographic Images

Legal guidelines and ethical responsibilities impact how digital radiographic images are captured and stored on computers; shared and transferred through the Internet;

and kept secure and confidential. For digital radiographic images to be of maximum benefit, digital systems must be able to interface with each other. **Digital Imaging and Communications in Medicine (DICOM)** sets standards for digital radiographic system compatibility that facilitates electronic transfer of digital radiographic images between systems. The American Dental Association Informatics Task Group has recommended that DICOM standards be used by dental imaging systems for storing and viewing digital radiographic images so that systems remain compatible with one another.

Similar to the DICOM standard application for storing and viewing digital radiographic images, standards are evolving for sharing images between the oral health care community and patients. Portable storage drives, such as compact discs (CDs), were the first mechanisms available to share digital radiographic images. There became a need for an alternative method for radiographic image sharing as file sizes increased with improved technology. Intraoral digital images in their original, uncompressed form, require between 290 and 16,000 kilobytes (KB) of storage space. The large variation in digital radiographic image size is dependent upon the spatial resolution of an image (see Chapter 8). The higher the spatial resolution, the larger the image file size creating difficulty in the ability to electronically store and send images. Although CDs are still used, their maximum storage capacity is approximately 750 megabytes (MB). Additionally, the method used to send CDs and other external portable devices containing confidential digital radiographic images to others in need of this information must be secure. Another concern with using CDs and external portable devices is that the receiver of the data may not have compatable image viewing software.

Online image exchange through **cloud file sharing systems**, which allow storage of documents and data as well as electronic access to image viewing software, provide an option for sharing large files, eliminating the need to securely ship digital images on external portable devices. DICOM has recently provided services to securely store and retrieve digital radiographic images online through the use of web browsers. Cloud file sharing systems, commonly referred to as *the cloud* are able to store images in a manner similar to a portable storage drive, with an increased space capacity and without the need to physically handle a device. Costs are usually associated with cloud file sharing systems when storage exceeds a predetermined amount of data. Duplicate copies of digital radiographic images can be transferrred securely through an online web browser between health care providers for consultation purposes; between an oral heath care practice and a patient who requests access to his/her radiographic images; and between a practice and a patient's dental insurance company (Figure 10–3 ■). Insurance companies have a right to request pretreatment radiographs prior to agreeing to pay for services. Most dental insurance companies accept digital radiographic images when sent through HIPAA-compliant cloud file sharing systems. As with film-based radiographs, only duplicate digital images should be sent electronically. Original digital

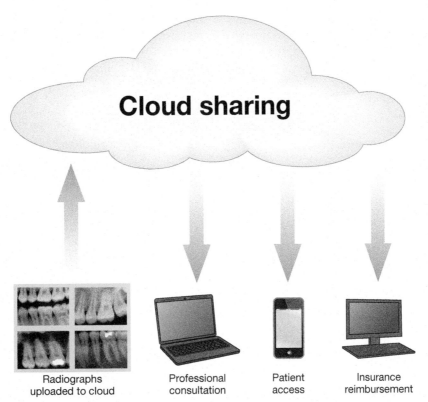

Cloud sharing

Radiographs
uploaded to cloud

Professional
consultation

Patient
access

Insurance
reimbursement

FIGURE 10–3 **Cloud file sharing system.** Digital radiographs can be uploaded to the cloud, where authorized professionals, patients, and third-party payers can access the images.

radiographic images must be backed up to a secure database prior to preparing an image copy for sending electronically. A copy image is "dropped off" on a secure cloud sharing site where it can be "picked up" by an approved user.

Radiographers should determine if the cloud file system being used is HIPAA certified to ensure system confidentiality and accountability. Cloud file sharing systems that are HIPAA compliant encrypt digital radiographic images to protect against unauthorized access. **Encryption** is a process of changing the digital image into a coded file that can be read only by individuals with the credentials for decoding the data. Encryption of digital radiographic images is necessary for optimal security of PHI and complies with the HIPAA standard for secure file transfer of patients' medical records.

The transfer of duplicate digital radiographic images through email presents another challenge; specifically, the privacy of legal records. A patient who requests a copy of digital radiographic images via email must be made aware of and accept possible risks to privacy. A dentist must weigh the risks of releasing PHI when it can be difficult to ensure confidentiality or to confirm the identity of the person receiving the email. Email could be misdirected in error, or forwarded to an unknown third party without proper controls. Due to the large file size of digital radiographic images, file compression is necessary to reduce image size for storing and sharing images electronically. However, converting images to the Joint Photographers' Expert Group (JPEG) for compression permanently changes the image by altering individual pixel values. Pixel size reduction through compressed

digital images can reduce optimal interpretation and compromise diagnoses. Compressing digital radiographic images is not recommended for storing original raw images because of this reduction in image quality. While it may sometimes be convenient to send a patient a copy of a digital radiographic image via a compressed email attachment, it should be noted that image quality will be significantly reduced and security could be compromised (Figure 10–4 ■). Encryption of compressed digital radiographic images is only possible with special software designed for JPEG files.

Digital images stored on computers, laptops, hard drives, or portable wireless devices are vulnerable to breaches of

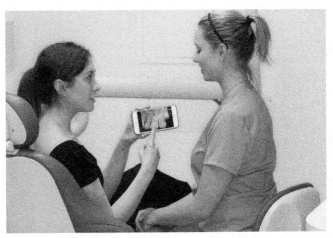

FIGURE 10–4 **Patient sharing digital images that were emailed to a mobile device.**

confidentiality so it is important to take steps that improve security. Devices should be password protected and encryption features should be enabled. Files containing PHI should be closed and access locked when leaving a treatment room or the area where the computer is located. Wireless devices should not be left alone with patients in treatment rooms. Portable devices such as a tablet computer or external hard drive should not be transported out of the facility unless the device can be securely protected against theft.

Ethics

In addition to the law, the ethics of a profession also guide the behavior of a health care practitioner. **Ethics** is defined as a sense of moral obligation regarding right and wrong behavior.

Digital Radiographic Images

Consider this example of ethical practice as it relates to digital radiographic images. Unlike film-based radiographs, digital radiographic images can be altered with software programs. The ability to manipulate a digital image aids in improving the diagnostic quality of an image. This same ability has the potential for misuse. A possible fraudulent manipulation to digital radiographic images is the use of software to create dental caries and dental restorations on images sent to insurance companies for payment of treatment rendered. To protect against fraud and unethical alteration of digital radiographic images, standard authentication procedures such as watermarking and the addition of icons that indicate image alteration are recommended to preserve and protect original digital radiographic images.

Ethical Responsibilities of a Radiographer

Professional ethics define a standard by which all members of a profession are obligated to conform. These professional rules of conduct are called a profession's **Code of Ethics**. Box 10–1 lists Web addresses for obtaining a profession's Code of Ethics. Managing risk, knowing the law, and applying ethics, a dental radiographer should strive for practice that is safe and professional, and places a patient's well-being first. This is achieved by setting goals. Such goals are closely related and all are equally important. Goals for a dental radiographer include the following:

- **Achieve excellence with each radiographic image.** Accomplished by careful attention to details. Each step in the radiographic process, whether image receptor placement, exposure technique, or processing and identification, is significant.
- **Perform confidently and with authority.** Patients are more likely to cooperate with someone who demonstrates self-confidence. Communicate with patients in a respectful manner.
- **Take pride in services rendered and professional advancement.** Obtain certification in radiation safety, whether or not required by law. Improve skills and update techniques by attending continuing education lectures and workshops, participating in professional association meetings, and reading professional journals and books.
- **Keep radiation exposure as low as reasonably achievable (ALARA).** Use protective devices that minimize radiation to a patient and follow strict protocols for self-protection during exposures. Maintain an environment that minimizes the risk of harm.
- **Avoid retakes.** Be familiar with and take precautionary steps to avoid common errors. Do not retake any exposure if not sure of the corrective action. If a patient cannot tolerate placement of an image receptor or cannot cooperate with the procedure, stop and get assistance, or try an acceptable alternative procedure.
- **Develop integrity, dedication, and competence** that promotes ethical behavior and high standards of care. Provide patients with information to assist them in making informed decisions regarding radiographic procedures. Serve all patients without discrimination.

REVIEW—Chapter summary

Be aware of laws and regulations pertaining to dental radiography. Both federal and state regulations control the manufacture and use of x-ray equipment.

State laws require that operators of x-ray equipment be trained and certified or licensed to take dental radiographs. Some states may require a registered dental hygienist and a certified dental assistant to take an additional examination or a continuing education course to be certified to take radiographs. Other states allow an "on-the-job" trained dental assistant with proper training to place and expose radiographs under the direct supervision of the dentist.

Risk management strategies and good patient relations reduce the risk of possible legal actions. Informed consent assists a patient in making decisions regarding dental imaging procedures. Disclosure informs a patient about the radiographic procedure and answers all questions the patient may have concerning the procedures. Both dentist and dental radiographer are liable for procedures performed by a dental radiographer.

Dental records, including radiographic images, are part of a patient's confidential medical record and considered to be protected health-related information (PHI). Patients may have access to duplicate copies of their radiographic images. Risk management and varying statutes of limitation suggest that radiographs be retained indefinitely.

Digital system manufacturers must adhere to DICOM and HIPAA standards for transfer of images between different systems. The security of CDs and other external portable devices and the ability of the reciever to access the data must be addressed when using these devices to share PHI. Cloud file sharing systems have large storage capacity and eliminate the need to securely ship digital images on external portable devices. Cloud file sharing systems that are HIPAA compliant encrypt digital radiographic images to protect against unauthorized access. The risks to confidentiality of releasing PHI via email must be weighed and understood. Compressing and saving original radiographic images using Joint Photographers' Expert Group (JPEG) files is not recommended because it can permanently change an image by altering individual pixel values. Computers, laptops, hard drives, or portable wireless devices are vulnerable to breaches of confidentiality so take steps to protect PHI stored on these devices. To protect against fraud and unethical alteration of digital radiographic images, standard authentication procedures such as watermarking and the addition of icons that indicate image alteration are recommended to preserve and protect original digital radiographic images.

A professional code of ethics guides the behavior of a radiographer. Suggested goals for a dental radiographer are to achieve excellence with each radiographic image, to perform radiographic examinations confidently and with authority, to take pride in services rendered and professional advancement, to keep radiation exposure ALARA, to avoid retakes, and to develop integrity, dedication, and competence that promotes ethical behavior and high standards of care.

RECALL—Study questions

1. Registration and inspection of dental x-ray machines is regulated by
   a. the federal government.
   b. the state government.
   c. the local government.
   d. any of the above.

2. Laws allowing individuals to place and expose dental radiographs vary from state to state.
   a. True
   b. False

3. Which of the following is a risk management strategy?
   a. The use of fast-speed film, film-holding devices, and collimation
   b. Monitoring a dental radiographer with radiation dosimeters
   c. Obtaining a copy of a new patient's radiographic images from a previous dentist
   d. All of the above

4. Which of these comments should be avoided when talking to a patient?
   a. "We have switched to digital radiographic imaging."
   b. "This exposure button sticks sometimes."
   c. "You must stay still during the exposure."
   d. "I'm certified to take your radiographs."

5. A patient has a legal right to refuse radiographs. This is called
   a. disclosure.
   b. informed consent.
   c. self-determination.
   d. liability.

6. If a patient expresses opposition to a radiographic examination, the best next step would be to
   a. ask the patient to sign a document to release the dentist of liability.
   b. consult a professional code of ethics about what to do next.
   c. postpone the procedure and ask the patient to return at a later date.
   d. explain why the radiographs are needed and what the benefits will be.

7. Each of the following is an aspect of informed consent prior to a dental radiographic examination EXCEPT one. Which one is the EXCEPTION?
   a. Amount of radiation exposure anticipated.
   b. Benefits expected from the examination
   c. Reason for the examination
   d. Possible risks of refusing the examination
   e. Identification of person who will expose the radiographs

8. Both dentist and dental radiographer are liable for procedures performed by the dental radiographer.
   a. True
   b. False

9. Each of the following regarding a dental radiographic examination should be documented in a patient's dental record EXCEPT one. Which one is the EXCEPTION?
   a. Number and type of radiographs exposed
   b. Film speed and size of image receptor
   c. Reason for taking radiographs
   d. Interpretive and diagnostic results.
   e. Number of retakes if any

10. A dentist must receive a signed release from a patient before sharing that patient's radiographs with another heath care professional *because* the patient owns his or her radiographs.
    a. Both statement and reason are correct and related.
    b. Both statement and reason are correct but NOT related.
    c. The statement is correct, but the reason is NOT.
    d. The statement is NOT correct, but the reason is correct.
    e. NEITHER the statement NOR the reason is correct.

11. How long should dental radiographs be retained by an oral health care practice?
    a. Until a time when the individual ceases to be a patient at the practice
    b. Until the pediatric patient reaches the age of majority.
    c. After determining a time line for state-mandated statute of limitations
    d. Indefinitely

12. Each of the following is an advantage of a cloud sharing system over a CD for storing and sharing dental radiographic images EXCEPT one. Which one is the EXCEPTION?
    a. Increased storage capacity
    b. Eliminates the need to secure a physical device
    c. Provides higher image spatial resolution
    d. Receiver can access compatable image viewing software

13. Which of the following qualifies a cloud file sharing system as HIPAA compliant?
    a. Meets or exceeds storage capacity requirements.
    b. Data is encrypted and requires a password to access.
    c. Provides services to share duplicate and original radiographic images.
    d. Utilizes Joint Photographers' Expert Group (JPEG) for compressing files.

14. Which of the following is a preferred method for sharing digital radiographic images?
    a. The cloud
    b. CD
    c. Email
    d. Thumb drive

15. Digital radiographic images that can be accessed only with a password are said to be
    a. encrypted.
    b. duplicated.
    c. compressed.
    d. digitized.

16. A professional code of ethics
    a. makes laws that govern the use of dental radiographs.
    b. establishes time frames for exposing dental radiographs.
    c. helps to define rules of conduct for its members.
    d. protects a dental radiographer in cases of legal action.

REFLECT—Case study

Consider the following scenario:

Following an initial oral examination on a new patient, a dentist prescribes a full mouth series of radiographs prior to beginning treatment. As the dental assistant is preparing for the exposures, the patient asks if someone can contact her previous dentist and have radiographs that were taken there sent to this practice. After placing a phone call, it is discovered that the previous dentist's office is closed for the day. The dental assistant informs the patient of this and states that the dentist needs radiographs in order to start treatment today. The patient agrees to have the new radiographs exposed today and the dental assistant proceeds with the examination. Reflect on this scenario and answer the following questions:

1. Has the dental assistant broken the law?

2. Did exposure of the new full mouth series endanger the patient?

3. Are there legal and/or ethical concerns the dental assistant and/or dentist face?

4. What alternative course of action might the dental assistant have taken?

5. Can you describe radiographic image sharing options that could have been investigated?

6. What information must be collected from the patient prior to requesting a copy of previous radiographic images?

7. What documentation should be noted in this patient's dental record regarding procedures performed today?

8. What, if any, follow-up should be made with the previous dental practice regarding this patient?

RELATE—Laboratory practice

Using the computer, visit the Web sites for the board of radiological health or the board of dentistry in all 50 states and the District of Columbia. Compile a listing of states with certification requirements for dental radiographers and answer the following questions.

1. How many states require individuals to be certified to perform radiographic procedures?

2. What states accept a registered dental hygienist's or certified dental assistant's credentials as certification for performing radiographic procedures?

3. Do any states require additional tests or continuing education classes for a dental assistant or dental hygienist to maintain radiographic certification?

4. Why do you think some states do not require certification for those individuals who place and expose dental radiographs?

5. Are there advantages for an oral health care practice to hire only certified radiographers?

RESOURCES

American Dental Association. (2007). *Dental records.* Council on Dental Practice Division of Legal Affairs. Chicago: Author.

American Dental Association Standards Committee for Dental Informatics. (2013). *Implementation requirements for DICOM in dentistry.* Technical report no. 1023–2005. Chicago: Author.

Darby, M. L., & Walsh, M. M. (2014). *Dental hygiene theory and practice* (4th ed.). St. Louis, MO: Elsevier.

Mendelson, D. S., Erickson B. J., & Choy, G. C. (2014). Image sharing: Evolving solutions in the age of interoperability. *Journal of the American College of Radiology, 11,* 1260–1269.

National Institute of Standards and Technology. (2016). *Computer security resource center.* Retrieved from NIST website: http://www.nist.gov/

U.S. Dept. of Health and Human Services. (2001). *Fact sheet: Protecting the privacy of patients' health information.* Retrieved from U.S. DHHS website: https://aspe.hhs.gov/basic-report/protecting-privacy-patients-health-information

Wenzel, A., & Moystad, A. (2010). Work flow with digital intra-oral radiography: A systematic review. *Acta Odontologica Scandinavica, 68,* 106–114.

Visit www.pearsonhighered.com/healthprofessionsresources to access the student resources that accompany this book. Simply select Dental Hygiene from the choice of disciplines. Find this book and you will find the complementary study tools created for this specific title.

11

Patient Relations and Education

CHAPTER OUTLINE

OBJECTIVES

Following successful completion of this chapter, you should be able to:

1. Define key terms.
2. Value the need for patient cooperation in producing quality radiographs.
3. List aspects of patient relations that help to gain confidence and cooperation.
4. Explain how professional appearance and first impression affect patient relations.
5. Explain how to project an attitude of professionalism.
6. State examples of facilitation skills.
7. Explain the relationship between verbal and nonverbal communication.
8. Demonstrate the patient management strategy Show-Tell-Do.
9. Explain the goals of active listening.
10. Explain the goals of patient education.
11. Describe methods of patient education.
12. Respond to questions frequently asked regarding a radiographic examination.

KEY TERMS

Active listening

Chairside manner

Empathy

Facilitation skills

Interpersonal skills

Nonverbal communication

Patient education

Patient relations

Professional appearance

Professionalism

Show-Tell-Do

Verbal communication

Introduction

Effective communication is essential to producing quality radiographic images. A radiographic examination requires that a patient understand and actively participate in the process. A radiographer must be able to effectively communicate specific directions for a successful outcome. Precise patient positioning, the challenge of placing of an image receptor intraorally, and use of ionizing radiation make clear communication and good patient management skills especially important. This chapter discusses how interpersonal skills influence the radiographic process and presents guidelines for effective communication and patient education.

Interpersonal Skills

Good **patient relations** require an understanding of patient needs and an ability to respond in a manner that builds confidence and trust. When a patient is told that he or she needs a dental radiographic examination, questions can arise regarding the procedure. A radiographer needs to be prepared to answer patient questions and address concerns in an informative and professional manner. Producing diagnostic quality radiographs requires both technical and **interpersonal skills**. Professional appearance, an attitude of professionalism, and an ability to facilitate a trusting relationship contribute to gaining patient confidence and cooperation, the outcome of which will be the production of quality radiographs.

Professional Appearance

A patient's first introduction to the person who will be performing the radiographic examination is important. A first impression is often formulated based on appearance. Maintaining a **professional appearance** will help to gain respect and acknowledgement that a radiographer is qualified to expertly perform a procedure (Figure 11–1 ■). Present a professional appearance by maintaining excellent health, good grooming, and appropriate attire. Pay careful attention to personal hygiene and grooming that may express an understanding of the importance of maintaining all aspects of infection control. A clean, neat appearance can convey competence to patients.

Attitude of Professionalism

Attitude is defined as the position assumed by the body in connection with a feeling or mood. An attitude of **professionalism** conveys skill and distinguishes a person as an expert. Attitude will play a significant role in gaining patient trust. A radiographer's attitude toward his or her own technical ability is conveyed to a patient. Because a demonstration of technical skill will build patient confidence, a radiographer should convey the attitude that his or her training and education provided adequate preparation for this role. Self-confidence fosters confidence in others.

A radiographer's attitude toward the radiographic procedure is conveyed to a patient. If a radiographer feels that a procedure is uncomfortable or unnecessary, a patient may sense these feelings. Be aware of this, and take steps to not project personal feelings onto a patient. Although a radiographer may have had a less than ideal experience with a certain procedure, this does not necessarily mean that a patient will undergo the same discomfort. For example, a radiographer may have experienced a gagging response when undergoing an intraoral radiographic examination. If this radiographer approaches a patient with an attitude of anxiety or dread that intraoral placement of an image receptor will excite a gag reflex, the outcome is likely to be just that. A fresh, positive attitude with each new patient will more likely ensure a cooperative and collaborative experience. This is especially true if a patient perceives that a radiographer has a nonjudgmental attitude.

Additionally, the unique close working relationship of the oral health care team requires that everyone work well together. Attitudes toward an employer and coworkers play a role in determining the degree of successful patient management. Patients can sense a professional's attitude by the way he or she walks, talks, and behaves. For example, a patient may easily sense a disgruntled dental assistant who had to interrupt what he or she was doing to take radiographs for a dental hygienist who was running behind in the schedule. Maintaining a pleasant, positive attitude will help generate the same from patients.

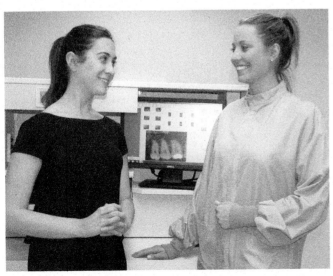

FIGURE 11–1 Professional appearance. Conveys authority and gains patient confidence.

Practice Point

Always greet a patient by name and address patients using a proper title (Miss, Mrs., Ms., Mr., Dr., etc.) and last name. If correct pronunciation of a patient's name is unknown, ask for it to be pronounced. Introduce yourself using both name and title. For example: "Good morning, Ms. Washington. My name is Maria Melendez. I'm the dental assistant who will be taking your radiographs today."

Facilitation Skills

Facilitation skills are used to enhance relationships with others. Respectfulness, courtesy, empathy, and patient, honest, and tactful communication are examples of facilitation skills that ease the way to good working relationships. When explaining a need for a radiographic examination, consider how a patient may feel and anticipate potential questions. If a patient has concerns regarding the need for x-ray exposure, respect those views. Statements such as, "Don't worry" and "Everything will be okay," may convey an attitude of apathy, or imply that the patient's apprehensions don't matter. If a patient complains that placement of an intraoral imaging receptor during the radiographic procedure is uncomfortable, show empathy. **Empathy** is defined as the ability to share in another's emotions or feelings. Be courteous and polite at all times even in difficult situations. If an uncomfortable situation must be tolerated to produce a necessary radiograph examination, empathetic, yet direct and tactful communication can help bring about the desired result.

Another important interpersonal skill is chairside manner. **Chairside manner** refers to the conduct of a radiographer while working clinically with a patient. Strive to develop a chairside manner that contributes to a patient's comfort and fosters a positive atmosphere. Working in a confident manner will help put a patient at ease. Avoid comments that indicate a lack of control, such as saying, "Oops!" Make a concentrated effort to provide praise and positive reinforcement during the procedure. Feedback that the procedure is going well helps to reassure a patient and foster continued cooperation. For example, complimenting a patient on his or her ability to hold an image receptor in place long enough to complete the exposure will help to motivate the patient to continue participating in a helpful manner. Conversely, showing frustration with a patient who is having difficulty managing a procedure will most likely only increase the patient's anxiety.

Practice Point

If it is necessary to position an intraoral image receptor into a particularly sensitive area, encourage a patient to cooperate and praise him or her for the willingness to tolerate a difficult placement. Express empathy, but let the patient know that the placement is correct and if he or she can tolerate the discomfort for the short time required for exposure, the result will be a diagnostic quality radiograph. Avoid asking, "Does that feel okay?" A patient will perceive this to mean that discomfort equals incorrect positioning and will feel obligated to inform you of any and all feelings associated with the procedure. The patient may now be acutely aware of the feeling of the image receptor in the mouth and continue to report on the "feeling" of each subsequent placement, possibly making the procedure more difficult. Saying, "Are you doing okay so far?" is a better way to let a patient know you are aware of his or her efforts to cooperate.

Box 11–1: Guidelines for Effective Communication

- Introduce self and show interest.
- Face the patient and make eye contact.
- Lean forward to demonstrate listening.
- Be honest to build trust.
- Show courtesy and respectfulness.
- Maintain positive attitude.
- Demonstrate empathy when appropriate.
- Use clear commands.
- Make nonverbal communication in agreement with verbal communication.

Communication

Communication is defined as the process by which information is exchanged between two or more persons. This may be accomplished verbally (with words) or nonverbally (without words). Effective communication is communication that works (Box 11–1). Verbal and nonverbal communication are essential to building patient confidence. Answer patient questions honestly, and clearly explain the need for cooperation; anticipate possible discomfort to gain assistance needed to produce a diagnostic quality examination. Honesty develops trust. When a patient trusts a dental radiographer, cooperation is more likely to result.

Verbal Communication

Effective use of words in **verbal communication** begins with facing a patient directly and maintaining eye contact. Because a face mask is recommended personal protective equipment (PPE) during radiographic procedures, it is important that verbal requests and commands used to communicate specific directions during radiographic procedures be understood by a patient. Once an intraoral image receptor is in place, give explicit directions to complete the procedure quickly. For example, once a receptor holding device is placed in the mouth, request that the patient bite firmly and hold completely still during exposure. The process will be hindered and prolonged if a patient does not understand the directions or the operator must repeat the commands.

Practice Point

Always give a command, do not use a question, to request that a patient hold still during exposure. For example, asking a patient, "Can you hold still, please?" will most likely cause the patient to attempt to move to answer you, defeating the purpose of your request. The command, "Hold still, please" is less likely to prompt a patient to move.

Box 11–2: Guidelines for Communicating with Children

- Use guidelines for effective communication.
- Use age-level appropriate language.
- Do not talk down or use baby talk.
- Avoid using words that sound threatening.
- Explain procedures simply and clearly.
- Use Show-Tell-Do.

Box 11–3: Guidelines for Communicating with Older Adults

- Use guidelines for effective communication.
- Address by person's title unless instructed otherwise.
- Avoid condescending salutations such as "Honey" and "Dear."
- Be aware of generational differences.
- Be aware of sensory or cognitive impairments such as hearing loss, effects of stroke.
- Encourage use of eyeglasses and hearing aids during procedures and when showing radiographs during patient education.

Choice of words and sentence structure are important in developing clear communication. Words used should be at a level a patient can understand. For example, young children may better understand that dental radiographs are "pictures of teeth made with an x-ray camera" (Box 11–2). An adult would appreciate having a more professional dialogue; however, too many highly technical words may lead to confusion and result in misunderstandings. Avoid words that imply negative images such as "zap," "shot," and "irradiate."

Nonverbal Communication

Nonverbal communication includes gestures, facial expressions, body movement, and listening. For example, a nod of the head indicates yes or agreement, and a shake of the head indicates no or disagreement. People usually interact using a combination of verbal and nonverbal communication. Nonverbal communication is very believable. When verbal and nonverbal communications are not in sync, it is often the nonverbal communication that conveys the strongest message—for example, telling a patient that it is okay to stop and take a break in between each radiograph placement, while performing an eye roll or tapping a foot while waiting. This patient will probably believe the actions over any words spoken. Facial expressions strongly convey attitude; a smile can contribute to relaxing a patient and reducing apprehension.

A patient management strategy called **Show-Tell-Do** is a combined verbal and nonverbal communication tool. Show-Tell-Do is especially useful when barriers to communication exist such as in the case of a language or cultural difference, a sensory disability, or a cognitive impairment

(Boxes 11–3 and 11–4). The nonverbal component of Show-Tell-Do consists of showing a patient the equipment that will be used to perform the radiographic examination; and demonstrating or practicing placement and positioning of the equipment, to familiarize a patient with what to expect. Prior to performing the procedure, verbal communication allows for an exchange of questions and answers to clarify the collaboration that will be needed between patient and radiographer for a successful outcome.

Active Listening

A skilled communicator possesses good listening skills. Careful attention to listening results in fewer misunderstandings. Be attentive and avoid formulating a response while a patient is talking. Concentrate on what is being said and do not impatiently rush to a reply. It is important to avoid selective hearing or stereotyping. Consider a patient who refuses to undergo a prescribed radiographic examination. It is important to ask and then actively listen to the patient's reason for feeling this way. Be mindful of maintaining eye contact and an attentive body posture that communicates warmth and caring.

Box 11–4: Guidelines for Communicating with People of Different Cultures

- Use guidelines for effective communication.
- Learn about cultures in the community.
- Be accepting and nonjudgmental.
- Be aware that gestures may be interpreted differently.
- Be aware that touch and personal space are sometimes considered differently by different cultures.
- If there is a language difference, speak slowly and avoid use of slang or uncommon terms.
- Verify that listener has understood what was said.

Practice Point

Sentence structure is important for the short, precise directions needed for radiographic procedures. For example, requesting that a patient bite down on an intraoral image receptor holder by saying, "Close slowly, please" may prompt the patient to close before the operator says the word *slowly*. Rearranging the words to say, "Slowly close, please," may be more likely to produce the desired result.

Active listening includes observing nonverbal communication. A patient may be embarrassed or reluctant to admit feelings of anxiety. Watch for physical signs of tension, such as nervous fidgeting and shallow breathing. Appropriately respond to nonverbal communication to avoid a medical emergency such as syncope (fainting). If a patient perceives a radiographic examination as stressful, then he or she may demonstrate irritability or impatience that is directed at a radiographer. Understanding that fear is the precipitator of these emotions will assist with responding with a management strategy that communicates empathy and reduces stress.

Patient Education

Good communication skills are necessary to educate patients on the importance of dental radiographs in comprehensive oral health planning and treatment. Many people have heard negative reports regarding effects of overexposure to radiation. A dental patient, when presented with a treatment plan that recommends radiographs, may rightfully question the necessity of being exposed to ionizing radiation. It is the responsibility of the entire oral health care team to provide clear, concise, and satisfactory answers regarding patient questions and concerns. Acceptance of a comprehensive oral health care treatment plan is more likely when a satisfactory explanation of radiographic need, and a description of ethical safeguards that reduce a risk of harm, are presented.

Identifying with a patient's concerns is the first step to open communication and meaningful **patient education**. Verbally agree with a patient that excess radiation exposure is a concern and explain that the oral health care practice has adopted a strict radiation safety program. Acceptance and confidence increase when a patient is made aware of the many safety protocols that are in place. Begin a conversation with a discussion of how a dentist uses evidence-based selection criteria guidelines to decide when, what type, and how many radiographs need to be exposed (see Chapter 6). These evidence-based guidelines are the single biggest factor in eliminating unnecessary radiographs.

Inform a patient that standard safety protocols as suggested by federal agencies are being followed, as well as state and local laws governing inspections, calibrations, and use of radiological equipment. Many people may not realize that x-ray equipment is strictly regulated by law. In some locations, laws regulate who can operate a dental x-ray machine. Where applicable, individuals must be educated and trained, and pass an examination prior to being certified to place and expose dental radiographs. A license or certificate achieved in radiation safety should be displayed for patients to see. Patient confidence increases when it is explained that the person who will be exposing his or her radiographs has passed a certification examination in safety protocols governing the use of x-radiation. Continuing education courses in radiology taken by a radiographer also boost patient confidence and elevate the practice as one that values competency.

Present a patient with an outline of the equipment the practice has chosen to use that is specially designed to reduce radiation exposure, such as a collimated position indicating device (PID), thyroid collar attached to a protective lead apron, and fast-speed film or digital sensor. A patient may not be aware of the reasoning behind the use of these devices, and the care with which the practice has selected them for use. An educated patient is more inclined to understand a need and accept a prescription for a radiographic examination. Such patient acceptance helps develop a spirit of confidence and mutual trust in an oral health care practice.

Methods of Patient Education

Patient education on the value of radiographs can be delivered through verbal discussion, printed literature, and electronic media. Backing up a verbal explanation with a printed brochure is an effective means of communication. Custom-developed and commercially available electronic mobile applications or video clips are another means of providing patient education. Literature and electronic applications may be obtained from professional organizations, commercial dental product companies, or shared with other professionals via the Web (Figure 11–2 ■). Take care to use reliable sources, and thoroughly review materials with all members of the oral health care team to be sure the message

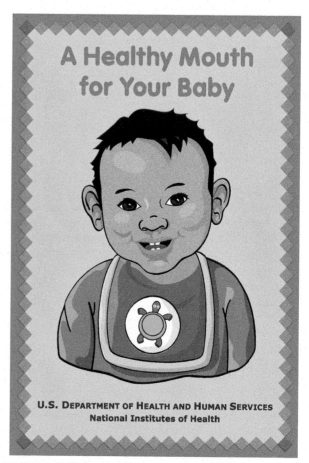

FIGURE 11–2 **Patient education brochure.** (Courtesy of National Institute of Dental and Craniofacial Research, NIH Publication No. 14-7340, July 2014.)

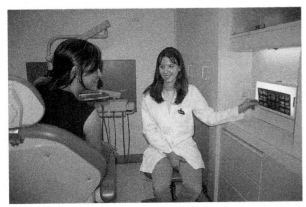

FIGURE 11–3 Patient education with film-based radiographs on a lighted view box.

meets the educational standards of the practice. A periodic review of media sources on the topic of dental radiographs can alert a radiographer to trends. Knowing what information is being disseminated, a radiographer can be prepared to respond to patient questions with factual information.

Sample radiographs placed in convenient mounts and digital radiographic images assembled into patient education electronic files can be effective media tools. Sample sets of radiographs can be used to explain types, sizes, and number of images; demonstrate interpretative ability of radiographs; and provide a basis for discussing a patient's oral health treatment plan. To enhance viewing, place film-based radiographs on a lighted view box (Figure 11–3 ■). Display digital images on a computer monitor, or use a tablet computer for convenient chairside viewing (Figure 11–4 ■; and see Figure 8–6). Use magnification to improve viewing. When using sample radiographs, be sure to eliminate labels that could identify the radiographs with another patient. When viewing a patient's own radiographs, remember that all members of the oral health care team can interpret radiographs, but it is the dentist's responsibility to make the final interpretation and diagnosis.

Frequently Asked Questions

Anticipate and be prepared to respond to frequently asked questions. Take the initiative to involve the entire oral health care team in developing a united and consistent

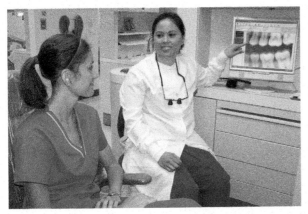

FIGURE 11–4 Patient education with digital radiographic images.

message to use in replying to the more common questions a patient may have regarding a radiographic examination. Establishing a team approach to patient education helps to reinforce patient confidence and aids in establishing trust. Consider the following questions frequently asked by patients and the suggested sample answers a radiographer may use to respond.

QUESTION: Why do I need dental x-rays?

ANSWER: Many diseases of the teeth and surrounding tissues cannot be seen through a visual examination alone. Finding and treating oral health problems at an early stage can save time, money, and unnecessary discomfort. An x-ray examination may reveal:

- Decay between teeth or under an existing filling, and at an early stage when it can be remineralized
- Damaged or loss of bone from periodontal disease or other abnormal condition
- Infection, such as an abscess or cyst, at an early stage before there are symptoms
- Developmental abnormalities such as tooth resorption or a tumor

QUESTION: How often should dental x-rays be taken?

ANSWER: Radiographs (dental x-rays) are prescribed by a dentist only when the examination is required to make a diagnosis and provide comprehensive treatment of an oral condition. Scheduling an x-ray examination is individualized for each patient. The dentist will review your medical and dental histories, examine your mouth, and then decide whether you need radiographs, how many, and what type. At recall appointments updated radiographs may be needed to detect new cavities, to determine the status of periodontal disease, or for evaluation of growth and development, and will vary according to your age, risk for disease, and signs and symptoms.

In general, adults who have had extensive dental work (fillings, crowns, bridges) may need more frequent radiographs to check for decay around or under the restorations. People who have a reduced salivary flow, a condition called xerostomia (dry mouth), are more prone to decay, prompting a need for more frequent radiographs. Smokers and people with periodontal disease may need more frequent radiographs to monitor bone loss; smokers are at an increased risk for periodontal disease. Children may need x-rays more often than adults, because the teeth are more likely to be affected by decay than those of adults, and jaws are still developing.

QUESTION: Why do I need so many different kinds of radiographs?

ANSWER: Intraoral radiographs, films, or digital sensors placed in the mouth record only a few teeth at a time. Teeth are positioned in the dental arches in an arc, or curve. This makes it necessary to expose multiple images at various angles to properly view all tooth surfaces. Additionally, some radiographs (bitewings) image tooth crowns when the goal is to detect decay; others (periapicals) record the entire tooth down to the root tip. Depending on the diagnostic goals, bitewings or periapicals or a combination of both will be exposed.

A panoramic radiograph, an extraoral procedure, provides a comprehensive view of all of the teeth plus the surrounding supporting structures. A panoramic and a combination of intraoral radiographs may be needed because although a panoramic radiograph records more tissues, periapical and bitewing radiographs provide more details needed to detect decay and periodontal bone changes. Radiographs are not prescribed indiscriminately. An accurate diagnosis depends on the different information that each radiograph can provide.

QUESTION: Can I refuse dental x-rays and still be treated?

ANSWER: No. Treatment cannot be rendered based on an incomplete diagnosis. Without necessary radiographs, a dentist could be held legally liable for failing to correctly diagnose a condition or for failing to provide adequate treatment.

QUESTION: Can you use radiographs taken by my previous dentist?

ANSWER: Yes, you can request a copy of your previous radiographs. Previous radiographs provide a history of disease activity. Unless they are less than six months old, previous radiographs are not likely to represent your current oral conditions, so you may require a new radiographic examination.

QUESTION: Are x-rays safe?

ANSWER: Exposure to all types of ionizing radiation, including naturally occurring background radiation, like sunlight and minerals in the soil, can damage body tissues and cells, possibly leading to the development of cancer. Therefore, dental radiographs are only prescribed after careful consideration, weighing risks and benefits. Modern dental x-ray equipment produces a small amount of radiation that is directed to a small restricted area of the body. Therefore, the risk of harmful effects from a dental x-ray examination is minimal. In fact, there are no recorded cases of a dental radiographic examination causing cancer in a patient.

QUESTION: What precautions will you take to minimize the amount of radiation I receive?

ANSWER: Most importantly, only necessary radiographs are taken. The x-ray beam is restricted to expose only a small region, less than 3 inches, only large enough to expose an image receptor. The image receptor requires a very small amount of radiation exposure to produce a diagnostic quality image. We continue to update to new equipment and products that allow for continued radiation exposure reductions as they become available. A lead/lead equivalent apron and thyroid shield will be placed on you during the exposure to absorb potential scatter radiation and protect other parts of your body from unnecessary radiation. Our practice has signed the Image Gently® pledge, stating that we are committed to implementing protocols and recommendations that help to reduce radiation exposure (see Chapter 27).

QUESTION: Why do you leave the room during x-ray exposure?

ANSWER: Remaining in the vicinity exposes a radiographer to unnecessary radiation that provides no benefit.

REVIEW—Chapter summary

Technical skills, effective communication, and good interpersonal relations with patients that build confidence and trust are essential to producing quality radiographs. Professional appearance and attitude facilitate a relationship of trust that assists with gaining patient confidence in, and cooperation with, a radiographic procedure. Professional appearance is conveyed by maintaining excellent health, good grooming, and appropriate attire. An attitude of professionalism conveys skill and distinguishes a person as an expert.

Attitudes can be conveyed to a patient. Maintain a positive, nonjudgmental attitude with each new patient. Be mindful to not project a negative attitude. A positive attitude can facilitate cooperation. Respectfulness, courtesy, empathy, and patient, honest, and tactful communication are examples of facilitation skills that ease the way to good working relationships. Be cognizant of the roles interpersonal skills and chairside manner play in producing quality radiographs.

Effective communication is communication that works. Verbal and nonverbal communication are essential to building patient confidence. Nonverbal communication is often stronger than verbal communication. Be sure actions match words spoken. Consider word choice and sentence structure to develop clear communication. Avoid overuse of highly technical words that may lead to confusion and result in misunderstandings. Show-Tell-Do, combining verbal and nonverbal communication, is effective when barriers exist such as a language or cultural difference, a sensory disability, or a cognitive impairment.

Active listening results in fewer misunderstandings. Be attentive when a patient is speaking; avoid formulating a response while a patient is still talking, and do not impatiently rush to a reply. Avoid selective hearing or stereotyping. Observe nonverbal signs of communication such as physical tension and shallow breathing to avoid a medical emergency. Manage patient fear that can precipitate irritability and lack of cooperation with a management strategy that communicates empathy to reduce stress.

Patient education plays a valuable role in securing acceptance of a comprehensive oral health care treatment plan. Acceptance of treatment is more likely when a satisfactory explanation of radiographic need and a description of radiation safeguards are presented. Explain that dental x-ray equipment must comply with safety regulations; individuals who place and expose dental radiographs must pass a radiation safety certification examination; and technique and equipment used is designed to reduce radiation exposure.

Deliver patient education through verbal discussion, printed literature, and electronic media. Methods of patient education include oral presentations and distribution of printed materials. Anticipate and be prepared to respond to frequently asked questions. Establish a team approach to patient education to reinforce patient confidence.

RECALL—Study questions

1. The key to producing quality radiographic images is
   a. gaining patient trust and cooperation.
   b. presenting a confident, caring image.
   c. communicating effectively.
   d. all of the above.

2. Which of the following does NOT contribute to a professional appearance?
   a. Establishing eye contact
   b. Good grooming
   c. Maintaining health
   d. Appropriate attire

3. A position assumed by the body in connection with a feeling or mood is called
   a. empathy.
   b. attitude.
   c. professionalism.
   d. chairside manner.

4. The conduct of a radiographer while working clinically with a patient is called chairside manner.
   A chairside manner can either put a patient at ease or increase a patient's anxiety.
   a. The first statement is true. The second statement is false.
   b. The first statement is false. The second statement is true.
   c. Both statements are true.
   d. Both statements are false.

5. What is the best choice of action if a patient complains that placement of an intraoral imaging receptor during the radiographic procedure is uncomfortable?
   a. Express empathy and complete the procedure as quickly as possible.
   b. Allow the patient to move the receptor into the most comfortable position.
   c. Tell the patient not to worry and explain that you are skilled at achieving a diagnostic quality image.
   d. Ask if the patient would like to have another team member expose the radiographs.

6. Each of the following will enhance verbal communication EXCEPT one. Which one is the EXCEPTION?
   a. Face the patient.
   b. Make eye contact.
   c. Use clear commands.
   d. Use slang words.

7. Which of the following words should be avoided when discussing the radiographic procedure?
   a. Picture
   b. Zap
   c. X-ray
   d. Radiograph

8. Nonverbal communication is very believable *because* when verbal and nonverbal communications are not in synch, nonverbal communication conveys the strongest message.
   a. Both the statement and reason are correct and related.
   b. Both the statement and reason are correct but NOT related.
   c. The statement is correct, but the reason is NOT.
   d. The statement is NOT correct, but the reason is correct.
   e. NEITHER the statement NOR the reason is correct.

9. Which of these does NOT contribute to active listening?
   a. Formulate a response while the patient is talking.
   b. Be attentive and maintain eye contact.
   c. Assume an attentive body posture.
   d. Avoid selective hearing

10. Use Show-Tell-Do to aid communicating with
    a. someone who speaks a different language.
    b. children.
    c. hearing-impaired patients.
    d. all of the above.

11. What is the value of patient education regarding dental radiographs?
    a. Reduces time required to expose radiographs
    b. Demonstrates a radiographer's positive attitude
    c. Enables patient to more likely accept treatment plan
    d. Increases patient requests for radiographs at each appointment

12. Patient education in radiography is necessary to
    a. increase the demand for oral health services.
    b. increase acceptance of oral health care recommendations.
    c. assure the patient that the radiographer is licensed.
    d. meet legally required mandates for it.

13. List four responses to a patient who asks, "Why do I need dental x-rays?"
    a. _____
    b. _____
    c. _____
    d. _____

REFLECT—Case study

A dentist has prescribed vertical bitewing and panoramic radiographs for a new patient who has the following questions and concerns regarding the examination. Together with a partner, role-play this scenario.

"Why do I need x-rays?"
"Why do I have to have bitewings and a panoramic x-ray?"

"How often should I have x-rays taken?
"Are you going to take the x-rays, or will the dentist take them?"
"I'm a little nervous about having this done."
"How long will it take?"
"What will you do to protect me from exposure?"

RELATE—Laboratory application

Produce a brochure for the purpose of educating patients regarding a dental radiographic examination. Provide the brochure with a title, for example, "Dental X-Rays for Your Health," or something similar. The narration should be simple and in language that is professional, yet not overly technical. Direct the brochure to a target population (e.g., children or a particular culture such as Spanish speakers). Illustrate the brochure with images or drawings.

REFERENCES

Bird, D. L., & Robinson, D. S. (2015). The professional dental assistant; communication in the dental office. *Modern dental assisting* (11th ed.). St. Louis, MO: Elsevier.

Colgate Oral Care Center. (2016). *X-ray.* Retrieved from Colgate-Palmolive Company website: http://www.colgate.com /en/us/oc/oral-health/procedures/x-rays

Visit www.pearsonhighered.com/healthprofessionsresources to access the student resources that accompany this book. Simply select Dental Hygiene from the choice of disciplines. Find this book and you will find the complementary study tools created for this specific title.

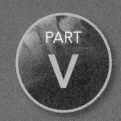

Dental Radiographic Techniques

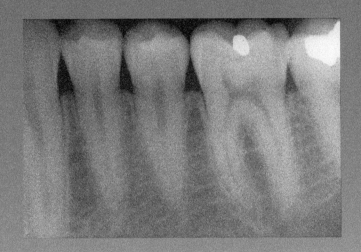

OUTLINE

Introduction to Radiographic Examinations

OBJECTIVES

Following successful completion of this chapter, you should be able to:

1. Define the key terms.
2. State the difference between intraoral and extraoral radiography.
3. Compare the three intraoral radiographic examinations.
4. Identify the two intraoral techniques.
5. List the five rules for shadow casting.
6. Determine conditions that affect the selection of image receptor size.
7. Select the type and number of image receptors required for a full mouth survey.
8. Explain horizontal and vertical angulation.
9. Explain point of entry.
10. List five contraindications for using the patient's finger to hold the image receptor during exposure.
11. Explain the basic design of image receptor positioners/holders.
12. Describe proper patient seating position.
13. Demonstrate a systematic and orderly sequence of the exposure procedure.

KEY TERMS

Angulation
Bisecting technique
Biteblock
Bitewing radiograph
Conecut error
Extraoral
Full mouth series (survey)

Horizontal angulation
Image receptor positioner or holder
Intraoral
Mean tangent
Midsaggital plane
Negative angulation
Occlusal plane
Occlusal radiograph

Paralleling technique
Periapical radiograph
Point of entry
Positive angulation
Rule of isometry
Shadow casting
Vertical angulation
Vertical bitewing radiograph

Introduction

Intraoral radiography (methods of exposing dental x-ray film, phosphor plates, or digital sensors within the oral cavity) is the focus of this chapter. **Extraoral** radiography (use of image receptors positioned outside the mouth) is discussed in Chapter 17. Producing diagnostic quality intraoral dental radiographs depends on knowledge of and attention to

- Positioning the patient
- Selecting a film, phosphor plate, or digital sensor of suitable size
- Determining how the image receptor is to be positioned and held in place
- Setting the radiation exposure variables
- Aiming the position indicating device (PID)

These considerations have specific applications for each of the three types of intraoral examinations and when utilizing the paralleling or the bisecting technique. This chapter will introduce the three types of intraoral examinations, explain the principles of producing intraoral images (shadow casting), and describe image receptor positioners or holding devices to set the stage for Chapters 13 through 16, where an in-depth explanation of the paralleling, bisecting, bitewing, and occlusal techniques will follow.

Intraoral Procedures

Each of the three types of intraoral radiographic examinations has a specific imaging objective.

1. **Bitewing examination.** Records the coronal portions of the teeth and the alveolar crests of bone of both the maxilla and mandible on a single radiograph (Figure 12–1 ■). **Bitewing radiographs** are especially useful in detecting caries (dental decay) of the proximal surfaces where adjacent teeth contact each other in the arch; and for examining crestal bone of patients with periodontal disease. The technique used to acquire bitewing radiographs is unique to the bitewing exam. However, because of the almost parallel

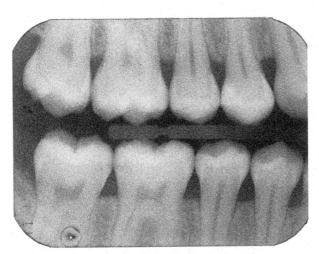

FIGURE 12–1 **Bitewing radiograph.**

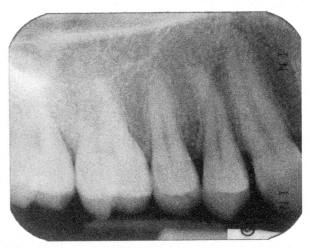

FIGURE 12–2 **Periapical radiograph.**

relationship of the image receptor to the teeth, the bitewing technique could be considered to be a modification of the paralleling technique used for exposing periapical radiographs.

2. **Periapical examination.** Uses **periapical radiographs** to image the apices of the teeth and surrounding bone (Figure 12–2 ■). The word *periapical* is derived from the Greek word *peri* (meaning around) and the Latin word *apex* (meaning tip or point). As the word suggests, the periapical radiograph images the entire tooth, including the root tip and surrounding bone. A periapical radiograph may be used to examine a single tooth or condition, or may be used in combination with other periapical and bitewing radiographs to image the entire dentition and supporting structures as in the case of a full mouth series (Figure 12–3 ■). Conditions prompting the exposure of a periapical radiograph include apical pathology (abscess), fractures, large carious lesions, extensive periodontal involvement, examination of developmental anomalies such as missing teeth and abnormal eruption patterns, and any unexplained pain or bleeding (Figures 12–4 ■ and 12–5 ■). Periapical radiographs may be taken utilizing either the paralleling or the bisecting technique.

3. **Occlusal examination.** Images the entire maxillary or mandibular arch, or a portion thereof, on a single radiograph (see Figure 16–1). **Occlusal radiographs** are most often taken with a larger size 4 intraoral film, making this examination useful in imaging large areas of pathology that may not be adequately recorded on a smaller periapical radiograph. Conditions that may prompt the exposure of occlusal radiographs include cysts, fractures, impacted or supernumerary (extra) teeth, and in locating the buccal or lingual position of foreign objects (see Chapter 30). The technique used to acquire occlusal radiographs is unique to the occlusal exam. However, because of the image receptor placement required, the occlusal technique could be considered a modification of the bisecting technique.

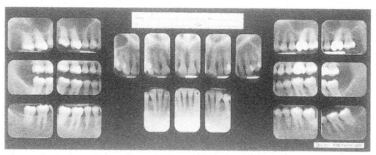

FIGURE 12–3 **Full mouth series.** This 20-film radiographic survey includes 4 bitewing radiographs and 8 anterior and 8 posterior periapical radiographs.

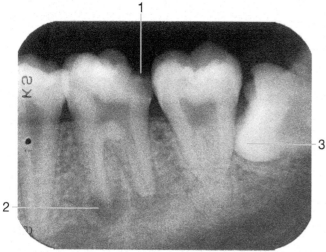

FIGURE 12–4 **Periapical radiograph.** Posterior periapical radiograph showing (**1**) extensive caries, (**2**) apical pathology, and (**3**) impacted third molar. Note the use of a size 2 film and the horizontal positioning of the long dimension of the film packet.

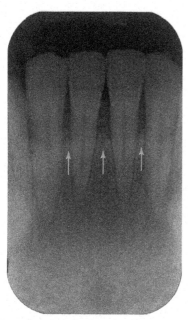

FIGURE 12–5 **Periapical radiograph.** Anterior periapical radiograph showing extensive periodontal involvement. Note the use of a size 1 film and the vertical positioning of the long dimension of the film packet.

Techniques

Two basic techniques are used in intraoral radiography: paralleling and bisecting. Either technique can be modified to meet special conditions and requirements. Although each technique will produce diagnostic quality radiographic images if the fundamental principles of the technique are followed, paralleling is the technique of choice because it is more likely to satisfy more of the shadow casting requirements.

The concept of the **bisecting technique** (formerly called the bisecting-angle or short-cone technique) originated in 1907 through the application of a geometric principle known as the **rule of isometry**. This theorem states that two triangles having equal angles and a common side are equal triangles (see Figure 14–1). The bisecting technique was the only method used for many years. However, because many radiographers experienced difficulties and obtained unsatisfactory results, the search for a less-complicated technique that would produce better radiographs more consistently resulted in the development of the paralleling technique in 1920. The **paralleling technique** (formerly called right-angle or long-cone technique) is considered to be the technique of choice because it produces better quality radiographs. The specific steps of each of these two techniques are discussed in detail in Chapters 13 and 14.

Fundamentals of Shadow Casting

X-rays produce an image on a film, phosphor plate, or digital sensor in a similar manner to light casting a shadow of an object. When an object is placed between a nearby light source, such as an electric bulb, and a flat object, such as a tabletop, a shadow of the object is seen on the tabletop. In dental radiography, x-rays cast a shadow of the teeth on to the image receptor.

The radiograph is essentially a shadow image. To produce an image that represents the teeth and supporting structures accurately, the x-ray beam must be directed at the structures and the image receptor at certain angles. The function of the image receptor is to record the shadow image. To produce the best image, it is important to understand the fundamentals of **shadow casting**. Shadow casting refers to the five basic rules for casting a shadow image as explained in Chapter 4.

1. Use the smallest possible focal spot.
2. The object (tooth) should be as far as practical from the target.

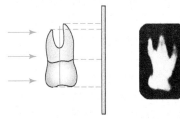

FIGURE 12–6 **Principle of the paralleling technique.** Positioning the recording plane parallel to the long axis of the tooth and directing the x-ray beam perpendicular to both the recording plane and the long axis of the tooth produces an image with less distortion. (Courtesy of Dentsply Sirona.)

3. The object (tooth) and the image receptor (film, phosphor plate, or digital sensor) should be as close to each other as possible.
4. The object (tooth) and the image receptor (film, phosphor plate, or digital sensor) should be parallel to each other.
5. The radiation (central rays) must strike both the object (tooth) and the image receptor (film, phosphor plate, or digital sensor) at right angles (perpendicularly).

Neither the paralleling nor the bisecting technique completely meets all five requirements for accurate shadow casting in all regions of the oral cavity on all patient types. With the bisecting technique, it is often not possible to position the image receptor parallel to the object, preventing the radiation from striking the object and the image receptor at right angles. With the paralleling technique, the distance between the object and the image receptor is often greater than ideal in some regions of the oral cavity. That being said, the paralleling technique is more likely to meet most of these requirements, in most regions, making this technique less likely to produce image distortion. For this reason, the paralleling technique is the recommended technique (Figures 12–6 ■ and 12–7 ■).

Although the paralleling technique produces superior diagnostic quality radiographs, not all patients present with conditions that allow for the use of this technique. When use of the paralleling technique is difficult, a reasonably acceptable quality radiograph may be produced using the bisecting technique. For this reason, a radiographer who is

skilled in both paralleling and bisecting techniques will be better prepared to produce quality radiographs in most all situations.

The Radiographic Examination

Size, Number, and Placement of Image Receptors

The size 4 image receptor is used exclusively for occlusal radiographs of adult patients, and the size 3 image receptor is used exclusively for horizontal bitewing radiographs of adult patients. Bitewing and periapical radiographs of adults, adolescents, and children can be made with any of the three intraoral image receptor sizes 0, 1, 2, or any combination of these sizes. The size of the image receptor selected for use depends on the:

- Age of the patient
- Size of the oral cavity
- Shape of the dental arches
- Presence or absence of unusual conditions or anatomical limitations
- Patient's ability to tolerate placement of the image receptor
- Image receptor positioner or holder and technique used

The bitewing survey may consist of two to eight radiographs. A complete set of seven or eight **vertical bitewing radiographs** may be exposed for the examination of a periodontally involved patient. This vertical bitewing set will include both posterior and anterior bitewings. When a patient does not require anterior bitewings, two or four posterior bitewing radiographs positioned either vertically or horizontally are usually taken (see Figure 15–6). When the periapical and bitewing examinations include a series of radiographs that image all the teeth, the term **full mouth series** or **full mouth survey** is used to describe the collection of radiographs (see Figure 12–3).

The number and size of image receptors used for a full mouth series of bitewing and periapical radiographs varies among oral health care practices. A minimum of four bitewing and 14 periapical radiographs make up a full mouth survey for most adult patients (Figure 12–8 ■). The four bitewing radiographs are used to image the following regions; one radiograph each for the right and left:

- Premolar regions
- Molar regions

The 14 periapical radiographs are used to image the following regions; one radiograph each for the:

- Maxillary and mandibular incisor regions
- Right and left maxillary and mandibular canine regions
- Right and left maxillary and mandibular premolar regions
- Right and left maxillary and mandibular molar region

Although most oral health care practices will use eight size 2 image receptors for the exposure of the posterior periapicals on an adult patient, the number and size of image receptors used for the exposure of the anterior teeth varies.

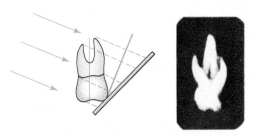

FIGURE 12–7 **Principle of the bisecting technique.** The x-ray beam is directed perpendicular to the imaginary line that bisects the angle formed by the recording plane and the long axis of the tooth. Because the tooth is a three-dimensional object, the part of the tooth farthest from the recording plane is projected in an incorrect relationship to the parts closest to the recording plane. (Courtesy of Dentsply Sirona.)

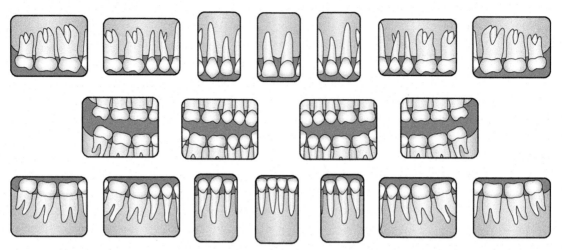

FIGURE 12–8 **Full mouth series.** Drawing of 18-image full mouth survey includes 14 periapical and 4 bitewing radiographs.

The general rule is to use the largest image receptor that can readily be positioned to minimize the number of exposures. For exposures of the anterior teeth, however, a size 1 image receptor is often used instead of the size 2 image receptor because it may fit better in this narrow region of the oral cavity. The use of the narrow size 1 image receptor may require additional exposures to completely record the region. Figure 12–9 ■ illustrates three examples of image receptor combinations for use in recording anterior periapical radiographs using size 1 and size 2 image receptors. See Table 12–1 ■ for a list of the various combinations of standard placements of the image receptor for each of the periapical radiographs of a full mouth series.

Orientation of the Image Receptor

With few exceptions, for exposure of the anterior regions of the oral cavity, the image receptor is placed with the longer dimension vertical (described as vertical placement; see Figure 12–5). For exposure of the posterior regions the image receptor should be placed with the longer dimension horizontal (described as horizontal placement; see Figure 12–4). The white, unprinted side of the film packet (front side) must face the source of radiation. Depending on the manufacturer, the plain side of the phosphor plate, or side without the cord attachment of the digital sensor, should be placed to face the source of radiation.

When placing a film packet for periapical radiographs, it is important to make note of where the identification

dot is located. The identification dot, embossed into the film by the manufacturer, will be used during interpretation of the radiograph to distinguish between the patient's right and left sides (see Chapter 20). There is a tendency for the embossed identification dot to distort images, so during film packet placement it is important to position the identification dot away from the area of interest. In the case of periapical radiographs, the identification dot should be positioned toward the incisal or occlusal edges, where it is least likely to interfere with diagnostic information.

Horizontal and Vertical Angulation

Angulation is the procedure by which the tube head and PID are aligned to obtain the optimum angle at which the radiation is to be directed toward the image receptor. The correct horizontal and vertical angulations are critical to producing a quality radiograph. Angulation is changed by rotating the tube head horizontally and vertically. The x-ray machine is constructed with swivel joints to support the yoke and tube head. One of these, located at the top and center of the yoke where it attaches to the extension arm, permits horizontal movement of the tube head to control the anterior–posterior dimensions. The other swivel joints are located at either side of the yoke. These permit the tube head to be rotated up or down in a vertical direction to control the longitudinal dimensions of the resulting image. Determining the correct direction of the x-ray beam in the horizontal and vertical planes requires practice.

Horizontal Angulation

Horizontal angulation is achieved by directing the central rays of the x-ray beam perpendicularly (at a right angle) toward the surface of the image receptor in a horizontal plane (Figure 12–10 ■). To change direction, swivel the tube head from side to side. The central rays, imagined as emanating from the middle of the PID, should be directed perpendicular to the curvature of the arch, through the contact points of the teeth. The horizontal angulation is

Practice Point

When using a film-holding device with a film slot, it is helpful to remember the phrase "dot-in-the-slot" to ensure correct positioning of the embossed identification dot away from the apices of the teeth where it could interfere with diagnosis. "Dot-in-the-slot" positions the identification dot toward the incisal or occlusal edges for both maxillary and mandibular periapical radiographs.

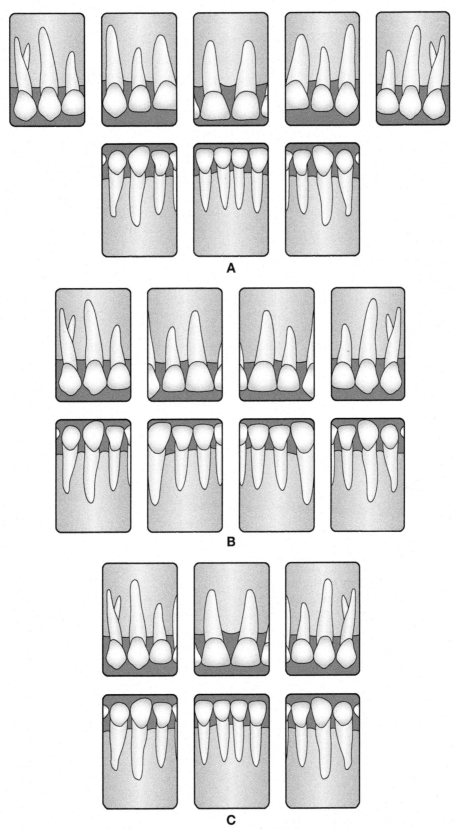

FIGURE 12–9 **Maxillary anterior image receptor placement.** (A) Eight-image survey using size 1 film; five maxillary and three mandibular radiographs. (B) Eight-image survey using size 1 film; four each maxillary and mandibular radiographs. (C) Six-image survey using size 2 film; three each maxillary and mandibular radiographs.

Table 12–1 Standard Image Receptor Placements for Periapical Radiographs of a Full Mouth Series

Periapical Radiograph	Image Receptor Placement
Maxillary central incisors (size 1 or size 2)	Center image receptor to line up behind central and lateral incisors; if using size 2 include mesial halves of canines
Maxillary central and lateral incisors (size 1)	Center image receptor to line up behind central and lateral incisors on one side; include distal half of central incisor on opposite side and mesial half of canine
Maxillary lateral incisor (size 1)	Center image receptor to line up behind lateral incisor; include distal half of central incisor and mesial half of canine
Maxillary lateral incisor and canine (size 1)	Center image receptor to line up behind lateral incisor and canine; include distal half of central incisor and mesial half of premolar
Maxillary canine (size 1 or size 2)	Center image receptor to line up behind canine; include distal half of lateral incisor and mesial half of first premolar
Mandibular central incisors (size 1 or size 2)	Center image receptor to line up behind central and lateral incisors; if using size 2 film include mesial halves of canines
Mandibular central and lateral incisors (size 1)	Center image receptor to line up behind central and lateral incisors on one side; include distal half of central incisor on opposite side and mesial half of canine
Mandibular canine (size 1 or size 2)	Center image receptor to line up behind canine; include distal half of lateral incisor and mesial half of first premolar
Maxillary and mandibular premolar (size 2)	Align anterior edge of image receptor to line up behind distal half of canine; include entire first and second premolars and mesial half of first molar
Maxillary and mandibular molar (size 2)	Align anterior edge of image receptor to line up behind distal half of second premolar; include entire first, second, and third molars

established by directing the central rays perpendicularly through the **mean tangent** of the embrasures between the teeth of interest. Incorrect alignment in the horizontal plane caused by incorrect angulation toward the mesial or the distal results in overlapping of adjacent tooth structures recorded on the radiograph. The steps in determining correct horizontal angulation are the same for both the

bisecting and paralleling methods and for exposing bitewing radiographs.

Vertical Angulation

Vertical angulation is achieved by directing the central rays of the x-ray beam perpendicularly toward the surface of the image receptor in a vertical plane (Figure 12–11 ■).

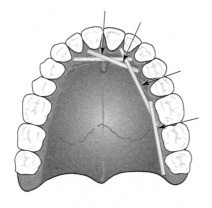 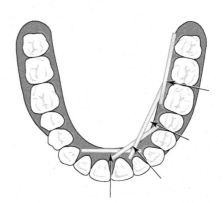

FIGURE 12–10 Horizontal angulation. Horizontal angulation is determined by directing the x-ray beam directly through the interproximal spaces perpendicular to the mean tangent of the teeth. The image receptor must be positioned parallel to the teeth of interest so that the central ray will also strike the image receptor perpendicularly.

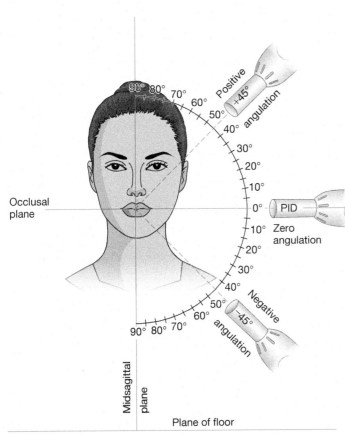

FIGURE 12–11 Vertical angulation. Patient positioned with midsagittal plane perpendicular to and occlusal plane parallel with the floor. Zero angulation is achieved when the PID is directed parallel with the floor. All angulations achieved with the PID pointed toward the floor are called positive, or plus (+) angulations. All angulations achieved with the PID pointed toward the ceiling are called negative, or minus (−) angulations.

Vertical angulation is customarily described in degrees. Dental x-ray machines often denote the vertical angles in intervals of 5 or 10 degrees on one or both sides of the yoke where the tube head is connected. The vertical angulation of the tube head and the PID begins at zero. In the zero position the PID is parallel to the plane of the floor. All deviations from zero in which the PID is tilted downward to direct the x-rays toward the floor are called **positive (plus) angulations**. Those in which the PID is tipped upward to direct the x-rays toward the ceiling are called **negative (minus) angulations**. Positive (+) angulation is used for exposure of bitewing radiographs and generally used for the exposure of periapical radiographs of the maxillary arch. Negative (−) angulation is generally used for the exposure of periapical radiographs of the mandibular arch. Although the vertical angulation setting for the exposure of bitewing radiographs for the adult patient is +10 for all regions of the oral cavity, the precise vertical angulation setting for periapical radiographs is determined differently depending on the technique used (see Chapters 13 and 14).

Points of Entry

The image receptor must be centered within the beam of radiation to avoid **conecut error**, where a portion of the image is not recorded on the radiograph. The **point of entry** for the central rays of the x-ray beam should be in the middle of the image receptor. An image receptor positioner with an external aiming device will assist the radiographer with determining the point of entry. The portion of the holder, or biteblock, that extends from the oral cavity can be used to estimate the center of the image receptor when using a holder without an external indicator. The open end of the PID should be placed as close to the patient's skin as possible without touching. Failure to bring the end of the PID in close to the patient will result in an underexposed radiograph because as the beam of radiation spreads out, less radiation is available to strike the image receptor and produce a diagnostic quality image.

Image Receptor Positioners

Film holders and holders designed to position a phosphor plate or digital sensor are collectively called **image receptor positioners** or **holders**. These devices are used to hold an image receptor in place to expose intraoral radiographs. When the bisecting technique was first introduced film holders did not yet exist, so a patient was directed to hold the film packet in his or her mouth using a finger or thumb. Asking a patient to hold the film packet in this manner has many disadvantages, and this practice is no longer acceptable (Box 12–1). Today, image receptor positioners and holders vary from simple disposable **biteblocks** to complex devices that position an image receptor at the correct angles for directing the x-ray beam in relation to the teeth and image receptor (Figures 12–12 ■ and 12–13 ■). Commercially manufactured image receptor holders may be designed specifically for use with either the bisecting or paralleling technique. Some holders may be slightly altered to accommodate both techniques (see Figure 14–5). Other

Box 12–1: Contraindications for Using a Patient's Finger to Hold an Image Receptor in Place

- Potential for bending image receptor
- Potential to move image receptor from correct position
- Increased patient instruction and cooperation required
- Potential patient objection to placing fingers in mouth
- Radiation exposure to patient's fingers
- No external aiming device to assist with aligning x-ray beam to correct position
- Potential to be viewed by patient as unprofessional and unsanitary

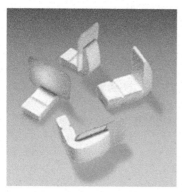

FIGURE 12–12 **Disposable image receptor positioners.** Note the film packet is inserted into the groove of the holder. (Courtesy of Flow Dental.)

manufactures offer interchangeable biteblocks to accommodate either technique and placement of a film packet, phosphor plate, or digital sensor (Figure 12–14 ■). It is important that a radiographer match the image receptor biteblock with the technique and type of receptor (film, phosphor plate, or sensor) for which it was designed to achieve optimal results.

It is beneficial to have a variety of image receptor positioners available, because one type of holder may not be suitable for all patients, or even all areas of the same patient's mouth. Additionally, an operator may have to alternate between the paralleling and bisecting technique to complete a full mouth series on a patient.

Preparations and Seating Positions

Preparation of the Dental X-ray Machine

Prior to placing an image receptor intraorally, the x-ray machine should be turned on and the exposure settings selected. It is helpful to place the tube head and PID in the approximate position for the exposure to limit the time

required for this step once the image receptor has been placed into the patient's oral cavity.

Patient Preparation

To help gain patient cooperation and confidence, it is important to explain the procedure. Include specific instructions regarding the need for patient cooperation and be honest about any difficulties anticipated (see Chapter 11). Perform a cursory oral inspection and ask the patient to remove any objects from the mouth that would interfere with the procedure, such as removable dentures or orthodontic appliances, and some oral and facial piercings. Ask the patient to remove eyeglasses. If metal or thick plastic parts of the eyeglasses remain in the path of the x-ray beam, these may block the x-rays from reaching the image receptor. Protect the patient with a lead/ lead equivalent apron and thyroid collar barriers.

Patient Seating Position

If the image receptor positioner has an external aiming device, usually a ring attached to an extension arm, the patient's head can be in any position. Without these aiming rings to indicate x-ray beam positions, a patient must be seated upright with his or her head straight so that the radiographer can estimate these angles using the occlusal and midsagittal planes. Correct patient positioning allows for consistent results in determining the best horizontal and vertical angulations of the x-ray beam and points of entry. Additionally, stabilizing the patient's head against the headrest is important to prevent movement during the exposure. Placing the headrest against the occipital protuberance (the back, base of the skull) provides the greatest stability.

The recommended position is to seat a patient upright and adjust the headrest so that the **occlusal plane** for the arch being examined is parallel to the floor (Figure 12–15 ■). The **midsagittal plane** that divides a patient's head into the

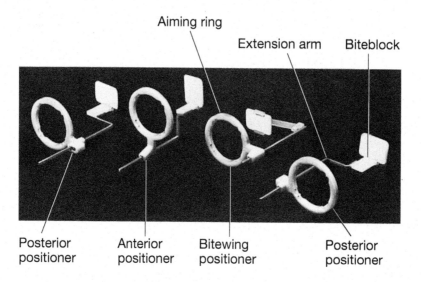

Aiming ring

Extension arm   Biteblock

Posterior positioner   Anterior positioner   Bitewing positioner   Posterior positioner

FIGURE 12–13 **Set of image receptor positioners.** Multiple parts to assemble for use in different regions of the oral cavity. External aiming ring on extension arm assists with locating the correct angles and points of entry. (Courtesy of Dentsply Sirona.)

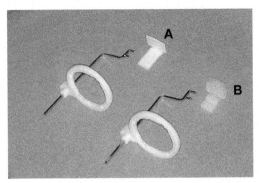

FIGURE 12–14 Paralleling and bisecting biteblocks. The same extension arm and aiming ring may be combined with (**A**) a biteblock suitable for the paralleling technique or (**B**) a biteblock suitable for the bisecting technique.

right and left side should be positioned perpendicular to the floor (Figure 12–16 ■). Although an experienced radiographer can expose radiographs with a patient either upright or supine, the use of predetermined head positions is recommended to standardize the procedure.

Sequence of Procedure

A definite sequence of positioning an image receptor should be followed to prevent omitting an area or exposing an area twice. Develop a set routine to prevent errors and save time.

Opinions differ as to which region should be exposed first when taking a full mouth series of periapical and bitewing radiographs. Some radiographers prefer to begin in the right maxillary molar region and continue in sequence to the left maxillary molar region, drop down to the left mandibular molar region, and finish in the right mandibular molar region.

Others begin with the anterior exposures, on the theory that an image receptor placement is more comfortable here and less likely to excite a gag reflex than when it is placed in the maxillary molar region, where the tissues may be more sensitive (see Chapter 29). If the first few placements produce no discomfort, a patient may become used to the feel of the image receptor and may more readily accept it as the procedure continues.

For an experienced radiographer who can place an image receptor skillfully and rapidly, it probably makes little difference which area is first exposed. However, the same

Practice Point

Seating a patient with his or her head against the headrest not only helps position the occlusal and midsaggital planes, but the patient is much less likely to move during the exposures when his or her head is firmly supported by the headrest. Additionally directing a patient's attention to the back of the head where it touches the headrest can serve as a distraction technique when needed, for example, when a hypersensitive gag reflex presents (Chapter 29).

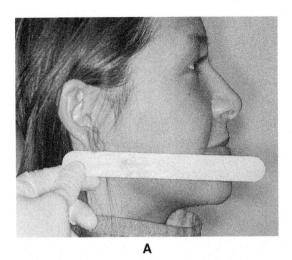

A

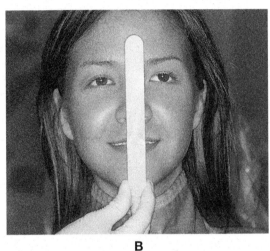

B

FIGURE 12–15 Patient positioning. Patient positioned with head supported and (**A**) occlusal plane parallel to the floor and (**B**) midsaggital plane perpendicular to the floor.

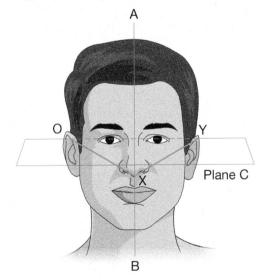

FIGURE 12–16 Head divided by midsagittal plane and occlusal plane. The midsagittal plane (**A–B**) should be perpendicular to the floor, and the occlusal plane (**C**) parallel with the floor unless using an image receptor positioner with an external aiming device. Lines **O–X** and **X–Y** represent another landmark plane called the ala–tragus line. The apices of the roots of the maxillary teeth are located close to this line.

order for placement of an image receptor should always be followed to make sure that all regions are exposed in an orderly and efficient manner. The following sequence of image receptor placements is suggested to help a student adopt a systematic routine:

- Maxillary anterior periapicals
- Mandibular anterior periapicals
- Maxillary posterior periapicals
- Mandibular posterior periapicals
- Anterior bitewings
- Posterior bitewings

Anterior image receptor placements are often more comfortable and allow a patient to become accustomed to the procedure. A bitewing examination could be performed last because patients tolerate these fairly well, and the radiographic procedure can end pleasantly (see Chapter 15). In addition, it may be helpful for a radiographer not to have to break the sequence of exposing periapical radiographs by switching to a bitewing holder and changing techniques in the middle of the procedure. Procedure 12–1 summarizes the steps for exposing a full mouth series of radiographs.

Procedure 12–1

Procedure for exposing a full mouth series of radiographs

1. Perform infection control procedures (see Procedure 9–2).
2. Prepare the dental x-ray machine. Turn on and set exposure factors.
3. Seat patient and explain the procedure.
4. Request that the patient remove objects from the mouth that can interfere with the procedure and remove eyeglasses.
5. Adjust chair to a comfortable working level.
6. Adjust the headrest to position the patient's head so that the occlusal plane of the arch being imaged is parallel to the floor and the midsagittal plane (midline) is perpendicular to the floor.
7. Place the lead/lead equivalent barrier apron and thyroid collar on the patient.
8. Perform a cursory inspection of the oral cavity and note possible obstructions (tori, shallow palatal vault, malaligned teeth) that may require an alteration of technique or number of exposures.
9. Place the image receptor into the positioner. When using film, place such that the embossed dot will be positioned toward the occlusal/incisal edge ("dot-in-the-slot"). Position anterior image receptors vertically and posterior image receptors horizontally.
10. Insert an image receptor and positioner into the patient's oral cavity and center the receptor behind the teeth of interest. (See Table 13–2 for the exact placements for each of the maxillary and mandibular periapical radiographs and Table 15–3 for placements for each of the posterior and/or anterior bitewing radiographs in the procedure.) Visually locate the contact points of the teeth of interest and place the image receptor perpendicular to the embrasures.
11. Hold the image receptor holder against the occlusal/incisal surface of the maxillary/mandibular teeth while asking the patient to bite firmly onto the biteblock of the holder. (Use a sterilized cotton roll for stabilization if needed; see Figure 13–9.)
12. Release the image receptor positioner when the patient has closed firmly, holding it in place.
13. Set the vertical angulation:
    a. For periapical radiographs: (See Table 13–2 for the recommended vertical angulation setting for the area being imaged.)
       1. Intersect the image receptor plane and the long axes of the teeth perpendicularly when utilizing the paralleling technique. If using an image receptor positioner with an external aiming device, align the open end of the PID with the indicator ring.
       2. Intersect the imaginary bisector of the receptor plane and the long axes of the teeth perpendicularly when utilizing the bisecting technique.
    b. For bitewing radiographs use +10 degrees.
14. Determine the correct horizontal angulation by directing the central rays of the x-ray beam perpendicular to the receptor in the horizontal plane through the contact point of the teeth of interest. (See Table 13–2 for the exact embrasure space through which to direct the central rays for each of the periapical radiographs and Table 15–3 for each of the bitewing radiographs in the procedure. Horizontal angulation is determined the same for both paralleling and bisecting techniques and for bitewing radiographs.) If using an image receptor positioner with an external aiming device, align the open end of the PID with the indicator ring.
15. Center the PID over the image receptor. If using an image receptor positioner with an external aiming device, align the open end of the PID with the indicator ring. (See Table 14–2 for point of entry recommendations when utilizing the bisecting technique.)
16. Make the exposure.

Procedure 12–1 *(continued)*

17. Remove the image receptor and positioner from the patient's oral cavity.
18. Repeat steps 9 through 17 until all radiographs in the series have been exposed.
19. Remove the lead/lead equivalent barrier apron and thyroid collar from the patient.
20. Perform infection control procedures following the examination (see Procedure 9–4).

REVIEW—Chapter summary

The three types of intraoral radiographic procedures are the bitewing, periapical, and occlusal surveys. Each of these examinations differs in purpose, and a variety of image receptor sizes may be used to achieve the desired result.

Both the bisecting and the paralleling techniques are used to produce a shadow image of the tooth onto the radiograph. Although neither technique completely satisfies all the requirements for accurate shadow casting, the paralleling technique is more likely to produce superior results. Each technique has advantages and disadvantages. A skilled operator, within the limits of the equipment available, must select the technique that fits the situation.

The size and number of image receptors used for exposure of a full mouth radiographic survey depends on several factors. A bitewing series may consist of two to eight radiographs. A minimum of 14 periapical radiographs are required for a full mouth series of an adult patient—additional images may be needed if narrow size 1 image receptors are used in the anterior regions. Exposures include the central incisor, canine, premolar, and molar areas of the right and left maxilla and mandible. The image receptor should be positioned with the long dimension vertical in the anterior region and horizontal in the posterior region. The embossed identification dot present on radiographic film should be placed toward the incisal/occlusal edges of the teeth when positioning the film packet for periapical radiographs.

The horizontal angulation is determined by directing the central rays of the x-ray beam perpendicular to the plane of the image receptor through the mean tangent of the embrasures between the teeth of interest. Both paralleling and bisecting techniques and bitewing procedures determine horizontal angulation in the same manner.

With negative vertical angulation, the PID is pointing down toward the floor. With positive vertical angulation, the PID is pointing up toward the ceiling. Vertical angulation is determined by directing the central rays of the x-ray beam perpendicular to the plane of the image receptor and the long axes of the teeth when utilizing the paralleling technique. When utilizing the bisecting technique, vertical angulation is determined by directing the central rays of the x-ray beam perpendicular to the imaginary bisector. The vertical angulation setting for exposing bitewings is +10. The point of entry is used to center the image receptor within the beam of radiation.

Before image positioners were developed, a patient would hold the film packet in the oral cavity with his or her fingers or thumb. With the variety of image receptor positioners currently on the market, this practice is unacceptable today. Image receptor positioners are designed for use with the paralleling or the bisecting technique or may be modified to use with both techniques.

Unless an image receptor positioner has an external aiming device to indicate the correct angulation, care must be taken to seat a patient so that the occlusal plane is parallel with the floor and that the midsaggital plane is perpendicular to the floor.

An exposure sequence is recommended to avoid error and be efficient. Anterior image receptor placements may be more comfortable for some patients. Beginning the exposure sequence in the anterior may assist in gaining patient cooperation with the procedure.

RECALL—Study questions

1. Which of these is NOT an intraoral radiograph?
   a. Bitewing
   b. Occlusal
   c. Panoramic
   d. Periapical

2. Which radiograph is used most often to detect proximal surface dental decay?
   a. Bitewing
   b. Occlusal
   c. Panoramic
   d. Periapical

3. Which intraoral technique satisfies more shadow casting principles?
   a. Bisecting
   b. Paralleling

4. Which intraoral technique is based on the rule of isometry?
   a. Bisecting
   b. Paralleling

5. Each of the following is a shadow casting principle EXCEPT one. Which one is the EXCEPTION?
   a. Object and image receptor should be perpendicular to each other.
   b. Object and image receptor should be as close as possible to each other.
   c. Object should be as far as practical from the target (source of radiation).
   d. Radiation should strike the object and image receptor perpendicularly.

6. Which of these factors does NOT need to be considered when deciding which image receptor size to use when exposing a full mouth series?
   a. Age of the patient
   b. Shape of the dental arches
   c. Previous accumulated exposure
   d. Patient's ability to tolerate the image receptor

7. What is the minimum image receptor requirement for an adult full mouth series of periapical radiographs?
   a. 12
   b. 14
   c. 16
   d. 18

8. How many size 2 image receptors are required by most health care practices for the exposure of posterior radiographs of a full mouth series?
   a. Five
   b. Six
   c. Seven
   d. Eight

9. Lining the image receptor up behind the right and left central and lateral incisors to include the mesial half of the right and left canines describes the image receptor placement for which of the following periapical radiographs?
   a. Central incisors
   b. Canines
   c. Premolars
   d. Molars

10. Anterior periapical image receptors are placed _____ in the oral cavity. Posterior periapical image receptors are placed _____ in the oral cavity.
    a. vertically; horizontally
    b. horizontally; vertically
    c. vertically; vertically
    d. horizontally; horizontally

11. Where should the film packet embossed identification dot be positioned when taking periapical radiographs?
    a. Toward the midline of the oral cavity
    b. Toward the incisal or occlusal edge of the tooth
    c. Toward the palate or floor of the mouth
    d. Toward the distal or back of the arch

12. The x-ray tube head must be swiveled from side to side to adjust the vertical angulation of the x-ray beam. To avoid overlap error the central rays of the x-ray beam must be directed perpendicular to the curvature of the arch through the contact points of the teeth.
    a. Both statements are true.
    b. Both statements are false
    c. The first statement is true. The second statement is false.
    d. The first statement is false. The second statement is true.

13. At which of the following settings would the PID be pointing to the floor?
    a. −30
    b. 0
    c. +20

14. An incorrect point of entry will result in
    a. overlapping.
    b. foreshortening.
    c. cutting off the root apices.
    d. conecutting.

15. List five contraindications for using the patient's finger to hold a film packet in position during exposure.
    a. _____
    b. _____
    c. _____
    d. _____
    e. _____

16. An image receptor positioner/holder must be used with
    a. the paralleling technique.
    b. the bisecting technique.
    c. the bitewing technique.
    d. all of the above techniques.

17. Which of the following is the correct seating position for the patient during radiographic examinations when an image receptor without an external aiming device is used?
    a. Occlusal plane parallel and midsaggital plane perpendicular to the floor
    b. Occlusal plane perpendicular and midsaggital plane parallel to the floor
    c. Occlusal and midsaggital planes parallel to the floor
    d. Occlusal and midsaggital planes perpendicular to the floor

18. Which of the following is the best sequencing for exposing a full mouth series of periapical radiographs?
    a. Mandibular anteriors, maxillary anteriors, mandibular posteriors, maxillary posteriors
    b. Maxillary anteriors, mandibular anteriors, maxillary posteriors, mandibular posteriors
    c. Mandibular posteriors, maxillary posteriors, mandibular anteriors, maxillary anteriors
    d. Maxillary posteriors, mandibular posteriors, maxillary anteriors, mandibular anteriors

REFLECT—Case study

A dentist has prescribed a full mouth series of periapical and bitewing radiographs for a patient who presents with several areas of decay and a suspected abscess. This oral health care practice uses an 18-image full mouth series configuration. Consider the following and write out your answers:

1. Prepare a list of the specific periapical and bitewing radiographs you intend to expose. Include what size image receptor you will use and why, and which specific teeth must be imaged on each of the projections.

2. Which radiographic technique for exposing periapical radiographs will you choose for this exam? Why?

3. How will your patient be seated for the exposures? Why?

4. Will you be using the patient's finger or a holder to position the image receptor within the oral cavity? Explain your choice.

5. Describe how the image receptor will be positioned in relation to the teeth and how you will be directing the central rays of the x-ray beam for the specific technique you plan to use.

6. Summarize the steps you will take to locate the vertical and horizontal angulations.

7. Prepare a sequence of exposures and explain your choice.

RELATE—Laboratory application

Set up a teaching manikin or skull in the radiography operatory. Position the occlusal plane parallel to the floor and the midsagittal plane perpendicular to the floor. Obtain an image receptor and holder. Using Table 12–1, Standard Image Receptor Placements for Periapical Radiographs of a Full Mouth Series, practice the standard image receptor placements for the periapical radiographs listed. Write out your answers to the following questions.

1. What size image receptors did you choose for each of the radiographs? List the considerations that prompted your decision.

2. Observe and describe the orientation of the image receptor in each position. Give a rationale for why the image receptor is positioned with the long dimension vertical or horizontal in different regions of the oral cavity.

3. If using intraoral film packets, where did you position the embossed dot? Why?

4. Explain the order you used to position each of the radiographs.

Next practice positioning the x-ray tube head in relation to each of the standard image receptor placements. Using the paralleling technique, determine the horizontal angulation by swiveling the tube head from side to side to direct the central rays of the x-ray beam perpendicular to the image receptor through the mean tangent of the embrasures between the teeth of interest. Determine the vertical angulation by moving the tube head up and down in the yoke to direct the central rays of the x-ray beam perpendicular to the image receptor.

5. List what teeth you used to determine where to horizontally direct the central rays of the x-ray beam for each of the standard image receptor placements. Why did you choose these teeth?

6. What error is most likely to occur if the horizontal angulation is not correctly aligned between the embrasures of the teeth of interest?

7. Observe the degrees of vertical angulation noted on the yoke of the x-ray tube head for each of the standard image receptor placements. Determine if using positive or negative angulation. Write down each of the settings.

8. Compare the vertical angulation settings you used for each of the standard image receptor placements with those noted in Table 14–2, Summary of Steps for Acquiring Periapical Radiographs–Bisecting Technique. Explain the difference between the vertical angulations you used for the paralleling technique with the vertical angulations recommended in Table 14–2 for use with the bisecting technique. What general statement can you make about the differences? Why?

RESOURCES

Eastman Kodak Company. (2002). *Successful intraoral radiography*. Rochester, NY: Author.

White, S. C., & Pharoah, M. J. (2014). Projection geometry. *Oral radiology: Principles and interpretation* (7th ed.). St. Louis MO: Elsevier.

Williamson, G. F. (2014). Intraoral radiography: Principles, techniques and error correction. Retrieved from the DentalCare.com website: http://www.dentalcare.com/en-US/dental-education/continuing-education/ce137/ce137.aspx?ModuleName=coursecontent&PartID=2&SectionID=-1.

The Periapical Examination— Paralleling Technique

CHAPTER OUTLINE

OBJECTIVES

Following successful completion of this chapter, you should be able to:

1. Define the key terms.
2. Discuss the principles of the paralleling technique.
3. List the advantages and limitations of the paralleling technique.
4. Identify, assemble, and position image receptor holders for use with the paralleling technique.
5. Explain the importance of achieving accurate horizontal and vertical angulation in obtaining quality diagnostic radiographs using the paralleling technique.
6. Identify vertical angulation errors unique to the paralleling technique.
7. Demonstrate the image receptor positioning, horizontal and vertical angulation, and points of entry for maxillary and mandibular periapical exposures using the paralleling technique.

KEY TERMS

Embrasure
Extension arm

External aiming device

Indicator ring

Table 13–1 **Advantages and Limitations of the Paralleling Technique**

Advantages	Limitations
• Produces images with minimal dimensional distortion • Minimizes superimposition of adjacent structures • Long axis of tooth and recording plane of image receptor can be visually located making it easier to direct x-rays appropriately • Many choices of image receptor holders available with external aiming devices specifically designed to make paralleling simple and easy to learn • With appropriate image receptor holding devices, takes less time than trying to locate position of imaginary bisector • Patient radiation dose may be reduced when using long PID (16 inches/41 cm)	• Parallel placement of image receptor may be difficult to achieve on certain patients: children; adults with small mouths, low palatal vaults, or presence of tori; patients with sensitive oral mucosa or hypersensitive gag reflex, edentulous regions • These same conditions may increase patient discomfort when image receptor impinges on oral tissues • Long PID has potential to be difficult to maneuver and stabilize (short PID—8 inches/20.5 cm—should not be used)

Introduction

Due to its ability to produce superior diagnostic quality radiographs, the paralleling technique should be the technique of choice when exposing periapical radiographs (Table 13–1 ■). This chapter presents step-by-step instructions for exposing a full mouth series of periapical radiographs using the paralleling technique.

Fundamentals of Paralleling Technique

The basic principles of the paralleling technique meet the following two shadow casting principles:

- The image receptor (film packet, phosphor plate, or digital sensor) is placed parallel to the long axis of the object (tooth) of interest.
- The central rays of the x-ray beam are directed to intersect both the image receptor and the object (tooth) perpendicularly (Figure 13–1 ■).

Oral structures, particularly the curvature of the palate and the outwardly inclined anterior teeth, make it difficult to place the image receptor parallel to the long axes of the teeth (Figure 13–2 ■). The paralleling technique must achieve parallelism by placing the image receptor away from the crowns of the teeth. Parallelism is accomplished by using an image receptor positioner or holder specifically designed to allow the patient to stabilize the image receptor in this position away from the crowns of the teeth. This position, however, does not meet the shadow cast principle that states that the image receptor (film, phosphor plate, or digital sensor) and the object (tooth) should be as close to each other as possible. To compensate for the increased object–image receptor distance needed to achieve parallelism, the target–image receptor distance should also be increased. The position indicating device (PID) length contributes to the target–image receptor distance and satisfies the shadow cast principle that states that the object (tooth) should be as far as practical from the target (source of radiation). Ideally, the target–image receptor distance used with

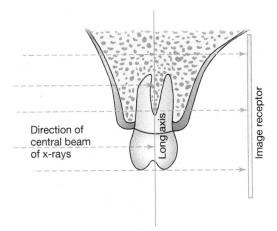

FIGURE 13–1 **Paralleling technique.** The x-ray beam is directed perpendicular to the recording plane of the image receptor, which has been positioned parallel to the long axis of the tooth.

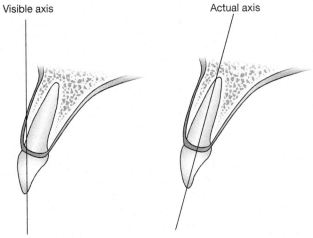

FIGURE 13–2 **Visible and actual long axis of the tooth.** The root portion of the tooth should be taken into consideration to accurately locate the long axis of the tooth.

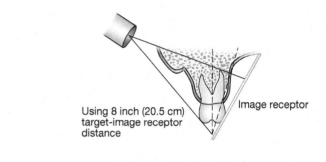

Using 8 inch (20.5 cm) target-image receptor distance

Image receptor

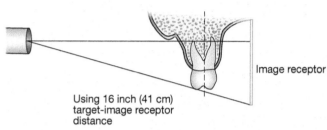

Using 16 inch (41 cm) target-image receptor distance

Image receptor

FIGURE 13–3 Comparison of the bisecting and paralleling techniques. With the bisecting technique, the image receptor is positioned adjacent to the tooth, making a target–image receptor distance of 8 inches (20.5 cm) acceptable. With the paralleling technique the image receptor is positioned near the center of the oral cavity, where it must be retained in a position parallel to the long axes of the teeth. This increased object–image receptor distance requires a longer (16 inches/41 cm) target–image receptor distance to produce a quality radiograph.

the paralleling technique is 16 inches (41 cm) or at least 12 inches (30 cm) (Figure 13–3 ■).

Holding the Periapical Image Receptor in Position

Image receptor positioners designed for use with the paralleling technique usually have a long biteblock for the purpose of achieving a parallel relationship between the recording plane of the image receptor and the long axes of the teeth, and an L-shaped backing to help support the image receptor and keep it in position (Figure 13–4 ■).

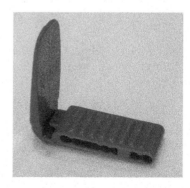

FIGURE 13–4 Paralleling biteblock. The bite plane is at a right angle (90 degrees) with the backing plate. The patient bites down far enough out on the bite extension to keep the image receptor and teeth parallel.

These instruments often have an **external aiming device** in the form of an **indicator ring** or rectangle attached to an **extension arm** to assist the radiographer in locating the correct angles and points of entry, making errors less likely. The external aiming device also eliminates the need to position a patient's head precisely.

There are many different styles of image receptor holders on the market (Figures 13–5 ■, 13–6 ■, and 13–7 ■). Manufacturers continue to reduce the size and weight of these holders by developing aiming rings and extension arms that are made of lightweight materials for the purpose of improving patient comfort. This is important because if placement of the image receptor is compromised due to patient discomfort, the aiming device will direct the x-ray beam to the wrong place. Image receptor positioners are usually available in sets with multiple parts that must be assembled to accommodate placements for exposure of periapical and bitewing radiographs in all regions of the oral cavity (see Figure 13–5). Often these parts are color coordinated to aid in correct assembly. As digital imaging sensors change with technology, more and more manufacturers are developing universal image receptor positioners that can accommodate many different styles of sensors (see Figure 13–7).

There are some image receptor positioners available that with slight modifications may be used with both the paralleling and the bisecting techniques. For example, it may be possible to shorten the long biteblock of a holder used with the paralleling technique to allow use of the holder with the bisecting technique (see Figure 14-5). Additionally, holders with a shortened biteblock designed for use with the bisecting technique may provide a parallel relationship between the recording plane of the image

A   B

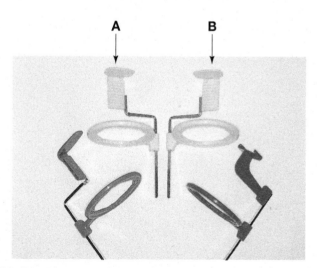

FIGURE 13–5 Set of image receptor positioners. Color-coded rings and biteblocks assist with assembly of multiple parts. Note the mirror-image assembly of (**A**) for exposures of the maxillary right and the mandibular left, and (**B**) for exposures of the maxillary left and the mandibular right. These biteblocks are used for positioning a film packet.

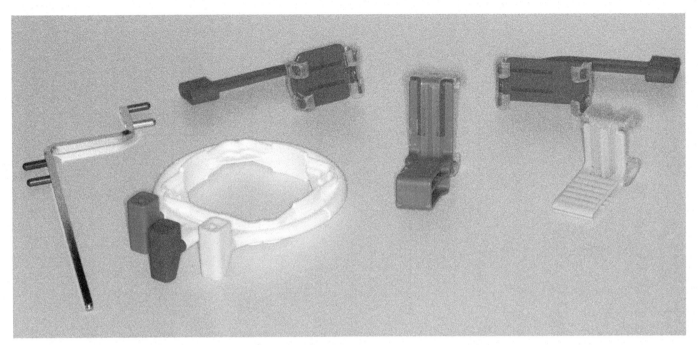

FIGURE 13–6 **Universal image receptor positioner.** One extension arm and one aiming ring with three color-coded openings allow this holder to be used in all regions of the oral cavity. These biteblocks are used for positioning a digital sensor.

receptor and the long axes of the teeth in certain regions of the oral cavity.

Although a radiographer should refer to the manufacturer's instructions for use, important key points regarding image receptor positioners are the:

- Patient must bite down on the biteblock as far away from the teeth as possible, utilizing the full extent of the biteblock. The exception to this rule is for the mandibular premolar and molar regions, where the image receptor can be close to the teeth and still remain parallel because of the nearly vertical position of the mandibular premolars and the slightly inward inclination of the mandibular molars (Figure 13–8 ■).

- Patient must bite down on the biteblock firmly enough to hold the image recptor in place. A sterilized cotton roll may be placed on the opposite side of the biteblock to provide stabilization and add to patient comfort (Figure 13–9 ■).
- Indicator ring must be slid all the way down the extension arm of the device to be as close to the patient's skin as possible without touching the patient.
- Open end of the PID must be aligned to the indicator ring as close as possible without touching to achieve correct horizontal and vertical angulations and correct point of entry.

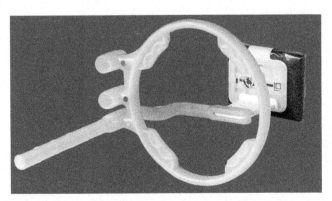

FIGURE 13–7 **Universal image receptor positioner.** One extension arm, one aiming ring, and one biteblock. Minor adjustments to this lightweight holder allow it to be configured for use in all regions of the oral cavity. This biteblock can accommodate a range of digital sensor sizes. (Courtesy of Dentsply Sirona.)

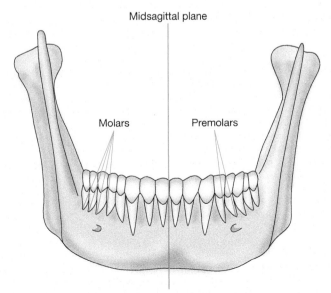

FIGURE 13–8 **Long axes of the premolar and molar teeth.**

Table 13–2   Summary of Steps for Acquiring Periapical Radiographs—Paralleling Technique

Periapical Radiograph	Placement	Vertical Angulation*	Horizontal Angulation	Point of Entry
Incisors (maxillary and mandibular) with image receptor size 1 or size 2 (Figures 13–12 and 13–13)	Center image receptor to line up behind central and lateral incisors; if using size 2 image receptor, include mesial halves of canines Align image receptor parallel to long axes of incisors and parallel to left and right central incisor embrasure	Direct central rays perpendicular to plane of image receptor and long axes of incisors PID pointed down for maxillary incisors PID pointed up for mandibular incisors	Direct central rays perpendicular to image receptor through left and right central incisor embrasure	Center image receptor within x-ray beam by directing central rays at center of image receptor
Canine (maxillary and mandibular) with image receptor 1 or 2 (Figures 13–14 and 13–15)	Center image receptor to line up behind canine; include distal half of lateral incisor and mesial half of first premolar Align image receptor parallel to long axes of canines and parallel to mesial and distal line angles of canine	Direct central rays perpendicular to plane of image receptor and long axis of canine PID pointed down for maxillary canine PID pointed up for mandibular canine	Direct central rays perpendicular to image receptor at center of canine	Center image receptor within x-ray beam by directing central rays at center of image receptor

Premolar (maxillary and mandibular) with image receptor size 2 (Figures 13–16 and 13–17)	Align anterior edge of image receptor to line up behind distal half of canine; include first and second premolars and mesial half of first molar Align image receptor parallel to long axes of premolars and parallel to first and second premolar embrasure	Direct central rays perpendicular to plane of image receptor and long axes of premolars PID pointed down for maxillary premolar PID pointed up for mandibular premolar	Direct central rays perpendicular to image receptor through first and second premolar embrasure	Center image receptor within x-ray beam by directing central rays at center of image receptor
Molar (maxillary and mandibular) with image receptor size 2 (Figures 13–18 and 13–19)	Align anterior edge of image receptor to line up behind distal half of second premolar; include first, second, and third molars Align image receptor parallel to long axes of molars and parallel to first and second molar embrasure	Direct central rays perpendicular to plane of image receptor and long axes of molars PID pointed down for maxillary molar PID pointed up for mandibular molar	Direct central rays perpendicular to image receptor through first and second molar embrasure	Center image receptor within x-ray beam by directing central rays at center of image receptor

* Patient must be seated in correct position, with occlusal plane of the arch being recorded parallel to the floor and the midsagittal plane perpendicular to the floor.

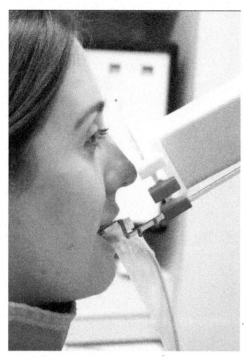

FIGURE 13–9 **Use of a sterile cotton roll** to aid in stabilizing the image receptor holder in position for the duration of the exposure.

Horizontal and Vertical Angulation

Horizontal Angulation

To rely on the image receptor positioner's indicator ring to accurately direct the central rays of the x-ray beam perpendicularly toward the surface of the image receptor in a horizontal plane, the image receptor itself must be positioned parallel to the teeth of interest in the horizontal dimension. The image receptor must be positioned parallel to the interproximal space or **embrasure**. To achieve this, locate and use two predetermined teeth. The teeth

Practice Point

When using a sterile cotton roll to aid in stabilizing the image receptor, be sure that the cotton roll is placed on the opposite side from the teeth of interest. For example, if the purpose of the radiograph is to image a maxillary tooth, the cotton roll should be placed under the biteblock so that the mandibular teeth contact the cotton roll when the patient occludes (see Figure 13–9). If the purpose of the radiograph is to image a mandibular tooth, the cotton roll should be placed on top of the biteblock so that the maxillary teeth contact the cotton roll when the patient occludes. Placing the cotton roll on the biteblock on the same side as the teeth being imaged will prevent the patient from occluding all the way onto the biteblock and will result in cutting off the apices of the teeth on the image.

Practice Point

If the image receptor is correctly positioned parallel to the teeth of interest and the central rays are accurately directed through the appropriate embrasure and overlapping of other adjacent teeth on the image occurs, it is usually attributed to crowded or malaligned teeth. Crowded or malaligned teeth will most likely require additional exposures to achieve a clear view of all proximal surfaces (see Chapter 29).

selected depend on the region being radiographed. Table 13–2 ■ lists the embrasure through which to align the image receptor and to direct the central rays for each projection. The particular embrasures listed for each exposure have been chosen because of the likelihood that if the image receptor is parallel to this space and the central rays of the x-ray beam are directed through this space, then the rest of the spaces should line up for a correct exposure, free of horizontal angulation errors. The central rays must be directed appropriately to avoid overlapping adjacent teeth on the resultant image.

Vertical Angulation

When utilizing the paralleling technique, the correct vertical angulation is achieved by directing the central rays of the x-ray beam perpendicular to the image receptor and perpendicular to the long axes of the teeth in the vertical plane. An image receptor holding device designed for use with the paralleling technique is used to position the image receptor parallel to the long axes of teeth so that directing the central rays perpendicular to the teeth will simultaneously direct the central rays perpendicular to the image receptor. To rely on a holder's indicator ring to accurately direct the central rays perpendicularly toward the surface of the image receptor in a vertical plane, the image receptor itself must be positioned parallel to the teeth of interest in the vertical dimension. Incorrect vertical angulation when utilizing the paralleling technique results in cutting off a portion of the area of interest from the image. When the vertical angulation is excessive (greater than perpendicular to the recording plane of the image receptor), the incisal or occlusal edges of the teeth will most likely be cut off, and when the vertical angulation is inadequate (less than perpendicular to the recording plane of the image receptor), the root apices of the teeth will most likely be cut off (Figure 13–10 ■).

Points of Entry

The point of entry for directing the central rays of the x-ray beam at the image receptor when utilizing the paralleling technique for periapical radiographs may be located using the external aiming device of the image receptor positioner. A round indicator ring will usually have demarcations such as four notches within the round

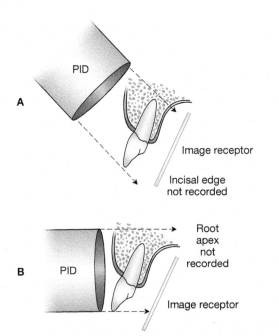

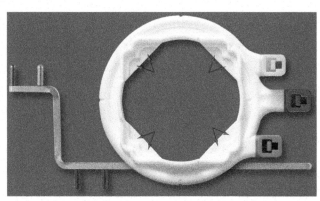

FIGURE 13–11 **Aiming ring to accommodate round and rectangular PID.** Round external aiming ring with notched edge to assist with aligning a rectangular PID. (Courtesy of Dentsply Sirona.)

FIGURE 13–10 **Vertical angulation error–paralleling technique.** (**A**) Excessive vertical angulation results in incisal/occlusal edges being cut off the image. (**B**) Inadequate vertical angulation results in the apices being cut off the image.

edge of the ring to assist with aligning the four corners of a rectangular PID (Figure 13–11 ■). Without an external indicator, care should be taken to center the image receptor within the beam of x-radiation. Use the portion of the holder, or biteblock, that extends from the oral cavity to estimate the center of the image receptor. Incorrect point

of entry, or not centering the image receptor within the x-ray beam, will result in conecut error (see Figures 18–8 and 18–9).

The Periapical Examination: Paralleling Technique

Figures 13–12 ■ through 13–19 ■ illustrate the precise positions and the required angulations for each of the periapical radiographs in a basic 14-image full mouth series utilizing the paralleling technique. See Table 13–2 for a summary of the four basic steps of the technique—placement, vertical angulation, horizontal angulation, and point of entry.

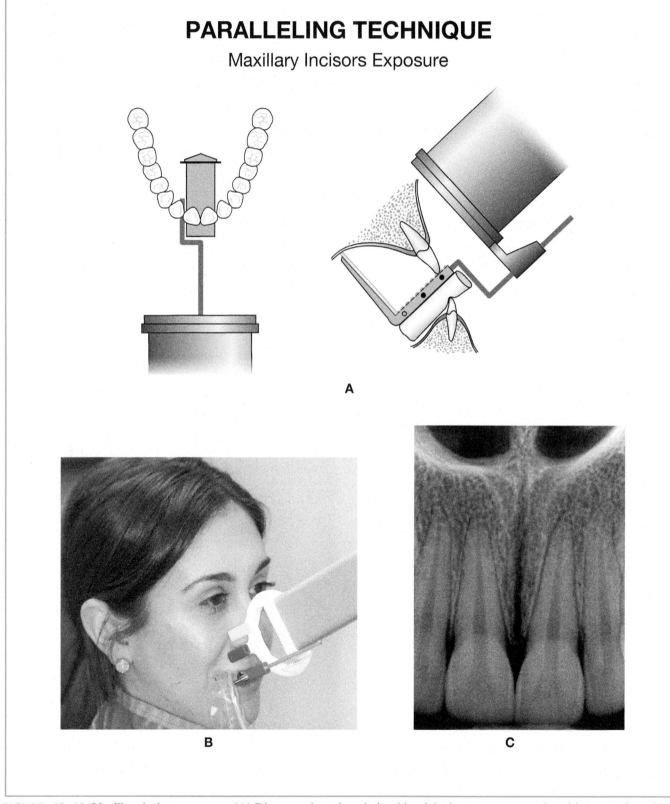

PARALLELING TECHNIQUE
Maxillary Incisors Exposure

A

B

C

FIGURE 13–12 **Maxillary incisors exposure.** (**A**) Diagrams show the relationship of the image receptor and positioner, teeth, and PID. As in all anterior regions, the image receptor is positioned with the long dimension vertically. Image receptor is parallel to the teeth with the biteblock inserted to its full length to position the image receptor back toward the region of the first molars to achieve parallelism with the long axes of the incisors. A sterile cotton roll may be placed on the biteblock on the opposite side from the image receptor to help stabilize the placement if needed. (**B**) Patient showing position of image receptor positioner and 16 inch (41 cm) rectangular PID. (**C**) Maxillary incisors radiograph.

PARALLELING TECHNIQUE
Mandibular Incisors Exposure

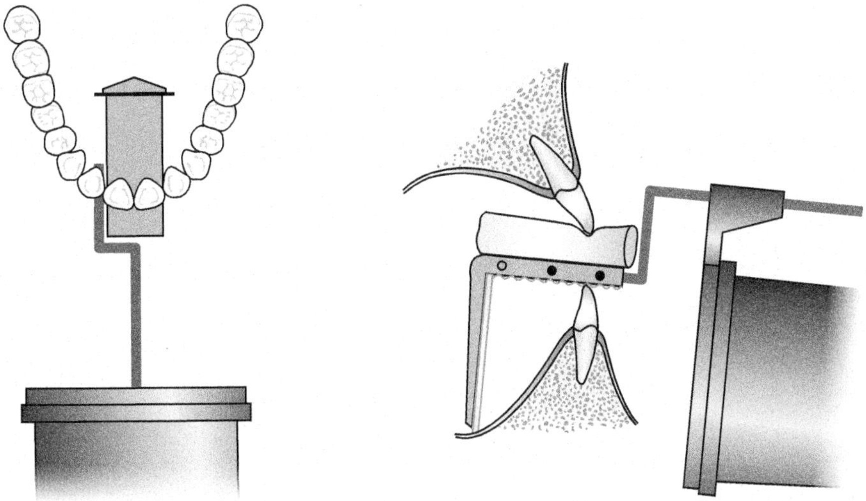

FIGURE 13–13 Mandibular incisors exposure. (A) Diagrams show the relationship of the image receptor and positioner, teeth, and PID. As in all anterior regions, the image receptor is positioned with the long dimension vertically. Image receptor is parallel to the teeth. A sterile cotton roll may be placed on the biteblock on the opposite side from the image receptor to help stabilize the placement if needed. This will aid in directing the biteblock down into position when the opposing teeth occlude. **(B)** Patient showing position of image receptor positioner and 16 inch (41 cm) rectangular PID. **(C)** Mandibular incisors radiograph.

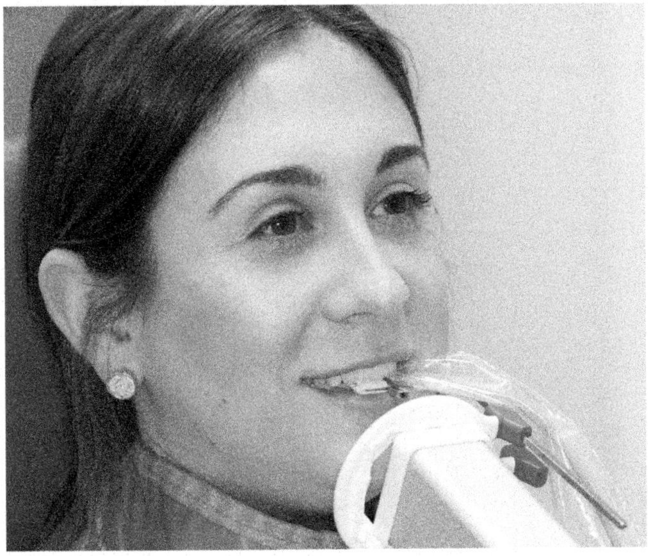

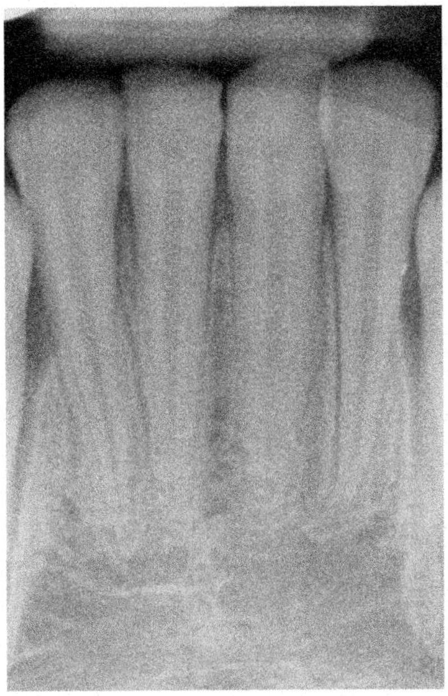

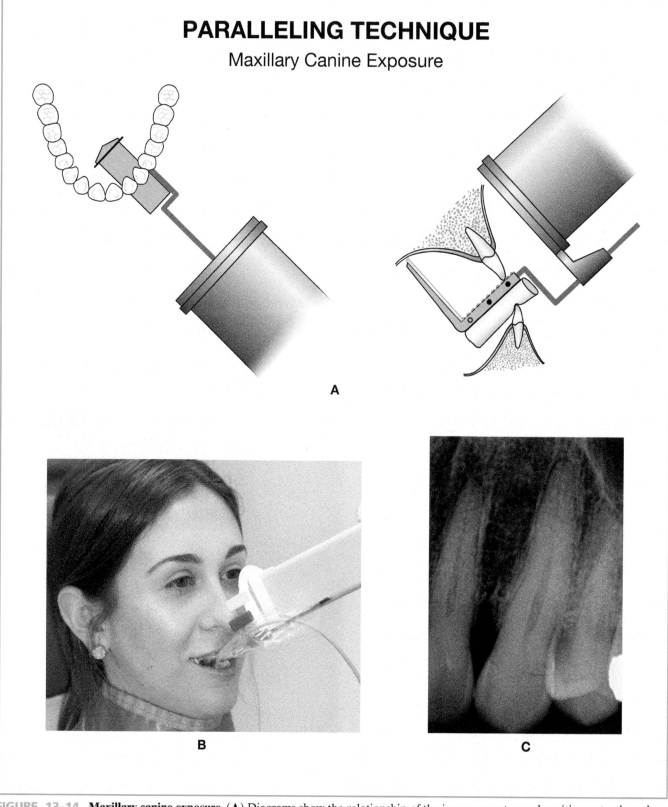

PARALLELING TECHNIQUE
Maxillary Canine Exposure

A

B

C

FIGURE 13–14 **Maxillary canine exposure.** (**A**) Diagrams show the relationship of the image receptor and positioner, teeth, and PID. As in all anterior regions, the image receptor is positioned with the long dimension vertically. Image receptor is parallel to the teeth with the biteblock inserted to its full length to position the image receptor up into the midline of the palate to take advantage of the highest point and achieve parallelism with the long axis of the canine. A sterile cotton roll may be placed on the biteblock on the opposite side from the image receptor to help stabilize the placement if needed. (**B**) Patient showing position of image receptor positioner and 16 inch (41 cm) rectangular PID. (**C**) Maxillary canine radiograph.

PARALLELING TECHNIQUE
Mandibular Canine Exposure

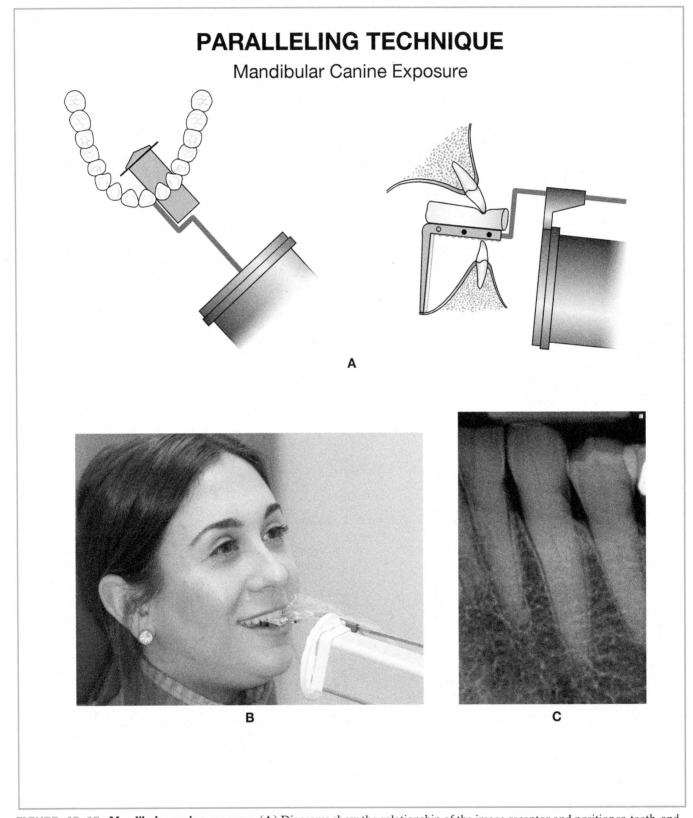

A

B

C

FIGURE 13–15 **Mandibular canine exposure. (A)** Diagrams show the relationship of the image receptor and positioner, teeth, and PID. As in all anterior regions, the image receptor is positioned with the long dimension vertically. Image receptor is parallel to the teeth. A sterile cotton roll may be placed on the biteblock on the opposite side from the image receptor to help stabilize the placement if needed. This will aid in directing the biteblock down into position when the opposing teeth occlude. **(B)** Patient showing position of image receptor positioner and 16 inch (41 cm) rectangular PID. **(C)** Mandibular canine radiograph.

PARALLELING TECHNIQUE
Maxillary Premolar Exposure

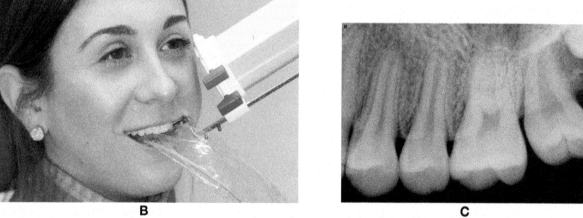

FIGURE 13–16 **Maxillary premolar exposure.** (**A**) Diagrams show the relationship of image receptor and positioner, teeth, and PID. As in all posterior regions, the image receptor is positioned with the long dimension horizontally. Image receptor is parallel to the teeth with the biteblock inserted to its full length to position the image receptor up into the midline of the palate to take advantage of the highest point and achieve parallelism with the long axes of the premolars. A sterile cotton roll may be placed on the biteblock on the opposite side from the image receptor to help stabilize the placement if needed. (**B**) Patient showing position of image receptor positioner and 16 inch (41 cm) rectangular PID. (**C**) Maxillary premolar radiograph.

PARALLELING TECHNIQUE
Mandibular Premolar Exposure

A

B

C

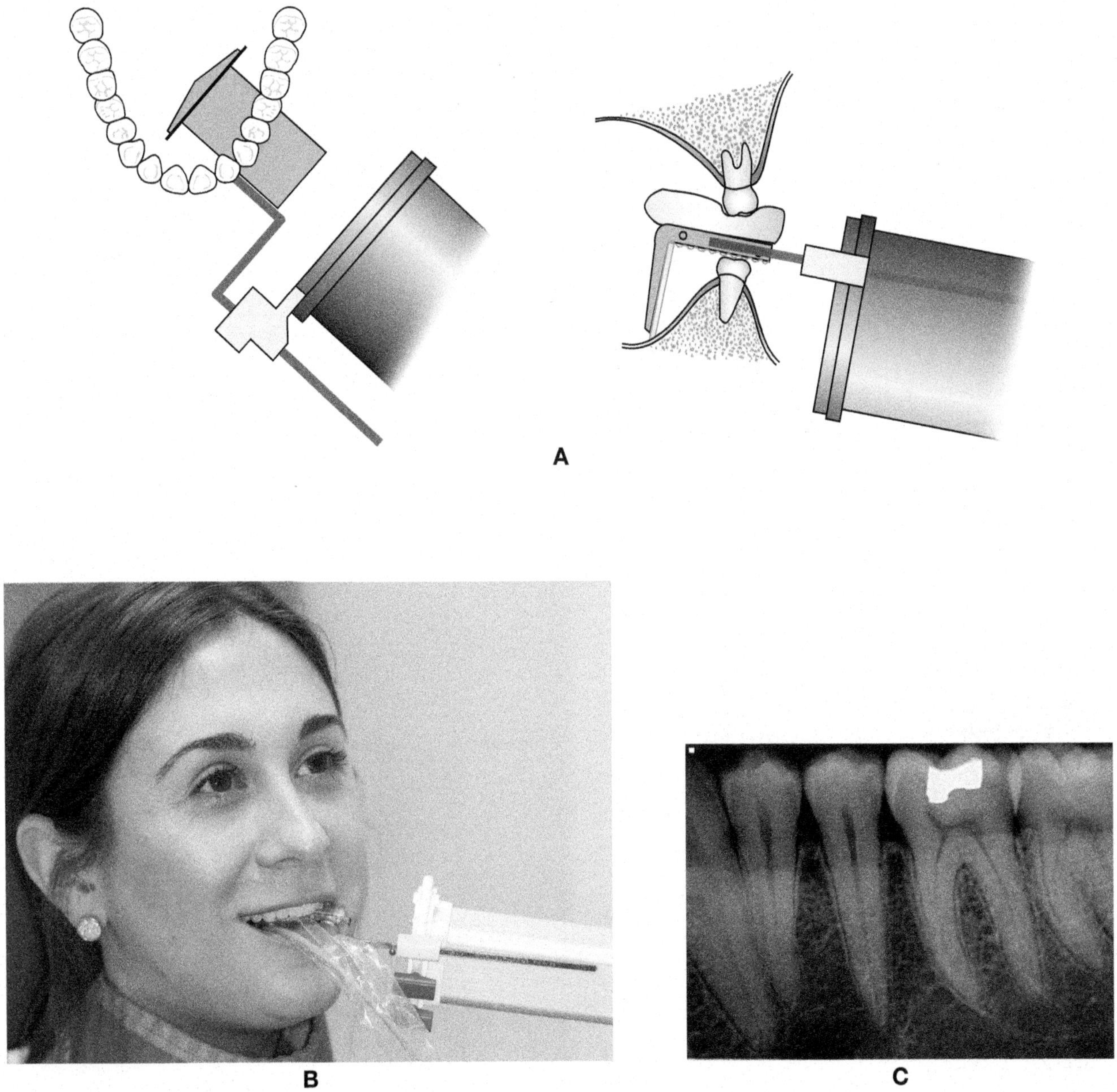

FIGURE 13–17 **Mandibular premolar exposure.** (**A**) Diagrams show the relationship of the image receptor and positioner, teeth, and PID. As in all posterior regions, the image receptor is positioned with the long dimension horizontally. Image receptor is parallel to the teeth. A sterile cotton roll may be placed on the biteblock on the opposite side from the image receptor to help stabilize the placement if needed. This will aid in directing the biteblock down into position when the opposing teeth occlude. (**B**) Patient showing position of image receptor positioner and 16 inch (41 cm) rectangular PID. (**C**) Mandibular premolar radiograph.

PARALLELING TECHNIQUE
Maxillary Molar Exposure

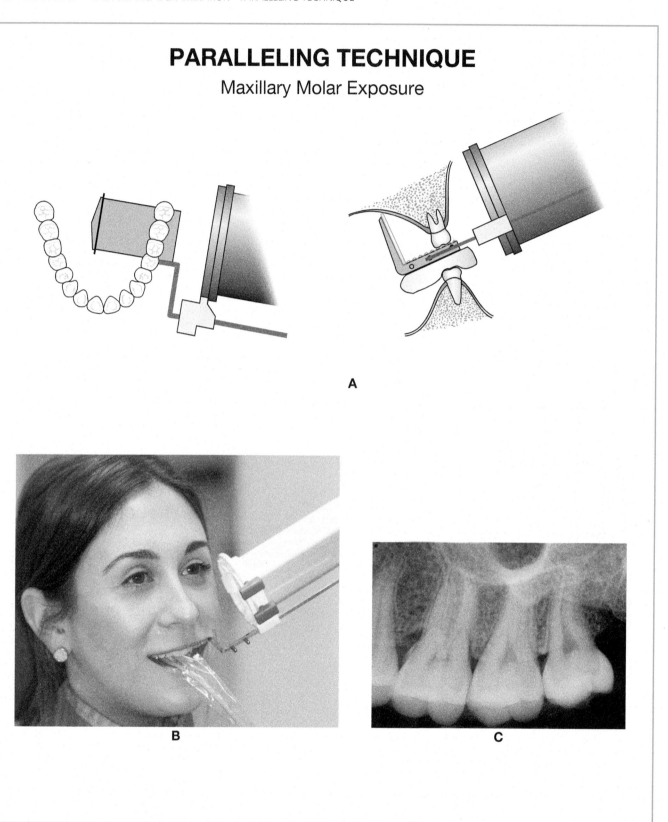

A

B

C

FIGURE 13–18 **Maxillary molar exposure. (A)** Diagrams show the relationship of the image receptor and positioner, teeth, and PID. As in all posterior regions, the image receptor is positioned with the long dimension horizontally. Image receptor is parallel to the teeth with the biteblock inserted to its full length to position the image receptor up into the midline of the palate to take advantage of the highest point and achieve parallelism with the long axes of the molars. A sterile cotton roll may be placed on the biteblock on the opposite side from the image receptor to help stabilize the placement if needed. **(B)** Patient showing position of image receptor positioner and 16 inch (41 cm) rectangular PID. **(C)** Maxillary molar radiograph.

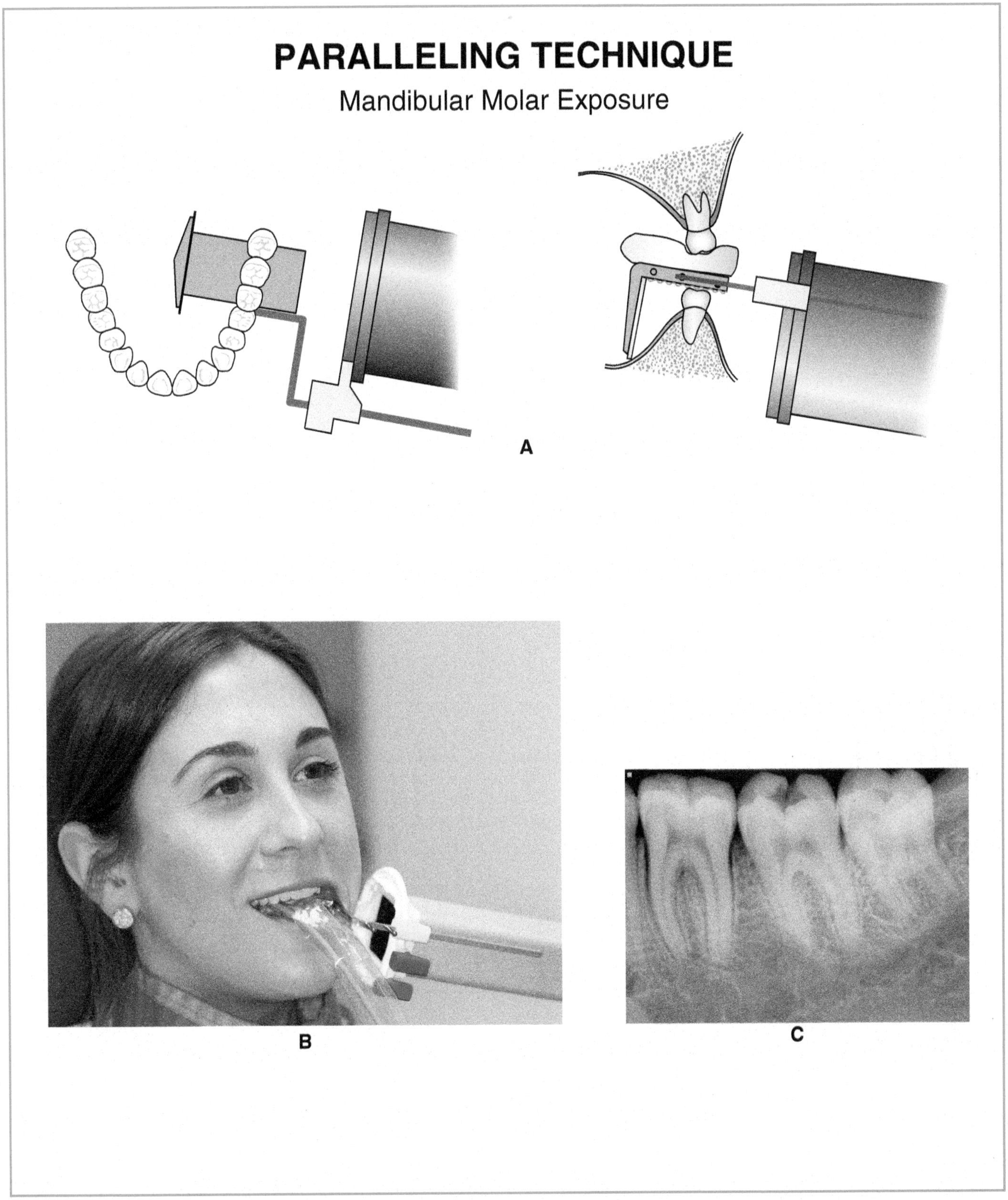

PARALLELING TECHNIQUE
Mandibular Molar Exposure

A

B

C

FIGURE 13–19 **Mandibular molar exposure.** (**A**) Diagrams show the relationship of the image receptor and positioner, teeth, and PID. As in all posterior regions, the image receptor is positioned with the long dimension horizontally. Image receptor is parallel to the teeth. A sterile cotton roll may be placed on the biteblock on the opposite side from the image receptor to help stabilize the placement if needed. This will aid in directing the biteblock down into position when the opposing teeth occlude. (**B**) Patient showing position of image receptor positioner and 16 inch (41 cm) rectangular PID. (**C**) Mandibular molar radiograph.

REVIEW—Chapter summary

The paralleling technique is the technique of choice when exposing periapical radiographs because of its ability to produce superior, diagnostic-quality radiographs. The paralleling technique satisfies two key shadow casting principles—an image receptor is placed parallel to the long axes of the teeth, and the central rays of the x-ray beam are directed perpendicular to both the recording plane of the image receptor and the long axes of the teeth. A long PID (16 inches/41 cm) compensates for the increased distance between the image receptor and the teeth required to achieve parallelism. A limitation of the paralleling technique is that a parallel object–image receptor relationship may be difficult to achieve on some patients.

Because the image receptor must be positioned farther from the teeth to achieve parallelism, an image receptor positioner or holder with a long biteblock and L-shaped backing is required. Image receptor positioners are readily available in sets with multiple parts that must be assembled to accommodate different regions of the oral cavity, and are designed for use with the paralleling or the bisecting technique or may be modified to use with both techniques. A positioner with an external aiming device, usually an indicator ring attached to an extension arm, assists in determining the correct horizontal and vertical angulations and with determining the precise point of entry if positioned correctly with the patient securely biting down on the biteblock extension. Round indicator rings have demarcations such as notched corners to allow

for aligning and centering a rectangular PID. To rely on the positioner's external aiming device, the image receptor must be positioned parallel to the long axes of the teeth (in the vertical dimension) and parallel to the embrasure of two predetermined teeth (in the horizontal dimension).

If an image receptor positioner without an external aiming device is used, the horizontal angulation is determined by directing the central rays of the x-ray beam perpendicular to the recording plane of the image receptor through the mean tangent of the embrasures between the teeth of interest. Specific embrasures are selected because of the likelihood that if the image receptor is parallel to these spaces and the central rays of the x-ray beam are directed through these spaces, then the rest of the spaces should line up for correct horizontal angulation. Vertical angulation is determined by directing the central rays of the x-ray beam perpendicular to the long axes of the teeth and perpendicular to the recording plane of the image receptor. The point of entry is determined by using that portion of the biteblock that extends beyond the oral cavity to direct the central rays of the x-ray beam to the center of the image receptor.

The four basic steps to exposing a periapical radiograph are placement, vertical angulation, horizontal angulation, and point of entry. Step-by-step illustrated instructions for exposing a full mouth series of periapical radiographs utilizing the paralleling techniques are presented.

RECALL—Study questions

1. What shadow casting principle is NOT likely to be met when utilizing the paralleling technique?
   a. Radiation should strike the object (tooth) and image receptor perpendicularly.
   b. Object (tooth) should be as far as practical from the target.
   c. Object (tooth) and image receptor should be parallel to each other.
   d. Object (tooth) and image receptor should be as close as possible to each other.

2. To compensate for the increased object–image receptor distance needed to achieve parallelism, the target–image receptor distance should be
   a. increased.
   b. decreased.

3. What PID length provides the best quality radiographic images when utilizing the paralleling technique?
   a. 8 inches (20.5 cm)
   b. 12 inches (30 cm)
   c. 16 inches (41 cm)

4. Which of the following is NOT an advantage of the paralleling technique?
   a. Produces images with minimal dimensional distortion.
   b. Minimizes superimposition of adjacent structures.
   c. Satisfies more shadow casting principles.
   d. Easy technique for children to tolerate.

5. The most important reason for using an image receptor positioner when utilizing the paralleling technique is to stabilize the image receptor in a position
   a. at a right angle to the teeth.
   b. at a longitudinal relationship to the teeth.
   c. parallel to the teeth.
   d. perpendicular to the teeth.

6. Image receptor positioners designed for use with the paralleling technique should have a
   a. short biteblock and L-shaped backing.
   b. long biteblock and L-shaped backing.
   c. short biteblock and no backing.
   d. long biteblock and no backing.

7. Which of the following would be a modification to a paralleling technique image receptor positioner for use with the bisecting technique?
   a. Shorten the long bite block.
   b. Ignore the color coding when assembling the holder.
   c. Use a sterile cotton roll to change the angulation.
   d. Remove the indicator aiming device.

8. Lining the image receptor up behind the distal half of the canine to include the first and second premolars and mesial half of the first molar describes the placement for which of the following periapical radiographs?
   a. Central incisors
   b. Canine
   c. Premolar
   d. Molar

9. To determine the horizontal angulation for the maxillary molar periapical radiograph, the central rays of the x-ray beam should be directed at the image receptor perpendicularly through the embrasures of the
   a. first and second molars.
   b. second premolar and first molar.
   c. first and second premolars.
   d. canine and first premolar.

10. To determine the horizontal angulation for the mandibular premolar periapical radiograph, the central rays of the x-ray beam should be directed at the image receptor perpendicularly through the embrasures of the
   a. first and second molars.
   b. second premolar and first molar.
   c. first and second premolars.
   d. canine and first premolar.

11. Directing the central rays perpendicular to the plane of the image receptor and perpendicular to the long axes of the teeth describes which step of the paralleling technique?
   a. Placement
   b. Vertical angulation
   c. Horizontal angulation
   d. Point of entry

12. Cutting off the root apex portion of the image on a periapical radiograph results from
   a. excessive horizontal angulation.
   b. inadequate horizontal angulation.
   c. excessive vertical angulation.
   d. inadequate vertical angulation.

REFLECT—Case study

You have recently accepted a position in a general practice dental office. This week you notice that the image receptor positioner for exposing a full mouth survey is the one pictured in Figure 13–7. You have always used the film-holding device pictured in Figure 13–5, and the new holder is unfamiliar to you. Based on what you have learned about image receptor holders designed for use with the paralleling technique, answer the following questions:

1. With which technique is the new positioner designed to be used? How can you tell?

2. How is the new positioner similar to the one you have been using? How is it different?

3. Which positioner would it be best to know how to use? Why?

4. What are the advantages/limitations of the new holder?

5. What are the advantages/limitations of the positioner you have been using?

6. What is your recommendation for this practice? Should they continue to use this positioner, or should they purchase the positioner you are familiar with? Explain your answers.

RELATE—Laboratory application

For a comprehensive laboratory practice exercise on this topic, see Thomson, E. M., & Bruhn, A. M. (2018). *Exercises in oral radiography techniques: A laboratory manual* (4th ed.). Hoboken, NJ: Pearson. Chapter 4, "Periapical radiographs—paralleling technique."

RESOURCES

Eastman Kodak Company. (2002). *Successful intraoral radiography.* Rochester, NY: Author.

White, S. C., & Pharoah, M. J. (2014). Intraoral projections. *Oral radiology: Principles and interpretation* (7th ed.). St. Louis, MO: Elsevier.

Williamson, G. F. (2014). Intraoral radiography: Principles, techniques and error correction. Retrieved from DentalCare. com website: http://www.dentalcare.com/en-US/dental-education/continuing-education/ce137/ce137.aspx?ModuleName=coursecontent&PartID=2&SectionID=-1

Visit www.pearsonhighered.com/healthprofessionsresources to access the student resources that accompany this book. Simply select Dental Hygiene from the choice of disciplines. Find this book and you will find the complementary study tools created for this specific title.

14

The Periapical Examination— Bisecting Technique

OBJECTIVES

Following successful completion of this chapter, you should be able to:

1. Define the key terms.
2. Discuss the principles of the bisecting technique.
3. List the advantages and limitations of the bisecting technique.
4. Identify, assemble, and position image receptor holders for use with the bisecting technique and distinguish these holders from those used with the paralleling technique.
5. Explain the importance of achieving accurate horizontal and vertical angulation in obtaining quality diagnostic radiographs using the bisecting technique.
6. List the recommended predetermined vertical angulation settings used with the bisecting technique.
7. Identify vertical angulation errors unique to the bisecting technique.
8. Locate facial landmarks used for determining the points of entry with the bisecting technique.
9. Demonstrate image receptor positioning, horizontal and vertical angulation, and points of entry for maxillary and mandibular periapical exposures using the bisecting technique.

KEY TERMS

Bisector
Elongated image

Foreshortened image

Isometric triangle

Introduction

Because it satisfies fewer shadow cast principles (see Chapter 12), the bisecting technique is less likely to produce superior diagnostic quality radiographs. However, some situations and conditions make the use of the paralleling technique difficult. When irregularities or obstructions of the oral tissues and the curvature of the palate prevent a parallel image receptor-to-long axes of the teeth placement, an acceptable diagnostic-quality radiograph may be obtained utilizing the bisecting technique (Table 14–1 ■). A radiographer who possesses a working knowledge of both the paralleling and the bisecting techniques will be prepared to meet and overcome conditions that challenge the ability to produce diagnostic radiographs. Although the bisecting technique is not often recommended because images produced contain inherent dimensional distortion, careful attention to the steps of the technique can produce acceptable results when needed. This chapter presents step-by-step instructions for exposing a full mouth series of periapical radiographs using the bisecting technique.

Fundamentals of Bisecting Technique

The bisecting principle is applied when the image receptor is not, or cannot, be placed parallel to the long axes of the teeth. This is often the case with children as their anatomy is smaller, with adults who have a shallow palatal vault or a large torus present, or when edentulous regions prohibit stabilizing the image receptor in place. If the image receptor is not positioned parallel to the long axes of teeth, it will not be possible to direct the central rays of the x-ray beam appropriately perpendicular to the long axes of the teeth and simultaneously perpendicular to the plane of the image receptor—two important shadow casting principles for producing an image free of magnification and distortion. It would seem that the central rays of the x-ray beam could either be directed perpendicular to the long axes of the teeth OR perpendicularly to the plane of the image receptor, but not perpendicular to both at the same time. So, the bisecting technique allows a radiographer to cast an accurate shadow representation of a tooth onto the image receptor by directing the central rays of the x-ray beam perpendicularly to a point in between these two planes, at essentially a halfway point. This point is called the imaginary **bisector** and is determined by using the geometric principle of **isometric triangles** (Figure 14–1 ■). Two triangles with the same side lengths and the same angles are said to be isometric to each other. The imaginary angle formed where the long axis of the tooth and the plane of the image receptor meet can be bisected producing two imaginary isometric triangles. First find the long axis of the tooth and then find the long axis of the image receptor as it is placed next to the tooth. After visualizing these two planes, imagine a line, the bisector, which bisects the angle where the long axis of the tooth and the long axis of the image receptor plane meet. The central rays of the x-ray beam are then directed perpendicular to this imaginary bisector to produce a radiographic image that should be reasonably free of magnification and distortion. In practice, this does not always result (see Figure 4–13). The quality of the image is usually compromised, with some dimensional distortion that is inherent when using the bisecting technique. However, meticulously following the steps to determine the correct angles will produce a radiograph from which a diagnosis can be ascertained despite the slight dimensional distortions.

TARGET–IMAGE RECEPTOR DISTANCE A shorter target–image receptor distance will limit magnification and distortion because the long axis of the tooth and the plane of the image receptor are not parallel. The shorter (8 inches/20.5 cm) position-indicating device (PID) facilitates a shorter target–image receptor distance and is generally recommended for use with the bisecting technique. Whereas the paralleling technique is better matched with a longer target–image receptor distance, typically a 12 inch (30 cm) or ideally a 16 inch (41 cm) PID to compensate for the greater object–image receptor distance, the bisecting technique should be matched with a shorter target–image receptor distance, typically an 8 inch (20.5 cm) PID, to compensate for the lack of parallelism between the long axis of the tooth and the plane of the image receptor.

Table 14–1 Advantages and Limitations of the Bisecting Technique

Advantages	Limitations
• Image receptor placement may be easier with certain patients: children, adults with small oral cavities, low or shallow palatal vaults, or presence of large tori; patients with sensitive oral mucosa or hypersensitive gag reflex, edentulous regions • Short PID has potential to be easy to maneuver and stabilize (8 inch/20.5 cm PID must be used with bisecting technique to minimize distortion)	• Produces images with dimensional distortion (some elongation or foreshortening will occur even when technique is performed correctly) • Often superimposes adjacent structures (necessary vertical angle increase often causes shadow of zygomatic process of maxilla to be superimposed over molar roots in maxillary regions) • Estimating location of imaginary bisector requires skilled radiographer • Patient radiation dose may be increased when using short PID (8 inches/20.5 cm)

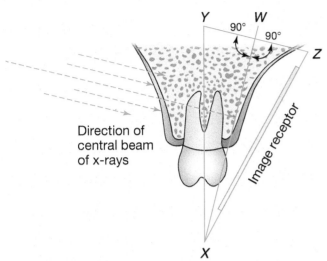

FIGURE 14–1 Rule of isometry applied to the bisecting technique. Line XY passes through the long axis of the tooth while the image receptor is positioned along line XZ. The central beam of radiation is directed perpendicularly through the apical area of the tooth toward the bisector XW. Because triangles WXY and WXZ are equal, the shadow image cast on the image receptor will be approximately equal to the length of the actual tooth, provided that the bisector line is correctly estimated.

OBJECT–IMAGE RECEPTOR DISTANCE It is important to note that when the image receptor is placed close to the teeth in both the anterior and the posterior regions of the maxilla and in the anterior region of the mandible, the bisecting technique must be utilized to compensate for the lack of parallelism between the image receptor and the long axes of the teeth. It is at this point that a radiographer has two choices: (1) reposition the image receptor further away from the teeth to achieve a parallel relationship, or (2) employ the bisecting technique. Ideally, an image receptor should be repositioned to achieve a parallel relationship, but if this is not possible, a skilled radiographer can obtain a reasonably

Practice Point

To aid in estimating the imaginary bisector, utilize the two *visible* planes: the teeth and the image receptor. Looking at the teeth, locate the long axes. Then align the x-ray beam to intersect the long axes of the teeth perpendicularly. Study the PID and make a mental note of this angle. Next look at the image receptor. Note the plane of the image receptor as it is placed against the teeth. Then shift the PID so that the x-ray beam is aligned to intersect the plane of the image receptor perpendicularly. Note this angle while recalling the angle at which the x-ray beam intersected the long axes of the teeth. If needed, repeat this process, shifting the PID to allow the x-ray beam to intersect the long axes of the teeth and then the image receptor plane perpendicularly until a position halfway in between these two angles can be estimated. This halfway point is the imaginary bisector.

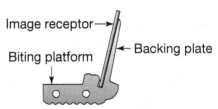

FIGURE 14–2 Bisecting technique biteblock. A 105° angle backing plate with short biteblock allows for close placement of the image receptor to the teeth.

diagnostic image using the bisecting technique. It should be noted that the mandibular posterior region, which includes the molars and premolars, usually allows for placement of the image receptor close to the teeth and still maintains a parallel relationship. In these regions of the oral cavity, the paralleling technique may be used successfully even with this short object–image receptor distance (see Figure 13–8).

Holding the Periapical Image Receptor in Position

Image receptor positioners or holders designed for use with the bisecting technique typically have a short biteblock and lack the L-shaped support backing of positioners used with the paralleling technique. If a support backing is present, it will be slanted to about 105 degrees (Figure 14–2 ■). Using this type of holder allows an image receptor to be placed close to the lingual surface of the teeth and is therefore unlikely to be parallel to the long axes of the teeth.

There are different styles available of image receptor positioners for use with the bisecting technique that can be used to position film, phosphor plates, or digital sensors (Figures 14–3 ■ and 14–4 ■). As noted in Chapter 12, there are paralleling image receptor positioners that can be slightly modified for use with the bisecting technique (see Figure 12–14 and Figure 14–5 ■). Additionally, image receptor positioners for use with the bisecting technique are available with external aiming devices with extension arms and indicator rings (Figure 14–6 ■).

Due to the variety of film, phosphor plate, and digital sensor positioners currently available and that continue to

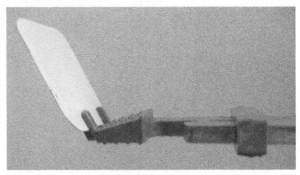

FIGURE 14–3 Image receptor positioner. Short biteblock and 105° angled backing indicate that this holder be paired with the bisecting technique. Note this holder is used with a film packet image receptor.

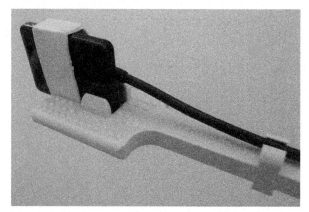

FIGURE 14-4 Image receptor positioner. Short biteblock and lack of L-shaped backing indicate that this holder be paired with the bisecting technique. Note this holder is used with a digital sensor image receptor.

come to market, it is important that a radiographer possess a working knowledge of the bisecting technique to better match the holder with the technique for optimal results.

Although a radiographer should refer to the manufacturer's instructions for use, important key points regarding image receptor positioners are to be sure that:

- The patient bites down on the biteblock as close to the teeth as necessary. This will most likely not position the image receptor parallel to the long axes of the teeth. The exception to this rule is in the mandibular premolar and molar regions, where the image receptor can be close to the teeth and still remain parallel because of the nearly vertical position of the mandibular premolars and the slightly inward inclination of the mandibular molars (see Figure 13–8).
- The patient bites down on the biteblock firmly enough to hold the image receptor in place. A sterilized cotton roll may be placed on the opposite side of the biteblock to provide stabilization and add to patient comfort (see Figure 13–9).
- If the image receptor positioner has an external aiming device, the indicator ring is slid all the way down the extension arm of the device to be as close to the patient's skin as possible without touching the patient.

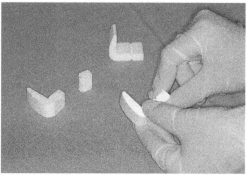

FIGURE 14-5 Image receptor positioner. Bite extension required for use with the paralleling technique may be broken off for use with the bisecting technique.

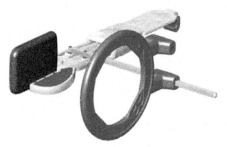

FIGURE 14-6 Image receptor positioner for use with the bisecting technique. Note the external aiming device with extension arm and indicator ring. (Courtesy of Dentsply Sirona.)

- The open end of the PID is aligned to the indicator ring as close as possible without touching to achieve correct horizontal and vertical angulations and correct point of entry.

Horizontal and Vertical Angulation

Horizontal Angulation

The steps for determining correct horizontal angulation are the same for both the bisecting and paralleling techniques. First, position the image receptor parallel to the interproximal space, or embrasure. Locate and use two predetermined teeth to achieve this. Next, the horizontal angulation is achieved by directing the central rays of the x-ray beam perpendicular to the mean tangent, or curvature of the arch, through the contact points of these teeth (Table 14–2 ■; see pages 182–183). The particular embrasures listed for each exposure have been chosen because of the likelihood that if the image receptor is parallel to this space and the central rays of the x-ray beam are directed through this space, then the rest of the spaces should line up for a correct exposure, free of horizontal angulation errors. The central rays must be directed appropriately to avoid overlapping adjacent teeth on the resultant image.

Vertical Angulation

With the bisecting technique the central rays of the x-ray beam cannot be directed perpendicular to both the long axes of the teeth and the plane of the image receptor simultaneously. When utilizing the bisecting technique, the correct vertical angulation is achieved by directing the central rays of the x-ray beam perpendicular to the imaginary bisector between the long axes of the teeth and the plane of the image receptor. If a patient is seated with correct head positioning, the occlusal plane parallel to the floor, and the midsaggital plane perpendicular to the floor, predetermined vertical settings may be utilized to position the PID at the correct vertical angulation (see Table 14–2). It is important to check that the occlusal plane of the arch being radiographed is parallel to the floor. Incorrect vertical angulation when utilizing the bisecting technique results in an image that appears foreshortened or elongated. When the vertical angulation is excessive (greater than perpendicular

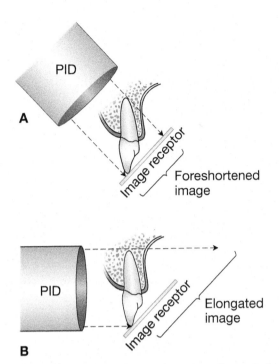

FIGURE 14–7 Vertical angulation error—bisecting technique. (**A**) Excessive vertical angulation results in a foreshortened image. (**B**) Inadequate vertical angulation results in an elongated image.

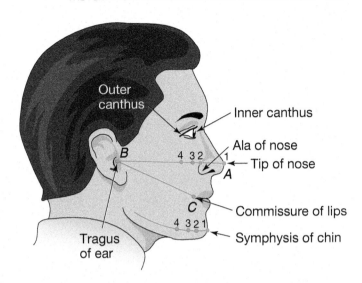

FIGURE 14–8 Points of entry. Facial landmarks provide a reference for positioning the PID and directing the central rays of the x-ray beam. Patient must be seated upright with midsagittal plane perpendicular to the floor and occlusal plane parallel to the floor to use these landmarks accurately. A–B represents the ala–tragus line landmark. Note that these numbers indicate the points of entry for each of the projections listed in Table 14–2.

to the imaginary bisector) a **foreshortened image** will result, and when the vertical angulation is inadequate (less than perpendicular to the imaginary bisector), the result is an **elongated image** (Figure 14–7 ■). Vertical angulation error is further explained in Chapter 18.

Points of Entry

An image receptor must be centered within the beam of x-radiation to avoid conecut error. The central rays of the x-ray beam should be directed through the apices of the teeth of interest. When utilizing the bisecting technique, if a patient is seated with the correct head position, the point

of entry may be estimated with the use of recommended landmarks (see Table 14–2 and Figure 14–8 ■).

The Periapical Examination: Bisecting Technique

Figures 14–9 ■ through 14–16 ■ illustrate the precise image receptor positions and the required angulations for each of the periapical radiographs in a basic 14–film full mouth series utilizing the bisecting technique. See Table 14–2 for a summary of the four basic steps of the technique—placement, vertical angulation, horizontal angulation, and point of entry.

Table 14–2 Summary of Steps for Acquiring Periapical Radiographs—Bisecting Technique

Periapical Radiograph	Placement	Vertical Angulation*	Horizontal Angulation	Point of Entry*
Maxillary incisors (image receptor size 1 or 2) (Figure 14–9)	Center image receptor to line up behind central and lateral incisors; if using size 2 image receptor, include mesial halves of canines Place image receptor as close as possible to lingual surfaces of incisors, parallel to left and right central incisor embrasure	Direct central rays toward imaginary bisector between long axes of incisors and plane of image receptor in vertical dimension at +40°	Direct central rays perpendicular to image receptor through left and right central incisor embrasure	Center image receptor within x-ray beam by directing central rays at a point near tip of nose (Figure 14–8 maxillary point 1)
Maxillary canine (image receptor size 1 or 2) (Figure 14–10)	Center image receptor to line up behind canine; include distal half of lateral incisor and mesial half of first premolar Place image receptor as close as possible to lingual surface of canine, parallel to mesial and distal line angles of canine	Direct central rays toward imaginary bisector between long axis of canine and plane of image receptor in vertical dimension at +45°	Direct central rays perpendicular to image receptor at center of canine	Center image receptor within x-ray beam by directing central rays at root of canine, at ala of nose (Figure 14–8 maxillary point 2)
Maxillary premolar (image receptor size 2) (Figure 14–11)	Align anterior edge of image receptor to line up behind distal half of canine; include first and second premolars and mesial half of first molar Place image receptor as close as possible to lingual surfaces of premolars, parallel to first and second premolar embrasure	Direct central rays toward imaginary bisector between long axes of premolars and plane of image receptor in vertical dimension at +30°	Direct central rays perpendicular to image receptor through first and second premolar embrasure	Center image receptor within x-ray beam by directing central rays at a point on ala–tragus line directly below pupil of eye (Figure 14–8 maxillary point 3)
Maxillary molar (image receptor size 2) (Figure 14–12)	Align anterior edge of image receptor to line up behind distal half of second premolar; include first, second, and third molars Place image receptor as close as possible to lingual surfaces of molars, parallel to first and second molar embrasure	Direct central rays toward imaginary bisector between long axes of molars and plane of image receptor in vertical dimension at +20°	Direct central rays perpendicular to image receptor through first and second molar embrasure	Center image receptor within x-ray beam by directing central rays at a point on ala–tragus line directly below outer canthus of eye (Figure 14–8 maxillary point 4)
Mandibular incisors (image receptor size 1 or 2) (Figure 14–13)	Center image receptor to line up behind central and lateral incisors; if using size 2 image receptor, include mesial halves of canines Place image receptor as close as possible to lingual surfaces of incisors, parallel to left and right central incisor embrasure	Direct central rays toward imaginary bisector between long axes of incisors and plane of image receptor in vertical dimension at −15°	Direct central rays perpendicular to image receptor through left and right central incisor embrasure	Center image receptor within x-ray beam by directing central rays at a point in middle of chin (symphysis), 1 inch (2.5 cm) above inferior border of mandible (Figure 14–8 mandibular point 1)

Mandibular canine (image receptor size 1 or 2) (Figure 14–14)	Center image receptor to line up behind canine; include distal half of lateral incisor and mesial half of first premolar. Place image receptor as close as possible to lingual surfaces of canine, parallel to mesial and distal line angles of canine	Direct central rays toward imaginary bisector between long axis of canine and plane of image receptor in vertical dimension at −20°	Direct central rays perpendicular to image receptor at center of canine	Center image receptor within x-ray beam by directing central rays at center of root of canine, 1 inch (2.5 cm) above inferior border of mandible (Figure 14–8 mandibular point 2)
Mandibular premolar (image receptor size 2) (Figure 14–15)	Align anterior edge of image receptor to line up behind distal half of canine; include first and second premolars and mesial half of first molar. Place image receptor as close as possible to lingual surfaces of premolars, parallel to first and second premolar embrasure	Direct central rays toward imaginary bisector between long axes of premolar and plane of image receptor in vertical dimension at −10°	Direct central rays perpendicular to image receptor through first and second premolar embrasure.	Center image receptor within x-ray beam by directing central rays at a point on chin, 1 inch (2.5 cm) above inferior border of mandible, directly below pupil of eye (Figure 14–8 mandibular point 3)
Mandibular molar (image receptor size 2) (Figure 14–16)	Align anterior edge of image receptor to line up behind distal half of second premolar; include first, second, and third molars. Place image receptor as close as possible to lingual surfaces of molars, parallel to first and second molar embrasure	Direct central rays toward imaginary bisector between long axes of molars and plane of image receptor in vertical dimension at −5°	Direct central rays perpendicular to image receptor through first and second molar embrasure	Center image receptor within x-ray beam by directing central rays at a point on chin, 1 inch (2.5 cm) above inferior border of mandible, directly below outer canthus of eye (Figure 14–8 mandibular point 4)

* Patient must be seated in correct position, with occlusal plane of the arch being recorded parallel to the floor and the midsagittal plane perpendicular to the floor.

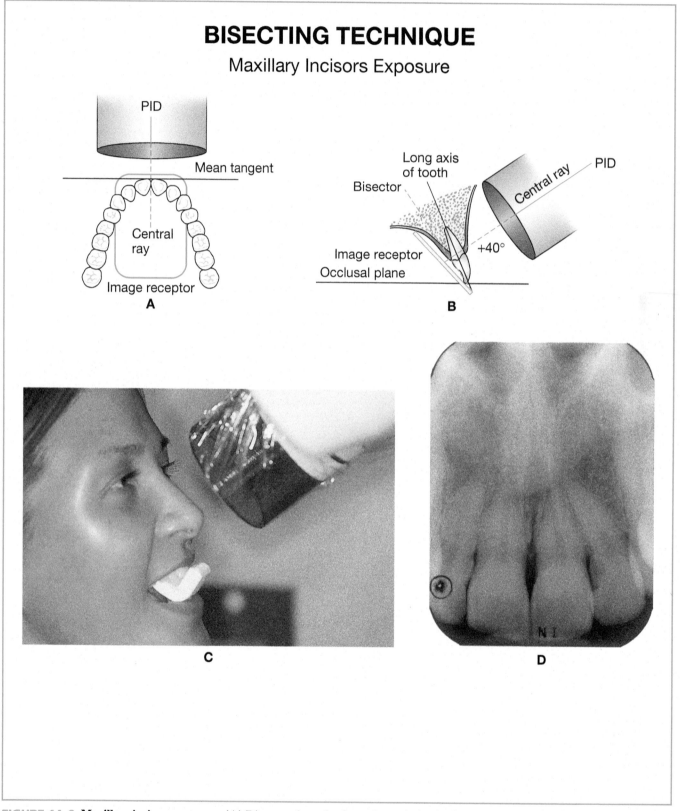

FIGURE 14–9 **Maxillary incisors exposure.** (**A**) Diagram shows horizontal angulation is directed through the central incisors embrasure and perpendicular to the mean tangent. (**B**) Vertical angulation is directed perpendicular to the bisector at approximately +40 degrees with the PID tilted downward. (**C**) Patient showing position of image receptor and positioner, and 8 inch (20.5 cm) circular PID. (**D**) Maxillary incisors radiograph.

BISECTING TECHNIQUE
Maxillary Canine Exposure

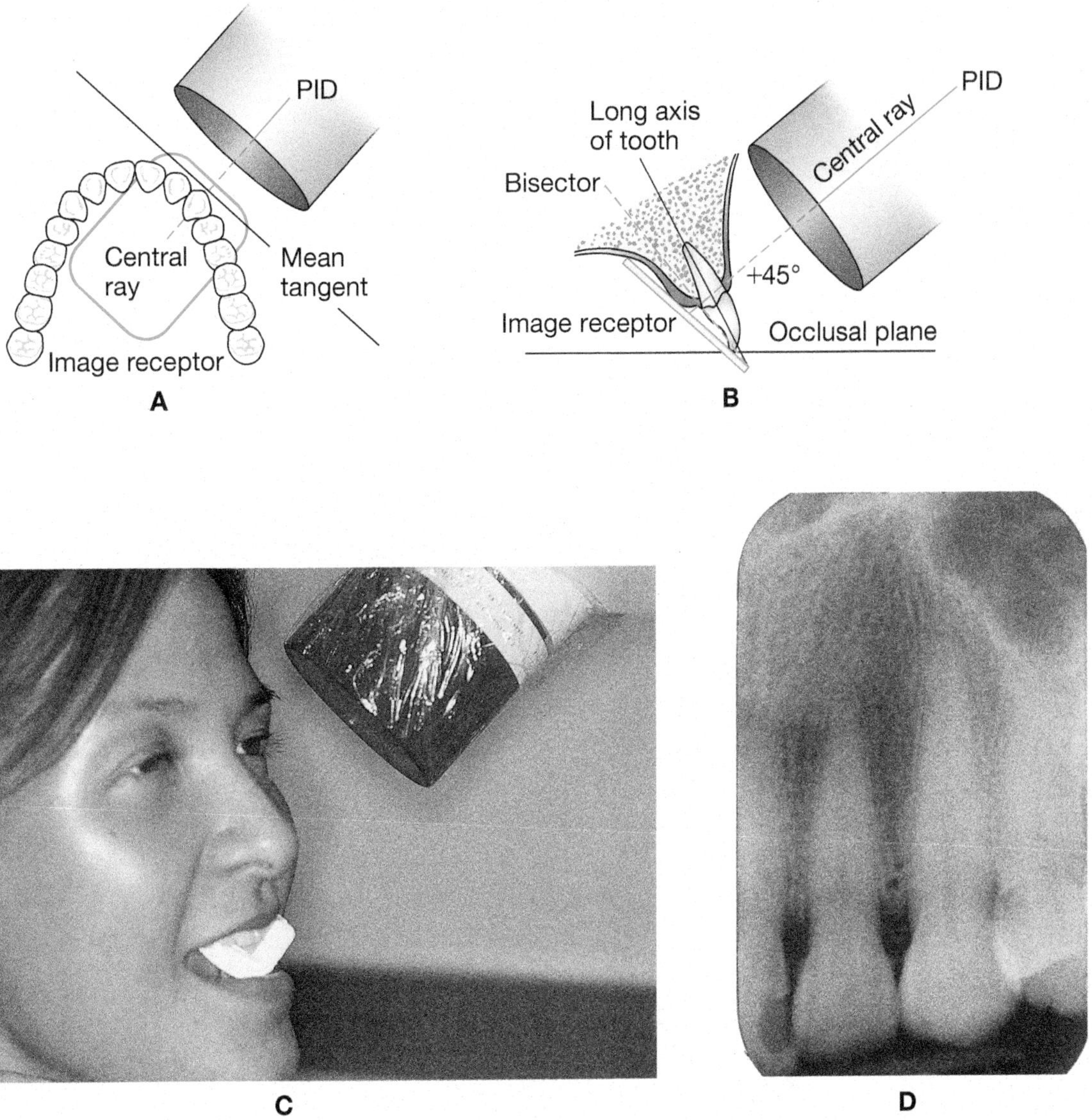

FIGURE 14–10 Maxillary canine exposure. (A) Diagram shows horizontal angulation is directed at the midline of the canine and perpendicular to the mean tangent. **(B)** Vertical angulation is directed perpendicular to the bisector at approximately +45 degrees with the PID tilted downward. **(C)** Patient showing position of image receptor and positioner, and 8 inch (20.5 cm) circular PID. **(D)** Maxillary canine radiograph.

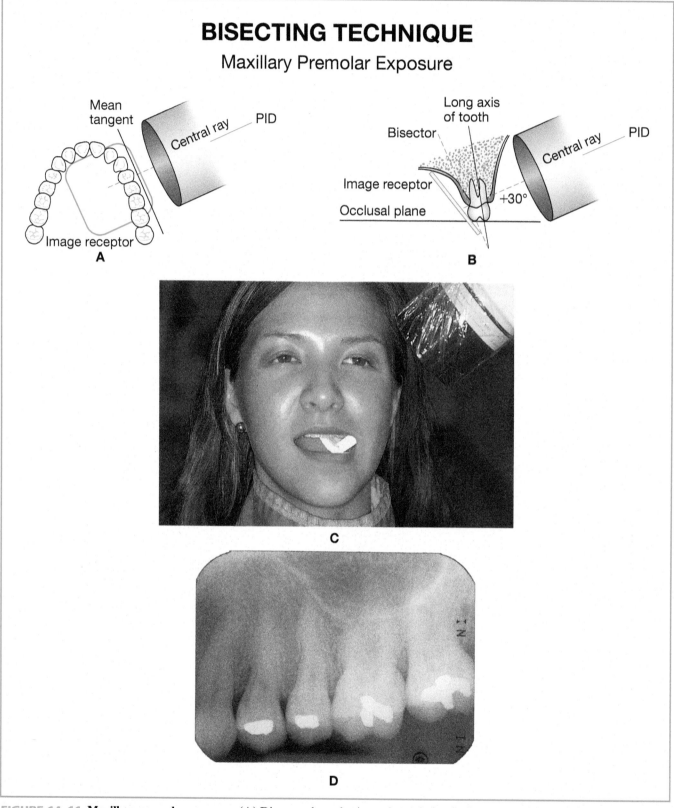

BISECTING TECHNIQUE
Maxillary Premolar Exposure

FIGURE 14–11 Maxillary premolar exposure. (**A**) Diagram shows horizontal angulation is directed through the premolars embrasure and perpendicular to the mean tangent. (**B**) Vertical angulation is directed perpendicular to the bisector at approximately +30 degrees with the PID tilted downward. (**C**) Patient showing position of image receptor and positioner, and 8 inch (20.5 cm) circular PID. (**D**) Maxillary premolar radiograph.

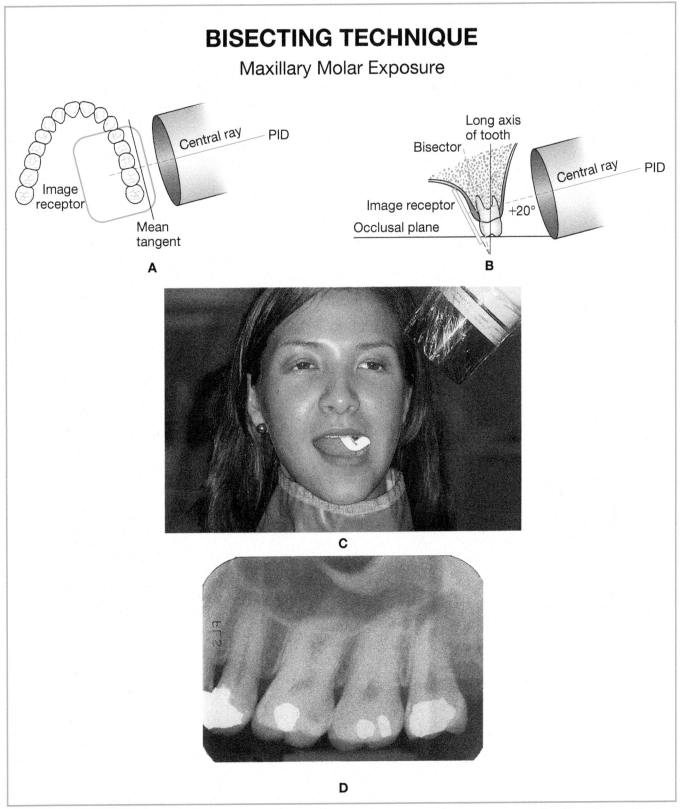

BISECTING TECHNIQUE
Maxillary Molar Exposure

A

B

C

D

FIGURE 14–12 **Maxillary molar exposure.** (**A**) Diagram shows horizontal angulation is directed through the first and second molar embrasure and perpendicular to the mean tangent. (**B**) Vertical angulation is directed perpendicular to the bisector at approximately +20 degrees with the PID tilted downward. (**C**) Patient showing position of image receptor and positioner, and 8 inch (20.5 cm) circular PID. (**D**) Maxillary molar radiograph.

BISECTING TECHNIQUE
Mandibular Incisors Exposure

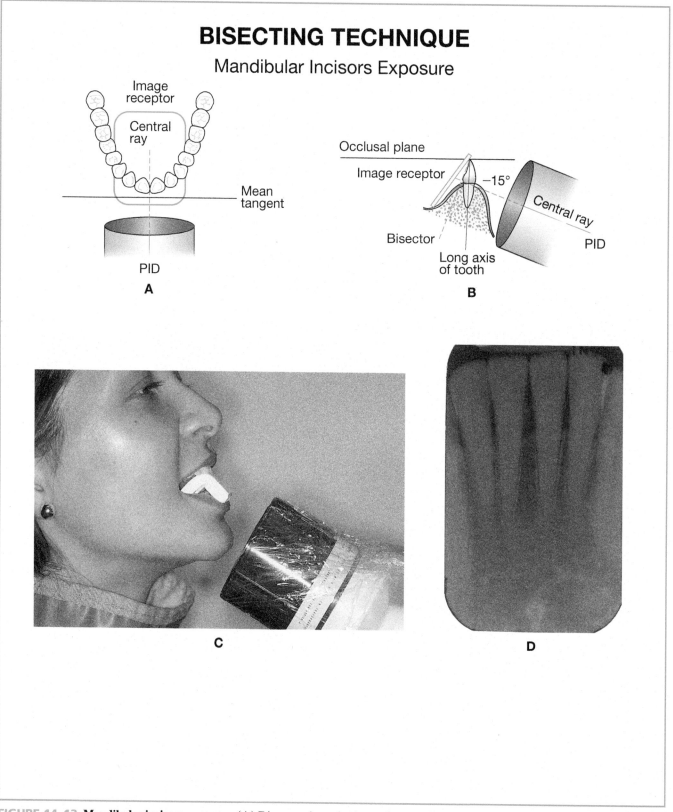

FIGURE 14–13 **Mandibular incisors exposure.** (**A**) Diagram shows horizontal angulation is directed through the central incisors embrasure and perpendicular to the mean tangent. (**B**) Vertical angulation is directed perpendicular to the bisector at approximately −15° with the PID tilted upward. (**C**) Patient showing position of image receptor and positioner, and 8 inch (20.5 cm) circular PID. (**D**) Mandibular incisors radiograph.

BISECTING TECHNIQUE
Mandibular Canine Exposure

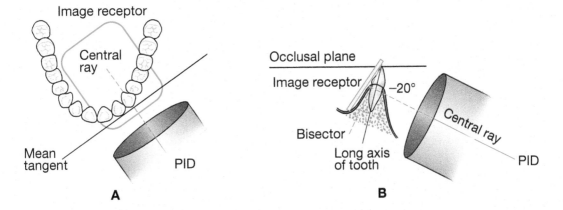

A

B

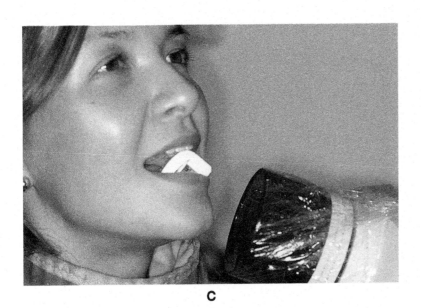

C

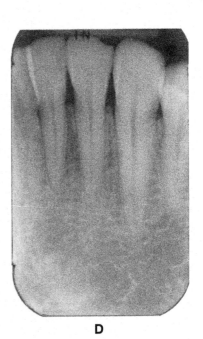

D

FIGURE 14-14 **Mandibular canine exposure.** (**A**) Diagram shows horizontal angulation is directed at the midline of the canine and perpendicular to the mean tangent. (**B**) Vertical angulation is directed perpendicular to the bisector at approximately −20° with the PID tilted upward. (**C**) Patient showing position of image receptor and positioner, and 8 inch (20.5 cm) circular PID. (**D**) Mandibular canine radiograph.

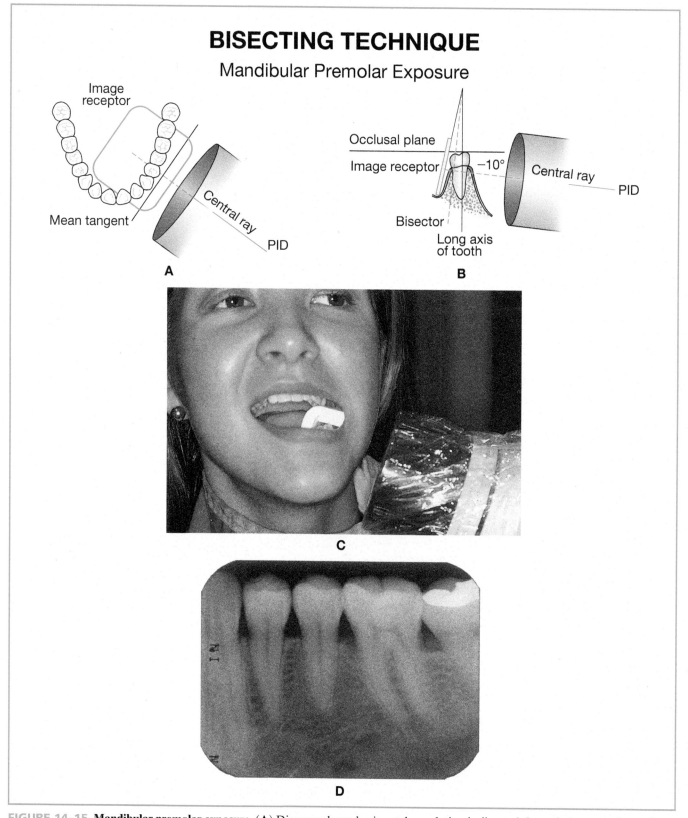

BISECTING TECHNIQUE
Mandibular Premolar Exposure

FIGURE 14–15 **Mandibular premolar exposure.** (**A**) Diagram shows horizontal angulation is directed through the premolar embrasure and perpendicular to the mean tangent. (**B**) Vertical angulation is directed perpendicular to the bisector at approximately −10° with the PID tilted upward. (**C**) Patient showing position of image receptor and positioner, and 8 inch (20.5 cm) circular PID. (**D**) Mandibular premolar radiograph.

BISECTING TECHNIQUE
Mandibular Molar Exposure

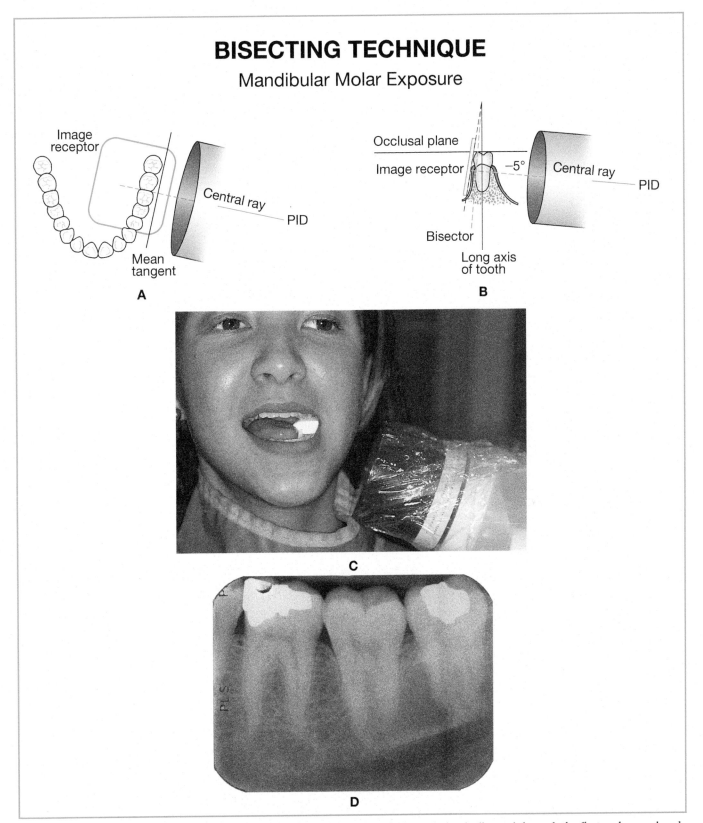

FIGURE 14–16 **Mandibular molar exposure.** (**A**) Diagram shows horizontal angulation is directed through the first and second molar embrasure and perpendicular to the mean tangent. (**B**) Vertical angulation is directed perpendicular to the bisector at approximately −5° with slight upward tilt of the PID. (**C**) Patient showing position of image receptor and positioner, and 8 inch (20.5 cm) circular PID. (**D**) Mandibular molar radiograph.

REVIEW—Chapter summary

Meeting fewer shadow casting principles than the paralleling technique, the bisecting technique is less likely to produce superior quality radiographs. However, when irregularities or obstructions of the oral tissues prevent a parallel image receptor placement, a radiographer who is skilled in the use of multiple techniques can produce an acceptable diagnostic-quality radiograph using the bisecting technique. When an image receptor is positioned close to the tooth, parallelism is not likely. The exception to this occurs in the mandibular posterior region, where the molars and premolars are positioned near vertical in the arch.

When parallelism cannot be established, to cast an accurate shadow representation of a tooth onto the image receptor, an understanding of geometric principles is needed. Two triangles with the same side lengths and the same angles are said to be isometric to each other. The bisecting technique is based on this geometric principle whereby an imaginary angle is formed where the long axis of the tooth and the plane of the image receptor meet. A radiographer must determine the point that bisects this angle. The imaginary bisector produces two imaginary isometric triangles. When the central rays of the x-ray beam are directed perpendicular to the imaginary bisector of this angle an image can be projected onto the image receptor that is reasonably free of magnification and exhibits little distortion. The images produced using the bisecting technique will have some amount of inherent magnification and distortion even when the technique is performed correctly.

A short target–image receptor distance (8 inches/20.5 cm PID) will limit magnification that is inherent when parallelism is not established. Image receptor positioners designed for use with the bisecting technique generally have a short biteblock and lack the L-shaped back support. A variety of image receptor positioners are available for use with the bisecting technique. Some positioners designed for use with the paralleling technique can be modified for use with bisecting technique.

The horizontal angulation is determined by directing the central rays of the x-ray beam perpendicular to the recording plane of the image receptor through the mean tangent of the embrasures between the teeth of interest. Both paralleling and bisecting techniques determine horizontal angulation in the same manner. The vertical angulation is determined by directing the central rays of the x-ray beam perpendicular to the imaginary bisector. If a patient's head position is correct, predetermined vertical angle settings may be used.

An image receptor must be centered within the beam of radiation. If a patient's head position is correct, predetermined landmarks may be used to estimate the points of entry. The four basic steps to exposing a periapical radiograph are placement, vertical angulation, horizontal angulation, and point of entry. Step-by-step illustrated instructions for exposing a full mouth series of periapical radiographs utilizing the bisecting technique are presented.

RECALL—Study questions

1. The bisecting technique satisfies more shadow casting rules than the paralleling technique.
   A better image results when the shadow casting rules are followed.
   a. The first statement is true. The second statement is false.
   b. The first statement is false. The second statement is true.
   c. Both statements are true.
   d. Both statements are false.

2. What shadow casting principle is most likely to be met when utilizing the bisecting technique?
   a. Object (tooth) and image receptor should be parallel to each other.
   b. Object (tooth) and image receptor should be as close as possible to each other.
   c. Object (tooth) should be as far as practical from the target.
   d. Radiation should strike the object (tooth) and image receptor perpendicularly.

3. What term describes the imaginary line between the long axis of the tooth and the plane of the image receptor?
   a. Tangent
   b. Median
   c. Midsagittal
   d. Bisector

4. When utilizing the bisecting technique, the image receptor is placed
   a. parallel to the tooth.
   b. parallel to the bisector .
   c. as close as possible to the tooth.
   d. as close as possible to the bisector.

5. When utilizing the bisecting technique, the central rays of the x-ray beam are directed
   a. perpendicular to the bisector.
   b. parallel to the bisector.
   c. perpendicular to the image receptor.
   d. parallel to the image receptor.

6. Which of these target–image receptor distances is recommended for use with the bisecting technique?
   a. 8 inches (20.5 cm)
   b. 12 inches (30 cm)
   c. 16 inches (41 cm)

7. Each of the following is a limitation of the bisecting technique EXCEPT one. Which one is the EXCEPTION?
   a. Produces images with dimensional distortion.
   b. Often superimposes adjacent structures.
   c. Estimating the location of the bisector may be difficult.
   d. May not be used with children or adults with small oral cavities.

8. Image receptor positioners designed for use with the bisecting technique will most likely have a
   a. short biteblock and L-shaped backing.
   b. long biteblock and L-shaped backing.
   c. short biteblock and 105-degree backing.
   d. long biteblock and 105-degree backing.

9. In which of the following regions of the oral cavity will positioning the image receptor close to the tooth most likely NOT require the use of the bisecting technique?
   a. Maxillary central incisors
   b. Maxillary premolers
   c. Mandibular canines
   d. Mandibular molars

10. Lining the image receptor up behind the distal half of the second premolar to include the first, second, and third molars describes the placement for which of the following periapical radiographs?
    a. Central incisors
    b. Canine
    c. Premolar
    d. Molar

11. To determine the horizontal angulation for the mandibular premolar periapical radiograph, the central rays of the x-ray beam should be directed at the image receptor perpendicularly through the embrasures of the
    a. canine and first premolar.
    b. first and second premolars.
    c. second premolar and first molar.
    d. first and second molars.

12. When utilizing the bisecting technique, the recommended vertical angle setting for the maxillary premolar periapical radiograph is
    a. +45 degrees
    b. +30 degrees
    c. −10 degrees
    d. −5 degrees

13. When utilizing the bisecting technique, the recommended vertical angle setting for the mandibular canine periapical radiograph is
    a. +40 degrees
    b. +20 degrees
    c. −15 degrees
    d. −20 degrees

14. With the bisecting technique, what is the effect on the radiographic image if the vertical angulation is significantly greater than necessary?
    a. Foreshortening
    b. Conecutting
    c. Elongating
    d. Overlapping

15. Elongation results from
    a. inadequate horizontal angulation.
    b. excessive horizontal angulation.
    c. inadequate vertical angulation.
    d. excessive vertical angulation.

16. Which of the following is the suggested point of entry for directing the central rays of the x-ray beam when exposing the maxillary incisors radiograph using the bisecting technique?
    a. The tip of the nose
    b. The ala of the nose
    c. A point on the ala–tragus line below the pupil of the eye
    d. A point on the ala–tragus line below the outer canthus of the eye

17. Which of the following points 1 inch (2.5 cm) above the inferior border of the mandible is the suggested landmark for directing the central rays of the x-ray beam when exposing the mandibular premolar radiograph using the bisecting technique?
    a. The middle (symphysis) of the chin
    b. The center of the root of the canine
    c. Directly below the pupil of the eye
    d. Directly below the outer canthus of the eye

REFLECT—Case study

Compare the paralleling (see Chapter 13) and the bisecting techniques. Include answers to the following questions in your discussion.

1. What are the major differences between the two techniques?

2. How are the two techniques similar?

3. What are the advantages/limitations of each of the two techniques?

4. When would use of the bisecting/paralleling techniques be appropriate?

5. Describe the characteristics of the image receptor positioners appropriate for use with the bisecting/paralleling techniques.

6. How does each of the four steps for exposing periapical radiographs (placement, vertical and horizontal angulation, and point of entry) differ between the two techniques? How are they similar?

7. Which technique do you anticipate being easier/more difficult to master?

8. Would you recommend that radiographers learn one technique over the other? Why/why not?

RELATE—Laboratory application

For a comprehensive laboratory practice exercise on this topic, see Thomson, E. M., & Bruhn, A. M. (2018). *Exercises in oral radiography techniques: A laboratory manual* (4th ed.). Hoboken, NJ: Pearson. Chapter 5, "Periapical radiographs—bisecting technique."

RESOURCES

Eastman Kodak Company. (2002). *Successful intraoral radiography.* Rochester, NY: Author.

Rinn Corporation. (1983). *Intraoral radiography with Rinn XCP/BAI instruments.* Elgin, IL: Dentsply Sirona.

White, S. C., & Pharoah, M. J. (2014). Intraoral projections. *Oral radiology: Principles and interpretation* (7th ed.). St. Louis, MO: Elsevier.

Visit www.pearsonhighered.com/healthprofessionsresources to access the student resources that accompany this book. Simply select Dental Hygiene from the choice of disciplines. Find this book and you will find the complementary study tools created for this specific title.

The Bitewing Examination

OBJECTIVES

Following successful completion of this chapter, you should be able to:

1. Define the key terms.
2. Describe the bitewing radiographic technique.
3. Match the bitewing examination with two ideal uses.
4. List the four sizes of image receptors that can be used for bitewing examinations, explaining advantages and limitations of each size.
5. Identify the size and number of image receptors best suited for a bitewing examination for a child with primary and/or mixed dentition.
6. Identify the size and number of image receptors best suited for a bitewing examination for an adult with and without periodontal disease.
7. Differentiate between horizontal and vertical bitewing radiographs.
8. Explain the role occlusion plays in aligning an image receptor for exposure of premolar and molar bitewing radiographs.
9. Explain the effect of incorrect horizontal angulation on the resultant bitewing image.
10. Identify positive and negative vertical angulations.
11. State the recommended vertical angulation for bitewing exposures.
12. Identify vertical angulation errors unique to the bitewing technique.
13. Demonstrate image receptor placement, horizontal and vertical angulation, and points of entry for horizontal and vertical posterior bitewing examinations.
14. Demonstrate image receptor placement, horizontal and vertical angulation, and points of entry for a vertical anterior bitewing examination.

KEY TERMS

Bitetab
Contact point
Film loop
Overlap
Proximal surface
Vertical bitewing radiograph

Introduction

Bitewing radiographs are probably the most frequently performed intraoral dental radiographic technique. Bitewings are most often exposed at the time of regularly scheduled recare or recall appointments. Bitewing radiographs record the crowns and alveolar bone of both the maxillary and mandibular teeth on a single radiograph. The name bitewing is descriptive. Traditionally, the bitewing film packet had a tab, or wing, that was either attached to the packet by the manufacturer or attached by the radiographer as a holder (Figures 15–1 ■ and 15–2 ■). The patient bites on this tab to hold the image receptor in place. This chapter presents step-by-step instructions for exposing bitewing radiographs.

Fundamentals of Bitewing Radiography

Bitewing radiographs, sometimes called interproximal radiographs, may be taken as a stand-alone series or in conjunction with a full mouth series of periapical radiographs or with an extraoral panoramic radiograph. Bitewing radiographs showing the crowns and alveolar bone crests of both the maxillary and mandibular teeth on the same image are ideal for detecting caries on the **proximal surfaces** of the teeth (where adjacent teeth contact each other in the arch) and for assessing periodontal bone levels supporting the teeth (Figure 15–3 ■). The true value of the bitewing radiograph is that it reveals caries in the very early stages when remineralization treatment may be possible. This is particularly important in the premolar and molar regions, where incipient (small) caries are often concealed from clinical detection by the wide bucco-lingual diameters of these teeth. Such caries are frequently unnoticed in a visual inspection. Bitewing radiographs do not image the entire tooth and therefore will not reveal apical conditions.

To expose a bitewing radiograph, the image receptor is positioned near and almost parallel to the teeth of both arches when the patient's teeth are occluded (closed). Bitewing image receptor placement is often closer to the teeth, and the central rays of the x-ray beam can be directed at a more ideal angle than for periapical radiographs (Figure 15–4 ■). With this ideal image receptor placement, the bitewing radiograph often images decay and the height of the alveolar bone crest better than periapical radiographs. It is because of this improved imaging for these conditions that bitewing radiographs are often taken in addition to periapical radiographs of the same area when exposing a full mouth series.

Size, Number, and Placement of Image Receptors

The size and number of image receptors to use depends on the type of survey required and the size and shape of the patient's oral cavity (Table 15–1 ■, page 198). An additional factor to be considered when deciding what size and how many image receptors to select is the length and curvature of the arches, which vary between individuals. A single image receptor placed on each side of the oral cavity often provides adequate coverage for children, prior to the eruption of the permanent second molars. Although an image receptor size 0 or 1 is often used for a child with primary teeth, the preferred size for mixed dentition is a size 2. However, tissue sensitivity or anatomical limitations must be taken into consideration, so size is often based on

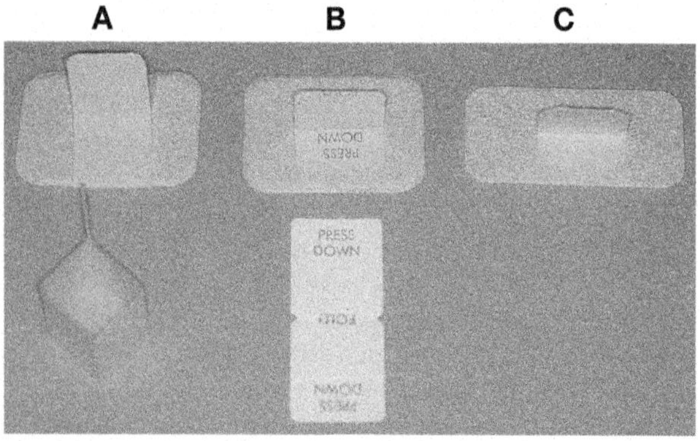

FIGURE 15–1 **Bitewing tabs and loops. (A)** Loop tabs; **(B)** stick-on tabs; **(C)** size 3 film packet with manufacturer-attached tab.

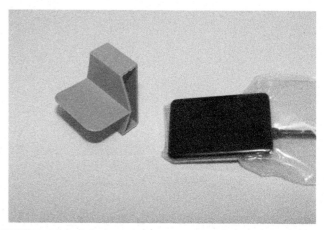

FIGURE 15–2 **Bitewing loop for digital sensor.**

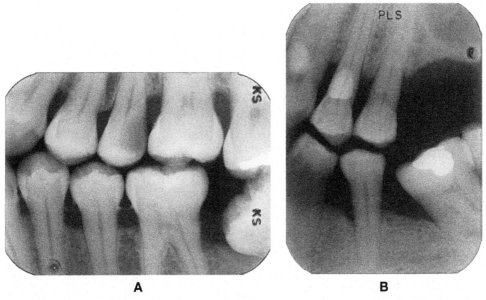

FIGURE 15-3 **(A) Horizontal and (B) vertical bitewing radiographs.** Bitewing radiographs are ideal at imaging the interproximal areas of the teeth to show caries and alveolar bone crests. Note the increased coverage of the alveolar bone imaged on the vertical bitewing radiograph.

the individual patient. The advantage to using the largest size image receptor possible is that the amount of structures recorded, including the developing permanent teeth, will be increased. For most adults, four size 2 image receptors (two on each side) are generally preferred.

Size 3 (extra-long) radiographic film packets with preattached tabs are especially made for taking horizontal bitewing radiographs. Phosphor plates used in digital imaging are also available in size 3 (see Figure 8–17). The advantage of these image receptors is that only one of them needs to be exposed on each side of the arch. Due to its length, size 3 image receptors can record both the premolars and the molars all on one image. When compared with the standard size 2 image receptor, however, the size 3 has two disadvantages. One being that most dental arches curve so that the horizontal angle required to clearly image the proximal surfaces of the premolars is not the same horizontal angle required to clearly image the proximal surfaces of the molars. There are two slightly divergent pathways of the posterior teeth. As the central rays pass through these divergent embrasures, it is not likely that all of the interproximal spaces will be recorded clearly without overlapping. The other disadvantage is that the long image receptor is narrower in the vertical dimension than size 2 and may reveal less of the periodontal crestal bone level (Figure 15–5 ■).

As discussed in Chapter 12, the bitewing examination may consist of two to eight images. The posterior bitewing examination consists of either two (one on the left and one on the right) or four (two on the left and two on the right) images (Figure 15–6A and B ■). The image receptor orientation in the oral cavity may be such that the longer dimension is placed horizontally or vertically. Traditionally, the image receptor has been placed horizontally in the

posterior region. This remains the placement of choice for children. However, if there is a need to image more of the supporting bone, as is the case in periodontally involved patients, a **vertical bitewing radiograph** is recommended. Some practitioners expose vertical bitewing radiographs on all adult patients, if the placement is well tolerated, regardless of periodontal status because of the increased anatomy recorded in the vertical dimension.

The anterior bitewing examination consists of either three (one just left of center, one centered behind the central incisors, and one just right of center; see Figure 15–6C)

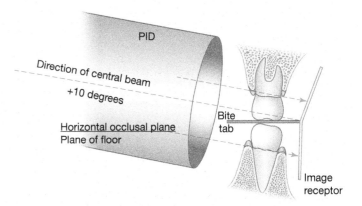

FIGURE 15-4 **Bitewing placement.** The bitewing image receptor placement, slightly angled to take advantage of the height of the midline of the palate when the patient occludes, is such that the coronal portion of both the maxillary and the mandibular teeth will be recorded on the image. The close relationship between the teeth and the image receptor and the ideal angle of the x-ray beam allow bitewings to accurately image caries and alveolar bone crests.

Table 15–1 Suggested Image Receptor Size and Number to Use for Bitewing Radiographs

Image Receptor Size	Recommended for Use with These Patients	Number and Orientation of Image Receptor
0	Child with primary dentition	2 horizontal posterior
1	Child with primary or mixed dentition	2 horizontal posterior
	Adult	3 or 4 vertical anterior
2	Child with mixed dentition, prior to eruption of permanent second molars	2 horizontal posterior
	Adolescent after eruption of permanent second molars	4 horizontal posterior
	Adult	4 horizontal posterior
	Adult with periodontal disease	4 vertical posterior
3	Adolescent after eruption of permanent second molars	2 horizontal posterior
	Adult	2 horizontal posterior

or four (two just left of center and two just right of center) images. The image receptor orientation in the anterior region of the oral cavity is usually such that the longer dimension is placed vertically. For ease of placement, especially when

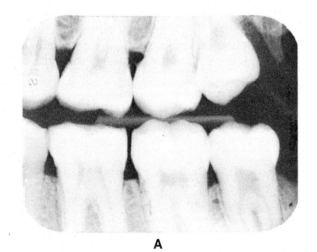

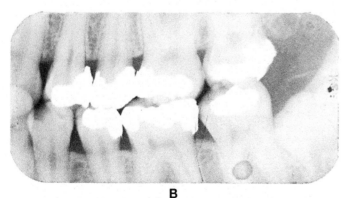

FIGURE 15–5 Comparison of size 2 and size 3 image receptors.
(A) Size 2 has a shorter horizontal dimension, taller vertical dimension. **(B)** Size 3 has a longer horizontal dimension, shorter vertical dimension.

using more rigid digital sensors and to avoid bending a film packet or phosphor plate, the narrow size 1 image receptor is usually selected, especially for use in the lateral-canine region. The central incisors region is usually wider and may allow selection of a size 2 image receptor for use here if the arch permits.

Bitewing image receptor placement is usually closer to the tooth than is possible with periapical image receptor placement. However, if the image receptor is placed too close to the lingual surfaces of the maxillary teeth, the top edge of the image receptor may contact the lingual gingiva or curvature of the palate when the patient occludes, pushing down on or causing the image receptor to slant away from the correct position (Figure 15–7 ▪). A sloping or slanting (tilted) occlusal plane is a frequent reason for having to retake bitewing radiographs. To avoid this error it is important to position the image receptor well into the oral cavity, a slightly increased distance from the lingual surfaces of the maxillary teeth, taking advantage of the midline where the palate is at its highest to accommodate the image receptor and facilitate correct stabilization and vertical alignment with the x-ray beam.

In the anterior region, use of a longer bitetab may facilitate positioning the image receptor further lingually to avoid contact with the anterior portion of the lingual gingiva or curvature of the palate when the patient occludes. This placement may prevent a film or phosphor plate from bending in the middle as the tab is pulled forward when the patient is asked to bite down, and may avoid pushing down on or causing the image receptor to slant in a way that compromises the vertical angulation. Two stick-on paper bitetabs may be attached to lengthen the bitetab for this purpose (Figure 15–8 ▪).

It is important to remember that each bitewing radiograph—molar, premolar, canine, and incisors—has a standard recommended placement. This means that a premolar bitewing taken at one oral health care practice will

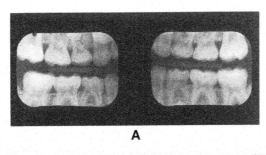

A

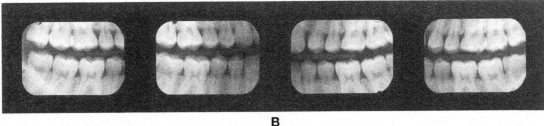

B

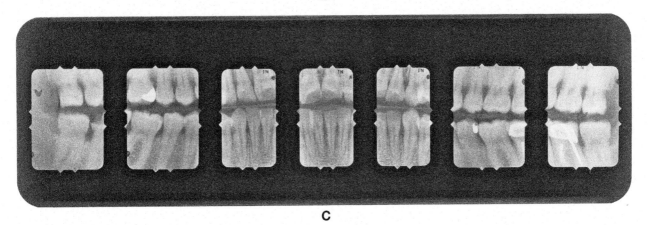

C

FIGURE 15–6 **Horizontal and vertical bitewing series.** (**A**) Set of two horizontal posterior bitewing radiographs. (**B**) Set of four horizontal posterior bitewing radiographs. (**C**) Set of seven vertical bitewing radiographs, including posterior and anterior images.

most likely image the same teeth as a premolar bitewing exposed in every other practice. This standardization is important to learn.

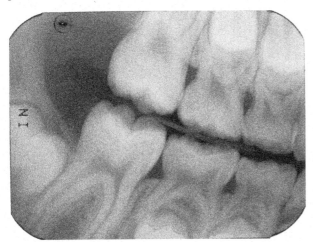

FIGURE 15–7 **Tilted image.** The slanted occlusal plane observed on this radiograph resulted from a failure to place the image receptor far enough lingually to avoid being pushed down by the palate when the patient occluded onto the bitetab.

The standard placements for the image receptor in the anterior region for incisors and canine radiographs are to center the teeth of interest in the middle of the image receptor. However, posterior anatomical considerations will not allow the radiographer to similarly center the premolar and molar teeth on the image receptor. Instead, focus on placing the anterior edge of the image receptor and allow the receptor, once in the correct position, to

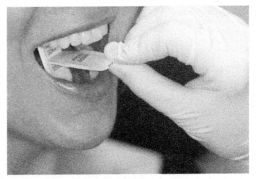

FIGURE 15–8 **Two stick-on bitetabs** lengthen the holder for use in the anterior region.

capture the images of the appropriate teeth. For example, when placing the image receptor for a premolar horizontal or vertical bitewing radiograph, try not to center the first and second premolars. Because of the curvature of the arches and the position of the canine, this is not usually possible. Focus on placing the anterior edge of the image receptor so that it lines up behind the distal half of the canine, and the rest of the teeth should be recorded correctly.

It is important to visually inspect the patient's occlusion to determine which canine, maxillary or mandibular, to use to align the image receptor for exposure of premolar bitewing radiographs. The premolar bitewing must record the distal portion of both the maxillary and the mandibular canines to record the mesial surface of the first premolar, one of the teeth of interest for this projection. Align the anterior edge of the image receptor behind the canine, either maxillary or mandibular, that is further forward in the mouth (the most mesial canine) when the patient occludes.

When placing the image receptor to image a molar horizontal or vertical bitewing radiograph, focus on placing the anterior edge of the image receptor so that it lines up behind the distal half of the second premolar. Again, a visual inspection of the patient's occlusion will determine whether to line up the image receptor with the maxillary or the mandibular second premolar.

Generally, in Class I and III occlusal relationships, choose to align the anterior edge of the image receptor behind the distal half of the mandibular canine for a premolar bitewing radiograph, and behind the distal half of the mandibular second premolar for a molar bitewing radiograph. When a Class II occlusal relationship presents, the most likely choice is to align the anterior edge of the image receptor behind the distal half of the maxillary canine for a premolar bitewing radiograph and behind the distal half of the maxillary second premolar for a molar bitewing radiograph (Figure 15–9 ■). It should be noted

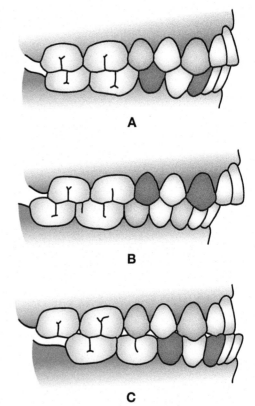

FIGURE 15–9 Occlusal relationships. (**A**) Class I occlusion demonstrating that the mandibular canine and second premolar (darker color) are located further forward in the oral cavity. (**B**) Class II occlusion demonstrating that the maxillary canine and second premolar (darker color) are located further forward in the oral cavity. (**C**) Class III occlusion demonstrating that the mandibular canine and second premolar (darker color) are located further forward in the oral cavity.

that patients often present with different occlusal relationships on the right and left sides or individual teeth that are malaligned or missing. It is important to perform a visual inspection prior to each placement.

Sequence of Placement

It is recommended to always follow a systematic order when exposing radiographs to prevent errors and for efficiency (Table 15–2 ■). See Chapter 12 for discussion about at what point to take bitewing radiographs when exposing a full mouth series. When exposing a set of four posterior bitewings alone, it is recommended that the premolar bitewing on one side be exposed first, followed by the molar bitewing on the same side. Placing the image receptor for exposure of the premolar may be more comfortable for the patient and less likely to excite a gag reflex, gaining the patient's confidence for the molar placements that may sometimes be more difficult. Then the premolar and molar bitewing on the opposite side should be exposed. Completing both the premolar and molar bitewing radiographs on one side first will avoid shifting the x-ray machine tube head back and forth across the patient.

Practice Point

Although contact with the lingual gingiva or curvature of the palate or other obstruction such as tori is the most likely cause of a tilted or slanting occlusal plane, other causes include (1) failure of the patient to maintain a steady pressure occluding on the bitetab, (2) patient swallowing while the exposure is being made, and (3) incorrect or slanted placement of the bitetab or image receptor positioner. The best corrective action is to position the image receptor far enough away from the lingual surfaces of the maxillary teeth to avoid premature and excessive contact with the palate. Other corrective actions include selecting the appropriately sized image receptor and providing the patient with specific instructions about securely biting on the bitetab and not swallowing during exposure.

Table 15–2 Recommended Sequence for Exposing Bitewing Radiographs

Bitewing Series	Recommended Sequence
2 posterior	1st: right* premolar 2nd: left premolar
4 posterior	1st: right* premolar 2nd: right molar 3rd: left premolar 4th: left molar
7 anterior and posterior	1st: central-lateral incisors 2nd: left* canine 3rd: right canine 4th: right premolar 5th: right molar 6th: left premolar 7th: left molar
8 anterior and posterior	1st: left* canine 2nd: left central-lateral incisors 3rd: right central-lateral incisors 4th: right canine 5th: right premolar 6th: right molar 7th: left premolar 8th: left molar

*Left-handed radiographers may choose to begin the exposures on the opposite side.

Holding the Bitewing Image Receptor in Position

There are many commercially made holders for stabilizing a film packet, phosphor plate, or digital sensor for bitewing exposures. Stick-on paper or plastic **bitetabs** have the most versatility because they can be fastened to the image receptor for both horizontal and vertical bitewings. The paper or plastic **film loop** into which a film packet or digital sensor can be slid may be limited to horizontal bitewings, although there are elastic loops available that may be stretched to accommodate both placements. Bitetabs and loops are easy to use, disposable, and readily tolerated by patients. Bitetabs must be attached to the white unprinted side (front) of the film packet or the plain side of the phosphor plate or digital sensor, over the plastic infection control barrier (see Chapter 9) so that this side will face the radiation source when placed intraorally.

Generally the bitetab or loop is visible extraorally after a patient bites down to stabilize the image receptor. This extension of the tab serves as a guide for directing the central rays of the x-ray beam toward the center of the image receptor. Without a significantly visible external aiming device, some operators find it difficult to determine the correct horizontal and vertical angulations and center the image receptor within the x-ray beam (Figure 15-10 ■).

Many image receptor positioners that are designed for positioning an image receptor for periapical radiographs

(see Chapters 12 and 13) can be used with a bitewing biteblock. Image receptor positioners with an extension arm and indicator ring assembly can assist with locating correct angles and points of entry, making errors less likely (Figure 15–11 ■). The external aiming device also eliminates the need to position a patient's head precisely. Biteblocks are available for both horizontal and vertical bitewings. Note that the biteblock on some image receptor positioners is wider or thicker than paper/plastic bitetabs and loops and may prevent a patient from biting down far enough to record the greatest amount of alveolar bone (Figure 15–12 ■). This is especially important when the goal of the bitewing image is to assess periodontal disease conditions. To overcome this limitation, a vertical bitewing biteblock attachment can be substituted.

Regardless of the image receptor positioner used, care should be taken to ensure that the image receptor is positioned in such a manner that it is evenly centered behind both the maxillary and mandibular teeth. Once the image receptor is satisfactorily positioned, the patient must close down on the tab or biteblock in an edge-to-edge relationship and hold it there for the duration of the exposure.

It is important to note that if an image receptor positioner with an external aiming device is not positioned correctly, the aiming device will indicate directing the x-ray beam to the wrong place. For this reason, it is important to develop the skills necessary to evaluate placement of the image receptor for correctness, regardless of the positioner used.

Horizontal and Vertical Angulation

The correct horizontal and vertical angulations are critical to producing a quality bitewing radiograph. Horizontal angulation is the positioning of the central rays of the x-ray beam in a horizontal (side-to-side) plane. While correct horizontal angulation is important in producing diagnostic quality periapical radiographs, it is of critical importance when exposing bitewing radiographs since assessing the proximal surfaces of the teeth is the most likely reason for exposing bitewing radiographs. The steps used for determining correct horizontal angulation are the same as those used for both the paralleling and bisecting techniques used to expose periapical radiographs (see Chapters 13 and 14). First, position the image receptor parallel to the interproximal space, or embrasure. Select two predetermined teeth to achieve this. Then direct the central rays of the x-ray beam perpendicular to the mean tangent, or curvature of the arch, through the contact points of these teeth to achieve horizontal angulation (see Figure 12–10). The particular embrasures listed for each exposure have been chosen because of the likelihood that if the image receptor is parallel to this space and the central rays of the x-ray beam are directed through this space, then the rest of the spaces should line up for a correct exposure, free of horizontal angulation errors. The goal of image receptor placement and directing the central rays of the x-ray beam perpendicular to the image receptor is to be sure that all contacts (mesial and distal surfaces) of all of the teeth of interest are recorded clearly on the resulting image. The

Practice Point

When using a stick-on tab holder, follow these steps for placement.

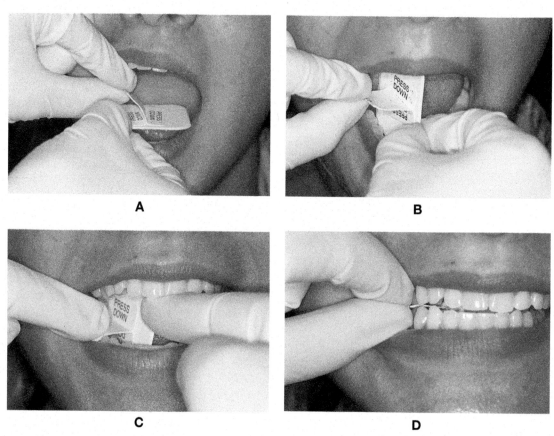

FIGURE 15–10 **Bitewing placement using a stick-on tab.** (**A**) Insert the image receptor completely into the patient's mouth. (**B**) Rotate until the image receptor is in a vertical position. Inserting in this manner allows the image receptor to move the tongue out of the way. (**C**) Using the index finger of one hand, hold the bitetab firmly against the occlusal surface of the mandibular teeth while the index finger of the other hand angles the top edge of the image receptor into the midline of the palate. (**D**) Instruct the patient to close so that the teeth occlude normally. Failure to hold the tab firmly while the patient closes may lead to a drift lingually and distally and increase the possibility that the tongue will move the image receptor out of the correct position.

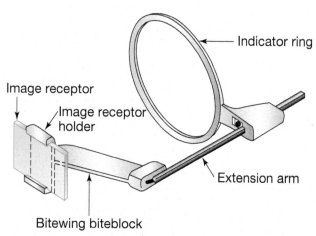

FIGURE 15–11 **Bitewing image receptor positioner** with extension arm and indicator ring assembly.

central rays must be directed appropriately to avoid **overlapping** adjacent teeth on the resultant image (Figure 15–13 ▪).

The contact points should appear open or separate from each other on the resultant radiograph. When the horizontal angulation is directed obliquely from the mesial, the overlapping will be more severe in the distal or posterior region of the image. When the horizontal angulation is directed obliquely from the distal, the overlapping will be more severe in the mesial or anterior region of the image (Figure 15–14 ▪). Because bitewing radiographs are taken to reveal information about the interproximal areas of the teeth, bitewing radiographs with overlapping error are undiagnostic.

It is important to note that even with correct horizontal angulation, the canine bitewing image will often exhibit significant overlap of the distal portions of the canines with the mesial portions of the first premolars. The anatomical positions of the canines, which are anterior teeth, and the

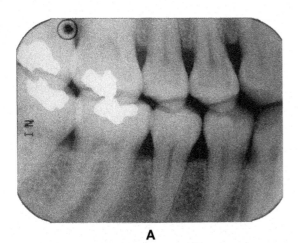

A

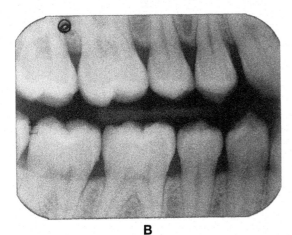

B

FIGURE 15–12 Image receptor positioner comparison.
(**A**) Bitewing radiograph taken using a disposable paper stick-on bitetab. (**B**) Bitewing radiograph taken using a thicker autoclavable image receptor positioner. Notice the wider space between the occlusal surfaces of the maxillary and mandibular teeth.

premolars, which are posterior teeth, is such that the lingual cusp of the first premolar is often superimposed over the distal edge of the canine. To minimize this occurrence correctly align the horizontal angulation to direct the central rays of the x-ray beam perpendicular to the image receptor at the center of the canine and then shift the x-ray machine tube head and position indicating device (PID) no more than 10 degrees toward the distal, which will slightly alter the horizontal angulation and minimize this inherent overlap (see Figure 29–7).

VERTICAL ANGULATION The correct vertical angulation for bitewing radiographs is +10 degrees. (A +5-degree vertical angulation is sometimes recommended for children; see Chapter 27.) Positioning the x-ray machine tube head and PID to point slightly downward will direct the central rays of the x-ray beam to more likely match the vertical slant of the image receptor when it is correctly placed into the oral cavity (see Figure 15–4). Because bitewing radiographs are placed to image both the maxillary and the mandibular teeth on one image, give consideration to the anatomic positions of the teeth in both arches. In general, the maxillary teeth have a slight buccal inclination, whereas the mandibular teeth often have a slight lingual inclination. This is more the

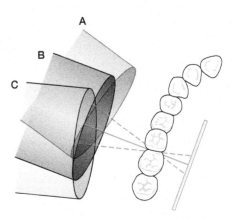

FIGURE 15–13 Horizontal angulation. (A) Mesiodistal projection of the x-ray beam shown here deviates from a right angle by about 15°, resulting in greater overlap of the contacts in the posterior region of the radiograph. (**B**) Correct horizontal projection of the x-ray beam produces no overlapping. (**C**) Distomesial projection of the x-ray beam shown here deviates from a right angle about 15°, resulting in greater overlap of the contacts in the anterior region of the radiograph.

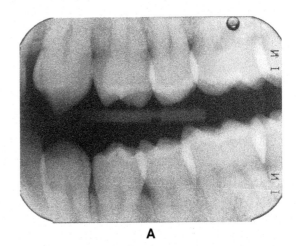

A

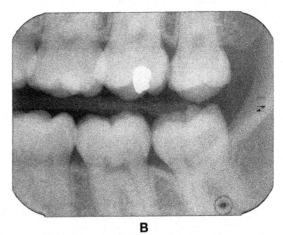

B

FIGURE 15–14 Horizontal overlap error. (A) When the PID is directed obliquely from the mesial (mesiodistal projection of the x-ray beam), the overlapping will be more severe in the distal or posterior region of the image. (**B**) When the horizontal angulation is directed obliquely from the distal (distomesial projection of the x-ray beam), the overlapping will be more severe in the mesial or anterior region of the image.

Practice Point

To avoid molar overlap follow these steps for placement (Figure 15–15 ■).

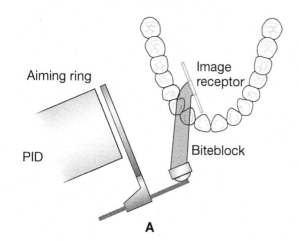

A

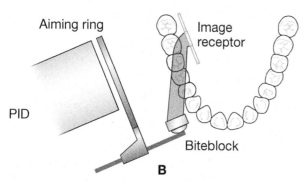

B

FIGURE 15–15 Avoiding molar overlap when using a holder with external aiming device. (**A**) Note the recommended premolar bitewing placement. (**B**) Because the proximal surfaces of the molar teeth are in a mesiodistal relationship to the sagittal plane, it is recommended that the image receptor be positioned perpendicularly to the embrasures, resulting in a diagonal placement similar to the premolar position.

case in the posterior regions than in the anterior regions. This anatomical relationship, when combined with the slight lingual tilt the image receptor takes on when a patient occludes, is the basis for using a +10 vertical degree angle to produce the best image. If using an image receptor positioner with an external aiming device, it is important that the patient occludes fully on the biteblock so that the indicator ring will direct the operator to the correct vertical angle.

Incorrect vertical angulation results in an unequal distribution of the arches on the radiograph. A quality bitewing radiograph should image an equal portion of the maxillary and mandibular teeth plus an equal portion of the supporting bone. When the vertical angulation is excessive (greater than +10 degrees), more maxillary teeth and bone are imaged, cutting off a portion of the mandibular structures. When the vertical angulation is inadequate (less than +10 degrees), more mandibular teeth and bone are imaged, cutting off a portion of the maxillary structures (Figure 15–16 ■).

Points of Entry

The points of entry for the central rays of the x-ray beam for all bitewing exposures are on the level of the incisal or occlusal plane (near the lip line) at a point opposite the center of the image receptor and through the interproximal spaces of the teeth of interest (see Figure 15–4). An image receptor positioner with an external aiming device will assist with determining the accurate point of entry. Incorrect point of entry, or not centering the image receptor within the x-ray beam, will result in conecut error, where the portion of the image receptor that was not in the path of the x-ray beam will be clear or blank on the resultant radiograph (see Figures 18–8 and 18–9).

The Bitewing Technique

Figures 15–17 ■ through 15–20 ■ illustrate the precise image receptor positions and required angulations for each of the horizontal and vertical bitewing radiographs discussed in this chapter. See Table 15–3 ■ for a summary of the four basic steps of the technique—placement, vertical angulation, horizontal angulation, and points of entry.

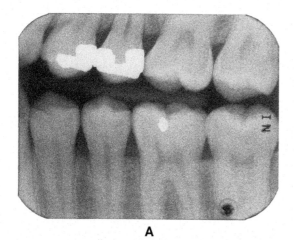

A

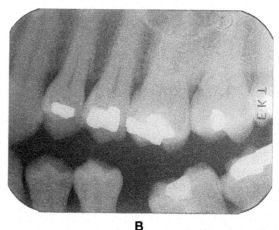

B

FIGURE 15–16 Vertical angulation error. (**A**) Inadequate vertical angulation results in imaging more of the mandible. (**B**) Excessive vertical angulation results in imaging more of the maxilla.

Table 15–3 Summary of Steps for Acquiring Bitewing Radiographs

Bitewing Radiograph	Placement	Vertical Angulation*	Horizontal Angulation	Point of Entry*
Incisors (vertical) (image receptor size 1 or 2) (Figure 15–17)	Center image receptor to line up behind central and lateral incisors; if using size 2 image receptor, include mesial halves of canines Align image receptor parallel to long axes of incisors and parallel to left and right central incisors embrasures	+10	Direct central rays perpendicular to image receptor through left and right central incisor embrasures	Center image receptor within x-ray beam by directing central rays at center of image receptor at a spot on incisal plane between maxillary and mandibular central incisors
Canine (vertical) (image receptor size 1 or 2) (Figure 15–18)	Center image receptor to line up behind maxillary and mandibular canines; include lateral incisors and first premolars Align image receptor parallel to long axes of canines and parallel to mesial and distal line angles of canines	+10	Direct central rays perpendicular to image receptor at center of canines To minimize distal overlap of canines with lingual cusps of first premolars shift PID horizontally to direct central rays no more than 10 degrees toward distal	Center image receptor within x-ray beam by directing central rays at center of image receptor at a spot on incisal plane between maxillary and mandibular canines
Premolar (horizontal or vertical) (image receptor size 2) (Figure 15–19)	Align anterior edge of image receptor to line up behind distal half of maxillary or mandibular canine; choose most mesially positioned canine; include first and second premolars and mesial half of first molars Align image receptor parallel to long axes of premolars and parallel to first and second premolars embrasures	+10	Direct central rays perpendicular to image receptor through first and second premolars embrasures	Center image receptor within x-ray beam by directing central rays at center of image receptor at a spot on occlusal plane between maxillary and mandibular second premolars
Molar (horizontal or vertical) (image receptor size 2) (Figure 15–20)	Align anterior edge of image receptor to line up behind distal half of maxillary or mandibular second premolar; choose most mesially located second premolar; include first, second, third molars (horizontal placement); include first, second molars (vertical placement) Align image receptor parallel to long axes of molars and parallel to first and second molars embrasures	+10	Direct central rays perpendicular to image receptor through first and second molars embrasures	Center image receptor within x-ray beam by directing central rays at center of image receptor at a spot on occlusal plane between maxillary and mandibular first molars

(continued)

Table 15–3 **Summary of Steps for Acquiring Bitewing Radiographs** (*continued*)

Bitewing Radiograph	Placement	Vertical Angulation*	Horizontal Angulation	Point of Entry*
Premolar-molar (image receptor size 3)	Align anterior edge of image receptor to line up behind distal half of maxillary or mandibular canine; choose most mesially located canine; include all premolars and molars Align image receptor parallel to long axes of second premolars and first molars and parallel to second premolars and first molars embrasures	+10	Direct central rays perpendicular to image receptor through second premolars and first molars embrasures	Center image receptor within x-ray beam by directing central rays at center of image receptor at a spot on occlusal plane between maxillary and mandibular second premolars
Molar (child) (horizontal) (image receptor size 1 or 2)	Align anterior edge of image receptor to line up behind distal half of maxillary or mandibular canine; choose most mesially located canine; include remaining erupted teeth Align image receptor parallel to long axes and parallel to embrasures of erupted teeth of interest	+5 to +10	Direct central rays perpendicular to image receptor through first and second primary molars embrasure; or, if erupted, first and second premolars embrasures	Center image receptor within x-ray beam by directing central rays at center of image receptor at a spot on occlusal plane between primary maxillary and mandibular first molars; or, if erupted, maxillary and mandibular second premolars

*Patient must be seated in correct position, with occlusal plane parallel to floor and midsagittal plane perpendicular to floor.

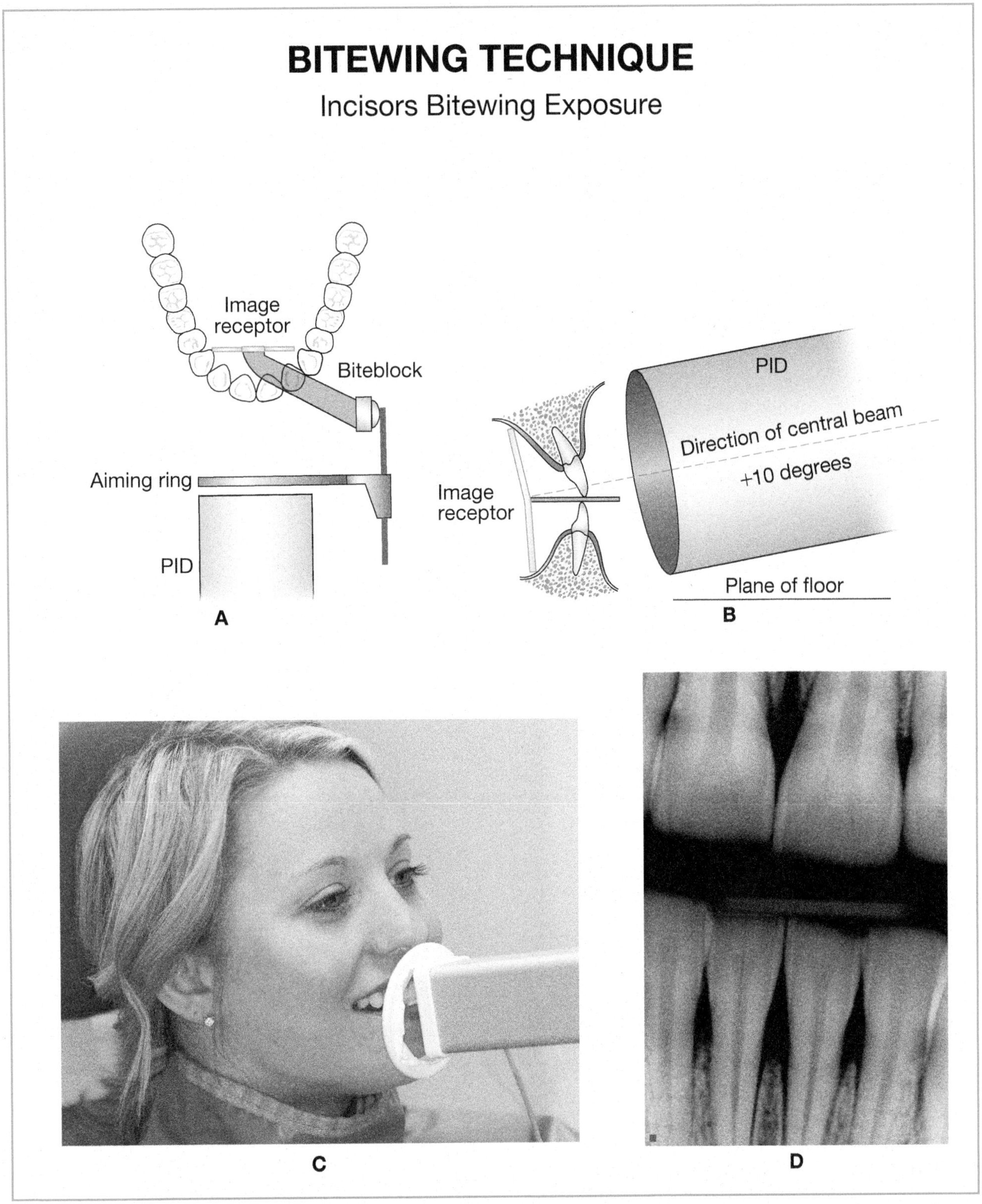

BITEWING TECHNIQUE
Incisors Bitewing Exposure

FIGURE 15–17 Incisors bitewing exposure. (A) Diagram showing relationship of image receptor and positioner, teeth, and PID. **(B)** Vertical angulation directed perpendicular to image receptor at approximately +10 degrees with PID tilted downward. Central rays of x-ray beam directed at center of image receptor at a spot on the incisal plane between maxillary and mandibular teeth. **(C)** Patient showing position of image receptor positioner and 16 inch (41 cm) rectangular PID. **(D)** Incisors bitewing radiograph. Image receptor positioned with long dimension vertical.

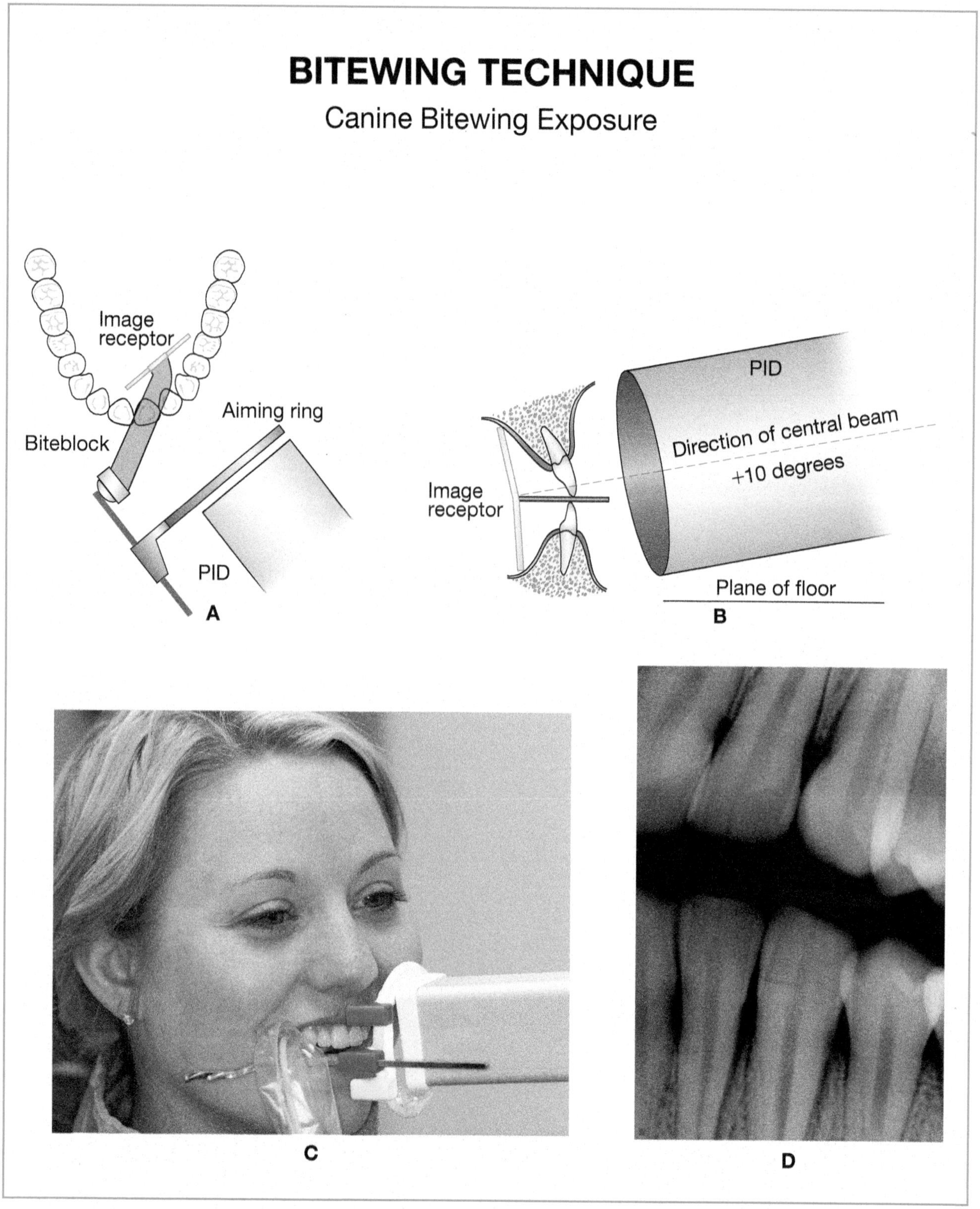

BITEWING TECHNIQUE
Canine Bitewing Exposure

FIGURE 15–18 **Canine bitewing exposure.** (**A**) Diagram showing relationship of image receptor and positioner, teeth, and PID. (**B**) Vertical angulation directed perpendicular to image receptor at approximately +10 degrees with PID tilted downward. Central rays of x-ray beam directed at center of image receptor at a spot on the incisal plane between maxillary and mandibular teeth. (**C**) Patient showing position of image receptor positioner and 16 inch (41 cm) rectangular PID. (**D**) Canine bitewing radiograph. Image receptor positioned with long dimension vertical.

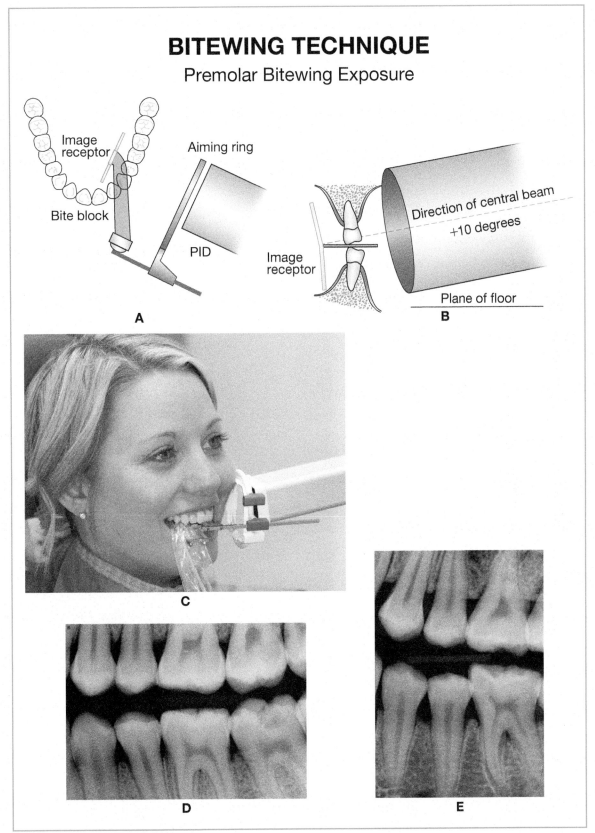

BITEWING TECHNIQUE
Premolar Bitewing Exposure

A

B

Image receptor

Bite block

Aiming ring

PID

Image receptor

Direction of central beam

+10 degrees

Plane of floor

C

D

E

FIGURE 15–19 **Premolar bitewing exposure.** (**A**) Diagram showing relationship of image receptor and positioner, teeth, and PID. (**B**) Vertical angulation directed perpendicular to image receptor at approximately +10 degrees with PID tilted downward. Central rays of x-ray beam directed at center of image receptor at a spot on the occlusal plane between maxillary and mandibular teeth. (**C**) Patient showing position of image receptor positioner and 16 inch (41 cm) rectangular PID. (**D**) Horizontal premolar bitewing radiograph. (**E**) Vertical premolar bitewing radiograph.

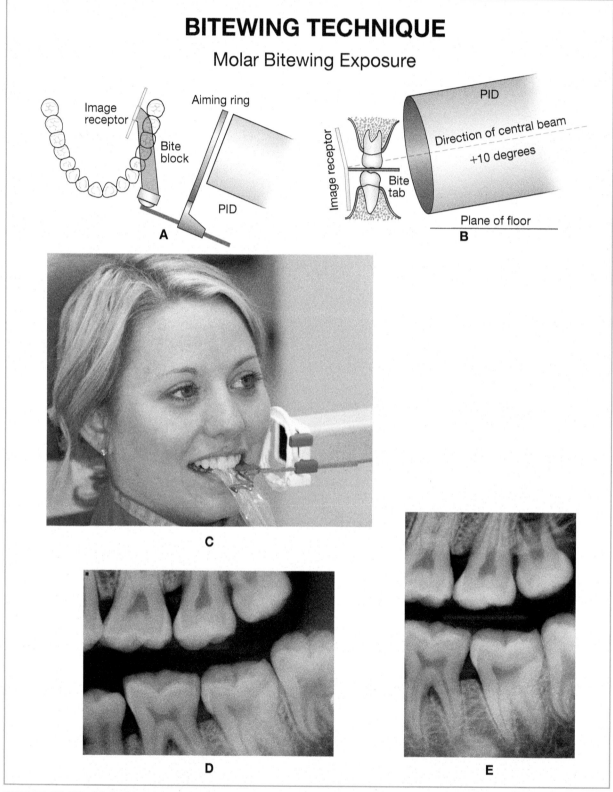

BITEWING TECHNIQUE
Molar Bitewing Exposure

FIGURE 15–20 **Molar bitewing exposure.** (**A**) Diagram showing relationship of image receptor and positioner, teeth, and PID. (**B**) Vertical angulation directed perpendicular to image receptor at approximately +10 degrees with PID tilted downward. Central rays of x-ray beam directed at center of image receptor at a spot on the occlusal plane between maxillary and mandibular teeth. (**C**) Patient showing position of image receptor positioner and 16 inch (41 cm) rectangular PID. (**D**) Horizontal molar bitewing radiograph. (**E**) Vertical molar bitewing radiograph.

REVIEW—Chapter summary

Bitewing radiographs image the coronal portion of both maxillary and mandibular teeth on one image receptor. Bitewing radiographs supplement and complete the full mouth survey because of their improved ability to image incipient caries in the tooth contact areas and early resorptive changes in the alveolar bony crest.

The size and number of images to expose depend on the type of survey required and the size and shape of a patient's oral cavity. The image receptor may be positioned with the long dimension horizontally or vertically. Traditionally posterior bitewing radiographs have been positioned horizontally; anterior bitewing radiographs are positioned vertically. Vertical positioning images more anatomical structures, especially periodontal bone. Image receptor placement is usually closer to the tooth than is possible with periapical image receptor placement. Be careful to avoid bending or slanting the image receptor as the patient occludes. Positioning the image receptor a slight distance away from the lingual surfaces of the maxillary teeth of interest will help avoid contact with the curvature of the palate, and avoid producing a sloping or slanted image that may result in a retake.

Each bitewing radiograph has a standard placement and can be expected to image particular teeth. Centering the teeth of interest is standard placement for anterior bitewing radiographs. Aligning the anterior edge of the image receptor behind the distal edge of the premolar or molar is standard placement for posterior bitewing radiographs. Use the patient's occlusal relationship to determine which arch to focus on during placement of the image receptor. Generally, the mandibular arch is used to align the anterior edge of the image receptor when a Class I or III occlusal relationship presents, and the maxillary arch is used when a Class II occlusal relationship presents. Use a systemic order of sequence in exposing bitewing radiographs to help avoid errors.

Image receptor positioners include stick-on or loop bitetabs and instruments with external aiming devices that assist with determining the correct horizontal and vertical angulations and the points of entry. If a holder without an external aiming device is used, the horizontal angulation is determined by directing the central rays of the x-ray beam perpendicular to the recording plane of the image receptor through the mean tangent of the embrasures between the teeth of interest. Vertical angulation for all bitewing radiographs is +10 degrees; +5 degrees vertical angulation is used for children. When the horizontal angulation is incorrectly directed obliquely from the mesial, overlapping will be more severe in the distal or posterior region of the image. When the horizontal angulation is incorrectly directed obliquely from the distal, overlapping will be more severe in the mesial or anterior region of the image. When the vertical angulation is excessive (greater than +10 degrees), more maxillary teeth and bone are imaged, cutting off a portion of the mandibular structures. When the vertical angulation is inadequate (less than +10 degrees) more mandibular teeth and bone are imaged, cutting off a portion of the maxillary structures. Directing the central rays of the x-ray beam at the level of the incisal/occlusal plane (at the lip line) will assist with directing the central rays of the x-ray beam to the center of the image receptor to avoid conecut error.

The four basic steps to exposing a bitewing radiograph are placement, vertical angulation, horizontal angulation, and point of entry. Step-by-step illustrated instructions for exposing anterior and posterior bitewing radiographs are presented.

RECALL—Study questions

1. Which of these conditions would NOT be visible on a bitewing radiograph?
   a. Proximal surface caries
   b. Overhanging restoration
   c. Apical abscess
   d. Alveolar bone resorption

2. How many standard size 2 image receptors are recommended for a posterior horizontal bitewing survey of an adult patient?
   a. Two
   b. Four
   c. Seven
   d. Eight

3. In which of the following situations would using a size 3 image receptor be acceptable?
   a. Horizontal bitewings on a pediatric patient who presented with a need for them
   b. Horizontal bitewings on an adult patient for caries detection
   c. Horizontal bitewings on an adult patient with periodontal disease
   d. Vertical bitewings on any patient who presented with a need for them

4. In which of the following conditions would vertical bitewing radiographs be recommended over horizontal bitewing radiographs?
   a. Child with rampant caries
   b. Adolescent with suspected third molar impactions
   c. Adult with malaligned teeth
   d. Adult with periodontal disease

5. The best rationale for taking vertical bitewings is that vertical bitewings
   a. image more alveolar bone than horizontal bitewings.
   b. result in less overlapping than horizontal bitewings.
   c. eliminate the need for periapical radiographs.
   d. are more easily tolerated by most patients.

6. Which size image receptor is used, and how is it positioned for exposure of an anterior bitewing radiograph of a small and narrow adult arch?
   a. Size 3 placed vertically
   b. Size 2 placed horizontally
   c. Size 1 placed vertically
   d. Size 0 placed horizontally

7. When taking a premolar horizontal bitewing radiograph, the anterior edge of the image receptor should be positioned behind the distal edge of the maxillary canine when presented with which occlusal relationship?
   a. Class I
   b. Class II
   c. Class III

8. A right-handed radiographer, when taking a set of eight vertical bitewing radiographs, would place and expose which of the following first?
   a. Left molar
   b. Left premolar
   c. Left canine
   d. Right premolar

9. An error in which of these results in overlapping?
   a. Placement of image receptor
   b. Point of entry
   c. Vertical angulation
   d. Horizontal angulation

10. What is the approximate vertical angulation for adult bitewing radiographs?
    a. –10 degrees
    b. 0 degrees
    c. +10 degrees
    d. +20 degrees

11. An error in vertical angulation will result in
    a. unequal distribution of the arches.
    b. overlapping.
    c. overexposure.
    d. conecut.

12. The image receptor placement for an adult horizontal molar bitewing is to align the receptor so that the
    a. central and lateral incisors are centered.
    b. canine is centered.
    c. anterior portion of the receptor lines up behind the distal half of the canine.
    d. anterior portion of the receptor lines up behind the distal half of the second premolar.

13. The image receptor placement for an adult vertical premolar bitewing is to align the receptor so that the
    a. central and lateral incisors are centered.
    b. canine is centered.
    c. anterior portion of the receptor lines up behind the distal half of the canine.
    d. anterior portion of the receptor lines up behind the distal half of the second premolar.

14. Through which interproximal space should the central rays of the x-ray beam be perpendicularly directed when exposing a molar bitewing on a child with primary teeth?
    a. Between the central and lateral incisors
    b. Between the lateral incisor and canine
    c. Between the canine and first molar
    d. Between the first and second molars

15. Through which interproximal space should the central rays of the x-ray beam be perpendicularly directed when exposing a premolar bitewing on an adolescent with permanent teeth?
    a. Between the central and lateral incisors
    b. Between the lateral incisor and canine
    c. Between the canine and first premolar
    d. Between the first and second premolars

REFLECT—Case study

Study the dental chart and patient record that follows. Note the dentist's written prescription for a radiographic examination. Decide the following:

1. What type of bitewings will most likely be exposed?

2. What size image receptor will best fit this patient?

3. How many image receptors will be required to complete the exam?

4. Write out a detailed procedure for exposing each of the required radiographs. Include:
   a. Specific image receptor placements
   b. Vertical angulation required
   c. How the horizontal angulation will be determined
   d. What the point of entry will be

Case:	New patient.		Social History:	Appears nervous of dental treatment
Age:	40-year-old.		Chief Complaint:	Gum disease
Medical History:	Hypertension.		Current Oral	Generalized 4–6 mm pockets
Dental History:	Extensive dental treatment as evidenced by extractions and restorations.		Hygiene Status:	Generalized moderate gingivitis
			Initial Treatment:	Bitewing radiographic examination.

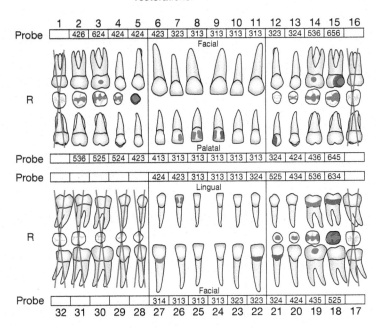

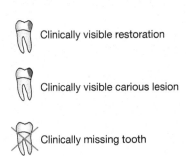

Clinically visible restoration

Clinically visible carious lesion

Clinically missing tooth

RELATE—Laboratory application

For a comprehensive laboratory practice exercise on this topic, see Thomson, E. M., & Bruhn, A. M. (2018). *Exercises in oral radiography techniques: A laboratory manual* (4th ed.). Hoboken,, NJ: Pearson. Chapter 6, "Bitewing radiographic technique."

RESOURCES

Eastman Kodak Company. (2002). *Successful intraoral radiography.* Rochester, NY: Author.

Rinn Corporation. (1989). *Intraoral radiography with Rinn XCP/ BAI instruments.* Elgin, IL: Dentsply/Rinn Corporation.

White, S. C., & Pharoah, M. J. (2014). Intraoral projections. *Oral radiology: Principles and interpretation* (7th ed.). St. Louis, MO: Elsevier.

Wilkins, E. M. (2012). Dental radiographic imaging. *Clinical practice of the dental hygienist* (11th ed.). Philadelphia, PA: Wolters Kluwer.

Visit www.pearsonhighered.com/healthprofessionsresources to access the student resources that accompany this book. Simply select Dental Hygiene from the choice of disciplines. Find this book and you will find the complementary study tools created for this specific title.

16

The Occlusal Examination

CHAPTER OUTLINE

OBJECTIVES

Following successful completion of this chapter, you should be able to:

1. Define the key terms.
2. State the purpose of the occlusal examination.
3. List the indications for occlusal radiographs.
4. Match the topographical and cross-sectional techniques with the condition to be imaged.
5. Compare patient head positions for the topographical and cross-sectional techniques.
6. Demonstrate the steps for the maxillary and mandibular topographical surveys.
7. Demonstrate the steps for the mandibular cross-sectional survey.

KEY TERMS

Cross-sectional technique

Occlusal radiograph

Topographical technique

Introduction

The occlusal examination allows for assessment of the large anatomical areas of the maxilla or the mandible with one intraoral radiograph. The image receptor is placed in the oral cavity between the occlusal surfaces of the maxillary and mandibular teeth. No image receptor positioner is required. The patient occludes lightly on the image receptor to stabilize it and the x-ray beam is directed to intersect the image receptor at precise angles. Occlusal radiographs play an important role in special situations and the oral health care professional skilled in this technique will be better prepared to respond to patients who present with these conditions.

This chapter discusses the use and explains the procedures for the occlusal examination and presents step-by-step instructions for two types of occlusal radiographic techniques.

Types of Occlusal Examinations

Occlusal radiographs are obtained by either the topographical or the cross-sectional technique.

Topographical Technique

The **topographical technique** that is used to expose occlusal radiographs produces an image that looks like a large periapical radiograph (Figure 16–1 ■). The topographical occlusal technique is similar to the bisecting technique used to produce periapical radiographs (see Chapter 14).

Topographical occlusal radiographs may be exposed in any area of the oral cavity; and the anterior and posterior regions of both the maxilla and the mandible. Topographical occlusal radiographs are best used to image conditions of the teeth and supporting structures when a larger area than that recorded by a periapical radiograph is required. Topographical occlusal surveys generally yield a greater amount of information in the alveolar crest and apical areas than periapical radiographs.

Cross-sectional Technique

The **cross-sectional technique** that is used to expose occlusal radiographs produces an image much like its name implies (see Figure 16–1). The shortened, elliptical or circular appearance of the teeth on the radiograph and the increased coverage of the sublingual area (under the tongue) allow the cross-sectional occlusal radiograph to yield more information about the location of impacted or malpositioned teeth and calcifications of soft tissues. Cross-sectional occlusal radiographs are used, if needed, almost exclusively for mandibular diagnoses and are not likely to be used to image any regions of the maxilla.

Fundamentals of Occlusal Radiographs

The occlusal examination may be made alone or to supplement periapical or bitewing radiographs or extraoral panoramic radiographs. The large size 4 occlusal image

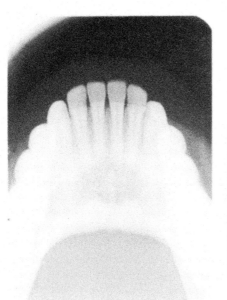
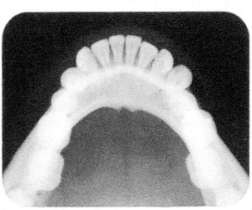

A   B

FIGURE 16–1 **A comparison of topographical and cross-sectional occlusal radiographs.** (**A**) The topographical occlusal radiograph of the anterior mandible closely resembles a periapical radiograph. Note how the large occlusal film images a larger portion of the region. (**B**) The cross-sectional occlusal radiograph of the mandibular anterior region reveals more information about the sublingual area (under the tongue) and conditions of the soft tissue than about the teeth and the supporting bone.

receptor is useful for recording information that cannot be adequately recorded on the smaller periapical image receptors. **Occlusal radiographs** are used to:

- Locate supernumerary, unerupted, or impacted teeth
- Locate retained roots of extracted teeth
- Detect the presence, locate, and evaluate the extent of disease and lesions (cysts, tumors, etc.)
- Locate foreign bodies in the jaw
- Reveal the presence of salivary stones (sialoliths) in the ducts of the sublingual and submandibular glands
- Aid in evaluating fractures of the maxilla or mandible
- Show the size and shape of mandibular tori
- Aid in examining patients with trismus (difficulty opening the mouth)
- Evaluate the borders of the maxillary sinus
- Examine a cleft palate
- Substitute for a periapical examination on young children who may not be able to tolerate periapical image receptor placement (see Chapter 27)

Topographical occlusal radiographs may be taken in any region of the oral cavity, whereas the cross-sectional occlusal radiograph is most often limited to imaging conditions of the mandible. This chapter focuses on five standard placements:

1. Maxillary topographical (anterior)
2. Maxillary topographical (posterior)
3. Mandibular topographical (anterior)
4. Mandibular topographical (posterior)
5. Mandibular cross-sectional

Image Receptor Requirements

The large 3 × 2.25 in. (7.7 × 5.8 cm) size 4 film or phosphor plate is used for occlusal radiographs on most adult patients. Currently this larger size 4 is not available as a digital sensor. Smaller size 2 intraoral image receptors may also be used with the occlusal technique, when the condition requiring an occlusal radiograph is localized or small enough to be recorded on the smaller image receptor. The standard size 2 image receptor may be substituted for the size 4 image receptor for exposing occlusal radiographs on children. Occlusal radiographs do not require the use of an image receptor positioner for stabilization in the oral cavity making it easy for a pediatric patient to tolerate. For this reason occlusal radiographs are sometimes used in place of periapical radiographs.

Orientation of the Image Receptor

When using a size 4 film, the packet is positioned with the white unprinted side (front side) against the arch of interest. When using a phosphor plate, the plain side is positioned against the arch of interest. When imaging the mandibular arch, the white, unprinted side of the image receptor will face the mandible. When imaging the maxillary arch, the white,

unprinted side of the image receptor will face the maxilla. The image receptor may be placed into the mouth with the long dimension positioned across the arches (buccal-to-buccal) or along the midline (anterior-to-posterior), centered over one small region of interest or over the entire right or left sides of the dental arches. The position used will depend on the type of occlusal radiograph needed and the area that needs to be examined.

In the correct position, the image receptor should be placed well back into the oral cavity, but with at least 0.25 inch (0.5 cm) protruding outside the mouth to avoid cutting off part of the image. Because the embossed identification dot (on a film packet) should be positioned away from the area of interest, positioning it toward the anterior should leave it outside the oral cavity and therefore prevent it from interfering with the image.

Patient Positioning

Because predetermined vertical angulations and points of entry are utilized in taking occlusal radiographs (just as they are for periapical radiographs using the bisecting technique), it is very important that a patient be seated with his or her head in the correct position for the area to be imaged. For occlusal radiographs taken on the maxilla, the patient should be seated with the occlusal plane parallel to the plane of the floor and the midsagittal plane perpendicular to the plane of the floor (see Figure 12–15). The head position for the mandibular exposures will depend on the type of occlusal radiograph to be produced. Topographical occlusal radiographs of the mandible may be taken with the head positioned the same as for maxillary exposures, with the occlusal plane parallel to the floor and the midsagittal plane perpendicular to the floor. Mandibular cross-sectional occlusal radiographs are taken with the patient reclined in the chair so that the head is tipped back, positioning the occlusal plane perpendicular to the plane of the floor (Figure 16–2 ■).

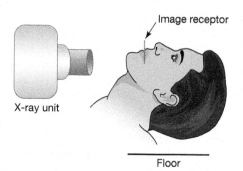

FIGURE 16–2 **Patient positioning for mandibular cross-sectional occlusal radiographs.** Patient reclined in the chair so that the head is tipped back, positioning the occlusal plane perpendicular to the plane of the floor. The central rays of the x-ray beam are directed toward the image receptor perpendicularly.

Exposure Factors

The exposure factors (kV, mA, and time) used for occlusal radiographs are usually the same as those settings used for periapical and bitewing radiographs of the same region. Be sure to consult the posted exposure settings chart prior to beginning the procedure.

Horizontal and Vertical Angulation

Horizontal Angulation

The correct horizontal angulation for topographical occlusal radiographs is determined in the same manner as for periapical and bitewing radiographs, by directing the central rays of the x-ray beam at the image receptor perpendicularly through the teeth embrasures (spaces). When exposing anterior topographical occlusal radiographs, the central rays of the x-ray beam are directed perpendicular to the image receptor through the interproximal embrasures of the anterior teeth. When exposing posterior topographical occlusal radiographs, the central rays of the x-ray beam are directed perpendicular to the image receptor through the interproximal spaces or embrasures of the posterior teeth. The horizontal angulation for the mandibular cross-sectional is also such that the central rays of the x-ray beam will intersect the image receptor perpendicularly. This alignment is best determined by positioning the open end of the position indicating device (PID) parallel to the image receptor.

Vertical Angulation

The vertical angulation for topographical occlusal radiographs follows the rules of the bisecting technique used for periapical radiographs, where the central rays of the x-ray beam are directed through the apices of the teeth perpendicularly toward the imaginary bisector (Figure 16–3 ■). To determine the correct vertical angulation when taking a topographical occlusal radiograph, observe the plane of the image receptor, then locate the long axes of the teeth of interest, and estimate the imaginary bisector of these two planes. If the patient's head is in the correct position, use predetermined vertical angulation settings (Table 16–1 ■).

The vertical angulation for the mandibular cross-sectional occlusal radiograph of the mandible is such that the central rays of the x-ray beam are directed toward the image receptor perpendicularly (see Figure 16–2). To achieve a perpendicular relationship between the plane of the image receptor and the central rays of the x-ray beam, the patient's head position must be such that the occlusal plane is perpendicular to the plane of the floor. In other words, the patient should be reclined and his or her chin tipped upward. In this position, the vertical angulation of the PID will most likely be set at 0 degrees, allowing the x-rays to strike the image receptor perpendicularly.

A patient may present with symptoms that require an assessment of the maxillary sinus, maxillary edentulous

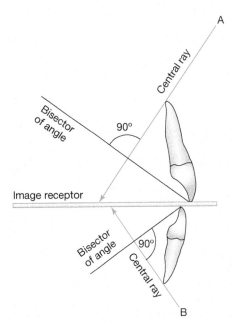

FIGURE 16–3 Angles for exposing topographical occlusal radiographs. The image receptor placement for occlusal radiographs is not parallel to the long axes of the teeth being imaged. Based on the bisecting technique, vertical angulation for (**A**) maxillary and (**B**) mandibular topographical radiographs is determined by directing the central rays of the x-ray beam perpendicular to the imaginary bisector between the plane of the image receptor and the long axes of the teeth of interest.

ridges, or other specific conditions of the maxilla. However, the significant amount of bony structures located here make cross-sectional occlusal radiographs of the maxilla difficult to image with clarity. Therefore maxillary cross-sectional occlusal radiographs are exposed less frequently.

Table 16–1 Recommended Vertical Angulation Settings for Occlusal Radiographs

Occlusal Radiograph	Vertical Angle Setting*
Maxillary topographical (anterior)	+65°
Maxillary topographical (posterior)	+45°
Mandibular topographical (anterior)	−55°
Mandibular topographical (posterior)	−45°
Mandibular cross-sectional	0°**

*Patient must be seated in correct position, with occlusal plane of arch being imaged parallel to floor and midsagittal plane perpendicular to floor.
**Patient must be seated in correct position, with occlusal plane of mandible perpendicular to floor and midsagittal plane parallel to floor.

Points of Entry

If a patient's head is in the correct position, predetermined points of entry may be used (Table 16–2 ■). Essentially, the central rays of the x-ray beam should strike the middle of the image receptor. The open end of the PID must be aligned as close as possible to the patient's skin at the correct point of entry. Because the technique used to expose occlusal radiographs is similar to the bisecting technique, like the bisecting technique a short 8-inch (20.5-cm) PID is recommended to minimize magnification and dimensional distortion. Also an 8-inch (20.5-cm) PID may be easier to maneuver into the increased vertical angulation positions required for this technique.

The Occlusal Examination

Figures 16–4 through 16–8 illustrate the image receptor positions and required angulations for each of the topographical and cross-sectional occlusal radiographs discussed in this chapter. See Table 16–2 for a summary of the technique.

Practice Point

When exposing an occlusal radiograph on the mandible, it may be necessary to modify placement of the lead/lead equivalent thyroid collar. Although it is important to use "as low as reasonably achievable" (ALARA) practices and the lead/lead equivalent thyroid collar to protect radiation-sensitive tissues in the head and neck region, the thyroid collar must not be placed in the path of the primary beam during mandibular topographical and/or cross-sectional techniques.

Place the lead/lead equivalent apron and thyroid collar on the patient in the usual manner. After adjusting the patient's head position, placing the image receptor, and aligning the PID into the correct horizontal and vertical positions, check the thyroid collar to ensure that it is not in the path of the x-ray beam. If the thyroid collar is in a position that will block the x-rays from reaching the image receptor, readjust the collar position prior to making the exposure. Failure to remove the thyroid collar from in front of the open end of the PID will most likely result in a retake of the radiograph.

Table 16–2 Summary of Occlusal Radiographic Technique

Occlusal Radiograph	Placement	Vertical Angulation*	Horizontal Angulation	Point of Entry*
Maxillary topographical (anterior) (Figure 16–4 ■)	Long dimension across oral cavity (buccal-to-buccal); white unprinted film side toward maxillary teeth	Perpendicular to imaginary bisector between long axes of teeth and image receptor in vertical dimension, +65°	Perpendicular to image receptor through maxillary central incisors embrasure	Through a point near bridge of nose toward center of image receptor
Maxillary topographical (posterior) (Figure 16–5 ■)	Long dimension along midline (anterior-to-posterior); white unprinted film side toward maxillary teeth	Perpendicular to imaginary bisector between long axes of teeth and image receptor in vertical dimension, +45°	Perpendicular to image receptor through maxillary posterior embrasures	Through a point on ala—tragus line below outer canthus of eye (see Figure 14–18) toward center of image receptor
Mandibular topographical (anterior) (Figure 16–6 ■)	Long dimension across oral cavity (buccal-to-buccal); white unprinted film side toward mandibular teeth	Perpendicular to imaginary bisector between long axes of teeth and image receptor in vertical dimension, −55°	Perpendicular to image receptor through mandibular central incisors embrasure	Through a point on middle of chin toward center of image receptor
Mandibular topographical (posterior) (Figure 16–7 ■)	Long dimension along midline (anterior-to-posterior); white unprinted film side toward mandibular teeth	Perpendicular to imaginary bisector between long axes of teeth and image receptor in vertical dimension, −45°	Perpendicular to image receptor through mandibular posterior embrasures	Through a point on inferior border of mandible directly below second mandibular premolar toward center of image receptor
Mandibular cross-sectional (Figure 16–8 ■)	Long dimension across oral cavity (buccal-to-buccal); white unprinted side toward mandibular teeth	Perpendicular to image receptor, 0°**	Align open end of PID parallel to plane of image receptor	Through a point 2 inches (5 cm) back from tip of chin toward center of image receptor**

*Patient must be seated in correct position, with occlusal plane of arch being imaged parallel to floor and midsagittal plane perpendicular to floor.
**Patient must be seated in correct position, with occlusal plane of mandible perpendicular to floor and midsagittal plane parallel to floor.

OCCLUSAL TECHNIQUE
Maxillary Topographical Occlusal Radiograph (Anterior)

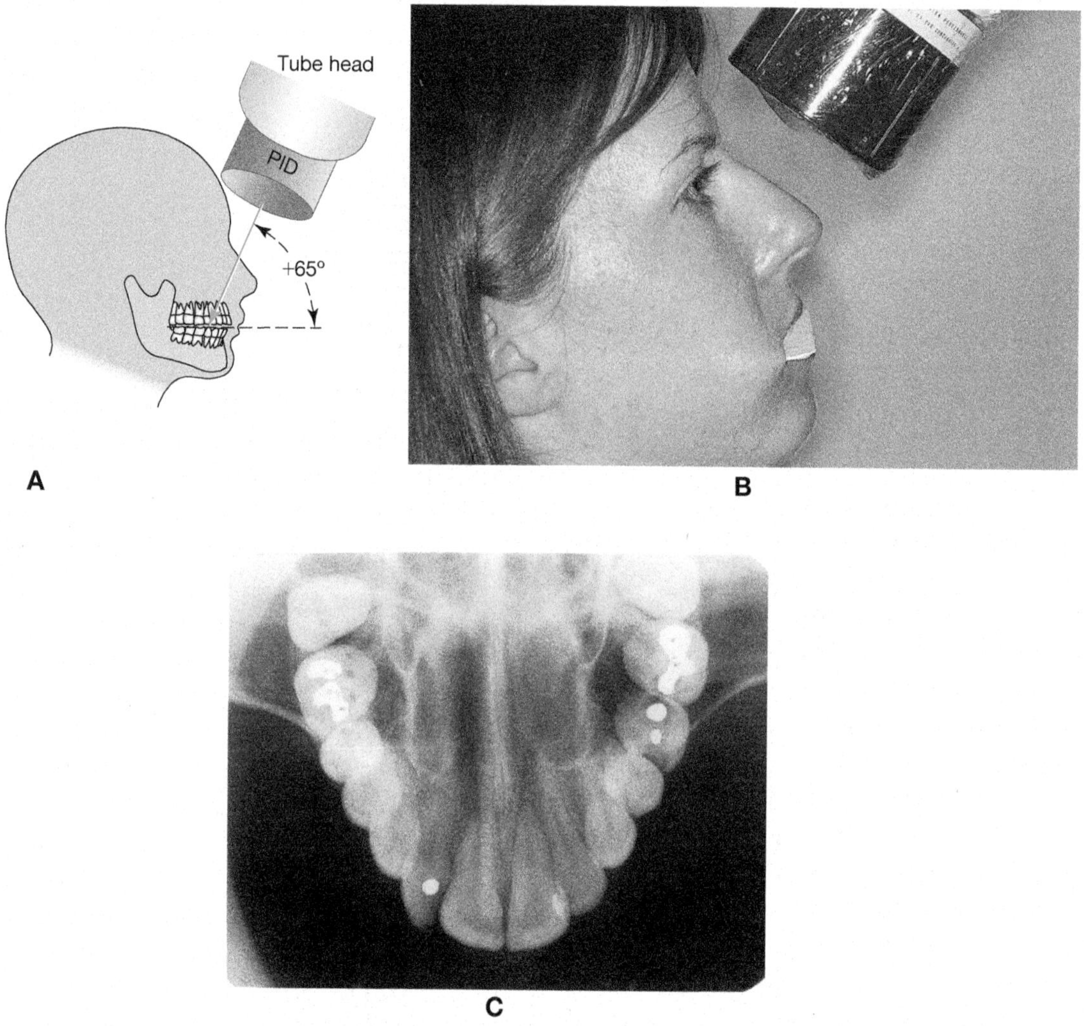

FIGURE 16–4 Maxillary topographical occlusal radiograph (anterior). (A) Diagram showing relationship of tube head and PID to image receptor and patient. Exposure side of image receptor faces maxillary arch with longer dimension buccal-to-buccal (across the arch). Central rays of x-ray beam are directed perpendicular in horizontal dimension to patient's midsagittal plane through the maxillary central incisors embrasure. Vertical angulation is directed approximately +65 degrees through a point near bridge of nose toward center of image receptor. **(B)** Patient showing position of image receptor and 8-inch (20.5-cm) circular PID. **(C)** Anterior maxillary topographical occlusal radiograph.

OCCLUSAL TECHNIQUE
Maxillary Topographical Occlusal Radiograph (Posterior)

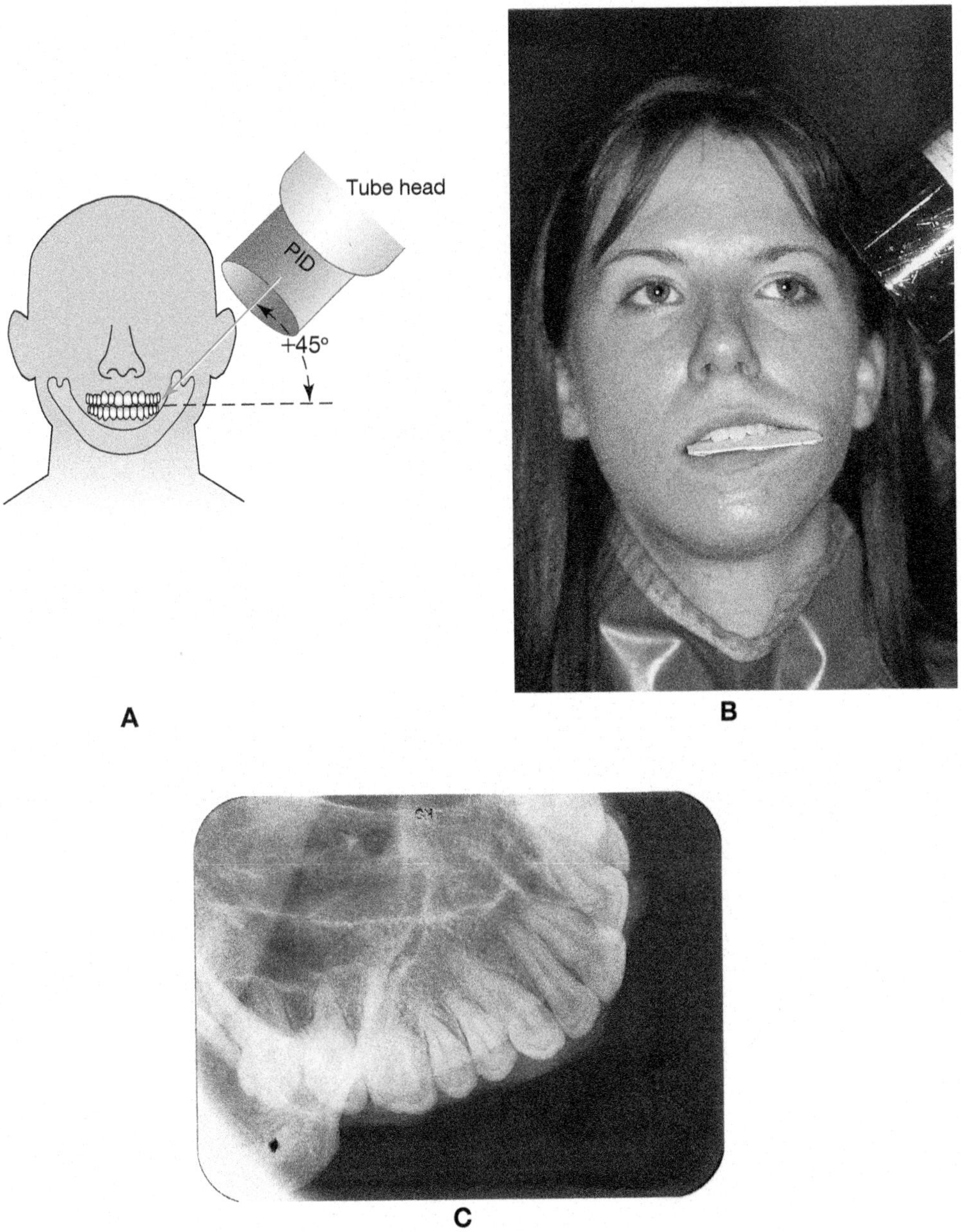

FIGURE 16–5 **Maxillary topographical occlusal radiograph (posterior).** (**A**) Diagram showing relationship of tube head and PID to image receptor and patient. Image receptor is positioned over left or right side, depending on area of interest. Exposure side of image receptor faces maxillary arch with longer dimension along midline (anterior-to-posterior). Central rays of x-ray beam are directed perpendicular in horizontal dimension to patient's midsagittal plane through maxillary posterior embrasures. Vertical angulation is directed approximately +45 degrees through a point on ala–tragus line below outer canthus of the eye toward center of image receptor. (**B**) Patient showing position of image receptor and 8-inch (20.5-cm) circular PID. (**C**) Posterior maxillary topographical occlusal radiograph.

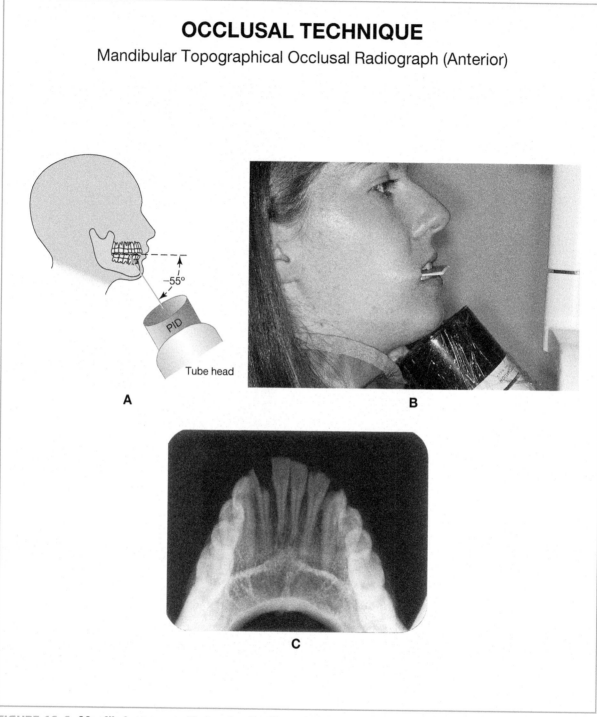

OCCLUSAL TECHNIQUE
Mandibular Topographical Occlusal Radiograph (Anterior)

A

B

C

FIGURE 16–6 **Mandibular topographical occlusal radiograph (anterior).** (**A**) Diagram showing relationship of tube head and PID to image receptor and patient. Exposure side of image receptor faces mandibular arch with longer dimension buccal-to-buccal (across the arch). Central rays of x-ray beam are directed perpendicular in horizontal dimension to patient's midsagittal plane through mandibular central incisors embrasure. Vertical angulation is directed approximately −55 degrees through a point in middle of chin toward center of image receptor. (**B**) Patient showing position of image receptor and 8-inch (20.5-cm) circular PID. (**C**) Anterior mandibular topographical occlusal radiograph.

OCCLUSAL TECHNIQUE
Mandibular Topographical Occlusal Radiograph (Posterior)

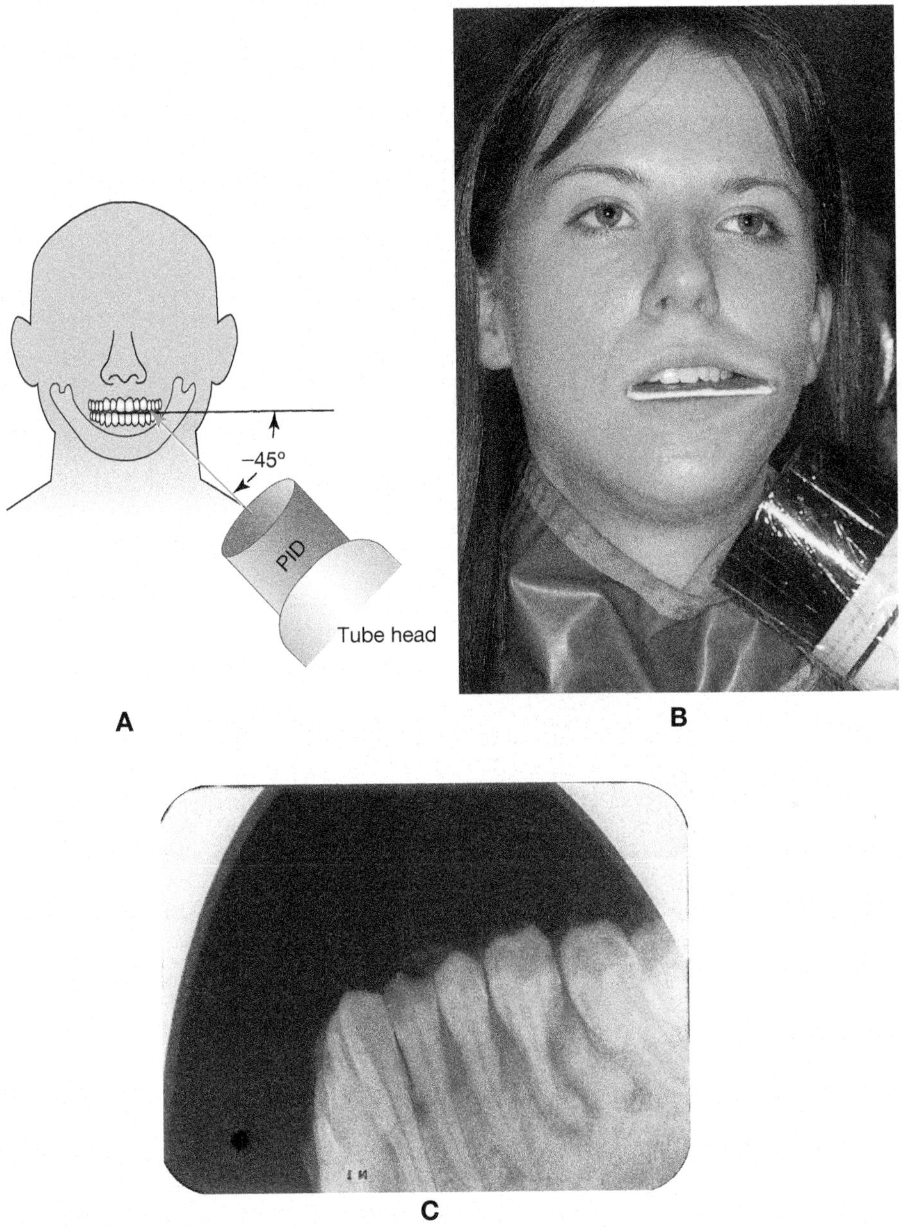

FIGURE 16–7 **Mandibular topographical occlusal radiograph (posterior).** (**A**) Diagram showing relationship of tube head and PID to image receptor and patient. Image receptor is positioned over left or right side, depending on area of interest. Exposure side of image receptor faces mandibular arch with longer dimension along midline (anterior-to-posterior). Central rays of x-ray beam are directed perpendicular in horizontal dimension to patient's midsagittal plane through mandibular posterior embrasures. Vertical angulation is directed approximately −45 degrees through a point on inferior border of mandible directly below second mandibular premolar toward center of image receptor. (**B**) Patient showing position of image receptor and 8-inch (20.5-cm) circular PID. (**C**) Posterior mandibular topographical occlusal radiograph.

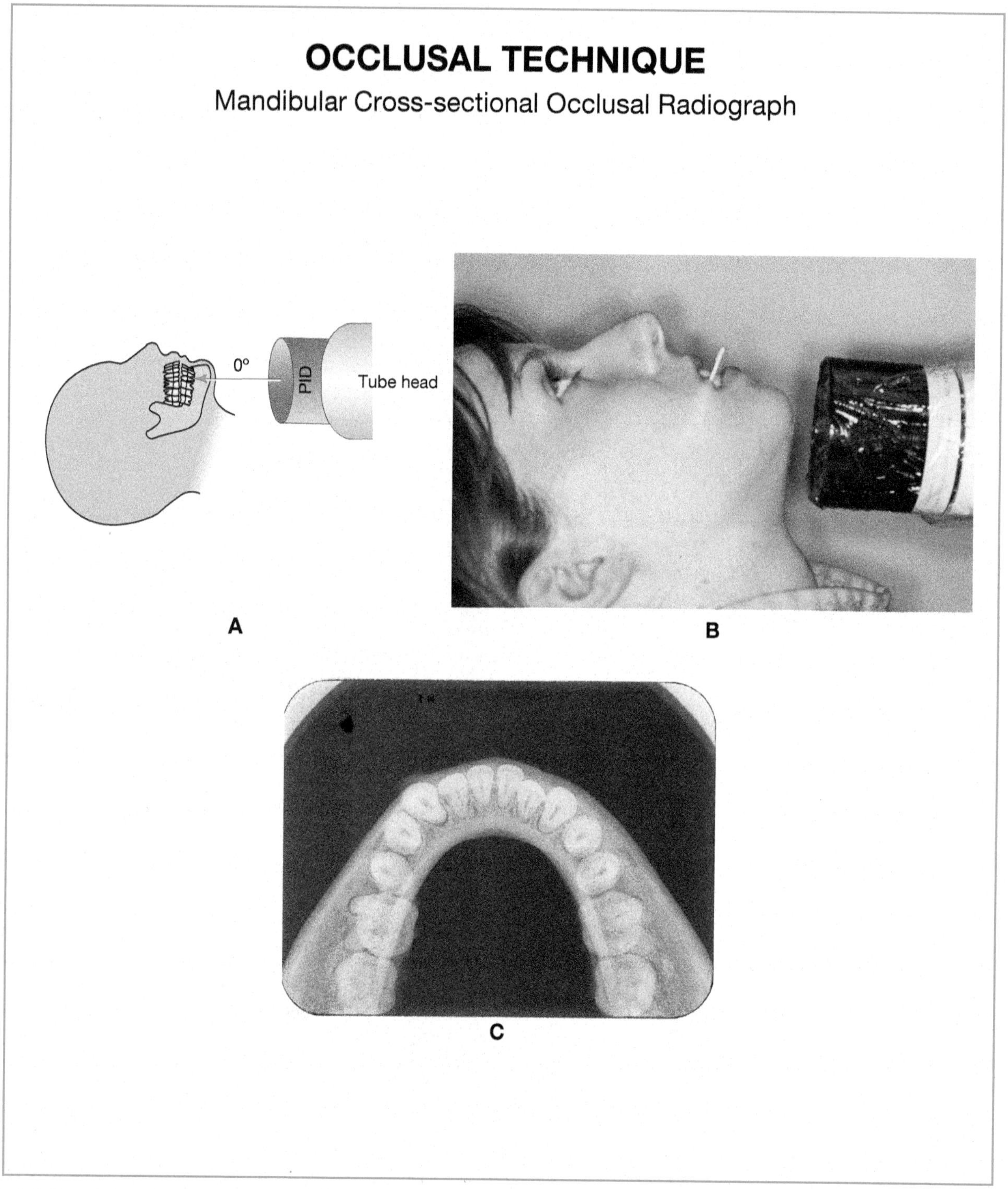

OCCLUSAL TECHNIQUE
Mandibular Cross-sectional Occlusal Radiograph

FIGURE 16–8 **Mandibular cross-sectional occlusal radiograph.** (**A**) Diagram showing relationship of tube head and PID to image receptor and patient. Exposure side of image receptor faces mandibular arch with longer dimension buccal-to-buccal (across the arch). Central rays of x-ray beam are directed perpendicular in both horizontal and vertical dimensions toward image receptor. Positioning open end of PID parallel to image receptor achieves required perpendicular alignment. Vertical angulation is directed approximately 0 degrees through a point 2 inches (5 cm) back from tip of chin toward center of image receptor. (**B**) Patient showing position of image receptor and 8-inch (20.5-cm) circular PID. (**C**) Mandibular cross-sectional occlusal radiograph.

REVIEW—Chapter summary

The purpose of occlusal radiographs is to record larger anatomical areas for diagnostic assessment of the maxilla or the mandible than can be done with periapical radiographs. The topographical occlusal radiograph resembles a large periapical radiograph. Topographical occlusal radiographs may be exposed in any area of the oral cavity. Cross-sectional occlusal radiographs produce shortened images of the teeth and are used to record conditions of the mandible and sublingual area. Cross-sectional occlusal radiographs are not usually used to examine conditions of the maxilla. Occlusal radiographs are used to view conditions of the teeth and supporting structures such as impactions, large apical lesions, calcifications in soft tissue, and fractures.

Size 4 image receptors are used for adult examinations. If indicated, a size 2 or smaller image receptor may be used with the occlusal technique, especially for children. An image receptor holder is not required; the patient lightly bites down on the image receptor to hold it in place. The image receptor may be positioned with the long dimension across the arches (buccal-to-buccal) or along the midline (anterior-to-posterior) with at least 0.25 inch (0.5 cm) protruding outside the mouth.

The patient's head should be positioned with the occlusal plane parallel and the midsagittal plane perpendicular to the floor when exposing maxillary and mandibular topographical occlusal radiographs. The patient's head should be tipped back into a position with the occlusal plane perpendicular to the plane of the floor and the midsaggital plane parallel to the floor when exposing a mandibular cross-sectional occlusal radiograph.

The topographical occlusal technique is based on the bisecting technique used to expose periapical radiographs. The horizontal angulation used to produce a topographical occlusal radiograph is determined in the same manner as for periapical and bitewing radiographs, where the central rays of the x-ray beam are directed perpendicularly to the image receptor through the embrasures of the teeth of interest. Aligning the open end of the PID parallel to the image receptor will assist in determining the correct horizontal angulation to produce a cross-sectional occlusal radiograph. The vertical angulation used to produce a topographical occlusal radiograph is determined in a similar manner to the bisecting technique used to produce periapical radiographs, where the central rays of the x-ray beam are directed perpendicular to the bisector between the long axes of the teeth and the plane of the image receptor. Determining the vertical angulation for exposure of a cross-sectional occlusal radiograph is assisted by positioning the open end of the PID parallel to the plane of the image receptor. Correct points of entry position are determined by directing the central rays of the x-ray beam at the center of the image receptor. If the patient's head is in correct position, predetermined vertical angulations and points of the entry may be used. Step-by-step illustrated instructions for exposing five standard occlusal radiographs are presented.

RECALL—Study questions

1. Each of the following is an indication for exposing occlusal radiographs EXCEPT one. Which one is the EXCEPTION?
   a. Evaluate periodontal disease.
   b. Examine sinus borders.
   c. Locate foreign bodies.
   d. Reveal sialoliths.

2. Which of the following will a mandibular cross-sectional occlusal radiograph best image?
   a. Cleft palate
   b. Fractured jaw
   c. Large periapical cyst
   d. Sublingual swelling

3. Which of these sizes is known as the occlusal image receptor?
   a. 1
   b. 2
   c. 3
   d. 4

4. The image receptor should be placed with the long dimension along the midline (anterior-to-posterior) for which of these occlusal radiographs?
   a. Maxillary topographical anterior
   b. Maxillary topographical posterior
   c. Mandibular topographical anterior
   d. Mandibular cross-sectional

5. Where should the embossed dot be positioned when placing an occlusal film packet intraorally?
   a. Toward the apical
   b. Toward the occlusal
   c. Toward the anterior
   d. Toward the posterior

6. The ideal patient head position when exposing a maxillary topographical occlusal radiograph is to position the occlusal plane _____ to the plane of the floor and the midsagittal plane _____ to the plane of the floor.
   a. parallel; perpendicular
   b. perpendicular; parallel
   c. parallel; parallel
   d. perpendicular; perpendicular

7. The ideal patient head position when exposing a mandibular cross-sectional occlusal radiograph is to position the examination chair head rest so that the chin is tipped _____ and the occlusal plane is _____ to the plane of the floor.
   a. down; perpendicular
   b. up; perpendicular
   c. down; parallel
   d. up; parallel

8. Assuming that the patient's head is in the correct position, which of the following is the correct vertical angulation setting for a maxillary anterior topographical occlusal radiograph?
   a. +65 degrees
   b. +45 degrees
   c. 0 degrees
   d. −55 degrees

9. Assuming that the patient's head is in the correct position, which of the following is the correct vertical angulation setting for a mandibular cross-sectional occlusal radiograph?
   a. +65 degrees
   b. +45 degrees
   c. 0 degrees
   d. −55 degrees

10. What is the point of entry for correctly exposing a posterior mandible topographical occlusal radiograph?
   a. The middle of the chin
   b. A point 2 inches (5 cm) back from the tip of the chin
   c. A point on the ala–tragus line below the outer canthus of the eye
   d. A point on the inferior border of the mandible directly below the second mandibular premolar

REFLECT—Case study

Consider the following cases. After determining the radiographic assessment for each of these three cases, write out a detailed procedure chart that a radiographer can follow to obtain the needed radiographs. Begin with patient positioning. Be sure to include the steps for determining the correct placement of the image receptor, x-ray beam angles, and landmarks for determining points of entry.

1. An adult patient presents with a sublingual swelling indicating the possibility of a blocked salivary gland. What type of occlusal radiograph will this patient most likely be assessed for?

2. An adult patient presents with the possibility of an impacted third molar. Pain and swelling limits the ability to open the mouth more than a few millimeters. What type of occlusal radiograph will this patient most likely be assessed for?

3. A pediatric patient presents with trauma to the maxillary anterior teeth after a fall off a bicycle. What type of occlusal radiograph will this patient most likely be assessed for?

RELATE—Laboratory application

For a comprehensive laboratory practice exercise on this topic, see Thomson, E. M., & Bruhn, A. M. (2018). *Exercises in oral radiography techniques: A laboratory manual* (4th ed.). Hoboken, NJ: Pearson. Chapter 12 "Supplemental Radiographic Techniques."

RESOURCES

Carroll, M. K. (1993). *Advanced oral radiographic techniques: Part I, occlusal and lateral oblique projections* (videorecording). Jackson, MS: Health Sciences Consortium, Learning Resources, University of Mississippi Medical Center.

Eastman Kodak Company. (2002). *Successful intraoral radiography.* Rochester, NY: Author.

White, S. C., & Pharoah, M. J. (2014). Intraoral projections. *Oral radiology: Principles and interpretation* (7th ed.). St. Louis, MO: Elsevier.

Visit www.pearsonhighered.com/healthprofessionsresources to access the student resources that accompany this book. Simply select Dental Hygiene from the choice of disciplines. Find this book and you will find the complementary study tools created for this specific title.

The Panoramic Examination

CHAPTER OUTLINE

OBJECTIVES

Following successful completion of this chapter, you should be able to:

1. Define the key terms.
2. List uses of panoramic radiography.
3. Compare the advantages and limitations of panoramic versus intraoral radiographs.
4. Explain how the panoramic technique relates to the principles of tomography.
5. Identify the three dimensions of the focal trough.
6. Identify and describe panoramic image receptors.
7. Explain the role of intensifying screens in producing a radiographic image.
8. Identify the intensifying screen type recommended ALARA.
9. Describe the purpose of a panoramic cassette.
10. List the components of a panoramic x-ray machine.
11. Demonstrate how to use each of the head positioner guides found on a panoramic x-ray machine.
12. Demonstrate the steps used to prepare a patient for exposure of a panoramic radiograph.
13. Explain the use of a cape-style lead/lead equivalent barrier or the use of an apron without an attached thyroid collar.
14. Match errors made in patient preparation procedures with the characteristic effect on the appearance of the panoramic radiograph.
15. Identify the anatomical landmarks and planes used to position the dental arches correctly within the focal trough.
16. Match errors made in patient-positioning procedures with the characteristic affect on the appearance of the panoramic radiograph.
17. List exposure and image receptor handling errors and describe how these will affect the appearance of the panoramic radiograph.

KEY TERMS

Ala–tragus line
Artifacts
Calcium tungstate
Cassette
Focal trough/layer
Frankfort plane
Ghost image
Head positioner guides
Intensifying screens
Negative shadows
Occult disease
Opportunistic screening
Panoramic radiograph
Rare-earth phosphors
Screen film
Tomography

Introduction

The panoramic radiograph is probably the most common extraoral examination used in general oral health care practice. Panoramic radiography refers to a technique for producing a broad view image of the entire dentition of both the maxilla and mandible with the surrounding alveolar bone, the sinuses, and the temporomandibular joints on a single radiograph. This chapter explains the fundamental concepts of panoramic radiography and presents step-by-step instructions for exposing a panoramic radiograph that is free of errors that compromise diagnostic quality.

Purpose and Use

The term panoramic means "wide view," and panoramic radiography is descriptive of the wide view of the maxilla and mandible produced on a single radiograph (Figure 17–1 ■). **Panoramic radiographs** play a valuable role in:

- Examining large areas of the face and jaws
- Locating impacted teeth or retained root tips
- Evaluating trauma, lesions, and diseases of the jaws
- Assessing growth and development

Panoramic image quality, especially with the introduction of digital imaging, continues to improve, suggesting that panoramic radiographs may also aid in the evaluation of caries and periodontal diseases. However, panoramic imagery is not as sharp and detailed as the images produced by intraoral radiographs. When specific conditions or diseases are suspected, intraoral radiographs are often prescribed in conjunction with panoramic radiographs (see Table 6–1).

Advantages and Limitations

The greatest advantage of a panoramic radiograph is that it images a larger area and provides an increased amount of diagnostic information, as compared to a full mouth series of individual radiographs, with a reduced amount of radiation dose to the patient (Box 17–1). A panoramic radiograph requires less time to expose than a full mouth series, and the procedure demands less patient cooperation; and because the image receptor is not placed intraorally, there is less potential for discomfort, making the panoramic procedure an acceptable substitute, under certain conditions, for patients who cannot tolerate intraoral procedures. In addition, the broad image produced by a panoramic radiograph is easy for patients to understand, aiding in the explanation of the diagnosis and the proposed treatment plan in a manner that is clear and understandable.

Although the steps to exposing a panoramic radiograph appear simple, producing quality results can be technically demanding. Additionally, because of the relative ease with which a panoramic radiograph may be obtained, there may be a tendency to overuse this diagnostic examination. It is

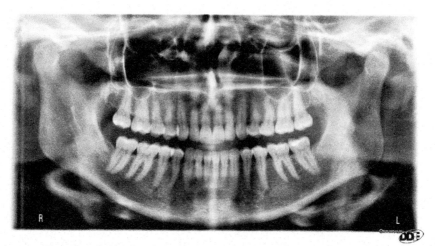

FIGURE 17–1 Panoramic radiograph. Provides a broad view of the dental arches. Note, however, the inherent distortion and ghost images. (Courtesy of Gendex Dental Systems/Imaging Sciences Intl.)

Box 17-1: Advantages and Limitations of Panoramic Radiographs

Advantages

- Increased recording area showing supporting structures of oral cavity

- Reduced patient radiation dose over a film-based intraoral full mouth series of radiographs

- Can be performed in less time than exposure of a full mouth series of radiographs

- Requires minimal patient instruction and cooperation

- May be substitute examination for patients who cannot tolerate placement of intraoral image receptor

- Infection control protocol minimized

- Aids in explaining treatment plan to patients

Limitations

- Increased image distortion; amount of vertical and horizontal distortion is not constant—varies from one part of radiograph to another

- Reduced image sharpness and detail that limits ability to detect disease in early stages

- Focal trough size and shape which limits recording with clarity only those structures that "fit" into image layer

- Increased occurrence of overlapping of proximal contact areas, especially in premolar regions

- Superimposition of structures (e.g., spinal column), soft tissue shadows, and ghost images that may make interpretation difficult

- Length of exposure time which may limit use on young children and other patients who cannot remain still throughout exposure cycle

- Perception of simple procedure that may lead to inappropriate overuse

important to note that research on the use of panoramic radiographs cautions against using panoramic images as a screening film for **occult disease** (diseases that may exist without signs or symptoms). However, research is continuing to validate the **opportunistic screening** potential of panoramic radiographs for markers of other diseases such as osteoporosis and calcification of the carotid arteries (see Chapter 26).

The greatest limitation of panoramic radiographs is lack of image detail. Magnification, distortion, and poor definition are inherent with panoramic techniques. **Ghost images, negative shadows,** and other **artifacts** can make interpreting panoramic images difficult (see Chapter 22). Further compromising the ability to obtain detailed images is the difficulty associated with positioning a patient within the **focal trough** (area of image sharpness). Manufacturers design panoramic x-ray machines to be able to adequately record the dental arches of an average patient. However, it may be difficult to record all structures with relative clarity when a patient's dental arches do not fit into the manufacturer's average range.

Fundamentals of Panoramic Radiography

Intraoral radiographs and other types of extraoral radiographs (see Chapter 30) are taken with a stationary x-ray source and image receptor. Structures such as the teeth and the supporting bone that lie along the same path travelled by the x-ray beam will be superimposed on the radiograph, limiting the ability of these radiographs to distinctly separate these structures. Panoramic radiography based on the principle of tomography provides a way to visually separate and represent these three-dimensional structures on a two-dimensional image. **Tomography** is a special radiographic technique used to record images of structures located within a selected plane of tissue, while blurring structures outside the selected plane making them less visible (Figure 17–2 ■). Panoramic x-ray machines operate on the basis of tomography with the patient positioned between the x-ray tube head and a cassette that holds the image receptor (Figure 17–3 ■). The exposure is made as the tube head and cassette rotate slowly around the patient's head during the operational cycle (usually about 15 to 20 seconds). The cassette with image receptor and the x-ray tube head move in directions opposite each other while the patient stands or is seated in a stationary position. The x-ray tube head moves around the back of the patient while the cassette with image receptor moves around the front. The x-ray beam enters the patient's tissues from the back of the head penetrating through to exit the front tissues and strike the image receptor (Figure 17–4 ■).

Through the use of a series of rotational points or centers (differing according to the unit manufacturer), the x-ray beam is directed toward the moving image receptor to record a select plane of dental anatomy. The rotational center, which is defined as the axis on which the x-ray tube head and the cassette rotate, is the functional focus of the projection. Most panoramic machines available today utilize a continuous moving rotational center to refocus the x-ray beam during movement to produce an image (Figure 17–5 ■). This type of rotational center will keep the inherent horizontal and vertical magnification of the image relatively constant. All panoramic images have between 10 and 30 percent image magnification, depending on where the structures are located in relation to the center of the slice of tissue being focused on. It is desirable to keep the inherent magnification even throughout the image. The elliptical pattern made by the rotational center very closely matches the arc of the teeth and jaws and is likely to keep image magnification relatively constant.

Unlike the concentric or rectangular beam of x-radiation of intraoral radiography, the x-rays of a panoramic

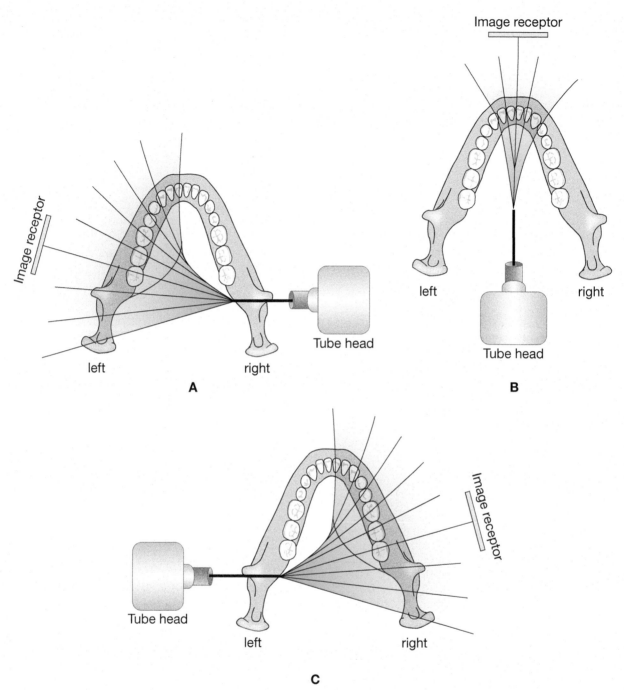

FIGURE 17–2 Principle of tomography. The x-ray beam is focused on imaging structures that are positioned closest to the image receptor. As the tube head and image receptor rotate, the x-ray beam is refocused to record the next section of anatomy. (**A**) Illustrated here, at this moment in the continuous exposure, the tube head is positioned on the right side, allowing the x-ray beam to penetrate the right side, then continue on to penetrate the left side and carry images of structures penetrated to the receptor. At this precise moment in the exposure sequence, the left side will be recorded on the image, while the right side will be blurred out as a ghost image. (**B**) As the tube head and image receptor rotate, the x-ray beam now penetrates the back of head (and the cervical vertebrae), then continues on to penetrate the anterior teeth. Because the anterior teeth at this moment are closer to the image receptor, the cervical vertebrae will most likely appear magnified and blurred out as a ghost image, while the anterior teeth will be more distinctly recorded onto the image. (**C**) As the tube head and image receptor continue to rotate to the opposite side, the x-ray beam now penetrates the left side first, blurring it out of the image. The right side is now closer to the image receptor, so it will be imaged more clearly.

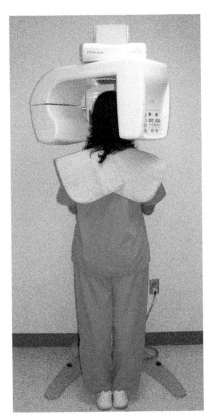

FIGURE 17–3 Panoramic x-ray machine. Patient positioned between the image receptor and the x-ray tube head of this digital panoramic x-ray machine.

machine emerge from a narrow vertical slit opening in the tube head and are constricted to form a narrow band. This narrow opening collimates (constricts) the x-ray beam so that a limited amount of tissue is irradiated at a time. The narrow vertical beam of radiation then passes through the patient and through a secondary collimator vertical slit in the cassette holder to expose the image receptor that is moving or rotating in the opposite direction (Figure 17–6 ■).

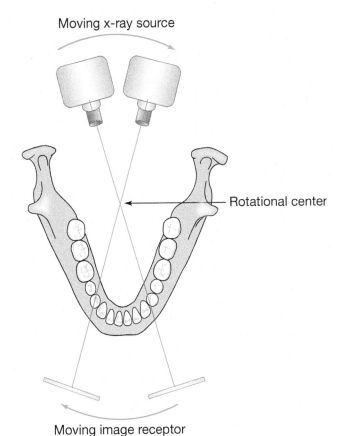

FIGURE 17–4 Panoramic radiography. Moving x-ray source passes through the rotational center in a horizontal plane toward the path of the moving image receptor. As the beam scans the object (dental arches), a continuous image is recorded on the moving image receptor.

Concept of the Focal Trough

The focal trough, or **focal layer,** is an estimated position between the x-ray source and the image receptor where the dental arches must be positioned to be recorded distinctly on the panoramic radiograph. Objects located at various distances from the center of the focal trough become less sharp the farther away they are located.

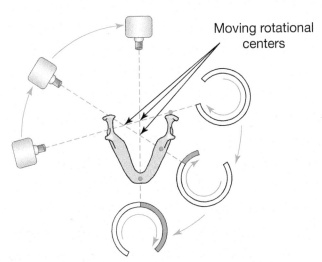

FIGURE 17–5 Moving rotational center allows the x-ray beam to continuously focus as the tube head and the image receptor simultaneously move.

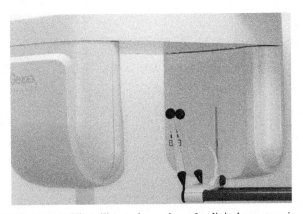

FIGURE 17–6 Slit collimated opening of a digital panoramic machine cassette holder. Note the lateral head positioner guides and bitepin.

The focal trough is three dimensional, and its actual shape varies depending on the manufacturer's equipment design. The three dimensions of the focal trough are (1) anterior–posterior, (2) lateral or left–right, and (3) superior–inferior or up–down (Figure 17–7 ■). The panoramic x-ray machine's moving center rotation system results in a focal trough that is naturally wider in the posterior regions and narrower in the anterior regions, making it imperative that the anterior teeth be positioned precisely to be recorded clearly. It is important to note that a mistake in positioning the arches in the anterior region of the focal trough by as little as 3 or 4 mm will make a significant difference in the degree of magnification on the resultant radiograph.

Panoramic Image Receptors

Digital Panoramic Sensor

The digital sensor image receptor used for panoramic radiography shares the same technology as the CCD and CMOS-APS solid-state sensors used in digital intraoral imaging (see Chapter 8). The major difference between intraoral digital sensors and those used for panoramic imaging is the arrangement of the pixels. Because the panoramic x-ray beam is collimated to expose only a narrow band of tissues at a time, the vertical portion of the sensor is only a few pixels wide. The x-ray source and sensor move in relation to each other to precisely expose this narrow vertical band of pixels.

The digital image receptor is usually built into the unit itself and therefore will appear as a contiguous part of, and indistinguishable from, the x-ray tube head carriage assembly (Figure 17–8 ■). Some panoramic machines have removable or interchangeable digital sensor/cassette combinations for the dual purpose of using the machine to expose panoramic radiographs or switching the image receptor out to expose another type of extraoral radiograph, such as a cephalometric image (see Chapter 30 and Figure 17–9 ■). Some manufacturers provide a film-to-digital conversion kit allowing a digital image receptor to be mounted in place of the film cassette holder.

PSP Imaging Plate

Panoramic photostimulable phosphor (PSP) imaging plates are available in sizes that approximate panoramic film sizes (5 × 12 inch [13 × 30 cm] and 6 × 12 inch [15 × 30 cm]) (Figure 17–10 ■). PSP panoramic technology functions in

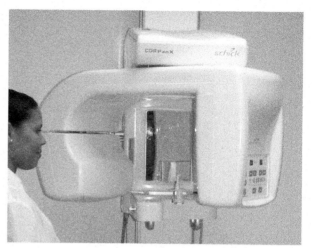

FIGURE 17–8 **Digital panoramic x-ray machine.** Tube head and cassette assembly. Note mirror to assist with positioning midsagittal plane.

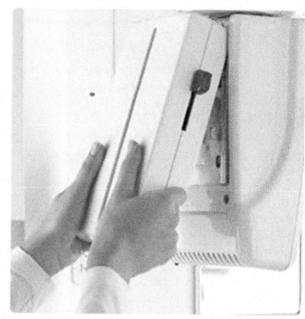

FIGURE 17–9 **Removable panoramic digital image receptor.** (Courtesy of Gendex Dental Systems.)

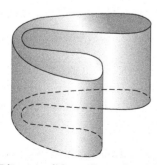

FIGURE 17–7 **Diagram of three-dimensional focal trough.**

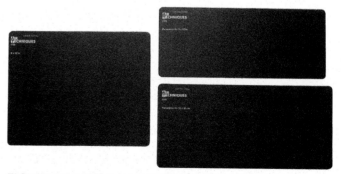

FIGURE 17–10 **Extraoral PSP plates.** (Courtesy of Air Techniques, Inc.)

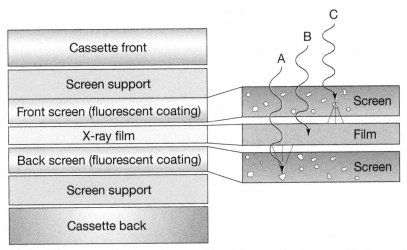

FIGURE 17–11 **Cross-section of cassette and image receptor assembly showing effect of x-ray and fluorescent light on image production.** X-ray **A** strikes a screen crystal behind, and x-ray **C** strikes a screen crystal in front of the image receptor, producing light that then strikes the image receptor. X-ray **B** strikes the image receptor directly. A latent image is produced by this combination of light exposure produced by the screen crystals and the x-ray exposure.

the same manner as PSP intraoral imaging (see Chapter 8). A panoramic PSP imaging plate is placed into a cassette to shield it from prolonged light exposure and attached to the cassette holder on the panoramic machine. The PSP plate captures the panoramic image and is then removed from the cassette and placed into a laser scanner, which converts analog data captured by the image receptor into digital information to be displayed as an image on a computer monitor.

Extraoral Film and Intensifying Screens

Panoramic extraoral film requires the use of **intensifying screens,** which transfer x-ray energy into visible light. This fluorescent light, along with the x-radiation, produces the radiographic image. Intensifying screens work in pairs. An intensifying screen is a smooth cardboard or plastic sheet coated with minute fluorescent crystals, also called phosphors, mixed into a suitable binding medium. Intensifying screens are based on the principle that crystals of certain salts—**calcium tungstate**, barium strontium sulfate, or **rare-earth phosphors** [lanthanum (La) and gadolinium (Gd)]—will fluoresce and emit energy in the form of blue (calcium tungstate) or green (rare earth) light when they absorb x-rays. **Screen film** is more sensitive to this type of fluorescent light than to radiation. When the film is sandwiched tightly between a pair of two intensifying screens, the x-rays cause the crystals on the screens to fluoresce and return the emitted light to the film emulsion to produce the radiographic image (Figure 17–11 ■).

As the name implies, intensifying screens "intensify" the effect of x-rays on the image receptor. What this means is that the amount of radiation required to cause the crystals of the intensifying screens to fluoresce is considerably less than the amount of radiation that would be required to directly expose the film alone. Additionally, rare-earth intensifying screens produce a latent image on the film with less radiation than calcium tungstate screens. ALARA dictates that

the fastest speed screen–film combination be used to reduce the amount of radiation exposure to the patient, so calcium tungstate screens are no longer recommended. In the same way that faster speed intraoral film produces images with slightly less image sharpness, the slight reduction in image clarity produced by rare-earth screens is considered acceptable to reduce the radiation dose to the patient.

Extraoral film for use with panoramic radiography comes in two sizes: 5 × 12 inch (13 × 30 cm) and 6 × 12 inch (15 × 30 cm) (see Figure 7-6). Film-based panoramic x-ray machines use extraoral film in conjunction with a pair of intensifying screens housed within a light-tight **cassette**. The cassette holds the intensifying screens in close contact with the film and protects the film from white light exposure. Cassettes are available as a rigid box or a flexible sleeve (Figures 17–12 ■ and 17–13 ■).

Extraoral radiographic film is extremely sensitive to light, especially in the blue-green spectrum. Extraoral film

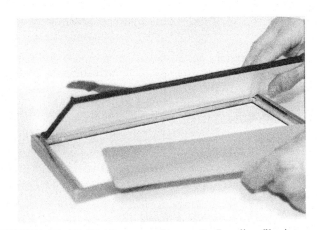

FIGURE 17–12 **Rigid panoramic cassette.** Loading film into cassette lined with intensifying screens.

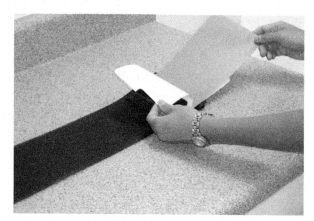

FIGURE 17–13 **Flexible sleeve cassette.** Loading film into cassette between pair of flexible intensifying screens.

is available with blue-light sensitive emulsion which must be paired with intensifying screens that emit blue light and green-light sensitive emulsion which must be paired with green-light-emitting intensifying screens. Inappropriately interchanging green- or blue-light sensitive film between green- and blue-light-emitting intensifying screens results in undiagnostic images.

Components of the Panoramic X-ray Machine

Although considerable differences exist in the size and configuration of panoramic x-ray machines, the operational procedures are similar (Procedure 17–1 and Figures 17–14 ■ and 17–15 ■). Many machines require that the patient stand during the exposure; others operate with the patient seated. The machine's design will determine whether the patient is positioned to face the radiographer and away from the machine or to face the machine and away from the radiographer.

All panoramic x-ray machines have four basic components:

1. Rotational x-ray tube head
2. Cassette holder (for film or PSP plate) or built-in digital image receptor
3. Head positioner guides to assist with locating the patient within the focal trough
4. Exposure control panel

The x-ray tube used in panoramic x-ray machines generates electrons to produce x-ray energy similar to x-ray units used for intraoral exposures. The PID used with the panoramic tube head is in a fixed vertical position pointing up slightly, about −8 degrees. Film-based panoramic machines and those using PSP technology require that the image receptor be loaded into a cassette that is then attached to the cassette holder opposite the PID so that it will rotate in relation with the tube head. Each machine manufacturer provides specific instructions for attaching the cassette to the unit (Figure 17–16 ■).

Because the focal trough is determined and set by the machine manufacturer, use the **head positioner guides** of

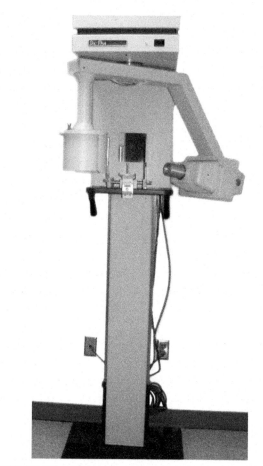

FIGURE 17–14 **Film-based panoramic x-ray machine.**

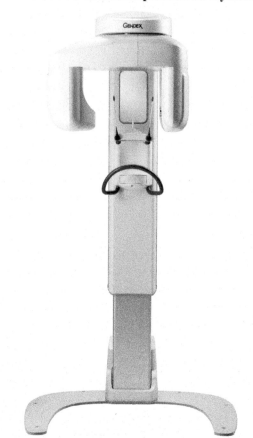

FIGURE 17–15 **Digital panoramic x-ray machine.** (Courtesy of Gendex Dental Systems/Imaging Sciences Intl.)

Procedure 17–1

Panoramic radiographic procedure*

Cassette and image receptor preparation

1. Examine cassette for proper function. Check hinge for wear. Check for light-tight seal.
2. Examine intensifying screens (if film based) or PSP plate for quality. Check for scratches and need of cleaning.
3. Obtain a box of extraoral film. Ensure that the film sensitivity matches the screen type used. (The image receptor is built into digital panoramic machines and will already be in place.)
4. In the darkroom, under safelight conditions, load film into the cassette. Load PSP plate in dimly lit conditions, into cassette without intensifying screens. Use clean, dry hands to handle image receptor. Avoid generating static electricity. Replace the cover on the box of extraoral film prior to turning on overhead white light and leaving the darkroom.

Panoramic machine preparation

1. Clean and disinfect with appropriate disinfectant all surfaces that will come in contact either directly or indirectly with the patient, such as the:
   a. Forehead rest
   b. Chin rest
   c. Side head positioner guides
   d. Patient support handles
   e. Chair (sit-down machine)
2. Attach the cassette onto the cassette holder of the panoramic machine according to the manufacturer's instructions. Ensure that the cassette is placed so that the exposure will begin at the appropriate edge of the image receptor.
3. Turn on the panoramic machine. Raise or lower the overhead assembly to the approximate height of the patient, and move to the patient-entry position or move assembly out of the way (if necessary) so that the way is clear for the patient to get into position.

Patient preparation

1. Inform the patient of the need for the panoramic radiograph. Explain the procedure, answer patient concerns/questions regarding the procedure, and obtain patient's consent.
2. Request that the patient remove items from the oral cavity and the head, neck, and shoulders that may interfere with the procedure such as removable dental appliances, eyeglasses, necklaces, hair barrettes, ear and facial jewelry (tongue, lip piercing adornments), and scarves or a hooded sweatshirt.
3. Place the lead/lead-equivalent cape or apron without a thyroid collar over the patient. Ensure that the lead apron will not impede the rotation of the tube head and image receptor assembly.
4. Select sterile or disposable biteblock or cotton roll for separating the arches into position.

Patient positioning

1. To position the arches into the focal trough's anterior/posterior dimension, instruct the patient to bite on the biteblock guide with the anterior teeth occluding edge to edge, or to place the chin completely forward into the chin rest or forehead against the forehead rest. If using a panoramic machine with light indicators, align the laser light beam at the interproximal space recommended by the machine manufacturer.
2. To position the arches into the focal trough's lateral (right–left) dimension, close the side head positioner guides or if using a panoramic machine with light indicators, align the laser light beam as recommended by the machine manufacturer. If using a panoramic machine with a mirror, instruct the patient to view reflection in the mirror to align the midsagittal plane perpendicular to the floor.
3. To position the arches into the focal trough's superior–inferior dimension, adjust the patient's chin up or down in the chin rest until the Frankfort plane is parallel to the plane of the floor or until the ala–tragus line is approximately positive 5 degrees to the plane of the floor. If available use the indicator lines engraved on the side head positioner guides or if using a panoramic machine with light indicators, align the laser light beam as recommended by the machine manufacturer.

Exposure

1. Select the appropriate kV and mA for the patient. Refer to posted exposure settings or the manufacturer's recommendations.
2. Instruct the patient to rest his or her tongue flat up against the hard palate and to close his or her lips around the biteblock or cotton roll. (Asking the patient to swallow or suck in the cheeks will assist with correct placement of the tongue and lips.)

Procedure 17–1 *(continued)*

3. Instruct the patient to remain still throughout the exposure cycle.

4. Take a position behind a protective barrier or an adequate distance away from the x-ray source and depress the exposure button for the duration of the cycle while watching to ensure that the patient does not move and that the rotation of the tube head assembly continues unhindered (see Figure 3-6). If patient movement occurs or the tube head assembly contacts the patient or protective barrier cape, release the exposure button to stop the process. The cassette should be removed and the procedure should start over, beginning with a new image receptor.

5. When the exposure cycle is complete, move the overhead assembly to the patient-exit position or move out of the way (if necessary) so that the way is clear for the patient to be released. Remove the protective barrier cape. Return patient's personal items that were removed prior to the procedure.

6. Return the head positioner and overhead assembly to the closed position and turn off the machine. Discard the disposable biteblock or prepare autoclavable biteblock for sterilization. Clean and disinfect with appropriate disinfectant all surfaces that came in contact either directly or indirectly with the patient (see Panoramic machine preparation, Step 1).

Processing

1. Observe the digital image on the computer screen for acceptable quality. If using film or PSP technology, remove the cassette from the cassette holder.

2. Proceed to the darkroom (with film) or to the laser scanner (with PSP plate). Under safelight conditions open the cassette and carefully remove the image receptor from between the intensifying screens with clean, dry hands. Avoid generating static electricity or scratching the screens or the image receptor.

3. Manually or automatically process the film or scan the PSP image receptor according to the manufacturer's instructions.

*The procedures for taking panoramic radiographs are similar on most panoramic machines; however, the complexity of the controls and head holder adjustments vary so be sure to read the manufacturer's instructions carefully before attempting to operate an unfamiliar machine.

---

the panoramic machine to position a patient correctly. These guides provide very specific and precise direction and will be discussed in detail in the section on patient positioning. The exposure control panel will usually allow for selection of the mA and kV as recommended by the manufacturer (Figure 17–17 ■). The size of the patient and density of the tissues to be imaged will determine what settings are used. The kV controls the penetrating ability of the beam, so it is often adjusted up when exposing larger patients or denser tissues, and adjusted down when exposing children and patients with significant edentulous regions. The exposure time is preset by the manufacturer and varies from 15 to 20 seconds to complete the cycle. To activate the exposure, depress the exposure button and hold for the duration of the cycle.

Patient Preparation

It is important to remember that the x-ray beam rotates around the patient from behind. Any objects made of metal or other dense material located here, such as a necklace, earrings, or hair adornments, will be in the path of the primary beam and result in radiopaque artifacts. These items, along with the patient's glasses, dental appliances, patient napkin chain, oral piercings, and other facial jewelry, must

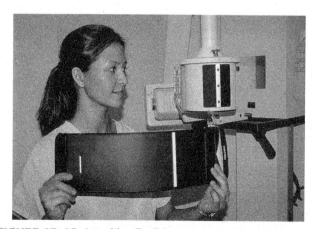

FIGURE 17–16 Attaching flexible cassette to the cassette holder carriage. Note markings on cassette that indicate correct direction for attaching the cassette to the holder.

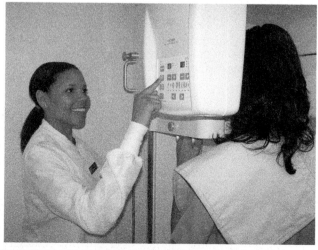

FIGURE 17–17 Using the control panel to set the exposure.

be removed prior to exposure. There are occasions when the clothing the patient is wearing may interfere with the rotation of the tube head. Thickly padded shoulders, scarves, and hooded sweatshirts need to be assessed to ensure that they won't impede the movement of the cassette and tube head during the rotational cycle. Lead/lead equivalent aprons are available without a thyroid collar, as are scoop-neck, cape-style aprons made especially for panoramic use (see Figure 6–12). Due to the position of the tube head and PID, the thyroid collar would get in the way of the primary beam and block the radiation from reaching the tissues.

Patient understanding of the procedure and cooperation are necessary to produce quality images. A patient must hold still, in position, throughout the exposure and he or she should rest the tongue against the palate and close the lips around the bite guide. The open air space between the tongue and the roof of the mouth (palatoglossal air space) will create a large radiolucency on the image that will obscure the root apices of the maxillary teeth (see Figures 22–13 and 22–14). Raising the flat, dorsal surface of the tongue to the palate utilizes the soft tissue image of the tongue to "fill in" this air space and create a more even density to the image. Closing the lips together around the biteblock will avoid recording an image of the lip line across the anterior teeth (Figure 17–18 ■). Open lips will create an image that can mimic caries of the anterior teeth (see Figure 22–11).

Practice Point

When asked to place the tongue against the roof of the mouth to reduce the radiolucency caused by the palatoglossal air space, a patient will sometimes incorrectly touch only the tip of the tongue to the palate. To assist with placing the entire dorsal surface of the tongue flat against the palate, ask the patient to swallow and note the position of the tongue. Another method used to get the tongue into the correct position is to ask the patient to suck in his or her cheeks, which automatically raises the tongue into a position flat against the palate. This directive works especially well when communicating with the pediatric patient.

Patient Positioning

Positioning a patient's head and dental arches within the focal trough is necessary for producing diagnostic images. Correct positioning will vary, depending on whether the area of interest is in the region of the temporomandibular joints, the sinuses, or the teeth and their supporting structures. Because the focal trough is predetermined by the panoramic machine manufacturer, refer to the manufacturer's instructions when positioning a patient. Panoramic x-ray machines have guides such as a biteblock or bite pin, forehead or chin rest, or beams of light that, when activated, shine on the patient's face to aid in positioning the patient within the focal trough (Figures 17–19 ■ and 17–20 ■). Each manufacturer provides an instruction manual that must be carefully read and followed. It is the radiographer's responsibility to position the patient's dental arches in relation to the focal trough to avoid images that are magnified, diminished, or blurred.

Because the focal trough or area of image sharpness is three dimensional (see Figure 17–7), the patient's dental arches must be positioned correctly: anterior–posterior (forward or back), lateral (left or right), and superior–inferior (up or down).

ANTERIOR–POSTERIOR POSITION. Most panoramic machines have a relatively narrow focal trough in the anterior region, requiring precision in locating the forward and backward dimension of image sharpness. Panoramic machines will have a forehead rest or may require a patient to bite on a biteblock or bite pin to position the arches correctly in this dimension. When using a biteblock the patient must bring both maxillary and mandibular central incisors into an edge-to-edge position on the biteblock. If using a machine with laser light beams, follow the manufacturer's recommendation for aiming the vertical beam of light at a predetermined tooth or interproximal space (Figure 17–21 ■).

LATERAL POSITION To correctly align the dental arches within the lateral dimension of the focal trough, the midsagittal plane (see Figure 12-16) that divides a patient's head into a right and left side must be positioned perpendicular to the floor. Panoramic machines will have a light beam

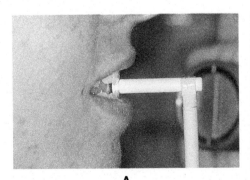
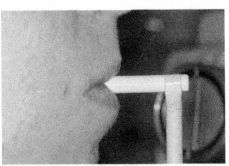

| A | B |

FIGURE 17–18 **Positioning of lips on the biteblock.** (**A**) Maxillary and mandibular central incisors in edge-to-edge position on biteblock. (**B**) Lips correctly positioned closed around biteblock.

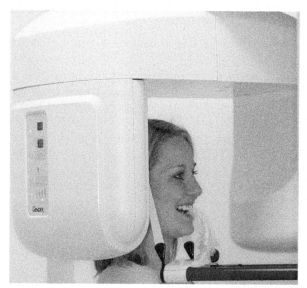

FIGURE 17–19 **Head positioner guides.** A biteblock aids in locating the correct anterior–posterior dimension; side positioner guides aid in locating the correct lateral dimension.

guide, side head positioners, or a mirror placed in front of the patient to assist with positioning the midsagittal plane correctly (see Figure 17–8).

SUPERIOR–INFERIOR POSITION Positioning the arches correctly in the superior–inferior dimension of the focal trough requires knowledge of two anatomical landmarks. The **ala–tragus line**—an imaginary plane or line from the ala (a winglike projection at the side of the nose) to the tragus

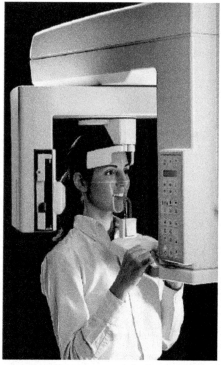

FIGURE 17–20 **Head positioner guides.** Beams of light shine on the patient's face to aid in positioning the arches in the focal trough. (Courtesy of Gendex Dental Corporation.)

(the cartilaginous prominence in front of the ear)—must be positioned approximately 5 degrees down toward the floor. When the ala–tragus line is positioned correctly, the **Frankfort plane**—an imaginary plane or line from the orbital ridge (under the eye) to the external opening of the ear—will be parallel to the floor. Some panoramic machines utilize guides that aid in locating the ala–tragus line, whereas others focus on the Frankfort plane. The radiographer should be able to utilize either landmark (Figure 17–22 ■).

In addition to positioning the patient into the three dimensions of the focal trough, the patient must stand or sit up straight, and avoid a slumped posture. When the arches are correctly positioned within the three dimensions of the focal trough, all teeth and supporting structures are recorded and there is less unequal magnification and unsharpness over all parts of the radiographic image (Figure 17–23 ■).

Exposure and Image Receptor Handling

Careful attention to exposure settings and handling of the image receptor will avoid errors that result in undiagnostic radiographs. Exposure settings should be posted near the control panel to avoid over- or underexposures. Because extraoral film is more sensitive than intraoral film, darkroom safelight filters that work with intraoral film handling may not be safe for extraoral film handling. The type of safelight required for extraoral film can usually be found written on the film package or by checking with the manufacturer.

Extraoral film should be handled with clean, dry hands. Latex or vinyl treatment gloves should be avoided and glove powder residue will produce radiolucent artifacts (black lines or smudges). Remove film slowly from its multipack box and place it into a cassette without sliding it across the intensifying screens to prevent a static discharge, which results in a white light spark that will expose the film, leaving radiolucent artifacts on the resultant image (Figure 17–24 ■). Generating static electricity will create artifacts on the films

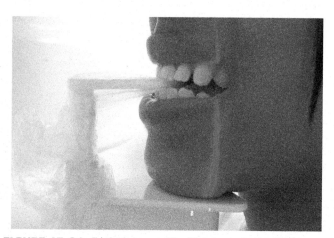

FIGURE 17–21 Light beam guide illuminated over the interproximal space of the canine and the premolar indicating correct anterior-posterior positioning.

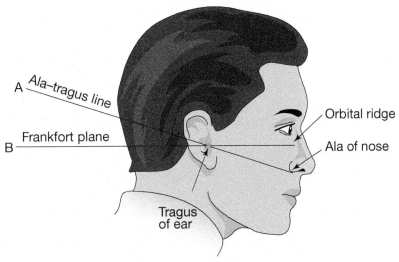

FIGURE 17–22 **Anatomical landmarks.** (**A**) When the ala–tragus line is positioned 5 degrees down, (**B**) the Frankfort plane will be in a position parallel to the plane of the floor.

inside the box as well as the one being removed. Additionally, film should be loaded into the cassette just prior to use; storing film inside cassettes until ready for use may increase

Practice Point

When standing straight is compromised due to a patient's stature or build/size, direct the patient to hold onto the handles of the machine with the arms crossed. Holding onto the right handle with the left hand and to the left handle with the right hand will bring the patient's shoulders in and usually out of the way of the machine rotation. For patients with a short neck, or short distance between the shoulders and chin, crossing the arms and holding onto the handles with the palms up will further round the shoulders in and out of the way during the rotational cycle of the exposure (see Figure 17–28).

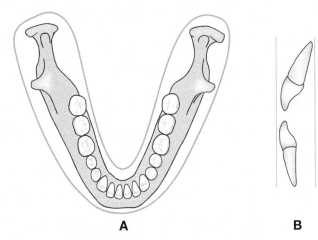

A   **B**

FIGURE 17–23 **Correct positioning.** Arches positioned correctly within the focal trough in all three dimensions: (**A**) Anterior–posterior and lateral (left–right); and (**B**) superior–inferior.

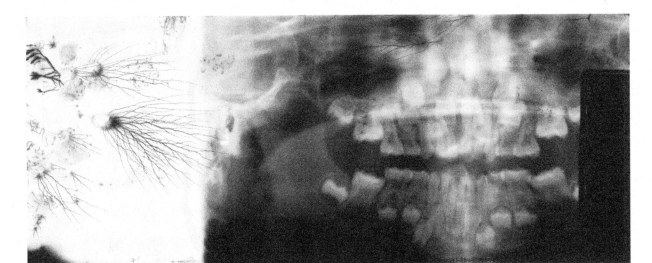

FIGURE 17–24 **Static electricity artifacts.** Blank area that resulted from incorrectly loading the image receptor into the cassette, showing static electricity artifacts.

the likelihood of generating artifacts. Load only one film into the cassette at a time unless using special film specifically made for duplication purposes.

Inspect cassettes to ensure a tight contact between film and intensifying screens. Blurry images result when the film and screens are not in tight contact. Intensifying screens must be free of scratches that would result in a loss of image and radiopaque artifacts. Protect PSP image receptors from bright light exposure and process by the laser scanner as soon as possible after exposure or a loss of data will occur. Carefully load flexible plastic sleeve cassettes to ensure that the film or PSP plate is seated all the way down at the fold. Failure to correctly load the image receptor into the cassette will result in a loss of part of the image (see Figure 17–24).

Panoramic Imaging Errors

Panoramic imaging errors may result from incorrectly preparing the patient for the procedure; incorrectly positioning the patient and dental arches in the focal trough; and incorrectly handling, exposing, and processing the image receptor. A radiographer should possess a working knowledge of the characteristic appearance of errors made in these steps to avoid producing undiagnostic radiographic images and to better implement appropriate corrective actions.

Figures 17–25 ■ through 17–28 ■ illustrate the appearance of the errors discussed in this chapter. See Procedure 17–1 for a summary of the basic steps of the panoramic technique.

ANTERIOR-POSTERIOR POSITIONING

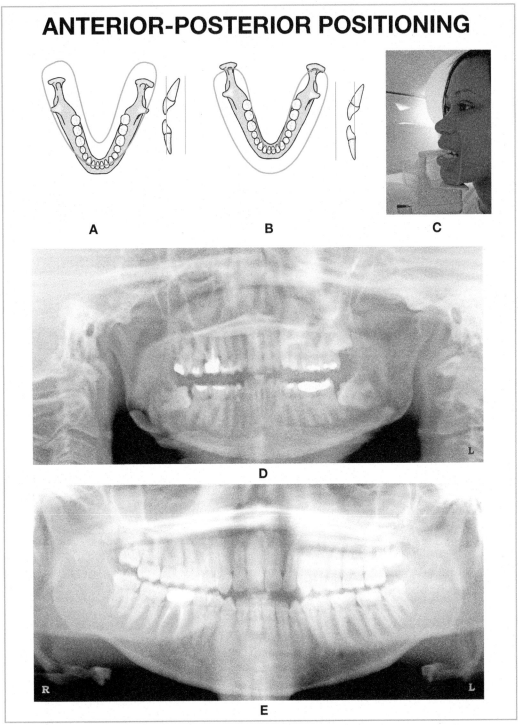

FIGURE 17–25 Incorrect anterior–posterior positioning. (A) Arches too far anterior positions anterior teeth incorrectly forward from center of focal trough. (B) Arches too far posterior positions anterior teeth incorrectly back from center of focal trough. (C) Example of patient positioned too far anterior. Compare this incorrect position of the laser light beam with the correct position in Figure 17–21. (D) Arches too far anterior results in blurred and diminished appearance of anterior teeth and prominent imaging of spinal column on both sides. (E) Arches too far posterior results in widened and magnified anterior teeth.

LATERAL (LEFT-RIGHT) POSITIONING

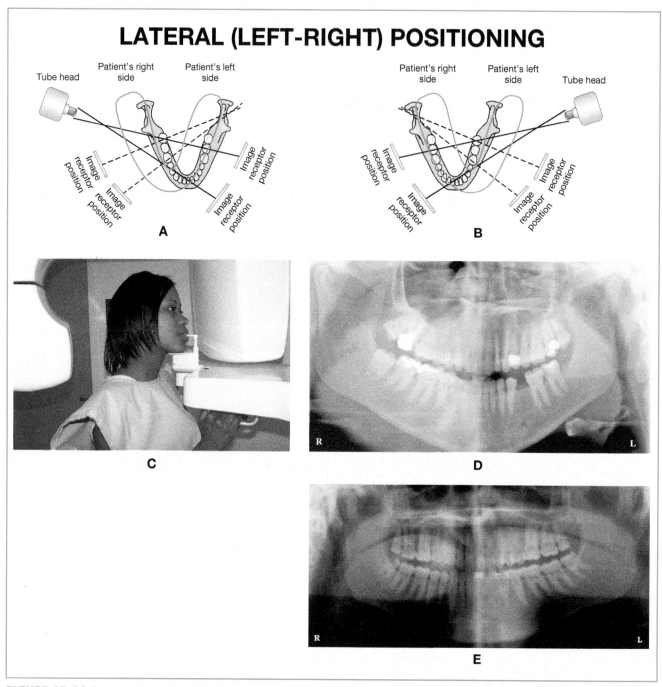

FIGURE 17–26 Incorrect lateral positioning. Arches tilted too far to one or the other side of focal trough results in a narrowed appearance of teeth on the side closer to the image receptor and a magnification of teeth on the side closer to the x-ray tube. **(A)** Arches too far left of center of focal trough. **(B)** Arches too far right of center of focal trough. **(C)** Example of patient with arches tilted left. **(D)** Arches tilted left results in a narrowed appearance of teeth and supporting anatomy on the left while teeth and anatomical structures on the right appear widened and magnified. **(E)** Arches tilted right results in a narrowed appearance on the right and magnification on the left.)

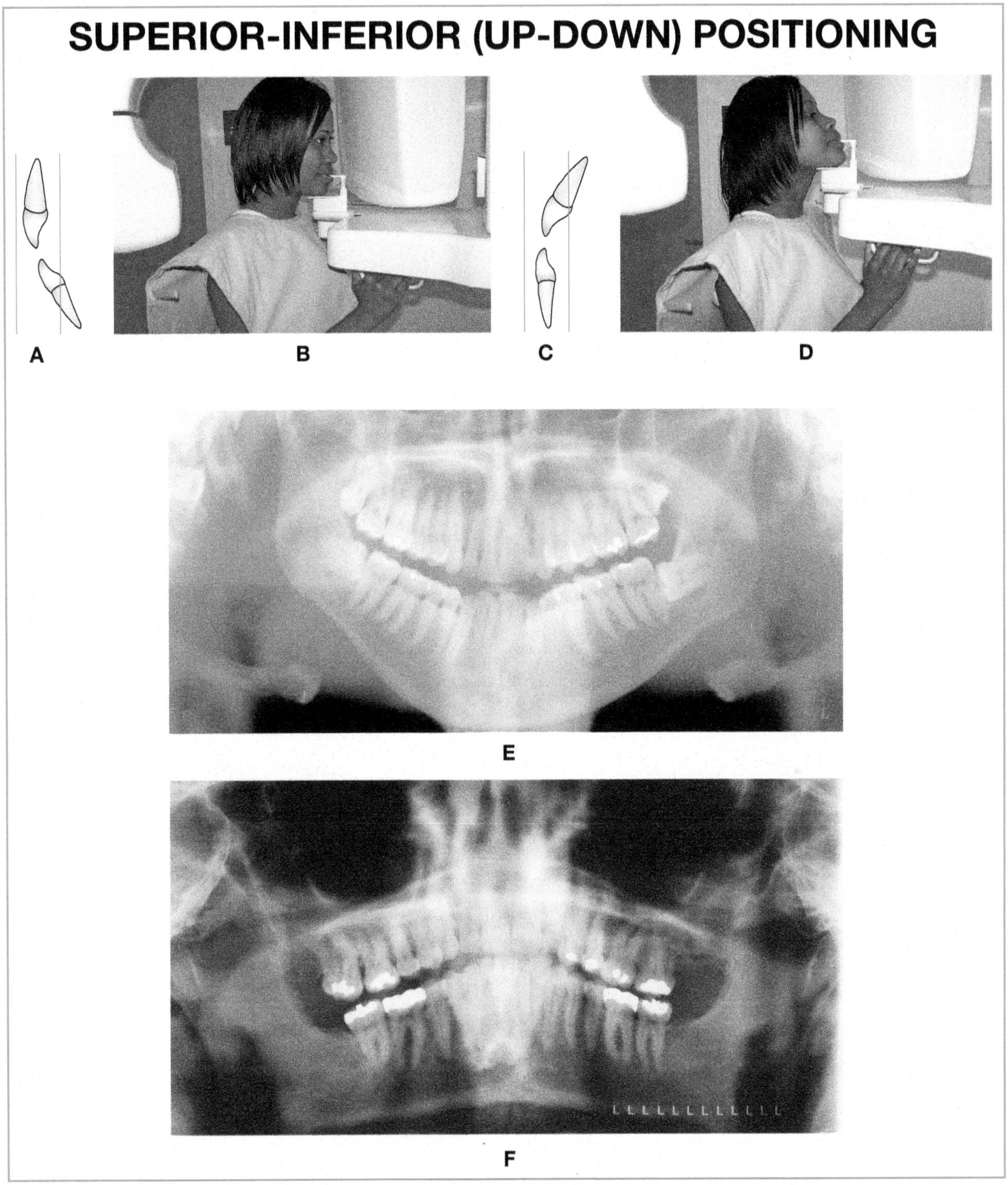

SUPERIOR-INFERIOR (UP-DOWN) POSITIONING

A B C D

E

F

FIGURE 17–27 **Incorrect superior–inferior positioning. (A)** Arches too inferior (chin tipped down) causes root apices of mandibular anterior teeth to slant out of focal trough. **(B)** Frankfort plane/ala–tragus line incorrectly aligned, positioning arches too inferior. **(C)** Arches too superior (chin tipped up) causes root apices of maxillary anterior teeth to slant out of focal trough. **(D)** Frankfort plane/ala–tragus line incorrectly aligned, positioning arches too superior. **(E)** Arches too inferior result in a characteristic exaggerated "smile" appearance, mandibular condyles slant inward, and nasopharyngeal air space appears larger and darker, reducing image quality. **(F)** Arches too superior result in a characteristic exaggerated "frown" appearance, and bottom of nasal cavity and hard palate widen into a radiopaque band that obscures root apices of maxillary teeth.

ACHIEVING CORRECT POSTURE POSITIONING

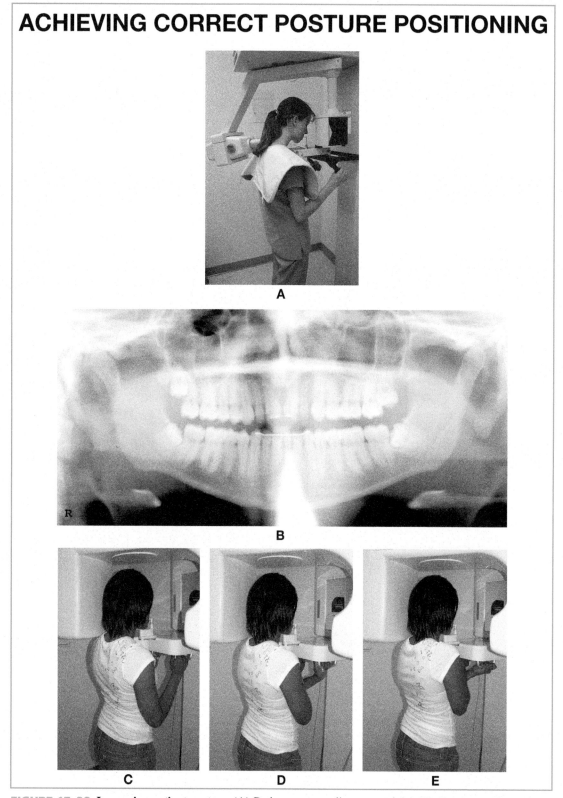

FIGURE 17–28 **Improving patient posture. (A)** Patient not standing up straight. **(B)** Compressed vertebrae in slumped position absorbs radiation and appears as a wide radiopacity at center inferior border of image. **(C)** Normal hand position on machine handles works for most patients. **(D)** Altered hand position with arms crossed, left hand holding right handle and right hand holding left handle assists with improving posture when needed. **(E)** Altered hand position with arms crossed, left hand holding right handle with palm facing up and right hand holding left handle with palm facing up further assists in overcoming a slumped posture.

REVIEW—Chapter summary

Panoramic radiography produces a broad view image of both the maxilla and the mandible on a single radiograph. Panoramic radiographs are valuable in examining large areas of the maxillofacial region; locating impacted teeth or retained root tips; evaluating trauma, lesions, and diseases of the jaws; and assessing growth and development.

The greatest advantage of the panoramic radiograph is that it can record a large region of structures and provide an increased amount of diagnostic information as compared to a full mouth series of intraoral radiographs. The greatest limitation of the panoramic radiograph is the image magnification and distortion that make interpreting the image for details difficult.

Panoramic imagery is based on tomography where a slice or layer of tissue is imaged with relative clarity, while blurring out other structures not of interest. During the panoramic exposure, the image receptor and x-ray tube head move slowly (a 15- to 20-second cycle) in opposite directions of each other around the patient's head. Through the use of a series of rotational points or centers, the x-ray beam is directed toward the moving cassette to record a select plane of dental anatomy.

The focal trough is the area between the x-ray source and the image receptor where structures will be imaged clearly on the radiograph. Structures positioned outside the focal trough will be blurred out of the image. The focal trough is three dimensional, and its size and shape is determined by the machine manufacturer. Each manufacturer provides instructions and head positioner guides to assist in positioning the patient within the focal trough.

Panoramic image receptors include digital sensors, PSP technology, and extraoral screen film. Extraoral screen film is used in conjunction with a pair of intensifying screens housed in a light-tight cassette. Intensifying screens transfer x-ray energy into visible light that in turn exposes screen film to produce an image. Intensifying screens intensify the effect of x-rays on the film,

resulting in a reduced dose of radiation required to produce an image. Rare-earth screens emit green light and must be paired with green-light sensitive film. In keeping with ALARA, calcium tungstate screens are no longer recommended.

All panoramic dental x-ray machines have (1) a rotational x-ray tube head, (2) a cassette holder for film or PSP plate or a built-in digital sensor, (3) head positioner guides, and (4) an exposure control panel. The PID is collimated to a narrow slit opening, allowing the x-ray beam to fan out to expose a narrow slice of tissue as the tube head rotates around a patient's head. The x-ray beam penetrates the patient from the back of the head.

Artifacts that compromise diagnostic quality result when metal or dense objects, such as a patient's personal items or clothing, or lead/lead equivalent thyroid collar are not removed prior to exposure. Instruct a patient to rest his or her tongue against the palate and to close the lips around the biteblock during exposure to minimize the appearance of these structures on the radiograph. Most panoramic dental x-ray machines have positioning guides to assist with determining the correct anterior–posterior, lateral (left–right), and superior–inferior position of the dental arches within the focal trough. The midsagittal, ala–tragus, and Frankfort planes are important anatomical landmarks to determine correct positioning.

Positioning the dental arches incorrectly in the focal trough results in characteristic image appearances: too far anterior produces blurred and narrowed anterior teeth and too far posterior produces blurred and widened anterior teeth; too far to one side (lateral dimension) results in narrowed teeth on the side closer to the image receptor and magnified teeth on the side closer to the x-ray tube head; too far inferior results in an image with an exaggerated "smile" and too far superior results in an image with an exaggerated "frown." Extraoral film is more sensitive than intraoral film. Careful handling is needed to avoid static electricity and other artifacts.

RECALL—Review questions

1. A panoramic radiograph is valuable when diagnosing each of the following EXCEPT one. Which one is the EXCEPTION?
   a. A cyst
   b. An impacted molar
   c. Recurrent caries
   d. A supernumerary tooth

2. Which of these is an advantage of a panoramic radiograph as compared to an intraoral radiograph?
   a. A larger region is recorded.
   b. The image is magnified.
   c. Distortion is eliminated.
   d. Definition is improved.

3. Which of these is a limitation of a panoramic radiograph as compared to a full mouth series of intraoral radiographs?
   a. Larger radiation dose to the patient
   b. Increased time required to obtain the radiographic image
   c. Superimposition of structures that may make interpretation difficult
   d. Requires an increase in patient instruction and cooperation with the procedure

4. What is the term given to the technique in which a slice of tissue is exposed distinctly, whereas structures outside the designated area are blurred out of the image?
   a. Ghost image
   b. Artifact
   c. Focal trough
   d. Tomography

5. All panoramic radiographs have 10 to 30 percent magnification.
   It is desirable to keep the magnification less in the anterior region than in the posterior region.
   a. The first statement is true. The second statement is false.
   b. The first statement is false. The second statement is true.
   c. Both statements are true.
   d. Both statements are false.

6. The panoramic PID is collimated to what shape?
   a. Round
   b. Rectangular
   c. Narrow slit
   d. Cone

7. What term is given to the area where structures will be imaged with relative clarity, whereas structures outside this area are blurred out of the image?
   a. Ghost image
   b. Artifact
   c. Focal trough
   d. Tomography

8. Which of the following is NOT a dimension of the focal trough?
   a. Intraoral–extraoral
   b. Anterior–posterior
   c. Lateral (right–left)
   d. Superior–inferior

9. Which of the following panoramic image receptors must be paired with intensifying screens to produce a radiographic image?
   a. PSP plate
   b. Digital sensor
   c. Film

10. Rare-earth intensifying screens require less radiation than calcium tungstate screens to produce a latent image on film *because* calcium tungstate intensifying screens produce visible blue light when exposed to radiation.
    a. Both the statement and reason are correct and related.
    b. Both the statement and reason are correct but NOT related.
    c. The statement is correct, but the reason is NOT.
    d. The statement is NOT correct, but the reason is correct.
    e. NEITHER the statement NOR the reason is correct.

11. Which of the following panoramic image receptors does NOT need to be placed into a cassette prior to exposure?
    a. PSP plate
    b. Digital sensor
    c. Film

12. Each of the following is a component of a panoramic x-ray machine EXCEPT one. Which one is the EXCEPTION?
    a. Rotational x-ray tube head
    b. Cassette holder or built-in digital sensor
    c. Head positioner guides
    d. Variable exposure timer

13. Prior to exposing a panoramic radiograph, a patient should be asked to swallow and rest his or her tongue flat against the palate.
    Expanding the tongue to fill in the oral cavity helps to eliminate a negative shadow on the resulting radiographic image.
    a. The first statement is true, the second is false.
    b. The first statement is false, the second is true.
    c. Both statements are true.
    d. Both statements are false.

14. Which of the following planes is used to position a patient correctly within the superior–inferior (up–down) dimension of the focal trough?
    a. Ala–tragus line
    b. Frankfort plane
    c. Midsaggital plane
    d. Both (a) and (b)

15. Which of the following positions within the focal trough results in anterior teeth that are blurry and narrowed in size?
    a. Too far to the left
    b. Too far to the right
    c. Too far forward
    d. Too far backward

16. When the dental arches are rotated to the left, the teeth on the right side will be positioned closer to the image receptor.
The teeth closer to the image receptor will appear blurry and magnified.
    a. The first statement is true. The second statement is false.
    b. The first statement is false. The second statement is true.
    c. Both statements are true.
    d. Both statements are false.

17. Which of the following positioning errors results in an exaggerated "smile" appearance of the arches?
    a. Chin tipped too far up
    b. Chin tipped too far down
    c. Midsagittal plane tipped to the left
    d. Midsagittal plane tipped to the right

18. Panoramic film should be loaded into the cassette just prior to use, *because* storing film inside cassettes until ready for use may increase the likelihood of generating artifacts.
    a. Both the statement and reason are correct and related.
    b. Both the statement and reason are correct but NOT related.
    c. The statement is correct, but the reason is NOT.
    d. The statement is NOT correct, but the reason is correct.
    e. NEITHER the statement NOR the reason is correct.

REFLECT—Case study

You have to expose a panoramic radiograph on the following patients. Each of these patients presents with a characteristic that will make positioning the patient for the procedure a challenge. Carefully review each of the patient descriptions and answer the following questions.

1. What patient positioning step do you anticipate to be a challenge?
2. What error is most likely to occur?
3. What will the image look like?
4. How can you prevent this error from occurring or minimize the result on the image?
5. What specific steps do you plan to take to produce a diagnostic quality image? Write out your answer.

Case A

A child who seems to be having difficulty paying attention to your directions

Case B

An adult with multiple facial piercings, including a tongue ring and several earrings

Case C

An adult with fashionable hair extensions gathered into a large ponytail

Case D

An adult who wears partial dentures that when removed reveal missing anterior teeth

Case E

An adult with osteoporosis who exhibits a pronounced stooped posture as a result of collapsed vertebrae

RELATE—Laboratory application

For a comprehensive laboratory practice exercise on this topic, see Thomson, E. M., & Bruhn, A. M. (2018). *Exercises in oral radiography techniques: A laboratory manual* (4th ed.). Hoboken, NJ: Pearson. Chapter 11, "Panoramic radiographic technique."

RESOURCES

Benson, B. W., Liang, H., & Flint, D. J. (2011, November-December). Panoramic radiography: Digital technology fosters efficiency. *Compendium, 32*(4), 6–8.

Eastman Kodak. (2000). *Successful panoramic radiography.* Rochester, NY: Eastman Kodak.

Ferrús-Torres, E., Gargallo-Albiol, J., Berini-Aytés, L., & Gay-Escoda, C. (2009). Diagnostic predictability of digital versus conventional panoramic radiographs in the presurgical evaluation of impacted mandibular third molars. *International Journal of Oral Maxillofacial Surgery, 38,* 1184–1187.

Horner, K., Drage, N., & Brettle, D. (2008). *21st century imaging.* London: Quintessence Publishing Co.

Rushton, V. E., & Rout, J. (2006). *Panoramic radiography.* London: Quintessence Publishing Co.

Scarfe, W. C., & Williamson, G. F. (2015). Practical panoramic radiography. Retrieved from Dental Care website: http://www.dentalcare.com/en-US/dental-education/continuing-education/ce71/ce71.aspx

Serman, N., Horrell, B. M., & Singer, S. (2003). High-quality panoramic radiographs. Tips and tricks. *Dentistry Today, 22*(1), 70–73.

Thomson, E. M. (2009). Focusing on the image. How to produce error-free radiographic images for the pediatric patient. *Dimensions of Dental Hygiene, 7*(2), 24–26, 27.

White, S. C., & Pharoah, M. J. (2014). Panoramic imaging. *Oral radiology: Principles and interpretation* (7th ed.). St. Louis, MO: Elsevier.

Visit www.pearsonhighered.com/healthprofessionsresources to access the student resources that accompany this book. Simply select Dental Hygiene from the choice of disciplines. Find this book and you will find the complementary study tools created for this specific title.

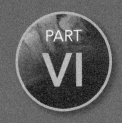

Radiographic Errors and Quality Assurance

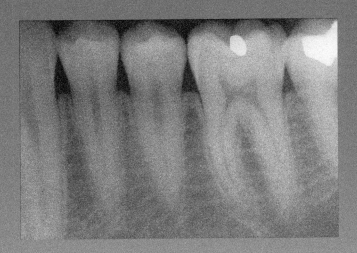

Identifying and Correcting Undiagnostic Radiographs

CHAPTER OUTLINE

OBJECTIVES

Following successful completion of this chapter, you should be able to:

1. Define the key terms.
2. Understand the need for a retake policy.
3. List the characteristics of a quality radiographic image.
4. Recognize errors caused by incorrect radiographic techniques.
5. Apply appropriate corrective actions for technique errors.
6. Recognize errors caused by incorrect radiographic processing.
7. Apply appropriate corrective actions for processing errors.
8. Recognize errors caused by incorrect radiographic image receptor handling.
9. Apply appropriate corrective actions for handling errors.
10. Identify causes of film fog.
11. Apply appropriate actions for preventing film fog.

KEY TERMS

Conecut error
Dead pixel
Distomesial overlap
Double exposure
Elongation
Film fog
Foreshortening
Herringbone error
Mesiodistal overlap
Noise
Overdevelopment
Overexposure
Retake policy
Static electricity
Underdevelopment
Underexposure

Introduction

Although radiographs play an important role in oral health care, it should be remembered that exposure to radiation carries a risk. Radiographers have an ethical responsibility to produce the highest diagnostic quality radiographs, in return for a patient's consent to undergo a radiographic examination. Less-than-ideal images diminish the usefulness of the radiograph. When an error is significant, a radiograph will have to be retaken. In addition to increasing a patient's radiation exposure, retake radiographs require additional consent and may reduce patient confidence in the operator and in the practice. The following is offered as a sample **retake policy** statement:

> *No radiograph should be retaken until a thorough investigation determines the exact cause of the error and the appropriate corrective action is identified and can be implemented.*

It is important to develop the skills needed to identify radiographic errors. Identifying common mistakes and knowing the causes will help to avoid these pitfalls. Being able to identify the cause of an undiagnostic image will allow a knowledgeable radiographer to apply the appropriate corrective action for retaking the exposure. This chapter investigates common radiographic errors, identifies probable causes of such errors, and presents appropriate corrective actions.

Recognizing Radiographic Errors

To recognize errors that diminish the diagnostic quality of a radiograph requires an understanding of what a quality image looks like (Table 18–1 ■). A radiograph must be an accurate representation of the teeth and supporting structures. The image should not be magnified, elongated, foreshortened, or otherwise distorted. Image density and

Practice Point

All errors reduce image quality; however, not all errors create a need to reexpose a patient. Consider these two examples. If a periapical radiograph exposed to image suspected pathology in the posterior region exhibits conecut error in the anterior region, then the radiograph would most likely not have to be retaken if the area of interest is adequately recorded.

When exposing a set of radiographs—bitewing or full mouth series—if an error prevents adequately observing a condition, then adjacent radiographs should be viewed for the possibility that the condition may be recorded in another image. Determining when a retake is absolutely necessary will avoid excess radiation exposure to a patient.

contrast should be correct for ease of interpretation: not too light, or too dark, or fogged.

The cause of a radiographic error must be identified to be able to take appropriate corrective action. Errors that diminish the diagnostic quality of radiographs usually fall into the following categories:

1. Technique errors
2. Processing errors
3. Handling errors

It is important to note that errors in any of these categories may produce the same or a similar result. For example, it is possible that a dark radiographic image may have been caused by overexposure (a technique error) or by overdevelopment (a processing error), or by exposing the film to white light (a handling error).

When utilizing direct digital imaging it may be possible to apply the corrective actions almost immediately, without removing the sensor from the oral cavity. Following exposure, observe the digital image on the computer monitor

Table 18–1 Characteristics of a Quality Radiograph

Bitewing Radiograph	Periapical Radiograph
• Image receptor placed correctly to record area of interest	• Image receptor placed correctly to record area of interest
• Equal portion of maxilla and mandible recorded	• Entire tooth plus at least 2 mm beyond incisal/occlusal edges of crowns and beyond root apex recorded
• Occlusal/incisal plane of teeth is parallel to edge of image receptor	• Occlusal/incisal plane of teeth is parallel to edge of image receptor
• Occlusal plane straight or slightly curved upward toward posterior	• Embossed dot (film) positioned toward incisal/occlusal edge
• Most posterior contact point between adjacent teeth recorded	• In full mouth survey, each tooth should be recorded at least once, preferably twice

before removing the sensor from the patient's mouth. Request that the patient remain still, and in position occluding on the biteblock of the image receptor holder while evaluating the image. If an error presents, it may be possible to immediately apply the corrective action. Being able to diagnose and correct a radiographic error while the image receptor sensor is still in place can increase the chances that a retake radiograph, with the corrective action applied, will be successful. For example, if mesiodistal overlap error is noted, the horizontal angulation of the tube head and position indicating device (PID) can be more accurately adjusted than if the tube head and PID and the image receptor are moved and repositioned.

Technique Errors

Technique errors include mistakes made in placing the image receptor, aiming the PID, and setting exposure factors. Additional technical problems result from movement of the patient, the image receptor, or the PID.

Incorrect Positioning of the Image Receptor

The most basic technique error is not imaging the correct teeth. A radiographer must know the standard image receptor placements for all types of projections and must possess the skills necessary to achieve these correct placements.

NOT RECORDING ANTERIOR STRUCTURES

- **Probable causes:** Image receptor was placed too far back in the oral cavity. Due to the curvature and narrowing of the arches in the anterior region, it is sometimes difficult to place the image receptor far enough anterior without impinging on sensitive mucosa. This is especially likely when tori are present. When using a digital sensor, the wire and/or infection control barrier may further compromise fitting the image receptor into the correct position.
- **Corrective actions:** To avoid placing a corner of the image receptor uncomfortably in contact with the soft tissues, and to make more room to fit a wired digital sensor, move the receptor in toward the midline of the oral cavity, away from the lingual surfaces of the teeth of interest. When positioning the image receptor for a premolar radiograph, the anterior edge of the receptor may be positioned to contact the canine on the opposite side to achieve the correct position. This slight change in horizontal positioning requires a corresponding change in the horizontal angulation of the PID (Figure 18–1 ■).

NOT RECORDING POSTERIOR STRUCTURES

- **Probable causes:** Image receptor was placed too far forward in the patient's oral cavity. When a patient presents with a small oral cavity or a hypersensitive gag reflex, it may be difficult to place the image receptor far enough posterior.

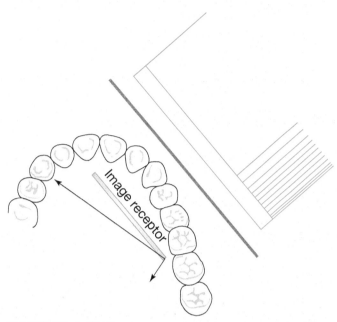

FIGURE 18–1 Tip for positioning the image receptor for exposure of a premolar radiograph. Positioning the anterior edge of the image receptor against the canine on the opposite side provides space to fit a wired digital sensor into the correct anterior position. A corresponding horizontal angle shift may be required.

- **Corrective actions:** Communicate with the patient to gain acceptance and assistance with placing the image receptor. Use tips for working with an exaggerated gag reflex (see Chapter 29).

NOT RECORDING APICAL STRUCTURES

- **Probable causes:**
  1. Image receptor was not placed high enough (on the maxillary arch) or low enough (on the mandibular arch) in the patient's oral cavity to image the root apices. This often occurs when a patient does not occlude completely and securely on the image receptor positioner biteblock or tab.
  2. Inadequate vertical angulation will result in less of the apical region being recorded onto the radiograph (Figure 18–2 ■).

- **Corrective actions:**
  1. Ensure that the image receptor is positioned correctly into the image receptor positioner and that the patient is biting down all the way on the biteblock or tab. Tip the image receptor and positioner assembly in toward the middle of the oral cavity where the midline of the palatal vault is the highest to facilitate the patient's ability to securely occlude on the biteblock. When placing an image receptor for a mandibular radiograph, use an index finger to gently massage the sublingual area to relax and move the tongue out of the way. Keep an index finger in place to shield the area while positioning

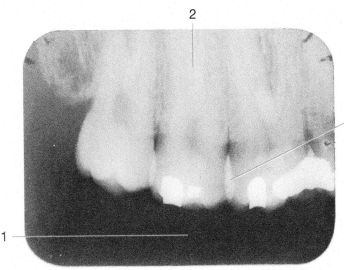

FIGURE 18–2 **Maxillary molar periapical radiograph.** Not recording the apical structures most likely resulted from a combination of not placing the image receptor correctly and inadequate vertical angulation. (**1**) Patient did not occlude completely and securely on the image receptor biteblock. (**2**) Inadequate vertical angulation did not record apical structures and caused elongation. (**3**) Incorrect distomesial horizontal angulation caused overlapped proximal surfaces; overlapping more severe in the anterior region and less severe in the posterior region.

the image receptor into a low enough position to record the mandibular teeth root apices.

2. Increase vertical angulation. If correctly directing the central rays of the x-ray beam perpendicular to the image receptor when using the paralleling technique (see Chapter 13) and perpendicular to the imaginary bisector when using the bisecting technique (see Chapter 14) does not adequately record the apical region, increase the vertical angulation slightly. An increase of no greater than 15 degrees will facilitate recording more apical structures without compromising radiographic quality.

NOT RECORDING CORONAL STRUCTURES

- **Probable causes:** Because this error appears to be the opposite of not recording the apical region, it would seem logical to assume that the image receptor was placed too high (on the maxillary arch) or too low (on the mandibular arch) in the oral cavity. However, the use of image receptor positioners will most likely make this impossible. When noted, the cause is more often the result of excessive vertical angulation (Figure 18–3 ■).
- **Corrective actions:** Decrease vertical angulation. If correctly directing the central rays of the x-ray beam perpendicular to the image receptor when using the paralleling technique and perpendicular to the imaginary bisector when using the bisecting technique does not record enough coronal structures, decrease the vertical angulation slightly. A decrease of no greater than 15 degrees will facilitate recording more coronal

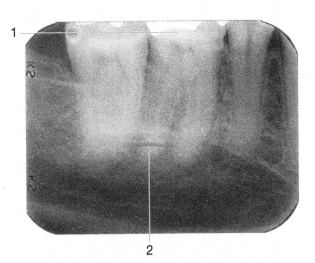

FIGURE 18–3 **Mandibular molar periapical radiograph.** (**1**) Excessive vertical angulation did not adequately record the occlusal structures. (**2**) Bending the film produced this radiolucent artifact.

structures without compromising radiographic quality (Figure 18–4 ■).

SLANTING OR TILTED INSTEAD OF STRAIGHT OCCLUSAL PLANE

- **Probable causes:** Edge of the image receptor was not parallel with the incisal or occlusal plane of the teeth, or the image receptor positioner biteblock or tab was not placed flush against the occlusal surfaces (Figure 18–5 ■). This error often results when the top edge of the image receptor contacts the lingual gingiva or the curvature of the palate when the patient occludes or when the image receptor is incorrectly placed on top of the tongue.
- **Corrective actions:** Straighten the image receptor by positioning away from the lingual surfaces of the teeth. Place the image receptor in toward the midline of the palate. Utilize this highest region of the palatal vault to stand the image receptor up parallel to the long axes of the teeth. For mandibular placements,

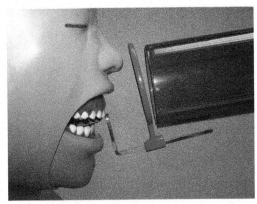

FIGURE 18–4 **Tip for recording incisal edges.** Decrease vertical angulation no more than 15 degrees.

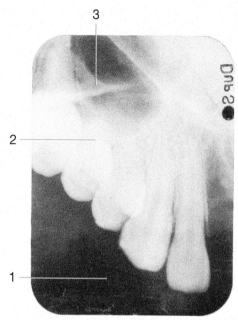

FIGURE 18–5 **Maxillary canine periapical radiograph.**
(**1**) Patient did not occlude completely and securely on the image receptor biteblock causing slanting or diagonal occlusal plane. (**2**) Excessive vertical angulation and incorrect image receptor position caused foreshortening. (**3**) Bent film produced this radiopaque artifact.

slide the image receptor in between the lingual gingiva and the lateral surface of the tongue. Ensure that the patient is biting down securely on the biteblock of the holder.

REVERSED FILM ERROR (HERRINGBONE ERROR)

- **Probable causes:** Image receptor film packet positioned so that the back side faced the teeth and the radiation source. The radiograph will be significantly underexposed. When placed on a viewbox and examined closely, a pattern representing the embossed lead foil that is in the back of a film packet can be detected. Historically film manufacturers used a herringbone pattern, and therefore some practitioners still call this a **herringbone error**. Film currently available has a pattern resembling a tire track or diamond pattern (Figure 18–6 ■).
- **Corrective actions:** Determine the front side of the film packet prior to placing into the image receptor holder. When in doubt, read the printed side of the film packet for direction. Once attached, examine the film and holder assembly to ensure that the tube side faces toward the teeth and the radiation source (Figure 18–7 ■). Due to the composition of photostimulable phosphor (PSP) plates and digital sensors, positioning the incorrect side of these image receptors toward the radiation source will result in failure to produce an image.

A cotton roll is sometimes utilized to help a patient bite down on an image receptor holder biteblock to secure it in place. Correct placement of a cotton roll is on the opposite side of the biteblock from where the teeth of interest occlude (see Figure 13–9). Placing a cotton roll on the same side as the teeth of interest will prevent the image receptor from being placed high enough (on the maxillary arch) or low enough (on the mandibular arch) in the mouth.

INCORRECT POSITION OF FILM IDENTIFICATION DOT

- **Probable causes:** Embossed identification dot positioned toward apical area where it can interfere with diagnosis.
- **Corrective actions:** Pay attention when placing the film packet into the film holding device to position the dot toward the incisal or occlusal region, where it is less likely to interfere with interpretation of the image. Some practitioners use the phrase "dot in the slot" to remind them to place the edge of the film packet where the dot is located into the slot of the film holding device. Placing the dot in the slot of a film holder will automatically position the dot toward the occlusal or incisal edges of the teeth and away from the apical regions.

Incorrect Positioning of the Tube Head and PID

Characteristic errors result from incorrect vertical and horizontal angulations and centering the x-ray beam over the image receptor. As discussed previously, incorrect vertical angulation can result in not recording the apices or the coronal edges of the teeth. **Elongation** (images that appear stretched out) and **foreshortening** (images that appear shorter than normal), with or without cutting off portions of the teeth, are dimensional errors that result from incorrect vertical angulation when using the bisecting technique. It is important to remember that it is impossible to create images that are elongated or foreshortened when the image receptor is positioned parallel to the teeth, as is the case when using the paralleling technique. If elongation or foreshortening errors result, it is important that the corrective action be to first try to position the image receptor parallel to the teeth of interest. Correctly positioning the image receptor parallel to the teeth will most likely prevent dimensional errors. If parallel placement of the image receptor to the teeth is not possible, then the bisecting technique must be carefully applied to avoid elongation and foreshortening of the image.

Conecut error results when the central rays of the x-ray beam are not directed toward the middle of the image receptor. **Conecut error** manifests as a white (clear) circular- or rectangular-bordered area indicating that part of the image receptor was beyond the range of the x-ray beam, and therefore received no exposure.

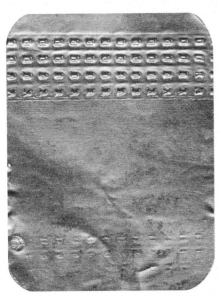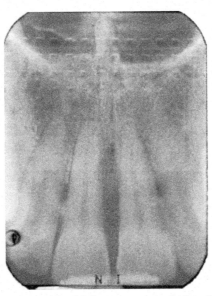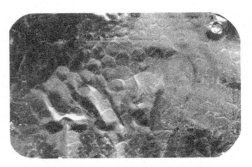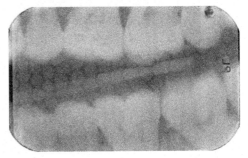

FIGURE 18–6 **Reversed film packet error.** Embossed lead foil patterns recorded on the images as a result of reversed film placement. Note the different patterns depending on the manufacturer and the film size.

ELONGATION/FORESHORTENING OF THE IMAGE (BISECTING TECHNIQUE ERROR)

- **Probable causes:** Insufficient vertical angulation with the PID not positioned steep enough away from 0 degrees results in elongation (see Figure 18–2). Excessive vertical angulation with the PID positioned too steep enough away from 0 degrees results in foreshortening (see Figure 18–5).
- **Corrective actions:** Direct the central rays of the x-ray beam perpendicular to the imaginary bisector between the long axes of the teeth and the plane of the image receptor (see Chapter 14). If relying on predetermined vertical angulation settings, ensure that the patient's occlusal plane is parallel, and that the midsagittal plane is perpendicular to the floor.

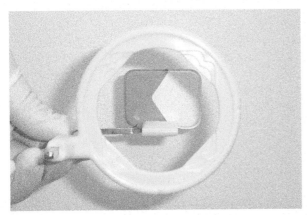

FIGURE 18–7 **Incorrect reversed film packet.** An examination through the ring of this image receptor holder assembly reveals that the back of the film packet will be positioned incorrectly toward the teeth and the x-ray source.

To correct elongation, increase the vertical angulation. To correct foreshortening, decrease the vertical angulation.

OVERLAPPED PROXIMAL CONTACTS

- **Probable causes:**
  1. Incorrect rotation of the tube head and PID in the horizontal plane. Superimposition of the proximal surfaces of adjacent teeth occurs when the central rays of the x-ray beam are not directed perpendicular through the interproximal spaces to the image receptor. Overlapped contacts result when the central rays of the x-ray beam are directed obliquely toward the image receptor from the distal or from the mesial. When the angle of the x-ray beam is directed obliquely from mesial to distal (**mesiodistal overlap**), the overlapping appears more severe in the posterior portion of the image. Conversely, when the angle of the x-ray beam is directed obliquely from distal to mesial (**distomesial overlap**), the overlapping appears more severe in the anterior portion of the image (see Figure 15–14).
  2. Not positioning the image receptor parallel to the interproximal spaces of the teeth of interest will prevent the central rays of the x-ray beam from being directed perpendicular through the contacts and perpendicular to the image receptor.

- **Corrective actions:**
  1. Examine the image to determine whether the overlap is more severe in the anterior or the posterior region of the image. To correct mesiodistal overlap, rotate the tube head and PID to direct the central rays of the x-ray beam more toward

Practice Point

Use the phrase "Move toward it to fix it" when correcting mesiodistal or distomesial overlap error. If the overlapping appears more severe in the posterior region (mesiodistal overlap), shift the tube head toward the posterior while rotating the PID to direct the x-ray beam from the distal toward the mesial. If the overlapping appears more severe in the anterior region (distomesial overlap), shift the tube head toward the anterior while rotating the PID to direct the x-ray beam from the mesial toward the distal.

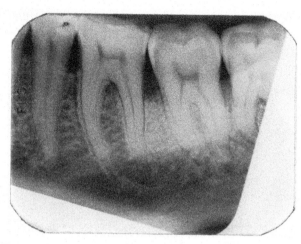

FIGURE 18–9 **Conecut error.** Rectangular PID.

the anterior teeth. To correct distomesial overlap, rotate the tube head and PID to direct the central rays of the x-ray beam more toward the posterior teeth. It should be noted that there are cases when mesiodistal and distomesial overlap cannot be readily distinguished from one another. When this happens, closely examine the teeth of interest to determine the precise contact points through which to perpendicularly direct the central rays of the x-ray beam.

2. Examine the teeth of interest to determine the contact points prior to positioning the image receptor. Place the image receptor parallel to the contact points of interest so that the central rays of the x-ray beam will intersect the image receptor perpendicularly through those contacts (see Figure 12–10).

CONECUT ERROR

- **Probable causes:**
  1. Central rays of the x-ray beam were not directed toward the center of the image receptor and therefore the beam diameter could not completely encircle and expose the entire surface area of the receptor (Figure 18–8 ▪).

2. Incorrectly assembled image receptor positioner that results in directing the central rays of the x-ray beam to the wrong place.

3. Not rotating a rectangular PID so that the long and short dimensions are appropriately aligned to match the long and short dimensions of the image receptor (Figure 18–9 ▪).

- **Corrective actions:**
  1. While maintaining correct horizontal and vertical angulations, move the tube head up, down, posterior, or anterior, depending upon which area of the radiograph shows a clear, unexposed region.

  2. After assembling the image receptor into the positioner, look through the external aiming ring to ensure that the image receptor is correctly in the center of the aiming device (Figure 18–10 ▪).

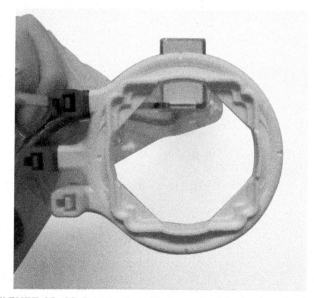

FIGURE 18–10 **Incorrect positioner assembly.** An examination through the ring of this image receptor holder assembly reveals that the digital sensor will be positioned incorrectly resulting in conecut error.

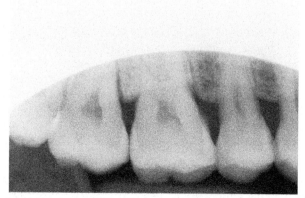

FIGURE 18–8 **Conecut error.** Circular PID.

3. A rectangular PID must be rotated to match the position of the image receptor. An image receptor will be placed with the long dimension vertical in the anterior region and horizontal in the posterior region. Switching between exposures requires careful adjustments to match the PID orientation. It is helpful to utilize the notched indicators on an external aiming ring (see Figure 13–11).

Incorrect Exposure Factors

Insufficient knowledge regarding the use of the control panel settings and exposure button can result in poor quality radiographic images. Digital imaging software may assist with adjusting incorrectly exposed images, but should not excuse careless disregard for exposure settings.

LIGHT/DARK IMAGES

- **Probable causes:**

  1. A light film-based image should first be examined closely for reversed film error. If an embossed pattern is not detected, an error in the selection of exposure factors should be suspected. Insufficient exposure time in relation to milliamperage, kilovoltage, and PID length will result in **underexposure**, whereas excessive exposure time in relation to these parameters results in **overexposure**. Failure to depress the exposure button for the full duration of the exposure cycle will also result in insufficient exposure (Figures 18–11 ■ and 18–12 ■).

  2. Exposing a PSP plate to prolonged or bright light prior to the laser processing step will result in a light or faded image.

  3. Under- or overexposure may rarely occur as a result of equipment malfunction.

- **Corrective actions:**

  1. An exposure chart posted near the control panel for easy reference can assist with preventing incorrect exposures. Increasing the exposure

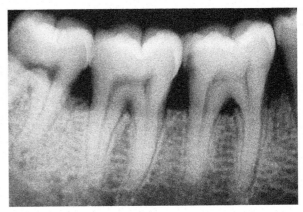

FIGURE 18–12 **Dark image.** Overexposed or overdeveloped radiograph.

time, milliamperage, kilovoltage, or a combination of these factors will correct underexposures, whereas decreasing these parameters will correct overexposures. If the PID length is changed, then a corresponding adjustment must be made to the exposure time to maintain image quality. The exposure button must be depressed for the full cycle, indicated by a red exposure light and audible signal on the control panel.

  2. Exposed PSP plates should be protected from prolonged or bright light exposure, by placing front side down on the counter or placing in a light-tight containment box until ready for the laser processing step (see Figure 8-14).

  3. If an under- or overexposure problem persists, check the accuracy of the timer for possible malfunction or the need for a professional calibration of the x-ray machine.

CLEAR OR BLANK IMAGE

- **Probable causes:**

  1. No exposure to x-rays, which results from failure to turn on the power to the x-ray machine, failure to maintain firm pressure on the exposure button during the exposure, failure to initiate exposure within the fixed time period required by a digital sensor.

  2. Incorrectly exposing the back side of a PSP plate or a digital sensor.

  3. A blank digital image may result from equipment malfunction.

- **Corrective actions:**

  1. Turn on the x-ray machine and maintain firm pressure on the exposure button for the full exposure cycle. Watch for the red exposure light and listen for the audible signal indicating that exposure has occurred. When utilizing digital sensor technology, do not activate the computer to receive the digital signal until ready to make the exposure to avoid being timed out.

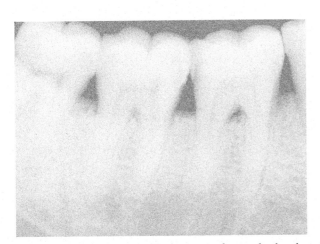

FIGURE 18–11 **Light image.** Underexposed or underdeveloped radiograph.

2. Become familiar with digital image receptors to determine the correct exposure side.

3. Check to ensure that there is a solid connection between a wired digital sensor and the computer or the universal serial bus (USB) interface box (see Figure 8–8). Unplug and reinsert the USB cord that connects the interface box with the computer into another port. Close all programs and restart the computer. Store digital sensors without crimping or folding the sensitive USB cord (Figure 18–13 ■). Check with manufacturer to determine if a damaged USB cord can be replaced.

DOUBLE IMAGE

- **Probable cause: Double exposure** resulting from accidentally exposing the same film or PSP plate twice.
- **Corrective actions:** Maintain a systematic order to exposing radiographs. Keep unexposed and exposed image receptors organized.

Miscellaneous Errors in Exposure

POOR DEFINITION

- **Probable causes:** Movement of the patient, slippage of the image receptor, or vibration of the x-ray machine tube head during exposure.

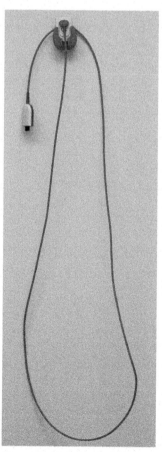

FIGURE 18–13 **Storage of digital sensor.** Hang digital sensors to avoid crimpling USB cord.

- **Corrective actions:** Stabilize the patient's head into position against the head rest of the examination chair and communicate the importance of remaining still throughout the duration of the exposure. Explain the procedure and gain the patient's cooperation to maintain steady pressure on the image receptor positioner biteblock. Do not use the patient's finger to stabilize the image receptor in the oral cavity. Ensure that the x-ray machine tube head is completely still and in position before activating the exposure.

ARTIFACTS Images other than anatomy or pathology that do not contribute to a diagnosis can be avoided with careful patient preparation prior to exposure.

- **Probable causes:** The presence of foreign objects in and near the oral cavity during exposure (e.g., appliances such as removable bridges, partial or full dentures, orthodontic retainers, patient glasses, and facial jewelry used in piercings). There may be occasions when the lead/lead equivalent thyroid collar could be in the path of the x-ray beam. These dense objects will result in radiopaque artifacts (Figures 18–14 ■ and 18–15 ■). The cord that connects a wired digital sensor with the computer may accidentally be placed within the path of the x-ray beam, resulting in a characteristic radiopaque artifact (Figure 18–16 ■).
- **Corrective actions:** Perform a cursory examination of the oral cavity to check for the presence of removable appliances. Ask the patient to remove any objects that may be in the path of the primary beam. Ensure that the lead/lead equivalent apron and thyroid collar and digital sensor cord do not block the x-rays from reaching the image receptor.

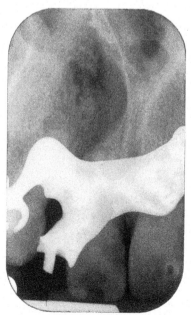

FIGURE 18–14 **Radiopaque artifact.** Partial denture accidentally left in place during exposure.

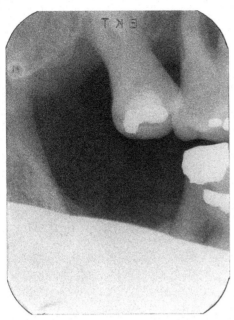

FIGURE 18–15 **Radiopaque artifact.** Lead thyroid collar accidentally within the path of the primary beam during exposure.

Processing Errors

Processing errors occur with both manual and automatic film processing, and include under- and overdevelopment, incorrectly following protocols, and failure to maintain an ideal darkroom. PSP plate image receptors are also subject to laser processing errors.

Development Error

LIGHT/DARK IMAGE

- **Probable causes: Underdevelopment** results when a film is not left in the developer for the required

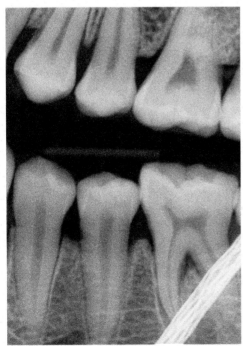

FIGURE 18–16 **Digital sensor cord artifact.** USB cord within the path of the primary beam during exposure.

time. **Overdevelopment** results when a film is left in the developer too long. The colder the developing solution, the longer the time required to produce an image of ideal density; the warmer the developing solution, the less developing time required. Images may be too light or too dark as a result of incorrectly mixing developer solution from concentrated chemicals. A weak developer mix produces light images; a strong mix produces dark images. Light images also result when the developer solution is old, weakened, or contaminated. A low solution level in the developer tank of an automatic processor that does not completely cover the rollers may also produce a light image.

- **Corrective actions:** When processing manually, check the temperature of the developer and consult a time-temperature chart before beginning the process. Ensure that an automatic processor indicates that the solutions have warmed up and the correct timed cycle is used. If weakened or old solutions are suspected, change the solutions. Maintain good quality control to replenish solutions to keep them functioning at peak conditions and at the appropriate levels in the tanks.

Processing and Darkroom Protocol Errors

BLANK/CLEAR IMAGE

- **Probable causes:** Film that is accidentally placed in the fixer before being placed in the developer will result in a blank or clear image. If allowed to remain in warm rinse water too long the emulsion may dissolve also resulting in a clear image.
- **Corrective actions:** When processing manually, and when filling automatic processor tanks during solution changes and cleaning procedures, check which tank contains the developer and which tank contains the fixer to avoid filling with the wrong solutions. Labelling the tanks prevents confusion. To prevent the emulsion from separating from the film base, promptly remove the film at the end of the washing period.

GREEN FILMS

- **Probable causes:** When films stick together in the developer the solution is prevented from reaching the (green) emulsion. The most common causes include failure to separate double film packets, placing additional films into the same intake slot of an automatic processor too close together resulting in overlapping of the two films, and attaching two films to one clip used in manual processing, or allowing films on adjacent film racks to contact each other.
- **Corrective actions:** Be skilled at separating double film packets under safelight conditions. Use alternating intake slots or wait 10 seconds before loading subsequent films into an automatic processor. Carefully

handle manual film hangers and clips to avoid placing films in contact with each other.

BROWN IMAGES

- **Probable cause:** Insufficient or improper washing. Films that have not been washed completely will appear normal immediately after drying, but will turn brown over a period of several weeks after processing as the chemicals that remain on the surface of the film erode the image.
- **Corrective actions:** When processing manually, rinse films in circulating water for at least 20 minutes. Always return a film to complete the fixing and washing steps after a wet reading. When processing automatically, ensure that the main water supply to the unit is turned on and that the water bottles of closed systems are full.

Handling Errors

The manner in which the image receptor is handled contributes to its ability to record a diagnostic quality image. Careless handling can produce artifacts and may damage the image receptor surface.

BLACK IMAGE

- **Probable cause:** Film was accidentally exposed to white light.
- **Corrective actions:** Unwrap a film packet only under safelight conditions. Prevent accidental white light from entering the darkroom by locking the door or use an "in-use" sign to prevent others from opening the door. When using an automatic processor, ensure that the film has completely entered the light-protected processor before turning on the white overhead light or before removing hands from the daylight loader baffles.

PRESSURE MARKS, SCRATCHES, AND ARTIFACTS

- **Probable causes:**
  1. Bending or excessive pressure can cause film emulsion to crack and can permanently damage PSP plates. Accidental damage can result when forcibly placing an image receptor into an image receptor positioner. Pressure marks and bending can appear either radiopaque or radiolucent (see Figures 18–3 and 18–5).
  2. Film emulsion and PSP plates are easily scratched, resulting in radiopaque artifacts (Figures 18–17 ■ and 18–18 ■).
  3. Handling film with damp fingers or latex treatment gloves, or with residual glove powder on the fingers will leave black smudges.
  4. Damaged digital sensors or sensors with **dead pixels** produce images with missing information in areas of the damage.

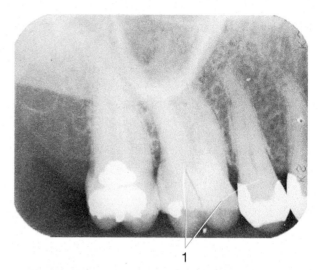

FIGURE 18–17 Damaged film emulsion. Scratches result in radiographic artifacts.

5. **Static electricity** may be produced when a film is pulled out of the packet wrapping quickly. Static electricity creates a white light spark that exposes the film resulting in radiolucent artifacts resembling smudges, fuzzy dots, or a unique lightning pattern (see Figure 17–24).

- **Corrective actions:**
  1. Use caution when assembling an image receptor and holding device. Do not bend an image receptor to make it fit the oral cavity. Instead, use a smaller size, the occlusal technique (see Chapter 16), or an extraoral procedure (see Chapter 30).
  2. Carefully handle all types of radiographic image receptors. Avoid cleansers and disinfectants that can damage PSP plates and digital sensors; use products only as recommended by the image receptor manufacturer. Check with the manufacturer regarding how often to clean, and

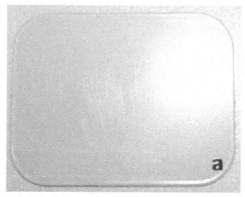

FIGURE 18–18 Damaged PSP plate. Scratches that will result in radiographic artifacts.

the necessity of vigorous rubbing to remove surface debris.

3. Avoid contact with the surface of film and PSP plates. Handle these image receptors carefully and only by the edges. Hands should be clean and free of moisture or glove powder. Use caution when separating double film packets for processing; avoid sliding films against one another. Mount dried radiographs promptly or enclose in a protective envelope.

4. Take care to store digital sensors to protect from damage. When dead pixels create artifacts, see manufacturer's instructions on recalibrating or replacing the sensor.

5. Take care opening film packets in a dry environment. Reduce the occurrence of static electricity by using antistatic products on protective clothing to prevent the buildup of static electricity.

Fogged Images and Decreased Contrast

Film fog and electronic **noise** (affecting digital images) diminish radiographic contrast by producing a thin, cloudy or grainy appearance that compromises the clarity of the image (Figure 18–19 ■). Fogged radiographs have a similar decreased contrast appearance, making it difficult to pinpoint the cause (Box 18–1). Careful attention to the exposure techniques and processing method used and darkroom and image receptor handling protocols will help reduce the occurrence of fogged images.

RADIATION FOG

- **Probable causes:** Not properly protecting the image receptor from stray radiation before or after exposure.
- **Preventive measures:** Store film in its original package at a safe distance from the source of x-rays. Exposing a film increases its sensitivity; therefore, it is

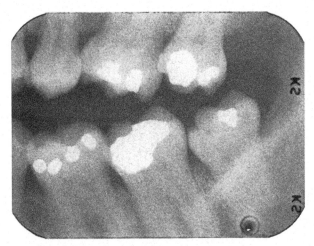

FIGURE 18–19 Film fog. Decreased image contrast.

Box 18-1: Causes of Film Fog

- Radiation
- Light
- Heat
- Humidity
- Chemical vapors
- Aging

very important that once a film has been exposed, it should be protected from the causes of film fog until processed.

WHITE LIGHT FOG

- **Probable causes:** White light leaking into the darkroom from around doors or plumbing pipes. White light leaking into the film packet through a tear in the outer wrapping.
- **Preventive measures:** Check the darkroom for white light leaks. Handle the film packet carefully to prevent tearing the light-tight outer wrapping.

SAFELIGHT FOG

- **Probable causes:** A safelight will fog film if the bulb wattage is stronger than recommended; the distance the safelight is located over the workspace area is too close; the filter is the incorrect type or color for the film being used; or the filter is scratched or otherwise damaged, allowing white light through. Even when adequate, prolonged exposure to the safelight will fog film.
- **Preventive measures:** Perform periodic quality control checks on the darkroom and safelight (see Chapter 19). Follow film manufacturer's guidelines when choosing filter color. Check the bulb wattage, check the distance away from the workspace, and examine the filter for defects. Open film packets aseptically within a two- to three-minute period to minimize the time films are exposed to the safelight.

MISCELLANEOUS LIGHT FOG

- **Probable causes:** Glowing light that reaches the film such as that from watches with fluorescent faces, indicator lights on equipment stored in the darkroom, and cell phones carried into the darkroom in a radiographer's pocket have the potential to create fog. This is especially true when processing sensitive extraoral films.
- **Preventive measures:** Watches with fluorescent faces should not be worn in the darkroom while processing

film unless covered with the sleeve of the operator's protective barrier gown or lab coat. Luminous dials of equipment located in the darkroom that glow in unsafe light colors should be masked with opaque tape. Cell phones should be powered off to avoid accidental illumination by an incoming call or message.

STORAGE FOG (HEAT, HUMIDITY, AND CHEMICAL VAPORS)

- **Probable causes:** Film fog will result from exposure to warm, damp conditions or in the vicinity of fume-producing chemicals.
- **Preventive measures:** Store film unopened, in its original package in a cool, dry area. Film should not be stored in the darkroom unless protected from heat, humidity, and fume-producing processing solutions.

CHEMICAL FOG

- **Probable cause:** Developing films too long, at too high a temperature, or in contaminated solutions will produce film fog.
- **Preventive measures:** Develop at the recommended time-temperature cycle. Avoid contamination of processing chemicals. Always replace the manual processing tank cover in the same position, with the side over the developer remaining over the developer and the side over the fixer remaining over the fixer to prevent contamination of the solutions. Thoroughly rinse films to remove developer before moving the film hanger into the fixer.

AGED FILM FOG

- **Probable cause:** Film emulsion has a shelf life with an expiration date (see Figure 7–17). As film ages, it can become fogged.
- **Preventive measures:** Consult dates on film boxes. Rotate film stock so that the oldest film is used before its expiration date. Do not overstock film. Thoroughly research a supplier before purchasing film, especially when buying in bulk or from an unfamiliar source.

DIGITAL RADIOGRAPHIC NOISE

- **Probable causes:**
  1. Exposure settings that are extremely low. When switching from film-based radiography to digital imaging, there is a tendency to set the exposure factors too low, launching a digital self-correction that can produce radiographic electronic noise.
  2. Digital sensors are especially sensitive to scatter radiation, possibly increasing the risk that a round collimator will allow more periphery radiation to add noise to the image.

- **Preventive measures:**
  1. Use correct exposure settings. After setting at manufacturer's recommendations, evaluate the images to determine the need for varying the settings to eliminate radiographic noise and obtain the desired image clarity and contrast.
  2. When switching from film-based radiography to digital imaging, some sensor manufacturers recommend switching from round to rectangular collimation to help reduce scatter radiation.

REVIEW—Chapter summary

Radiographic errors may require retakes. A sound retake policy states that no radiograph should be retaken until a thorough investigation determines the exact cause of the error and the appropriate corrective action is identified and can be implemented. A dental radiographer must be able to recognize criteria for a quality diagnostic radiograph, identify common mistakes and their causes, and apply appropriate corrective actions. Errors produced when utilizing direct digital imaging can be corrected almost immediately, without removing the sensor from the oral cavity. Undiagnostic radiographs result from technique errors, processing errors, and handling errors.

Technique errors include mistakes made in placement of the image receptor, positioning the tube head and the PID, and choosing the correct exposure factors. Processing errors include development mistakes, not following protocols for processing and darkroom use, and chemical contamination. Handling errors include damaged image receptors and fogged images.

Investigate probable causes and corrective actions for not recording the entire tooth and supporting structures, producing a slanted occlusal plane, herringbone error, and for incorrectly positioning the embossed identification dot. Investigate probable causes and corrective actions for elongation and foreshortening, overlapping teeth contacts, and conecut error. Investigate probable causes and corrective actions for light/dark, clear/blank, and double-exposed images, and for images with poor definition, the presence of artifacts, and pressure marks. Investigate probable causes and corrective actions for over- and underdevelopment; clear, green, and brown images.

Fogged radiographs result from exposure to stray radiation, light, heat, humidity, chemical vapors, and contamination. Film has a shelf life, and aging may result in film fog. Electronic noise, the digital equivalent of film fog, results when radiation exposure settings are set extremely low and when excess scatter radiation reaches the digital sensor.

RECALL—Study questions

1. Each of the following should be included in a policy statement on retaking undiagnostic radiographs EXCEPT one. Which one is the EXCEPTION?
   a. The cause of the error must be identified.
   b. The solution to the problem must be established.
   c. The corrective action can be implemented.
   d. The radiation exposure can be reduced.

2. Which of the following is NOT a characteristic of a quality periapical radiograph?
   a. Embossed dot is positioned toward the apical region.
   b. At least 2 mm beyond teeth crowns and root tips is recorded.
   c. Occlusal/incisal edges of teeth are parallel to edge of the image receptor.
   d. Image is free of magnification, distortion, and film fog or digital noise.

3. Each of the following may be a possible corrective action for retaking a periapical radiograph that did not image the roots of the teeth of interest EXCEPT one. Which one is the EXCEPTION?
   a. Move the image receptor in toward the midline of the oral cavity.
   b. Request that the patient bite down securely on the image receptor holder biteblock.
   c. Decrease the vertical angulation not more than 15 degrees.
   d. Ensure that the image receptor is not resting on the tongue.

4. What does herringbone error indicate?
   a. Embossed dot was positioned incorrectly.
   b. Lead foil was processed with the film.
   c. Film packet was placed in the oral cavity backwards.
   d. Rectangular collimated PID was used.

5. When using the bisecting technique, which of these errors results from inadequate vertical angulation?
   a. Elongation
   b. Foreshortening
   c. Conecut
   d. Overlapping

6. Which of the following errors can be avoided by correctly using the paralleling technique?
   a. Cutting root apices off the image
   b. Elongating the image of the tooth
   c. Overlapping proximal contacts
   d. Conecutting in the occlusal/incisal region

7. What error causes more severely overlapped proximal surface contacts between the first and second molar than between the first and second premolar?
   a. Excessive vertical angulation
   b. Inadequate vertical angulation
   c. Distomesial projection of horizontal angulation
   d. Mesiodistal projection of horizontal angulation

8. Which of these errors results from a failure to direct the central rays of the x-ray beam toward the middle of the image receptor?
   a. Overlapping
   b. Conecutting
   c. Occlusal plane slanting
   d. Foreshortening

9. Which of these images indicates an overexposed radiograph?
   a. Clear
   b. Light
   c. Dark
   d. Brown

10. Each of the following will result in radiographs that are too light EXCEPT one. Which one is the EXCEPTION?
    a. Hot developer solution
    b. Old, expired film
    c. Underexposing
    d. Underdeveloping

11. Which of these image receptors will get lighter in response to prolonged white light exposure?
    a. Intraoral film
    b. Extraoral film
    c. Digital sensor
    d. PSP plate

12. Each of the following will result in radiographs that are blank (clear) EXCEPT one. Which one is the EXCEPTION?
    a. No exposure to x-rays
    b. Placing films in the fixer first
    c. Extended time in warm water rinse
    d. Accidental white light exposure

13. Which of the following describes films that stick together inside an automatic processor?
    a. Green
    b. Brown
    c. Black
    d. White

14. Which of these indicates that a film was not properly washed?
    a. Image appears light
    b. Fogging results
    c. Film turns brown
    d. White spots form

15. Each of the following will result in black artifacts on the radiograph EXCEPT one. Which one is the EXCEPTION?
    a. Static electricity
    b. Bent film
    c. Fixer splash
    d. Glove powder

16. Rectangular collimation is recommended when using digital sensors, *because* a rectangular PID reduces more scatter radiation than a circular PID.
    a. Both the statement and reason are correct and related.
    b. Both the statement and reason are correct but NOT related.
    c. The statement is correct, but the reason is NOT.
    d. The statement is NOT correct, but the reason is correct.
    e. NEITHER the statement NOR the reason is correct.

17. Each of the following is a cause of film fog EXCEPT one. Which one is the EXCEPTION?
    a. Exposure to scatter radiation
    b. Double exposing the film
    c. Use of old, expired film
    d. Chemical fume contamination

REFLECT—Case study

A full mouth series of periapical and bitewing radiographs exhibits the following errors:

1. Maxillary right molar periapical radiograph did not image the third molar.

2. Maxillary right canine periapical radiograph appears elongated with the root tip cut off.

3. Proximal contacts of adjacent premolar teeth in the right premolar bitewing radiograph are overlapped. The overlapping appears most severe in the posterior portion of the image and less severe in the anterior region.

4. Left molar bitewing film was bent when it was placed into the image receptor holder.

5. Mandibular incisors periapical radiograph appears very light, with a hint of a diamond-like pattern superimposed over the image of the teeth.

6. Film that should have been a left mandibular molar periapical radiograph is blank, with no hint of an image.

7. Left maxillary premolar periapical radiograph appears to have been double exposed.

Consider these seven radiographs with the errors noted and answer the following questions:

a. What is the most likely cause of this error? How did you arrive at this conclusion?

b. Could there be multiple causes for this error? What other errors would produce this result?

c. Why do you think this error occurred?

d. What corrective action would you take when retaking this radiograph? Be specific.

e. On what are you basing your decision to reexpose the patient?

f. What steps or actions would you recommend to prevent this error from occurring in the future?

RELATE—Laboratory application

For a comprehensive laboratory practice exercise on this topic, see Thomson, E. M., & Bruhn, A. M. (2018). *Exercises in oral radiography techniques: A laboratory manual* (4th ed.). Hoboken, NJ: Pearson. Chapter 8, "Identifying and correcting radiographic errors."

REFERENCES

Carestream Health, Inc. (2007). *Kodak Dental Systems: Exposure and processing for dental film radiography.* Pub. N-414, Rochester, NY: Author.

Eastman Kodak Company. (2002). *Successful intraoral radiography.* N-418 CAT No. 103. Rochester, NY: Author.

Kalathingal, S. M., Shrout, M. K., et al. (2010). Rating the extent of surface scratches on photostimulable storage phosphor plates in a dental school environment. *Dentomaxillofacial Radiology, 39,* 179–183.

Thomson, E. M., & Bruhn, A. M. (2018). Identifying and correcting radiographic errors. *Exercises in oral radiographic techniques: A laboratory manual* (4th ed.). Hoboken, NJ: Pearson.

White, S. C., & Pharoah, M. J. (2014). Film imaging. Projection geometry. *Oral radiology: Principles and interpretation* (7th ed.). St. Louis, MO: Elsevier.

Williamson, G. F. (2014, December 9). Digital imaging techniques and error correction. Retrieved from Dental Care website: http://www.dentalcare.com/media/en-US/education/ce462/ce462.pdf

Quality Control and Environmental Safety in Dental Radiography

OBJECTIVES

Following successful completion of this chapter, you should be able to:

1. Define the key terms.
2. State the objectives of dental radiographic quality control.
3. Explain the role a competent radiographer plays in quality assurance.
4. Describe quality control tests for monitoring a dental x-ray machine.
5. Describe quality control tests for monitoring a darkroom and processing equipment.
6. Describe quality control tests for monitoring radiographic image receptors.
7. Describe quality control tests for monitoring viewboxes and computer monitors used to view radiographic images.
8. List precautions to put in place that protect digital radiographic images.
9. List data supplied by Safety Data Sheets (SDS) for radiographic processing chemistry.
10. Describe safe handling procedures for radiographic processing chemicals and materials.
11. Describe environmentally sound options for disposal of radiographic processing chemistry and materials.

KEY TERMS

Biodegradable
Eyewash station
Fresh-film test
Hazardous waste
Reference film
Safety Data Sheet (SDS)
Silver thiosulphate complex
Step-wedge
Waste stream

Introduction

Quality assurance is defined as the planning, implementation, and evaluation of procedures used to produce high-quality radiographs with maximum diagnostic information (yield) while minimizing radiation exposure. Quality control is the term given to the tests that ensure an acceptable level of quality (Table 19–1 ■). Establishing a quality assurance program for radiographic procedures should include safe handling of materials and products used in dental radiography that may have an impact on the environment. This chapter presents quality control tests that can be used to monitor operator competency, evaluate dental x-ray machine operation, maintain efficacy of processing systems, and guide safe handling and disposal of potentially hazardous radiographic materials.

Quality Administration

A quality assurance program should include an assessment of current practices, identification of where and how problems may be occurring, development of a written plan that identifies responsibilities and personnel training needs, record keeping, and periodic evaluation of the plan. Begin a needs assessment by periodically reviewing patient radiographs for problems that affect image quality. Based on the needs assessment findings, develop a written plan that lists the equipment that requires monitoring; tests that will be performed and at what time intervals; authority and responsibility assignments for performing these tests; and record-keeping logs needed for documenting quality assurance test results, retake radiographs, and personnel training (Box 19–1).

Table 19–1 Suggested Quality Control Tests

Quality Control Test	Suggested Time Interval
Automatic processor	Daily
Processing solutions	Daily
PSP plate sensors	Daily
CCD/CMOS-APS sensors	Monthly
Tube head stability	Monthly
Darkroom safelighting	Semiannually
Viewboxes	Semiannually
X-ray machine output consistency	Annually
Cassettes and screens	Annually
Digital image storage	Annually

Box 19–1: Objectives of Quality Control

- Maintain high standard of image quality.
- Identify problems before image quality is compromised.
- Keep patient and occupational exposures to a minimum.
- Reduce occurrence of retake radiographs.

Although the dentist is ultimately responsible for quality administration, each oral health care team member can be given authority to carry out specific aspects of a quality control program. Assigning authority and clearly defining specific tasks and/or maintenance procedures helps to ensure that the procedures are being performed. Each oral health care team member must be informed of how and why the tasks are to be performed and be offered training opportunities to ensure competency. A monitoring schedule list of quality control tests, identification of the person responsible for each test, and the frequency of testing should be generated and posted. Checkoff lists can be used to record maintenance and inspections.

A quality control test log should include test dates and results, actions taken as a result of testing, and the name of the person who conducted the test. A log of all radiographs retaken should be recorded to identify recurring problems. The oral health care team should meet periodically to evaluate the logs. Careful planning and thoroughly carrying out a quality assurance program can increase the likelihood of producing high-quality radiographs while minimizing radiation exposure.

Radiographer Competency

Essential to a quality assurance program is the ability of the radiographer. Operator errors that result in undiagnostic radiographs generate a need for retakes, which results in increased radiation exposure for the patient and lost time. A radiographer must be competent not only in obtaining radiographic images, but also in identifying when errors occur. Even competent radiographers encounter situations where less-than-ideal radiographic images result. It is important, therefore, to be able to recognize problems, identify the cause, and apply the appropriate corrective action.

Operator errors and retakes should be recorded to identify and correct recurring problems. Each radiographic exposure should be recorded in a log that can be reviewed periodically for the purpose of identifying problems. This will also help monitor the skills of the radiographer. Continuing education and opportunities for on-the-job-training can assist in brushing up on skills, improving in an area of deficiency, and/or staying apprised of new technology.

Quality Control for the Dental X-ray Machine

Periodic comprehensive testing of the x-ray machine is essential to a quality assurance program. Quality control tests include radiation output, accuracy of exposure settings, focal spot size, filtration, collimation, beam alignment, and tube head stability (Procedure 19–1). State and local health departments may provide or require x-ray machine testing as part of registration or licensing programs. In this case, a qualified health physicist will conduct these tests prior to renewing registration or license. However, the radiographer who uses the equipment on a daily basis should pay attention to the control panel indicator lights, audible alerts, and stability of the tube head to detect when the equipment is not functioning at peak performance.

Quality Control for the Darkroom

Quality control tests for the darkroom include assessment of safelighting; checking for white light leaks; processing chemistry maintenance; and detection of conditions that create film fog. The darkroom should be checked to determine that it is adequately ventilated, free from chemical fumes, within the prescribed temperature and humidity range recommended by the film manufacturer, beyond the reach of stray radiation, and light-tight. Essential for a quality darkroom is the elimination of white light leaks and an appropriate safelight.

Safelight Monitoring

Whether the darkroom is light-tight can be determined by closing the door and turning off all lights, including the safelight. Light leaks, if present, become visible after about five minutes when the eyes become accustomed to the dark. Possible sources of light leaks include around the entry door or around the pipes leading into the darkroom. Drop ceiling tiles and ventilation screens may also allow white light to enter the darkroom. While eyes are still adjusted to the dark, white light leaks may be marked with tape or chalk to allow them to be located when the white overhead lights are turned back on. Light leaks should be sealed with tape or weather stripping. A coin test can be performed to evaluate safelighting conditions (Procedure 19–2). Periodically

---

Procedure 19–1

X-ray Machine Output Consistency Test

1. Place an image receptor on the counter or examination chair within reach of the dental x-ray machine tube head.
2. Place a **step-wedge** on top of the image receptor (Figure 19–1 ■).
3. Position the x-ray machine tube head over the image receptor and step-wedge, placing the open end of the position indicating device (PID) directly against the counter with the image receptor centered in the middle.
4. Set the exposure factors to those used for an adult patient maxillary anterior periapical radiograph. Make the exposure.
5. Process, label, date, and save the image in a quality control log.
6. After a desired time interval (for example: 24 hours, 1 week, 1 month) repeat steps 1 to 5 with a second image receptor.
7. Repeat step 6 with a third image receptor after an additional time interval.
8. Observe and compare the three images for consistency in density and contrast. A failed test will produce images that are different from each other, indicating that the radiation output varied over time (Figure 19–2 ■).

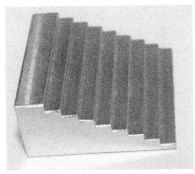

FIGURE 19–1 **Step-wedge.** Metal pyramid of steps of increasing thickness used in radiographic quality control tests.

FIGURE 19–2 **Evaluating step-wedge outcomes.** Compare step-wedge exposures side by side for consistency.

Procedure 19–2

Coin Test for Safelight Adequacy

1. Obtain a size 2 intraoral film packet and a coin.
2. Place the film packet on the counter or examination chair within reach of the x-ray tube head.
3. Position the x-ray machine tube head over the film packet. Direct the central rays of the x-ray beam perpendicularly toward the film packet at a distance of about 12 inches (30 cm) above the film packet.
4. Set the exposure factors to the lowest possible setting and make the exposure. (Because films that have already been exposed are more sensitive to conditions that cause film fog, using a film preexposed in this manner will provide a more realistic test.)
5. Take the preexposed film and a coin to the darkroom. Turn off the overhead white light and turn on the safelight.
6. Unwrap the film packet. Place the film on the counter and place the coin on top of the unwrapped film.
7. Wait approximately two or three minutes.
8. Remove the coin from the film and process the film in the usual manner.
9. When processing is complete, place the radiograph on a viewbox and observe for evidence of an outline of the coin. (The image will have an overall gray appearance or slight fogging from the preexposure in step 4.)
10. A failed test will show evidence of an outline of the coin.

examine the safelight for correct bulb wattage, filter color, scratches or cracks, and distance away from working area.

Additional sources of inappropriate light include illuminated dials or fluorescent objects worn or carried into the darkroom by personnel. Illuminated dials on equipment located in the darkroom must be red or masked with tape if necessary. Fluorescent wristwatch faces should not be worn in the darkroom unless covered by the sleeve of the operator's lab coat. Operators who carry a cell phone, even in a pocket, must completely shield any light or shut off the phone to prevent accidental illumination.

Processing System Monitoring

The key to peak performance of an automatic film processor is maintenance. Manufacturers recommend daily, weekly, monthly, and quarterly maintenance and cleaning procedures to ensure quality performance. A schedule of set maintenance procedures, and a log of when those procedures need to be performed, should be posted for easy reference. These two tests are helpful in daily monitoring of the automatic processor:

1. Process an unexposed film under safelight conditions. The film should come out of the return chute of the automatic processor clear (slightly blue tinted) and dry.
2. Process a film that has been exposed to white light. This film should come out of the return chute of the automatic processor black and dry after processing.

A failed test should prompt a check of the processing solution tanks, the water supply, and film dryer. The solution levels should be checked and must be replenished and changed on a regular basis. The processor should maintain the correct temperature. The water supply must be turned on and the dryer operating correctly to produce a dry film.

Manufacturers of processing chemicals recommend extending the life of solutions with regular replenishment

and changing out expired chemistry at regular intervals. Therefore it is important to monitor the strength of the processing solutions on a daily basis, before undiagnostic radiographs result. The developer solution is the more critical of the processing solutions and demands careful attention. When the developer solution deteriorates and loses strength, underdeveloped, lightened radiographic images result. A **reference film**, processed in fresh chemistry, representing ideal image density and contrast, can assist with monitoring processing solution strength (Procedure 19–3).

Image Receptor Quality Control

A **fresh-film test** can be used to monitor radiographic film. When a new film box is opened for use, immediately process one of the films without exposing it. The processed film should appear clear with a slight blue tint. If film fog is noted, the remaining films in the box should not be used. Film should be properly stored, protected, and used before the expiration date.

Photostimulable phosphor (PSP) plates should be examined for scratches and bending prior to preparing for use intraorally. The universal serial bus (USB) cord attached to a solid-state digital sensor should be examined for crimping or damage that results in separation of the cord from the body of the sensor (Figure 19–3 ■). Pay attention to the indicator lights on the USB interface module to detect digital computer equipment malfunction (see Chapter 8).

Extraoral cassettes should be checked for warping and light leaks that can result in fogged radiographs. Defective cassettes should be repaired or replaced. Intensifying screens should be examined for cleanliness and scratches. Specks of dirt, lint, or other material will absorb the light given off by the screen crystals and produce white or clear artifacts on the resultant radiographic image. Dirty screens should be cleaned as needed with solutions recommended

Procedure 19–3

Reference Film to Monitor Processing Solutions

1. Obtain several size 2 intraoral film packets from the same package.
2. Place one of the film packets on the counter or examination chair within reach of the dental x-ray machine tube head.
3. Place a step-wedge on top of the film packet (see Figure 19–1).
4. Position the x-ray machine tube head over the film packet and step-wedge, placing the open end of the PID directly against the counter with the image receptor centered in the middle.
5. Set the exposure factors to those used for an adult patient maxillary anterior periapical radiograph. Make the exposure.
6. Place the exposed film in a protected area away from film fog–causing elements.
7. Immediately repeat steps 2 through 6 with the rest of the films.
8. Process one of the exposed films in fresh chemistry. Mount this reference film on a viewbox.
9. Each day immediately after replenishing processing chemistry, retrieve one of the stored exposed films and process as usual. Compare this film to the reference film. Look for similar density and contrast indicating that the processing solutions are functioning at peak levels (see Figure 19–2).
10. Repeat step 9 each day to monitor the processing solutions.

by the screen manufacturer. Overuse of chemical cleaning should be avoided. Scratched or damaged screens should be replaced.

Quality Control for Equipment Used to View and Store Radiographic Images

VIEWBOX. If functioning properly, the viewbox should give off a uniform, subdued light. Flickering light may indicate bulb failure. The surface of the viewbox should be wiped clean as needed.

COMPUTER MONITOR. Periodically performing manufacturer recommended quality control calibrations on the monitor used to view digital radiographic images will ensure proper resolution and gray scale. The location of the monitor where images are viewed should be evaluated to ensure that bright ambient light is not producing glare off the monitor surface that will compromise viewing the images (Figure 19–4 ■). With the computer turned off, take the usual operator position in front of the monitor, either seated or standing. Observe the monitor for reflected images indicating that the monitor should be moved to a position that eliminates glare.

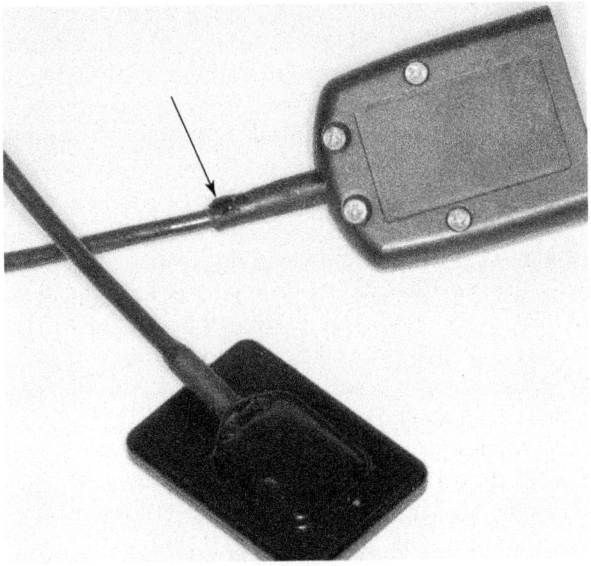

DIGITAL IMAGE STORAGE. Digital images stored on computers, laptops, hard drives, or portable wireless devices are vulnerable to threats from computer viruses, software malfunction, and misplaced or stolen equipment. Original digital image data should be appropriately backed up. Computer and virus software must be kept up to date, and operating system firewall protection should be enabled and functioning. Wireless devices with access to patient records and digital images should not be taken out of the oral health care practice setting. Handheld wireless devices connected to computer networks with protected health-related information (PHI) that are taken out of the practice setting are

FIGURE 19–3 **Digital sensor with damaged USB cord.**

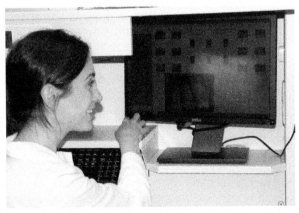

FIGURE 19–4 **Monitor surface glare.** Ambient light will compromise viewing images.

more vulnerable to be lost or stolen as compared to in-office desktop computers. All computers and digital radiographic image storage devices should be password protected. Do not write or display a password or username near the device itself. Digital radiographic image storage devices with PHI must be physically secured and locked when not in use.

Safe Handling of Radiographic Chemicals and Materials

Dental radiography quality control should include a plan for careful handling and special disposal considerations of products and chemicals that impact the environment and are used in obtaining and processing dental radiographs. One of the roles of the Occupational Safety and Health Administration (OHSA) is to present recommendations and regulations regarding safe handling of chemicals and materials and the management of potentially **hazardous wastes** used in dental radiography (Box 19–2). OSHA requires that manufacturers of chemical products such as developer and fixer used in processing dental radiographs supply **Safety Data Sheets (SDS)**, formally known as Material Safety Data Sheets, to oral health care practices that purchase these products. SDS list the properties of, and the potential effects, the product may have on the health of the person using the product (Box 19–3; Figure 19–5 ■).

Dentists are required by OHSA to obtain and keep on file a SDS for every chemical product used in the practice. The SDS should be reviewed by all personnel who work with the product; and be kept for easy reference and periodic review. All personnel should receive training with the use of, and practice safe handling of, the product and be able to respond appropriately to an emergency.

Box 19–2: General Recommendations for Safe Handling of Potentially Hazardous Chemicals

- Read SDS.
- Provide personnel training on use of product.
- Wear recommended personal protective equipment (PPE) when working with product.
- Avoid direct contact with product; wash hands thoroughly after handling.
- Use only with adequate ventilation; avoid breathing mist or vapor.
- Properly label container; store in original container; keep container tightly closed.
- Do not store product in same area where food or drinks are stored or consumed.
- Dispose of container appropriately; do not reuse container.

Box 19–3: Information Found on SDS

- Identification of product ingredients and common name
- Manufacturer's contact information and emergency phone number
- Requirements for safe handling and storage
- Exposure controls and PPE required when working with product
- Potential hazards associated with working with product
- First aid response measures and toxicological information
- Accidental spill and fire fighting protocols
- Disposal and ecological considerations and regulatory information

Chemical product manufacturers must identify a product container with a label that meets OSHA's recently updated Hazard Communication Standard. In addition to identification of the product and the manufacturer's contact information, the label must contain a signal word, such as DANGER, and easily recognized pictograms (Figure 19–6 ■). Labeling products assists in safe management of potentially harmful chemicals and aids in establishing proper work practices and in taking steps to reduce exposure and the occurrence of work-related illnesses and injuries. All containers must be labeled. This includes the developer and fixer tanks, even those inside an automatic processor; tubs used to clean the processor rollers; and any containers used for disposing absorbent towels used to clean up a spill.

Fixer and Developer

Safe handling of dental film processing chemicals begins with a well-ventilated darkroom and the use of PPE (see Chapter 9). Under normal conditions, processing chemicals should not cause respiratory difficulty in most individuals. If heated sufficiently or if an accidental mixing of fixer and developer occurs, an irritating sulphur dioxide gas may be released (Figure 19–7 ■). Prolonged exposure to this gas may cause some hypersensitive or asthmatic individuals discomfort. If uncomfortable symptoms occur, move to a well-ventilated area. If symptoms persist, seek medical attention.

The use of PPE should protect a radiographer from direct contact with processing chemicals (Figure 19–8 ■). In the event of accidental skin contact, immediately wash off with soap and water. A sink and **eyewash station** should be available in the darkroom or in close proximity to where processing equipment and chemistry is handled (Figure 19–9 ■). Developer has a high pH, meaning that it is alkaline or caustic, capable of burning biological tissues on contact. It is this caustic property that makes developer a more serious eye irritant than fixer. An accidental eye

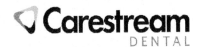

SAFETY DATA SHEET

Issuing date 2014-04-30   **Revision Date** 2014-04-30   **Version** 1

1. IDENTIFICATION OF THE SUBSTANCE/MIXTURE AND OF THE COMPANY/UNDERTAKING

Product name: READYPRO Developer

Product code: 1176262DEV

Supplier Carestream Health, Inc., 150 Verona Street, Rochester, New York 14608

Emergency telephone number
CHEMTREC: +1-703-527-3887 (INTERNATIONAL)
1-800-424-9300 (NORTH AMERICA)

For other information contact: 800-328-2910

Product Use: Photographic chemical.

2. HAZARDS IDENTIFICATION

Classification

Serious eye damage/eye Irritation	Category 2A
Skin Sensitization	Category 1
Germ cell mutagenicity	Category 2
Carcinogenicity	Category 2

Label elements

<table>
<tr><td colspan="2" align="center">Emergency Overview</td></tr>
<tr><td>**Signal word**</td><td align="center">Warning</td></tr>
<tr><td colspan="2">
hazard statements
Causes serious eye irritation
May cause an allergic skin reaction
Suspected of causing genetic defects
Suspected of causing cancer

</td></tr>
</table>

Contains Hydroquinone

Appearance aqueous solution   **Physical state** liquid   **Odor** Odorless

FIGURE 19–5 Sample SDS. Pages 1 and 2 of 10-page SDS for developer. (Courtesy of Carestream Health, Inc.)

(continued)

Precautionary Statements - Prevention
Obtain special instructions before use. Do not handle until all safety precautions have been read and understood. Wash face, hands and any exposed skin thoroughly after handling. Avoid breathing dust/fume/gas/mist/vapors/spray. Contaminated work clothing should not be allowed out of the workplace. Wear protective gloves/protective clothing/eye protection/face protection.

Precautionary Statement - Response
IF exposed or concerned: Get medical advice/attention.
Eyes
IF IN EYES: Rinse cautiously with water for several minutes. Remove contact lenses, if present and easy to do. Continue rinsing. If eye irritation persists: Get medical advice/attention.
Skin
IF ON SKIN: Wash with plenty of soap and water. If skin irritation or rash occurs: Get medical advice/attention. Wash contaminated clothing before reuse.

Precautionary Statement - Storage
Store in a closed container.

Precautionary Statements - Disposal
Dispose of contents/container to an approved waste disposal plant.

Hazards not otherwise classified (HNOC)
• Not applicable

Other Information
Toxic to aquatic life. Contact with strong acids liberates sulfur dioxide. May cause respiratory irritation.
<1%% of the mixture consists of ingredient(s) of unknown toxicity

3. COMPOSITION/INFORMATION ON INGREDIENTS

Chemical Name	CAS-No	Weight %	Trade Secret
Water 7732-18-5	7732-18-5	80-90	*
Sodium sulfite 7757-83-7	7757-83-7	1-5	*
Hydroquinone 123-31-9	123-31-9	<2.5	*
Sodium bicarbonate 144-55-8	144-55-8	1-5	*
Sodium borate 1330-43-4	1330-43-4	0.1-1	*
Sodium bromide 7647-15-6	7647-15-6	<1	*

*The exact percentages (concentrations) have been withheld as trade secrets.

4. FIRST AID MEASURES

First Aid Measures

General advice   If symptoms persist, call a physician.

Eye contact   Rinse immediately with plenty of water, also under the eyelids, for at least 15 minutes. Get medical attention immediately if symptoms occur.

Skin contact   Wash off immediately with plenty of water for at least 15 minutes. Remove and wash contaminated clothing before re-use. Get medical attention immediately if symptoms occur. Wash off immediately with soap and plenty of water while removing all contaminated clothes and shoes. May cause an allergic skin reaction.

FIGURE 19–5 Sample SDS. Pages 1 and 2 of 10-page SDS for developer. (Courtesy of Carestream Health, Inc.)

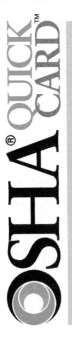

OSHA® QUICK CARD™

Hazard Communication Standard Labels

OSHA has updated the requirements for labeling of hazardous chemicals under its Hazard Communication Standard (HCS). All labels are required to have pictograms, a signal word, hazard and precautionary statements, the product identifier, and supplier identification. A sample revised HCS label, identifying the required label elements, is shown on the right. Supplemental information can also be provided on the label as needed.

For more information:

OSHA® Occupational Safety and Health Administration

U.S. Department of Labor   www.osha.gov   (800) 321-OSHA (6742)

OSHA 3492-01R 2016

SAMPLE LABEL

Product Identifier

CODE
Product Name _____

Supplier Identification

Company Name _____
Street Address _____
City _____ State _____
Postal Code _____ Country _____
Emergency Phone Number _____

Hazard Pictograms

Signal Word
Danger

Hazard Statements
Highly flammable liquid and vapor.
May cause liver and kidney damage.

Precautionary Statements
Keep container tightly closed. Store in a cool, well-ventilated place that is locked.
Keep away from heat/sparks/open flame. No smoking.
Only use non-sparking tools.
Use explosion-proof electrical equipment.
Take precautionary measures against static discharge.
Ground and bond container and receiving equipment.
Do not breathe vapors.
Wear protective gloves.
Do not eat, drink or smoke when using this product.
Wash hands thoroughly after handling.
Dispose of in accordance with local, regional, national, international regulations as specified.

In Case of Fire: use dry chemical (BC) or Carbon Dioxide (CO2) fire extinguisher to extinguish.

First Aid
If exposed call Poison Center.
If on skin (or hair): Take off immediately any contaminated clothing. Rinse skin with water.

Supplemental Information

Directions for Use
_____
_____
_____

Fill weight: _____ Lot Number: _____
Gross weight: _____ Fill Date: _____
Expiration Date: _____

FIGURE 19–6 **Sample Hazard Communication Standard Label.** (Courtesy of Occupational Safety and Health Administration (OSHA®).)

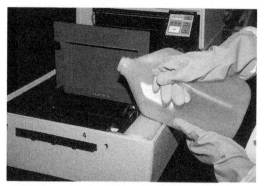

FIGURE 19–7 Barrier placed to separate the developer and fixer tanks when adding chemicals to avoid accidental mixing of chemicals.

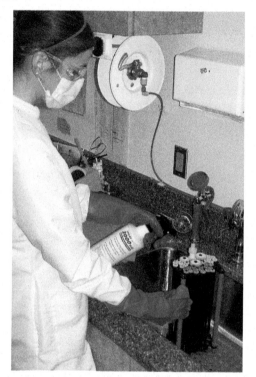

FIGURE 19–8 **PPE used when cleaning processing equipment.**

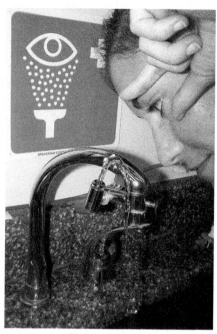

FIGURE 19–9 **Eyewash station.** Radiographer preparing to use the eyewash station in response to accidental contact with a potentially hazardous chemical. Note the recognizable label on the wall stating location of the eyewash station.

exposure requires an immediate flushing with water at an eyewash station for a minimum of 15 minutes (Procedure 19–4). Seek medical attention following accidental eye contact with developer.

Lead Foils

Routine handling of intact lead foil used in intraoral film packets and lead sealed in aprons and thyroid collars will not present a hazard to the radiographer. In years past, lead-lined containers or film packet dispensers were available in which to store film protected from stray radiation until ready for use. Improvements made to fast-speed film have made these lead-lined boxes unnecessary. These lead-lined

---

Procedure 19–4

Use of an Emergency Eyewash Station

1. Eyewash station
   a. Must be clearly labeled with appropriate signage that is easily recognized.
   b. Must be within 55 feet of where potentially hazardous chemicals are being used.
   c. Personnel must be able to get to the station within 10 seconds from where they are handling potentially hazardous chemicals.
2. Remove caps covering the eyewash faucets. Caps should be easy to remove.
3. Turn on water flow to a rate of about 0.5 gallon per minute.
4. Water temperature should be tepid, between 60°F and 95°F.
5. Hold the eyelids open with an index finger and thumb. Do not touch the eyeballs.*
6. Maintain water contact with the eyes for the recommended rinsing time listed on the SDS.
7. Seek medical attention at completion of the recommended rinse time.

*If easy to do, contact lens should be removed. Rinse fingers well. Do not use the same finger to hold open the eyelids unless thoroughly washed of possible chemical contamination.

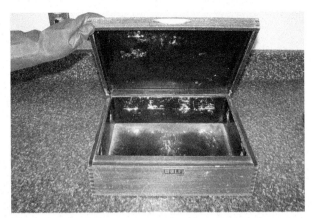

FIGURE 19–10 **Old lead-lined storage box showing signs of flaking.**

Box 19–4: Options for Management of Radiographic Wastes

- Contract with waste management company to provide container and pickup service.
- Contract with lead or silver reclaiming company for recycling.
- Establish agreement with supplier to take back used fixer/unused radiographic film.
- Collect used products and transport to designated local facility.
- Utilize silver recovery or reclaiming system.

containers should not be used either for storage of film or any other storage or dispensing purpose. The lead lining is subject to flaking off in a powder form with the potential for inhalation or ingestion (Figure 19–10 ■). Old radiographic storage containers suspected of being made of lead should be appropriately discarded.

Management of Radiographic Wastes

Disposal of potentially hazardous wastes generated by an oral health care practice should be done in accordance with federal, state, and local waste management regulations. In many areas, it is against the law to discard used fixer into the municipal sewer system or to discard lead foil at municipal landfills. Know what laws apply in the practice area. Equally important is the ethical responsibility to recycle or properly dispose of wastes that may be harmful to the environment.

Often, the best way to appropriately dispose of potentially hazardous materials used in dental radiography is to contract with a waste disposal company. Many practices already employ a waste management company to dispose of biohazard materials. These same companies usually offer a hazardous waste service that can manage radiographic wastes as well. Product SDS sometimes use vague language regarding proper disposal of a product, often stating to "dispose of according to state or local regulations." Therefore is it important to know what the regulations are for the practice area and that the qualifications of the contractor selected for disposal of hazardous wastes or recycling be thoroughly investigated. If materials are disposed of inappropriately, it is possible that the oral health care practice would be partly liable for fines and costs incurred by faulty handling of materials by the disposal service (Box 19–4).

Used Fixer Waste

Both developer and fixer are **biodegradable**, meaning that they can be broken down into harmless products by a wastewater treatment facility. During processing, fixer functions to remove unexposed and undeveloped silver halide crystals from the emulsion of radiographic film. Used fixer solution contains silver in the form of a stable **silver thiosulphate complex**. Thus bonded, there are virtually no

free silver ions present in used fixer, prompting experts to conclude that used fixer poses very little threat to the environment if discharged into wastewater treatment facilities. However, some state and local municipalities have regulations regarding the amount and/or the concentration of used fixer that can be discharged to a wastewater treatment facility. There are environment-friendly options to responsibly dispose of used fixer. Collecting used fixer for the purpose of extracting the silver ions will conserve a resource and prevent adding this metal to the **waste stream**.

Silver recovery or reclaiming systems are available that attach to an automatic processor fixer and/or rinse water drain line (Figure 19–11 ■). These systems can be adapted

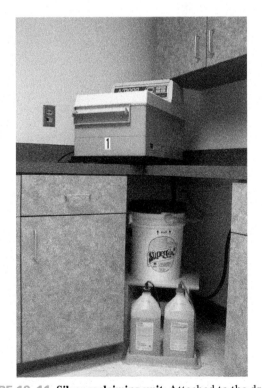

FIGURE 19–11 **Silver reclaiming unit.** Attached to the drain tube of an automatic processor. Note the appropriately labeled bottles of developer and fixer attached to the unit for automatic chemical replenishment.

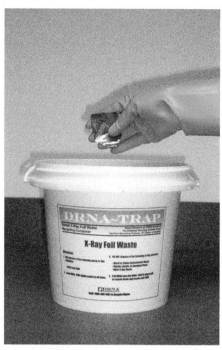

FIGURE 19–12 Lead foil waste. Collecting lead foil from film packets for proper disposal by a licensed waste management contractor.

for use with manual and chairside processing as well. When attached to an automatic processor, as the processor operates and when the fixer tank is drained for cleaning and changing the chemistry, the used fixer is circulated through the silver recovery unit. Silver recovery systems that use metallic replacement technology remove silver ions from the used fixer before allowing the solution to go down the drain. Once the cartridge inside the silver recovery unit is saturated with silver ions, it can be removed by a commercial waste disposal company and replaced with a fresh cartridge.

Lead Waste

Lead foil from inside intraoral film packets should be separated from the outer moisture-proof wrap and black paper to keep it out of the waste stream (Figure 19–12 ■). Many states or local municipal landfills have regulations regarding disposal of this heavy metal. Other lead-containing products that are no longer serviceable, such as damaged lead aprons or thyroid collars, and lead-lined film storage boxes or dispensers, should also have the lead recovered or recycled prior to disposing of these items into the waste stream.

Radiograph Waste

Oral health care practices are advised to keep dental radiographs indefinitely (see Chapter 10). However, circumstances do present when radiographs may no longer be needed. Additionally, unused radiographic film that has been damaged or contaminated or past its expiration date may need appropriate disposal. Dental radiographic film, whether exposed and processed or still in an unused condition, contains silver that should be recovered or recycled prior to disposal into the waste stream. The amount of silver remaining in dental radiographic film will depend on whether it has been processed, and on the density of the radiographic image. Film that has been processed will have had some of the silver ions removed during fixation, and radiographs of an increased density will have more of the silver ions remaining on the radiograph base material. Options for proper disposal of radiographic film and lead foils include contacting the company that the product was purchased from to see if they will take back the product or contracting with a licensed waste management company.

Digital Equipment Waste

The move away from film-based radiography to digital imaging will reduce and may eventually eliminate many of the potentially hazardous wastes currently associated with dental radiography. However, electronic equipment poses a new set of considerations for disposal and recycling. As technology advances, older equipment becomes obsolete. Computers, monitors, solid-state digital sensors, and PSP plates continue to improve, phasing out older systems (see Chapter 8). Solid-state sensors and PSP plates that become damaged or are no longer working will need to be disposed of properly. This electronic equipment contains both potentially hazardous materials such as lead, mercury, cadmium, and beryllium, and valuable metals such as gold, palladium, platinum, and silver. Computers and monitors also contain glass, plastic, and aluminum that are readily recycled. Proper recycling and disposal of electronic equipment can preserve precious resources and keep potentially hazardous materials out of municipal landfills.

A radiographer must possess a working knowledge of safe handling and disposal of the products and materials used in dental radiography. It is equally important to be familiar with laws regulating the handling and disposal of hazardous wastes, and to adopt an ethical responsibility to the environment in reducing, reusing, and recycling materials to avoid adding to the waste stream.

REVIEW—Chapter summary

Quality assurance requires planning, implementation, and evaluation of procedures used to produce radiographs with maximum diagnostic yield while minimizing radiation exposure. Quality control refers to tests that ensure

an acceptable level of radiographic quality. A health care team with a quality assurance program will assess current practices, identify problems, develop a plan that outlines responsibilities and personnel training needs, provide record-keeping logs, and perform periodic evaluation of the plan. Each oral health care team member must understand the role quality assurance plays in obtaining radiographic excellence, be given authority to perform quality control, and be offered continuing education and training opportunities to ensure competency.

Quality control monitoring schedules and checklists are used to record maintenance and inspections; testing schedules, results, and corrective actions; radiographic errors and retakes. Quality control tests for the dental x-ray machine include radiation output, accuracy of exposure settings, focal spot size, filtration, collimation, beam alignment, and tube head stability. Quality control tests for the darkroom include assessment of safelighting, checking for white light leaks, processing chemistry maintenance, and detection of conditions that create film fog. The coin test and checking for white light leaks are used to assess darkroom safelighting. Daily processing of two radiographic films (one unexposed and one exposed) and a reference film are used to monitor film processing chemistry. The fresh-film test is used to monitor an intraoral film supply. Examine digital image receptors, extraoral cassettes, and intensifying screens for defects prior to use. Quality assurance includes monitoring the efficacy of radiographic view-boxes, computer monitors, and the safety of digital image storage.

All personnel who will work with radiographic chemistry and materials must be familiar with and have ready access to the SDS for those products, and must be able to safely handle and respond appropriately to emergency exposure situations. Container labels that comply with OSHA Hazard Communication Standard identify the chemical ingredients, list manufacturer's emergency contact phone number, and present a signal word and pictograms indicating potential hazards. Avoid direct contact with processing chemicals by careful handling of products and the use of PPE. Following accidental fixer or developer skin contact, immediately wash with soap and water; use an eyewash station in response to accidental contact with eyes.

Radiographic wastes that require appropriate disposal include used fixer; lead foils from intraoral film packets; other lead products such as protective aprons, thyroid collars, and film dispenser boxes; radiographic films; and equipment used in digital imaging. Options for management of dental radiographic wastes include to contract with a reputable waste management or reclaiming/recycling company, to purchase from dental radiographic suppliers who take back unused products, to collect used products and transport to a designated local facility, and to utilize in-office equipment to reclaim silver from used fixer.

RECALL—Study questions

1. Each of the following is an objective of quality control in dental radiography EXCEPT one. Which one is the EXCEPTION?
   a. Maintain a high standard of image quality.
   b. Identify problems promptly after image quality is compromised.
   c. Keep patient and occupational exposures to a minimum.
   d. Reduce the occurrence of retake radiographs.

2. To whom may a dentist delegate authority to carry out specific aspects of a quality control program?
   a. Dental assistant
   b. Dental hygienist
   c. Practice manager
   d. All of the above

3. Which of the following is NOT a skill of a competent radiographer?
   a. Recognizes problems before they compromise radiographic quality
   b. Identifies causes of poor quality radiographs.
   c. Applies corrective measures that will produce quality radiographs.
   d. Takes sole responsibility for radiographic quality control

4. Which of the following is NOT a quality control test for a dental x-ray machine?
   a. Consistency of radiation output
   b. Accuracy of exposure settings
   c. Number of exposures per day
   d. Tube head stability

5. Use of the coin test will monitor darkroom safelight conditions.
   When an image of the coin appears on the radiograph, the safelight is adequate.
   a. The first statement is true. The second statement is false.
   b. The first statement is false. The second statement is true.
   c. Both statements are true.
   d. Both statements are false.

6. A film processed under ideal conditions and used to compare subsequent radiographic images is called a
   a. fresh film.
   b. fogged film.
   c. periapical film.
   d. reference film.

7. When an automatic processor is functioning properly, an unexposed film will exit the return chute dry and
   a. black.
   b. clear.
   c. green.
   d. with the image of a coin.

8. Security of digital radiographic image storage is enhanced through each of the following EXCEPT one. Which one is the EXCEPTION?
   a. Back up original images.
   b. Store images on a handheld wireless device.
   c. Use passwords for access.
   d. Update virus protection regularly.

9. Each of the following may be found on a Safety Data Sheet (SDS) EXCEPT one. Which one is the EXCEPTION?
   a. Date of manufacture
   b. Chemical ingredients
   c. Requirements for safe handling
   d. Disposal considerations

10. After processing dental x-ray film, used fixer solution contains silver in the form of a silver thiosulphate complex.
    A silver recovery/reclaiming device can be used to heat used fixer solution to release sulphur dioxide gas.
    a. The first statement is true. The second statement is false.
    b. The first statement is false. The second statement is true.
    c. Both statements are true.
    d. Both statements are false.

11. In general, what is the emergency recommendation if fixer or developer splashes into the eyes?
    a. If an irritation develops, then move to a well-ventilated area.
    b. Keep eyes securely closed and seek medical attention immediately.
    c. Wait 5 minutes to determine the severity of the exposure. Then seek medical attention.
    d. Immediately flush with a steady stream of tepid water for a minimum of 15 minutes.

12. Which of the following is LEAST likely to require special consideration prior to discharging into the waste stream?
    a. Lead foils from intraoral film packets
    b. Used fixer
    c. Used developer
    d. Digital imaging equipment

REFLECT—Case study

Develop a quality control plan for a new dental office facility. Include the following:

1. List of equipment that will need monitoring

2. Description of tests that will be needed

3. Recommended time interval for performing test

4. Name of the person assigned to perform the test

5. Description of what a failed test and a successful test would look like

6. Action required if a failed test results

Now develop a sample quality administration log that can be used to document this plan.

RELATE—Laboratory application

For a comprehensive laboratory practice exercise on this topic, see Thomson, E. M., & Bruhn, A. M. (2018). *Exercises in oral radiography techniques: A laboratory manual* (4th ed.).

Hoboken, NJ: Pearson. Chapter 13, "Radiographic quality assurance."

RESOURCES

American Dental Association Council on Scientific Affairs. (2003). Managing silver and lead waste in dental offices. *Journal of the American Dental Association, 134*, 1095–1096.

Carestream Dental. (2007). *Kodak dental systems: Exposure and processing for dental film radiography.* Pub. N-414. Rochester, NY: Author.

Carestream Dental. (2010). Environmental health and safety support. Health, safety and environment frequently asked questions. Retrieved from Carestream Dental website: http://carestreamhealth.com/ehs-faqs.html

National Council of Radiation Protection and Measurements. (1988). *Quality assurance for diagnostic imaging equipment: Recommendations of the National Council on Radiation Protection and Measurements.* NCRP Report no. 99. Bethesda, MD: NCRP Publications.

Thomson, E. M., & Bruhn, A. M. (2018). Radiographic quality assurance. *Exercises in oral radiographic techniques: A laboratory manual* (4th ed.). Hoboken, NJ: Pearson.

Thomson-Lakey, E. M. (1996). Developing an environmentally sound oral health practice. *Access, 10*(4), 19–26.

U.S. Environmental Protection Agency. (2016, March 10). eCycling. Retrieved from EPA website: http://www.epa.gov/epawaste/conserve/materials/ecycling/index.htm

Visit www.pearsonhighered.com/healthprofessionsresources to access the student resources that accompany this book. Simply select Dental Hygiene from the choice of disciplines. Find this book and you will find the complementary study tools created for this specific title.

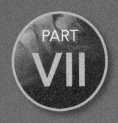

Viewing and Interpreting Dental Radiographic Images

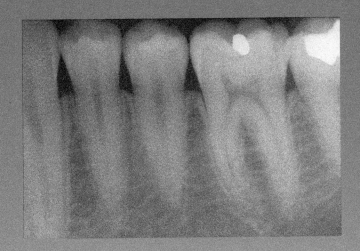

OUTLINE

Image Orientation and Introduction to Interpretation

OBJECTIVES

Following successful completion of this chapter, you should be able to:

1. Define the key terms.
2. List advantages of mounting film-based radiographs.
3. Identify anatomic landmarks that assist with distinguishing radiographs of the maxilla and mandible.
4. Describe characteristics of a quality film mount.
5. Discuss the use and importance of the embossed film identification dot.
6. Compare labial and lingual methods of film mounting.
7. List steps to an orderly mounting procedure.
8. List anatomic generalizations that aid in image orientation.
9. Describe actions that will assist in correctly orienting digital images.
10. Explain the difference between interpretation and diagnosis.
11. Describe equipment used to view radiographic images.
12. Demonstrate image viewing according to the suggested steps presented.
13. Describe the use and care of radiographic images during and after patient care.

KEY TERMS

Diagnosis
Film mount
Identification dot
Interpretation
Labial mounting method
Lingual mounting method
Viewbox

Introduction

Mounting film-based radiographs and organizing digital radiographic images is recommended prior to interpretation. Dental radiographic images must be properly oriented in the correct anatomic order to allow for a thorough and systematic interpretation. A working knowledge of the appearance of normal anatomical landmarks of the maxillofacial region and of the teeth is needed to correctly mount and orient radiographic images. Orientation and interpretation of dental radiographic images are interrelated; that is, recognition of landmarks guides mounting, and mounting facilitates further examination of these landmarks. This chapter describes step-by-step procedures for image orientation and viewing dental radiographic images. To aid in this process, basic key points regarding anatomic landmarks are presented.

Mounting Film-based Radiographs

Film mounting is the placement of film-based radiographs into a holder arranged in anatomical order (Figure 20–1 ■). A working knowledge of the radiographic appearance of the dentition and maxillofacial anatomy will assist in correctly orienting radiographic images (Table 20–1■). The advantages of film mounting include:

- Ease of viewing when radiographs are in the correct anatomical position
- Facilitation of comparison between radiographs in side-by-side position
- Masking out of distracting side light, enhancing viewing and interpretation
- Decreased chance of confusing right and left sides
- Protection against handling to avoid damage to emulsion
- Provision of a means for labeling (i.e., patient's name, date of exposure, name of the practice)
- Provision of a means of filing and storage

- Enhancement of patient education and consultations
- When mounted labially, that radiographic findings can be easily transferred to a dental chart

Film mounting generally refers to intraoral films. Large extraoral radiographs may be labeled with radiopaque letters or tape to identify the right and left sides, and these larger radiographs are often placed in an envelope so patient name and date of exposure can be written on the outside.

Occasionally, single intraoral radiographs are not mounted, but are placed into a small envelope and attached to the dental record. However, it is better to mount even a single or a small group of radiographs. A full mouth series should always be mounted for accurate viewing.

Film Mounts

Film mounts are cardboard or plastic holders with frames or windows for attaching, and through which to view radiographs (Figure 20–2 ■). Attaching radiographs to a film mount is called film mounting. Film mounts are available in many sizes and with numerous combinations of windows or frames to fit films of different sizes. Mounts may be large enough to accommodate a full mouth series of radiographs or hold only a few or even a single radiograph. Standard commercially made mounts are available, and manufacturers offer custom mounts to suit special needs. Black plastic or gray cardboard mounts are often preferred over clear plastic mounts because the former can block out extraneous light from the viewbox, enhancing viewing and interpretation.

Identification Dot

An embossed **identification dot** near the edge of a film appears convex or concave, depending on the side from which the film is viewed. If a film packet was placed in the patient's oral cavity correctly, the raised portion of the identification dot (the convexity) automatically faces the x-ray

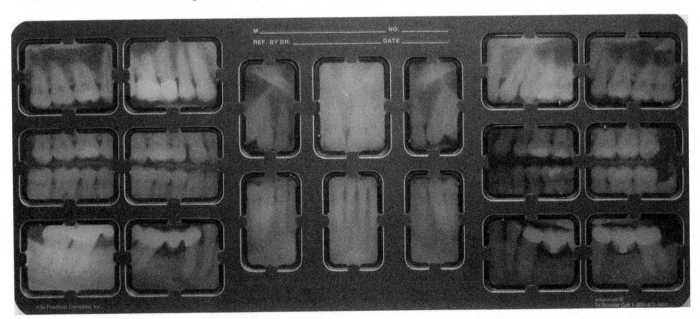

FIGURE 20–1 **Full mouth series mounted in an opaque mount.**

Table 20–1 Anatomical Landmarks Distinguishing Maxillary Radiographic Images from Mandibular Radiographic Images

Area	Maxillary Anatomical Landmarks	Mandibular Anatomical Landmarks
Incisor	Incisive foramen Median palatine suture Nasal fossa Nasal septum Anterior nasal spine	Lingual foramen Genial tubercles Nutrient canals Mental ridge Mental fossa
Canine	Inverted Y Lateral fossa	
Premolar	Maxillary sinus	Mental foramen
Molar	Maxillary sinus Zygomatic process of maxilla Zygoma Maxillary tuberosity Hamulus Coronoid process of mandible	Mandibular canal Oblique ridge Mylohyoid ridge Submandibular fossa

tube and source of radiation. When a processed radiograph is viewed, the identification dot may be relied on to determine which is a patient's left and right sides. Because a radiograph may be viewed from either side, it is important to understand the role the identification dot plays in film orientation.

Film Mounting Methods

Because a radiograph may be viewed from either side, two methods of film mounting can be used. The first method, considered by most to be obsolete but still in use by some practitioners, is the lingual method. With the **lingual mounting method**, radiographs are mounted so that the embossed dot is concave. In this position, the viewer is reading the radiograph as if standing behind a patient (Figure 20–3 ▪). What the viewer observes on the right side of the radiograph will correspond to the patient's right side. Essentially, the viewer's right is the patient's right.

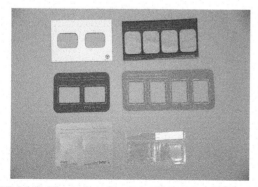

FIGURE 20–2 **Examples of various film mounts.** Film mounts are available in a variety of sizes and combinations.

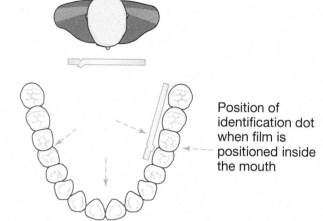

Viewer's orientation is looking at the teeth from inside the mouth

Position of identification dot when film is positioned inside the mouth

FIGURE 20–3 **Lingual method of film mounting.** When the identification dot is viewed in the concave position, the viewer's orientation is from behind the patient. The patient's left is the viewer's left.

The method recommended by the American Dental Association and the American Academy of Oral and Maxillofacial Radiology is the **labial mounting method**. Using this method of film mounting, radiographs are mounted so that the embossed dot is convex. In this position, the viewer is reading the radiograph as if standing in front of, and facing, a patient (Figure 20–4 ▪). What the viewer observes on the right side of the radiograph will correspond to the patient's left side. Essentially, the viewer's right is the patient's left. This also corresponds to the order in which teeth and anatomical structures are drawn on most dental and periodontal charts.

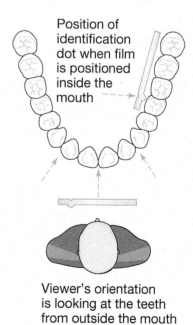

Position of identification dot when film is positioned inside the mouth

Viewer's orientation is looking at the teeth from outside the mouth

FIGURE 20–4 **Labial method of film mounting.** When the identification dot is viewed in the convex position, the viewer's orientation is in front of and facing the patient. The patient's left is the viewer's right.

Film Mounting Procedure

Film-based radiographs should be mounted immediately after processing. Handle radiographs by the edges to avoid smudging or scratching the emulsion. Label film mounts to prevent loss or mixing up with other patient radiographs. An orderly sequence to the mounting procedure is suggested. This is especially important for a beginner. Although the sequence for mounting is often a matter of preference, the first step in orienting radiographs should be to place the embossed identification dot the same way for all films. When mounting films using the labial method, orient so that the embossed dot is convex.

When orienting a full mouth series of periapical and bitewing radiographs, it is helpful to use film size to assist with the process. Size 1 film is often used to record the anterior region; size 2 film is used to record the posterior region. Additionally, films are usually placed into the anterior region with the long dimension of the image receptor positioned vertically, and into the posterior region with the long dimension of the image receptor positioned horizontally. Periapical radiographic images should be oriented and placed into a film mount so that the roots are pointing up for the maxilla and down for the mandible; bitewing radiographic images should be oriented so that the occlusal plane presents as a slight upward curve or "smile." To aid in determining correct image orientation, consider the following generalizations:

- Maxillary anterior teeth have larger crowns and longer roots than mandibular teeth.
- Canine teeth have longest roots as compared to adjacent teeth.

- Maxillary molars have three roots; the palatal root makes it difficult to visualize three distinct roots.
- Mandibular molars have two divergent roots, distinctly observed with bone visible in between the roots.
- Roots of most all teeth curve distally.
- Large radiolucencies denoting nasal fossa or maxillary sinus indicate a maxillary radiographic image.
- Body of mandible has distinct upward curve toward ramus in molar area.

Digital Image Orientation

Digital radiographic images acquired with either direct digital sensors or indirect digital photostimulable phosphor (PSP) plates must be manipulated into their respective orientation within imaging software on computer monitors. Do not assume that digital images will be automatically placed into the correct orientation immediately after exposure or after the laser scanning step. Digital images can be flipped upside down, transposed into a mirror image, and rotated varying degrees within imaging software programs. Additionally, depending on the position or orientation of the sensor when placed into the oral cavity, and which window of the template was selected, the image may end up in the wrong place (Figure 20–5 ■). The same working knowledge and generalizations regarding the radiographic appearance of the dentition and maxillofacial anatomy used to mount film-based radiographs will apply when determining correct orientation of digital radiographic images.

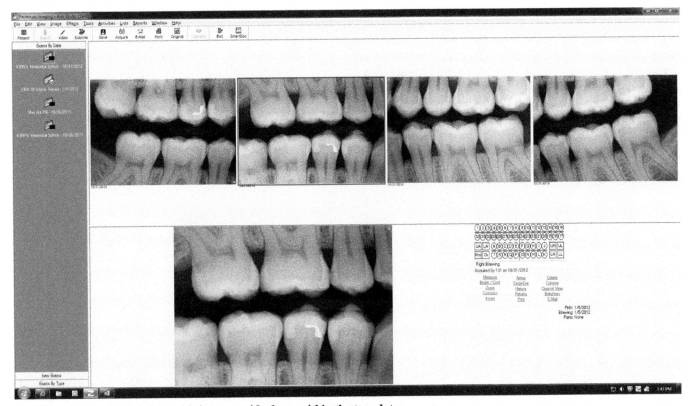

FIGURE 20–5 Digital radiographic image upside down within the template.

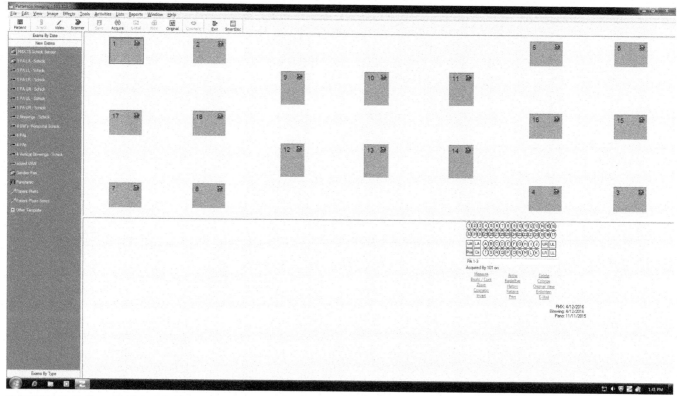

FIGURE 20–6 **Sample digital radiographic imaging system template.**

Direct Digital Imaging Orientation

Digital imaging systems come with template software. Templates are the digital equivalent of film mounts. Pay careful attention to which template configuration is selected prior to exposing radiographic images to avoid errors in orientation of the images. The digital system default template may be selected for use, or one can be set up within the system's imaging software that is specific to individual preference. Most digital imaging system templates can accommodate any configuration and many combinations as to where right and left side images are located; how many and what types of images are displayed; and what default settings are preferred (Figure 20–6 ■).

To assist with arranging an image in the correct position within a selected template, follow the digital system manufacturer's instructions. Direct digital imaging usually requires that the window of the template be selected first, prior to making the exposure. Using a computer mouse or monitor touch screen, click the template window that corresponds to the radiographic image to be taken. Position the sensor, make the exposure, and the digital software will position the image into the selected window. Assess the image for correct orientation. Reposition as needed using the computer mouse to drag-and-drop or copy-and-paste images; or follow the software prompts to flip or rotate images.

Indirect Digital Imaging Orientation

Indirect digital imaging systems use PSP plates that must be processed by a laser scanner connected to a computer (see Chapter 8). To assist with getting the scanned images into their respective correct positions within a selected template, follow the manufacturer's instructions. Indirect digital imaging systems come with guides that help orient the plates as they are being fed into the scanner (see Figure 8–16). Careful attention to how the plates are placed into these guides can assist with correct orientation of images into the appropriate windows of the template. Some PSP plates are imprinted with a small letter or icon in the lower left corner as an aid to determining the correct image orientation, similar to radiographic film's embossed identification dot (Figure 20–7 ■).

Viewing Radiographic Images

Correct mounting and orientation is essential prior to reading and interpreting dental radiographic images.

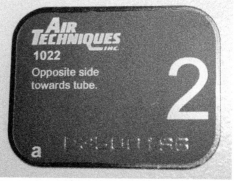

FIGURE 20–7 **PSP plate with imprint to aid in orientation.**

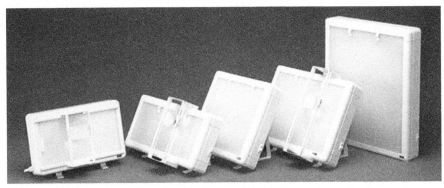

FIGURE 20–8 **Viewboxes.** A variety of sizes are available. (Courtesy of Dentsply Sirona.)

Interpretation is enhanced when optimal viewing conditions are in place and a proper sequence of viewing images is followed.

Interpretation and Diagnosis

Dental radiographic images are viewed by any trained professional (dentist, dental hygienist, or dental assistant) with knowledge of normal anatomic landmarks of the maxilla, mandible, and related structures. While radiographic images may be interpreted by all members of the oral health care team, the dentist is responsible for the final interpretation and diagnosis. **Interpretation** is explanatory and may be defined as reading a radiographic image and explaining what is observed in terms a patient can understand. Items that a dental hygienist or dental assistant may interpret are radiographic errors such as overlapped contacts or elongated images; artifacts that may have appeared on the radiograph such as the recording of a direct digital sensor cord; and normal radiographic anatomy such as the absence of a developing permanent tooth under a primary tooth or the presence radiographically of unerupted third molars. **Diagnosis** is defined as the determination of the nature and the identification of an abnormal condition or disease. Identifying an unerupted third molar is an example of interpretation; determining that the third molar is impacted is a diagnosis. Referring a patient to a dentist for evaluation of a radiolucent finding on the proximal surface of a tooth is interpretation; identifying that radiolucency as caries is a diagnosis. Dental hygienists and dental assistants are trained to identify deviations from normal and can point out these abnormalities for further evaluation by a dentist. These members of the oral health care team play a valuable role in a preliminary diagnosis, by interpreting deviations from normal radiographic anatomy and calling these to the attention of a dentist. The more professionals there are to evaluate radiographic images, the more the patient will benefit.

Viewing Equipment

A **viewbox** and magnifying glass are required for optimal viewing of film-based radiographs. Holding a radiograph up to overhead room light will not provide adequate conditions in which to observe subtle details.

- **Viewbox.** Several different types and sizes of viewboxes are available (Figure 20–8 ■). Viewbox lighting must be of uniform intensity and be evenly diffused for enhanced interpretation conditions. The viewing surface should be large enough to accommodate a full set of intraoral radiographs as well as typical dental extraoral radiographs (i.e., panoramic radiographs). A film mount or a cardboard template should be used to mask out distracting light around the mount. Blocking out excess sidelight reduces glare and facilitates viewing by reducing eye fatigue. The use of gray or black cardboard or frosted plastic film mounts helps to reduce glare. Subdued room lighting will allow the eyes to adapt to the light level of the radiographs.

- **Magnification and enhancement.** Some viewboxes are equipped with a magnifying device. Otherwise, use a handheld magnifying glass to aid in viewing films (Figure 20–9 ■). Digital radiographic systems offer magnification and other software tools that enhance image viewing and interpretation (Figures 20–10 ■ through 20–12 ■).

- **Computer monitor.** Applying film-based interpretation skills to digital images requires practice, especially for those who are new to digital imaging. A

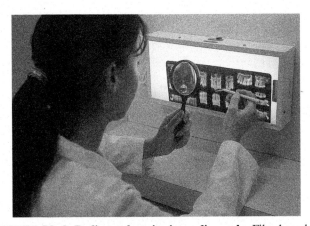

FIGURE 20–9 **Radiographer viewing radiographs.** Film-based radiographs should be viewed in subdued room lighting, using a viewbox and a magnifying glass. Note the black film mount that blocks distracting light around the films.

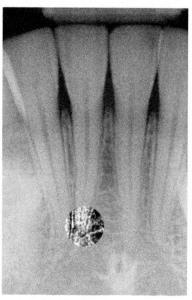

FIGURE 20–10 **Digital image magnification.** Digital imaging software can be used to spotlight an image to enhance viewing.

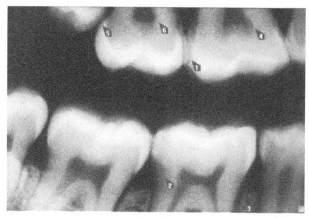

FIGURE 20–12 **Charting software tools.** Interpretation notes can be placed directly on the image.

consideration not encountered with film-based radiographs is the need for multiple mouse clicks to view digital radiographic images side-by-side or to locate images exposed on different days and stored in different files on the computer. Viewing digital images is usually restricted to the area where the computer and monitor are located, although the use of wireless tablet devices eliminates this restriction. Dim overhead room lighting to reduce the potential for glare that may reflect off a computer monitor screen and hinder interpretation (see Figure 19–4).

Interpretation Sequence

Interpretation is a skill that requires a great deal of practice. Beginning radiology students are sometimes frustrated by not being able to "see" what an expert easily identifies. To help develop this skill, a solid working knowledge of normal radiographic anatomy is needed. First identify normal radiographic anatomy, then systematically progress through a sequence of evaluation, naming each radiopaque and radiolucent structure observed.

Practice Point

The rule follows that when viewing radiographs, *give everything observed a name.* Every radiopaque and radiolucent object recorded on a radiograph should be identified as an anatomical landmark. Is the observation in question the mental foramen, the submandibular fossa, or the periodontal ligament space? When all possibilities of what a finding could be are exhausted, it then becomes a deviation from the normal, requiring a dentist's evaluation.

Following a systematic sequence for viewing radiographic images will assist in producing a thorough interpretation. Examine each radiographic image for a specific condition, and then repeat the examination process for the next condition. For example, examine each radiographic image to determine what teeth are present. Next, start the process over, reexamining each radiograph again noting what dental materials are present. Continue reexamining each radiograph for one condition at a time. Depending on training and responsibility, proceed to make a preliminary interpretation that can be presented to a dentist, who will make the final diagnosis regarding any findings. A thorough

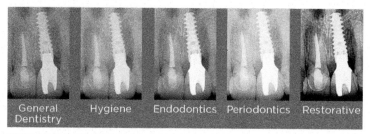

FIGURE 20–11 **Digital image enhancement.** Digital imaging software can be used to change image density and contrast to enhance viewing. (Courtesy of Sirona Dental, Inc., Long Island City, NY.)

Procedure 20–1

Suggested sequence for viewing a full mouth series of radiographic images

1. Orient images correctly.
2. Dim overhead lights and turn on viewbox light or computer monitor. Use magnification and/or software enhancement tools.
3. Begin examination in the maxillary right posterior region; continue clockwise to the maxillary left posterior; drop down to the mandibular left posterior; continue to the mandibular right posterior; end with an examination of the right and then the left bitewings (Figure 20–13 ■).
4. Repeat step 3 for the following conditions:
   a. Presence or absence of teeth
   b. Tooth morphology and eruption patterns
   c. Deviations from normal and/or suspected pathology
   d. Presence, type, and condition of dental materials
   e. Caries
   f. Periodontal conditions and risk factors
5. Document findings on a preliminary radiographic interpretative form or electronic record.
6. Collaborate with dentist regarding findings.
7. After confirmation and diagnosis of findings by dentist, record findings on the permanent dental record.
8. Assist dentist in explaining findings and treatment plan to patient using the radiographic images.

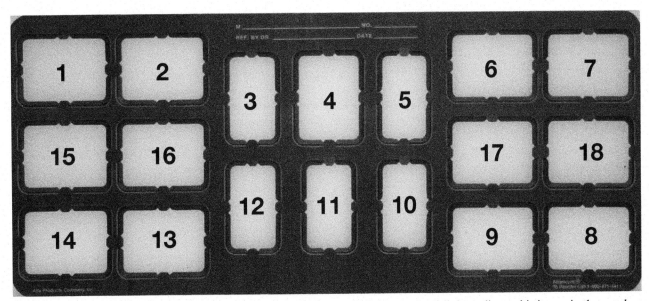

FIGURE 20–13 Recommended sequence for viewing radiographic images. Begin with the radiographic image in the number 1 position and proceed clockwise through to the number 18 position.

examination is best accomplished when a specific sequence of analysis is used (Procedure 20–1).

If multiple radiographic images are available, such as a set of bitewings or a full mouth series, teeth and supporting structures will usually be recorded more than once. While maintaining a systematic order of interpretation, compare these duplicated structures in all of the views.

Radiographs exposed in slightly different positions, with differing angulations of the x-ray beam, may reveal more information than that found on one radiograph alone. For example, a periapical radiographic may image a different alveolar bone height from a bitewing radiograph of the same region. Comparing adjacent images will add to a thorough interpretation.

Using Radiographic Images

Process and mount radiographic images as soon as possible for easy reference during treatment. At each subsequent appointment the radiographic images should be available, where they can be easily accessed as needed.

At the end of patient care, thoroughly interpret radiographic images during time set aside for this purpose. Unless only one or two radiographic images were taken, there may not have been enough time during the appointment to thoroughly review each image for all possible conditions. Note all radiographic findings in a patient's dental record after confirmation by a dentist. Although all professionals may record findings, the final interpretation and diagnosis is the responsibility of a dentist.

Once interpretation is complete, store the radiographic images appropriately and keep indefinitely as part of a patient's permanent dental record. Although radiographic images are said to lose value after more than six months to one year due to changes in a patient's oral conditions, they are valuable for comparing present with previous conditions. The need for an orderly filing system and electronic backup of digital image data cannot be overstressed. Misplaced or deleted radiographic images can result in unnecessary retakes, or inappropriate treatment being rendered.

REVIEW—Chapter summary

A working knowledge of the appearance of normal anatomical landmarks of the maxillofacial region and of the teeth is needed to correctly mount and orient radiographic images. Mounting film-based images is recommended for its many advantages. Film mounts vary in size and number of frames, and have space for documenting information such as patient's name and date of exposure.

Radiographic film has an embossed identification dot used to determine a patient's left and right sides. Lingual mounting places the identification dot in a concave position, so that the patient's left side is the viewer's left side. Labial mounting places the identification dot in a convex position, so that the patient's left side is the viewer's right side. Labial mounting method is the recommended method.

Mount film-based radiographs immediately after processing. In addition to recognition of anatomic landmarks, use generalizations regarding teeth size, and root shapes and directions to aid in correctly orienting radiographic images. Digital imaging systems come with templates, the digital equivalent of film mounts. Default and custom-designed templates can be used. Follow the manufacturer's guidelines for positioning digital images correctly within the selected template. If incorrectly oriented within the template window, use the computer mouse to drag-and-drop or cut-and-paste to correct. Using scanner guides can assist with correctly orienting PSP plates.

Interpretation or reading radiographic images is explanatory. Diagnosis uses radiographic images to determine the nature and identification of disease or abnormality. Dental radiographic images may be interpreted by a dentist, dental hygienist, or dental assistant; a dentist is responsible for the final diagnosis.

Viewing film-based radiographs is facilitated with the use of a viewbox with magnification. Digital imaging software provides interpretation enhancement tools such as magnification and the ability to adjust density and contrast. Locate a computer monitor away from ambient lighting that can cause glare. Use a systematic order to interpret radiographic images. Compare the appearance of structures that may be imaged twice in radiographs that were exposed with slightly different angles. Interpret radiographic images thoroughly after patient care as necessary. Note radiographic findings in a patient's dental record after confirmation by a dentist. Accurately label radiographic images to be used to compare present with previous conditions, and keep indefinitely.

RECALL—Study questions

1. List four advantages of mounting film-based radiographs.
   a. _____
   b. _____
   c. _____
   d. _____

2. Which of these landmarks would be likely to appear on a maxillary radiograph?
   a. Genial tubercles
   b. Mental fossa
   c. Oblique ridge
   d. Zygoma

3. Which of these is NOT a characteristic of a quality film mount?
   a. Provides space to document patient name and date of exposure
   b. Constructed of clear plastic that does not mask light around radiograph edges
   c. Supports and protects radiographs from scratches that may occur during handling
   d. Contains enough windows to secure the number of radiographs exposed

4. Which of these helps to determine whether a radiograph was exposed on a patient's left or right side?
   a. Slight "smile" appearance
   b. Distally curved roots
   c. Large crowns
   d. Embossed film dot

5. Labial method film mounting positions the identification dot concave.
   Labial method is the recommended film mounting method.
   a. The first statement is true. The second statement is false.
   b. The first statement is false. The second statement is true.
   c. Both statements are true.
   d. Both statements are false.

6. Lingual method film mounting positions the identification dot convex.
   When utilizing the lingual method, the viewer's right is the patient's left.
   a. The first statement is true. The second statement is false.
   b. The first statement is false. The second statement is true.
   c. Both statements are true.
   d. Both statements are false.

7. Which of the following should be done first when mounting film-based radiographs?
   a. Orient all identification dots the same way.
   b. Separate bitewing from periapical films.
   c. Separate anterior from posterior films.
   d. Orient the teeth roots to point in the correct direction.

8. Each of the following will aid in correctly orienting radiographic images EXCEPT one. Which one is the EXCEPTION?
   a. Anterior image receptors are positioned with the long dimension vertically.
   b. Canine teeth generally have the longest roots.
   c. Maxillary molars usually have three roots.
   d. Roots and crowns of mandibular teeth are usually larger than maxillary teeth.

9. Which of these is NOT a consideration when viewing digital radiographic images?
   a. Glare off a computer monitor must be managed to enhance interpretation.
   b. Image must be checked to ensure exposure was placed into correct template window.
   c. A magnifying glass is required for optimal viewing and interpretation.
   d. Multiple mouse clicks may be required to view a full mouth series of radiographs.

10. Reading and explaining what is observed on a radiographic image is
    a. diagnosing.
    b. interpreting.
    c. viewing.
    d. mounting.

11. Viewing correctly oriented radiographic images in a systematic sequence can help prevent errors in interpretation.
    Digital imaging software provides special features such as magnification enhancements that aid in interpretation.
    a. The first statement is true. The second statement is false.
    b. The first statement is false. The second statement is true.
    c. Both statements are true.
    d. Both statements are false.

12. In which region is it best to begin the interpretation process when viewing a full mouth series of radiographs?
    a. Maxillary right posterior
    b. Maxillary left posterior
    c. Mandibular right posterior
    d. Mandibular left posterior

13. Following a dentist's diagnosis, radiographic findings must be recorded in the patient's record by
    a. a dental assistant.
    b. a dental hygienist.
    c. a dentist.
    d. any of the above.

REFLECT—Case study

The four radiographs shown have just exited an automatic processor. Correctly mount each of these by writing the corresponding number in the correct frame of the film mount. Assuming the identification dots are all positioned convex, label the film mount indicating the left and right sides. Then address the following:

1. Describe how the left and right sides were determined.

2. List the steps followed to mount these radiographs.

3. What generalizations aided the mounting process?

4. Order the radiographs as to where to begin and end the interpretation process.

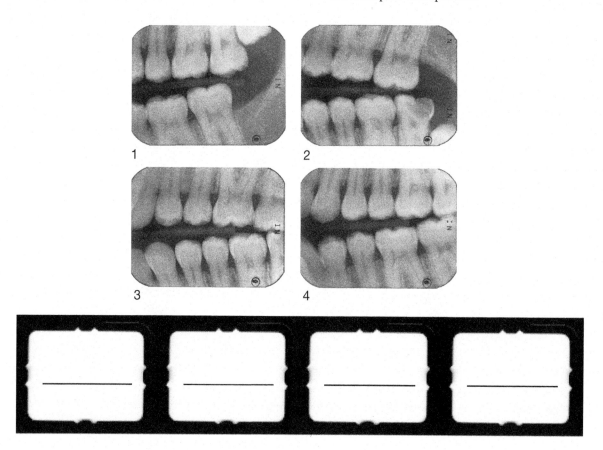

RELATE—Laboratory application

For a comprehensive laboratory practice exercise on this topic, see Thomson, E. M., & Bruhn, A. M. (2018). *Exercises in oral radiography techniques: A laboratory manual* (4th ed.). Hoboken, NJ: Pearson. Chapter 7, "Mounting and radiographic landmarks."

RESOURCES

Horner, K., Drage, N., & Brettle, D. (2008). *21st century imaging.* London: Quintessence Publishing Co.

Langland, O. E., & Langlais, R. P. (2002). Processing and film mounting procedures. *Principles of dental imaging* (2nd ed.). Philadelphia: Lippincott Williams & Wilkins.

White, S. C., & Pharoah, M. J. (2016). Principles of radiographic interpretation. *Oral radiology: Principles and interpretation* (7th ed.). St. Louis, MO: Elsevier.

Recognizing Normal Radiographic Anatomy—Intraoral Radiographs

OBJECTIVES

Following successful completion of this chapter, you should be able to:

1. Define the key terms.
2. Explain how two-dimensional radiographs present a challenge to developing interpretation skills.
3. List facial and cranial bones important to radiographic interpretation.
4. Differentiate between the radiographic appearance of cortical and cancellous bone.
5. Differentiate between the radiographic appearance of the lamina dura and the PDL space.
6. List and identify the radiographic appearance of the structures of the teeth.
7. Demonstrate use of a systematic method for interpreting dental radiographs.
8. Categorize bony landmarks as to whether they will appear radiopaque or radiolucent on a dental radiograph.
9. Identify significant anatomy recorded on dental radiographs of the maxilla and mandible.

KEY TERMS

Alveolar process
Alveolus
Cancellous (trabecular) bone
Cementum
Cortical bone
Dentin
Enamel
Inverted Y
Lamina dura
Periodontal ligament (PDL)
Torus mandibularis (lingual torus)
Trabeculae

Introduction

Basic knowledge of the radiographic appearance of normal head and neck anatomy is essential for correct orientation and mounting of dental radiographs. This chapter builds on the basic skills presented in Chapter 20 to assist in developing the ability to read radiographs. A working knowledge of the radiographic appearance of normal anatomy must be mastered before developing the skills needed to recognize deviations and abnormalities such as periodontal disease, caries, and growth and development anomalies. This chapter reviews the structures comprising the anatomy of the head and neck and describes the radiographic appearance of these anatomical structures as they appear on dental radiographs. An organizational flow chart to interpretation is presented to assist the beginning radiographer by providing a framework on which to learn the terms associated with head and neck radiography. This flow chart can be used as a basis for continuing to build on these basic interpretative skills.

Interpretation Fundamentals

Learning to identify the radiographic appearance of anatomical structures and their specific landmarks takes practice. Radiographs provide a two-dimensional representation of three-dimensional structures. Depending on the placement of the image receptor, patient position, and angle of the x-ray beam, certain landmarks may or may not be recorded on dental radiographs. Furthermore, the angle of the x-ray beam may distort the appearance of the structure so that it doesn't appear exactly as illustrated in a textbook. Additionally, bilateral landmarks may take on a different appearance when comparing the right and left sides. When imaging the oral cavity, multiple structures are usually recorded superimposed on top of each other, all adding to the difficulty of correctly identifying anatomical structures. Achieving competence in reading and interpreting dental radiographs requires a working knowledge of what structures are likely to be imaged based on an understanding of where the path of the x-ray beam is directed (Figure 21–1 ▪).

Although most anatomical landmarks observed on intraoral radiographs are located on the maxilla and the mandible, the radiographer should be able to recognize and identify the major bones and anatomical landmarks of the cranium and face. Some of these structures are more likely to be visible on larger occlusal and extraoral radiographs. Nevertheless, it is helpful to consider the general location of these anatomic features prior to learning how and where each will be recorded on a dental radiograph (see Chapter 22).

Radiographic Appearance of Bone

The bones of the skull that are of primary interest for intraoral dental radiographs are the maxilla and mandible. The teeth are located within the alveolar processes of the maxilla and the mandible, so most dental radiographs record portions of these bones. The compact and dense bone that lines

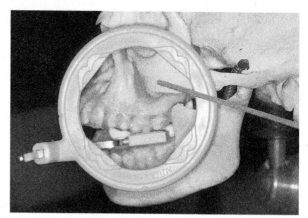

FIGURE 21–1 **Superimposed structures.** Note the position of the image receptor holder when exposing a maxillary posterior periapical radiograph. The zygomatic arch will most likely be recorded on this radiograph.

the outside layers of the maxilla and the mandible is called **cortical bone,** which appears radiopaque. **Cancellous bone** (or spongy bone) forms the bulk of the inner bone (Figure 21–2 ▪). Small, interconnected **trabeculae** (bars or plates of bone) form a multitude of various-sized compartments that account for the honeycomb appearance of cancellous bone. These trabecular bone spaces are usually filled with fat, blood, or bone cells, which accounts for the difference in the radiographic appearance of bone. Cancellous bone varies in radiopacity, appearing to have various shades of gray according to the size and number of the trabecular spaces. Some bony regions may normally appear almost radiolucent if these spaces are very large or if the bone is thin. A thinner dimension of bone in the area of the submandibular fossa typically presents radiolucent (Figure 21–3 ▪).

Lamina Dura

The **alveolar process** is that portion of the maxilla and the mandible that surrounds and supports the teeth. It is composed of a base of supporting cancellous bone and the

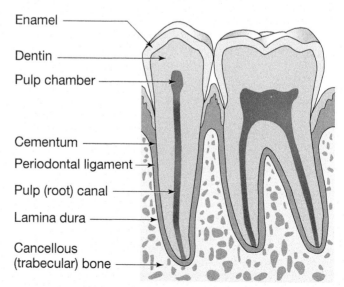

Enamel

Dentin

Pulp chamber

Cementum

Periodontal ligament

Pulp (root) canal

Lamina dura

Cancellous (trabecular) bone

FIGURE 21–2 **Composition of teeth and supporting bone.**

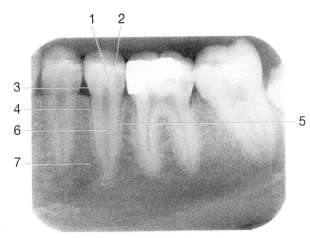

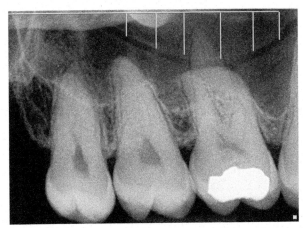

FIGURE 21–4 **Nutrient canal observed in maxillary sinus wall.**

FIGURE 21–3 **Mandibular premolar radiograph.** (**1**) Dentin, (**2**) enamel, (**3**) pulp chamber, (**4**) PDL space, (**5**) lamina dura, (**6**) root canal, and (**7**) cancellous bone. Note the radiolucent appearance of the submandibular fossa.

lamina dura. The cancellous supporting bone varies in density in the different parts of the alveolar process. The lamina dura is the hard, cortical bone that lines the **alveolus** (tooth socket). On radiographs, the lamina dura appears as a thin radiopaque border that outlines the shape of the alveolus. The lamina dura appears radiographically to follow the outline of the tooth root (see Figures 21–2 and 21–3).

Periodontal Ligament Space

The teeth are attached to the lamina dura by the fibers of the **periodontal ligament (PDL).** The PDL itself is made up of soft tissues and therefore will not be recorded on a radiograph. However, the space in which the PDL lies is often visible radiographically as a thin radiolucent border between the lamina dura and the roots of the teeth (see Figures 21–2 and 21–3).

Nutrient Canals

Nutrient canals are thin radiolucent lines of fairly uniform width that sometimes exhibit radiopaque borders. Nutrient canals contain blood vessels and nerves that supply the teeth, bone, and gingivae. Nutrient canals are not commonly recorded on a radiograph, but can sometimes be observed in the anterior regions of the mandible and in edentulous areas and in the walls of the maxillary sinus (Figure 21–4 ■). Nutrient canals open at the surface of the bone, appearing radiographically as a tiny radiolucent dot called the nutrient foramen. It is important to distinguish nutrient canals and nutrient foramina (plural) as normal radiographic anatomy.

Radiographic Appearance of the Dentition

Identification of the normal radiographic appearance of the dentition provides the basis upon which to build interpretative skills. There are 20 primary teeth that are gradually lost and replaced with 32 permanent teeth. When recorded on a radiograph, primary teeth may appear in

various stages of resorption in response to the developing permanent dentition (see Chapter 27). Developing permanent teeth may appear in various stages of development with incomplete crown and root formation (Figure 21–5 ■). Interpretation of radiographs to determine timely exfoliation (shedding) of primary teeth and normal formation and eruption patterns of the permanent teeth is an important use of the radiographic examination.

Teeth are composed of enamel, dentin, cementum, and pulp. **Enamel** covers the tooth crown and because of its density (the hardest in the human body) appears radiopaque; the less dense underlying **dentin** appears also radiopaque, but slightly less so than enamel; and the **cementum** that covers the roots is even less dense. Because

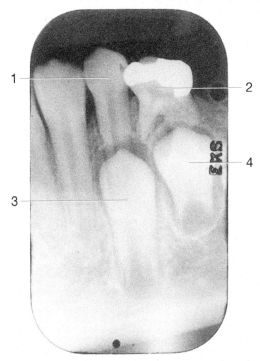

FIGURE 21–5 **Mandibular canine radiograph.** (**1**) Primary canine, (**2**) primary first molar with partially resorbed roots, (**3**) permanent canine, and (**4**) permanent first premolar with incomplete root formation.

only a thin layer of cementum covers the tooth root, it is generally indistinguishable radiographically from the underlying dentin. Although all three of these dense, calcified tooth structures vary in radiopacity in direct proportion to their thickness, for descriptive purposes all are considered radiopaque. The tooth pulp that occupies the pulp chamber and the root canals is composed of noncalcified blood and nerve tissues. As these tissues offer only minimal resistance to the passage of x-rays, the tooth pulp chamber and root canal appear radiolucent (see Figures 21–2 and 21–3).

Steps to Interpreting Normal Radiographic Anatomy

Just as it is helpful to follow a systematic order when mounting radiographic images, a radiographer will benefit from organizing the identification of anatomical landmarks into specific steps. Memorizing the structures that make up the head and neck region can be an overwhelming task, so the following organizational flow chart is offered to assist a beginning radiographer in learning to identify structures commonly recorded on intraoral radiographs.

As illustrated in Figure 21–6 ■, differentiating among which structures will most likely be recorded on radiographs in which regions of the oral cavity will help organize the anatomy terms and narrow the possible choices. When beginning the interpretation process, first determine if the intraoral radiograph is a maxillary view or a mandibular view (see Chapter 20). Once the correct arch is identified, determine if the view is of the anterior or the posterior region. Certain anatomical structures are more likely to be visible on radiographs of the anterior region; others are more likely to be visible in the posterior region. Prior to deciding which anatomical structure is being observed, it is helpful to recall which structures appear radiopaque and which structures appear radiolucent. Bone and its dense features such as a ridge, spine, or tubercle will appear radiopaque; less dense features such as a foramen, canal, or suture will appear radiolucent (Table 21–1 ■).

In keeping with the organizational system presented in Figure 21–6, anatomical landmarks in this chapter are organized by the region of the oral cavity where they are most

Table 21–1 Radiopaque and Radiolucent Generalizations

Radiopaque	Radiolucent
• Bone	• Canal
• Border (wall)	• Foramen
• Process	• Fossa
• Ridge	• Meatus
• Spine	• Sinus
• Tubercles	• Space (PDL)
• Tuberosity	• Suture

Table 21–2 Anatomical Landmarks

Area	Maxillary Anatomical Landmarks	Mandibular Anatomical Landmarks
Incisor	Incisive foramen Median palatine suture Nasal fossa Nasal septum Anterior nasal spine	Lingual foramen Genial tubercles Nutrient canal Mental ridge Mental fossa
Canine	Inverted Y Lateral fossa	
Premolar	Maxillary sinus	Mental foramen
Molar	Maxillary sinus Zygomatic process of maxilla Zygoma Maxillary tuberosity Hamulus Coronoid process of mandible	Mandibular canal Oblique ridge Mylohyoid ridge Submandibular fossa

likely to be observed on a dental radiograph (Table 21–2 ■). The following descriptions offer guidance for learning these structures.

Radiographic Appearance of Bony Landmarks

Maxillary Anterior Region (Figures 21–7 ■ through 21–14 ■)

RADIOPAQUE FEATURES

1. **Nasal septum.** Dense cartilage structure that separates the right nasal fossa from the left; usually appears as a vertical radiopaque line separating the paired radiolucencies of the nasal cavity.
2. **Anterior nasal spine.** V-shaped projection from the floor of the nasal fossa in the midline; usually appears as a triangular radiopacity.
3. **Inverted Y.** Important landmark seen in the canine–premolar area, made up of the lateral wall of the nasal fossa and the anterior–medial wall of the maxillary sinus. The intersection of these two radiopaque lines often cross each other forming the letter Y that appears upside down or turned on its side.
4. **Soft tissue of the nose.** A magnified outline representing the soft tissue tip of the nose may be recorded onto intraoral anterior radiographs (see Figures 21–13 and 21–14). This is another example of how multiple structures along the same path of the x-ray beam can be superimposed on top of each other. The tip of the nose is at an increased distance from the intraoral image receptor, resulting in magnification (see Chapter 4).

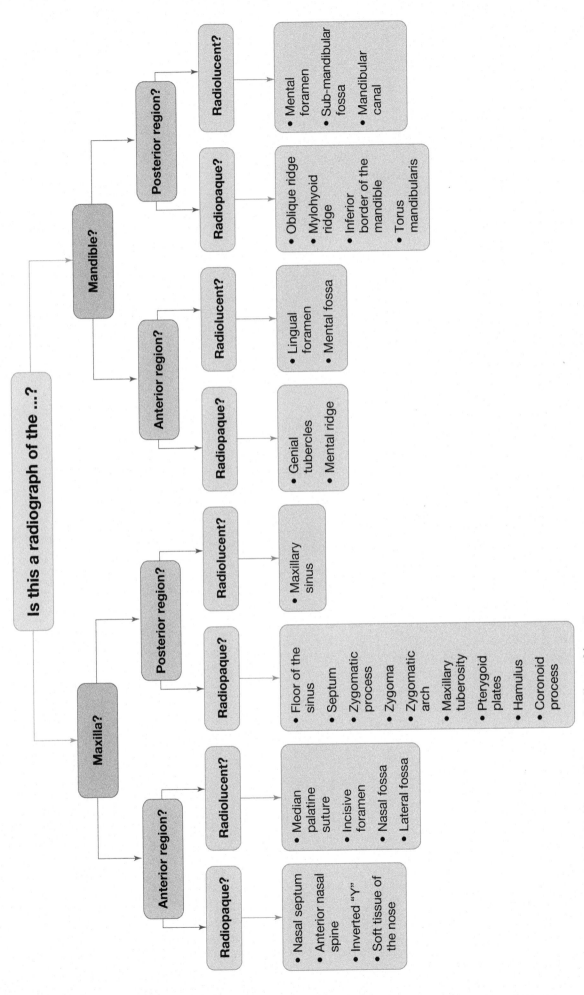

FIGURE 21-6 Sequence for interpreting normal radiographic anatomy.

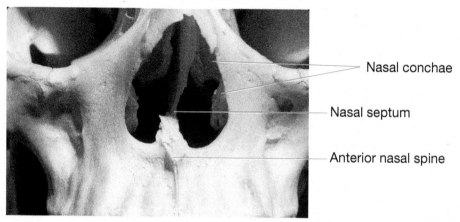

FIGURE 21-7 Front skull view of maxillary anterior region.

- Nasal conchae
- Nasal septum
- Anterior nasal spine

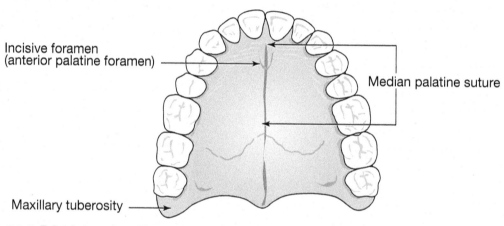

- Incisive foramen (anterior palatine foramen)
- Median palatine suture
- Maxillary tuberosity

21-8 Palatal view of maxilla.

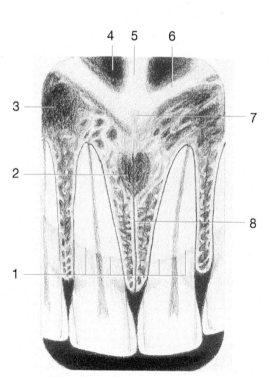

FIGURE 21-9 Maxillary incisors view. (**1**) Outline of nose, (**2**) incisive foramen, (**3**) lateral fossa, (**4**) nasal fossa, (**5**) nasal septum, (**6**) border of nasal fossa, (**7**) anterior nasal spine, and (**8**) median palatine suture.

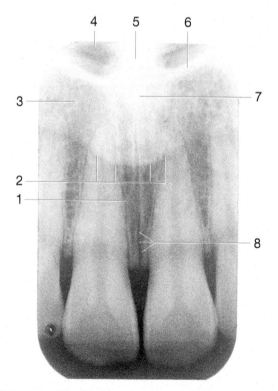

FIGURE 21-10 Maxillary incisors radiograph. (**1**) Incisive foramen, faint pear-shaped, radiolucency, (**2**) outline of the nose, (**3**) lateral fossa, (**4**) nasal fossa, (**5**) nasal septum, (**6**) border of nasal fossa, (**7**) anterior nasal spine, and (**8**) median palatine suture.

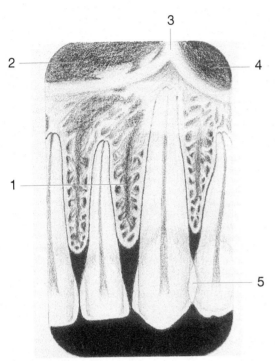

FIGURE 21–11 **Maxillary canine view. (1)** Lateral fossa, **(2)** nasal fossa, **(3)** inverted Y landmark, and **(4)** maxillary sinus. **(5)** Note the dense radiopaque area caused by superimposition of the mesial surface of the first premolar and the distal surface of the canine. This overlapping is often noted on radiographs taken in this region because of the curvature of the arch.

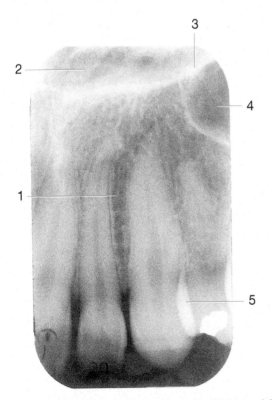

FIGURE 21–12 **Maxillary canine radiograph. (1)** Lateral fossa, **(2)** nasal fossa, **(3)** inverted Y landmark, **(4)** maxillary sinus, and **(5)** superimposition of the mesial surface of the first premolar and the distal surface of the canine.

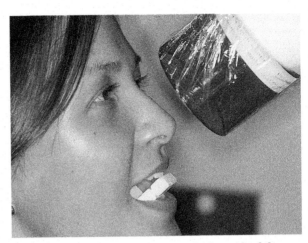

FIGURE 21–13 **Soft tissue of the nose in the path of the x-ray beam.**

RADIOLUCENT FEATURES

1. **Median palatine suture.** Radiolucent thin line that delineates the midline of the palate and the junction of the right and left maxillae; frequently seen between the central incisors, this structure should not be mistaken for a fracture.
2. **Incisive foramen** (anterior palatine foramen). Round or pear-shaped radiolucent opening that varies greatly in size; allows the passage of nerves and blood vessels. Often visible near or between the apices of the central incisors; this foramen should not be mistaken for an abscess, cyst, or other pathological condition.

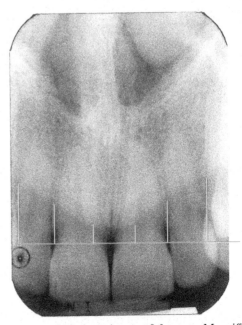

FIGURE 21–14 **Soft tissue image of the nose.** Magnified outline interpreted as the soft tissue tip of the nose.

3. **Nasal fossa** (cavity). Large air space divided into two paired radiolucencies by the radiopaque nasal septum, often visible above the roots of the incisors. The radiolucency of the nasal cavities will vary depending on the angle of the x-ray beam. At times, the x-ray beam may have to penetrate the nasal conchae, thin bony extensions of the nasal wall, and result in a less radiolucent appearance of the nasal fossa itself (see Figure 21–7).

4. **Lateral fossa.** Radiolucency between the maxillary lateral incisor and the maxillary canine representing the decreased thickness in bone in this area.

Maxillary Posterior Region (Figures 21–15 ■ through 21–20 ■)

RADIOPAQUE FEATURES

1. **Sinus walls** or borders. Dense bony walls of the maxillary sinuses appear to outline the radiolucent sinus cavities. Due to its large size, the anterior wall of the maxillary sinus is often recorded as far anterior as the canine region where it joins with the posterior wall of the nasal cavity to form the inverted Y landmark.

2. **Septum.** Radiopaque wall, or partition, may be seen separating the maxillary sinus into two or more compartments. Septa (plural) are not always visible on all patients.

3. **Zygomatic process** of the maxilla. Appears as a broad U-shaped band often recorded superior to, or superimposed over, the roots of the first and second molars.

4. **Zygoma** (malar or cheekbone). Extends laterally and distally from the zygomatic process of the maxilla; appears as a wide radiopacity at the edge or corner of an intraoral radiograph.

5. **Zygomatic arch.** Continuous with the zygoma extending distally. Radiographs are a two-dimensional picture of three-dimensional structures; therefore, it is often difficult to distinguish radiographically where the zygomatic process, zygoma, and zygomatic arch end and begin.

6. **Maxillary tuberosity.** Extension of the alveolar bone distal to the molars marking the posterior limits of the maxillary arch. The maxillary tuberosity is usually referred to as radiopaque. Depending on the size of the trabeculae located here, the radiopacity will vary.

7. **Pterygoid plate** of the sphenoid bone. Usually appearing only on the most posterior positioned intraoral radiograph, look for the posterior outline of the maxilla, distal to the maxillary tuberosity to distinguish this structure from the maxilla. A radiolucent suture may be detected separating the lateral pterygoid plate from the maxilla, or the pterygoid plate may appear to be superimposed onto the maxilla.

8. **Hamulus** (hamular process). Downward projection of the medial pterygoid plate, appears as a radiopaque

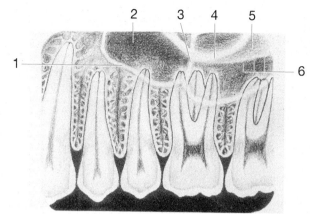

FIGURE 21–15 **Maxillary premolar view. (1)** Border of maxillary sinus, (**2**) maxillary sinus, (**3**) septum in maxillary sinus, (**4**) zygomatic process of maxilla, (**5**) zygoma, and (**6**) border of zygomatic arch.

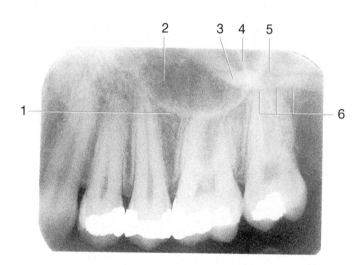

FIGURE 21–16 **Maxillary premolar radiograph. (1)** Border of maxillary sinus, (**2**) maxillary sinus, (**3**) zygomatic process of maxilla, (**4**) septum in maxillary sinus, (**5**) zygoma, and (**6**) border of zygomatic arch.

pointed, sometimes hooklike, structure that serves as a muscle attachment. The hamulus is usually observed on only the most posterior intraoral radiographs.

9. **Coronoid process** of the mandible. Sometimes seen as a triangle or large pointed radiopacity superimposed over the maxillary tuberosity. Although this structure is a feature of the mandible, it is often in the path of the x-ray beam when aligning the position indicating device (PID) for images of the maxillary posterior region (see Figures 21–19 and 21–20).

RADIOLUCENT FEATURES

1. **Maxillary sinus.** Large air chamber inside the maxilla is visible in almost all periapical radiographs from the region of the canines posterior to the molars. The thin, radiopaque sinus wall can be observed outlining the radiolucent sinus.

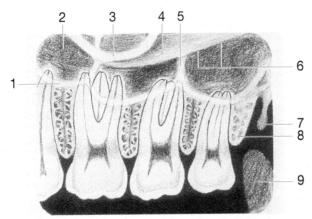

FIGURE 21-17 Maxillary molar view. (**1**) Border of maxillary sinus, (**2**) maxillary sinus, (**3**) zygomatic process of maxilla, (**4**) zygoma, (**5**) septum in maxillary sinus, (**6**) border of zygomatic arch, (**7**) hamulus, (**8**) maxillary tuberosity, and (**9**) coronoid process of mandible.

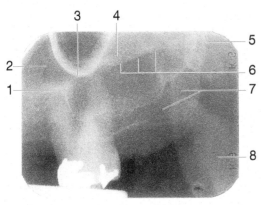

FIGURE 21-18 Maxillary molar radiograph. (**1**) Border of maxillary sinus, (**2**) maxillary sinus, (**3**) zygomatic process of maxilla, (**4**) zygoma, (**5**) lateral pterygoid plate, (**6**) border of zygomatic arch, (**7**) maxillary tuberosity, and (**8**) coronoid process of mandible.

Mandibular Anterior Region (Figures 21–21 ■ through 21–26 ■)

RADIOPAQUE FEATURES

1. **Genial tubercles.** Made up of four small, bony crests on the lingual surface of the mandible that serve for muscle attachments. Generally visible as a round radiopaque "doughnut" at the midline below the apices of the central incisors.
2. **Mental ridge.** Located on the lateral surface of the mandible, appears as a horizontal radiopaque line extending from the premolar region to the symphysis (the midline of the mandible where the left and right sides of bone are fused together).

RADIOLUCENT FEATURES

1. **Lingual foramen.** Very small, circular radiolucency in the middle of the radiopaque genial tubercles. May not be recorded on a radiograph because of its small size.

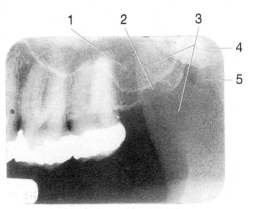

FIGURE 21-19 Maxillary molar radiograph. (**1**) Maxillary sinus, (**2**) maxillary tuberosity, (**3**) coronoid process of mandible, (**4**) lateral pterygoid plate, and (**5**) hamulus.

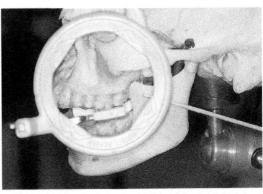

FIGURE 21-20 Coronoid process of the mandible in the path of the x-ray beam. Note the position of the image receptor holder when exposing a maxillary posterior periapical radiograph.

2. **Mental fossa.** Depression on the labial aspect of the mandibular incisor area, representing an accentuated thinness of the mandible, often appears as a generalized radiolucent area around the incisor apices.

Mandibular Posterior Region (Figures 21–27 ■ through 21–31 ■)

RADIOPAQUE FEATURES

1. **Oblique ridge** or external oblique ridge. Continuation of the anterior border of the ramus that extends downward and forward on the lateral surface of the mandible; appears as a radiopaque horizontal line of varied width superimposed across the molar roots.
2. **Mylohyoid ridge.** An irregular crest of bone for muscle attachments on the lingual surface of the mandible in the molar region; appears as a horizontal radiopaque line parallel and always inferior to (below) the oblique ridge. The mylohyoid ridge will most likely be imaged inferior to the teeth roots.
3. **Inferior border of the mandible.** Heavy layer of cortical bone imaged only if the radiograph is deeply depressed in the floor of the mouth or the vertical angle of the x-ray beam is excessive. The inferior border of the mandible will appear as a distinct, thick radiopaque border.

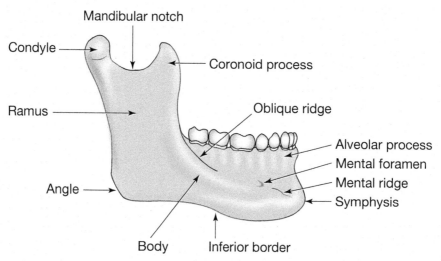

FIGURE 21–21 **Lateral view of detached mandible.**

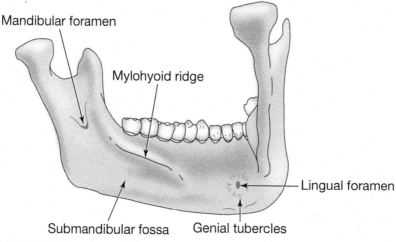

FIGURE 21–22 **Lingual view of detached mandible.**

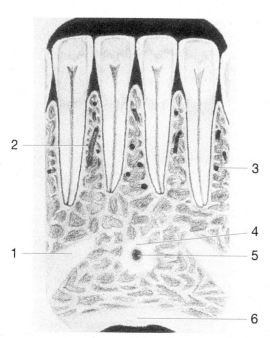

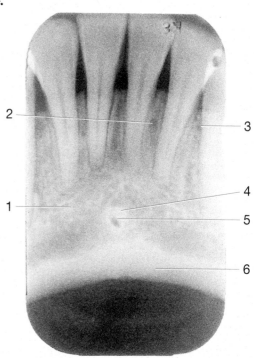

FIGURE 21–23 **Mandibular incisors view.** (**1**) Mental ridge, (**2**) nutrient canal, (**3**) nutrient foramen, (**4**) genial tubercles surrounding the (**5**) lingual foramen, and (**6**) inferior border of mandible.

FIGURE 21–24 **Mandibular incisors radiograph.** (**1**) Mental ridge, (**2**) nutrient canal, (**3**) nutrient foramen, (**4**) genial tubercles surrounding the (**5**) lingual foramen, and (**6**) inferior border of the mandible (radiopaque band of dense cortical bone).

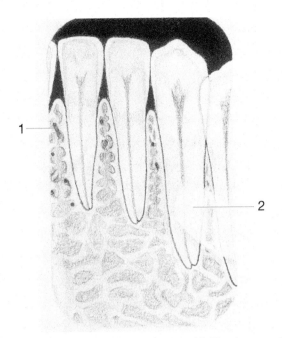

FIGURE 21–25 **Mandibular canine view.** (**1**) Nutrient canal, and (**2**) torus mandibularis.

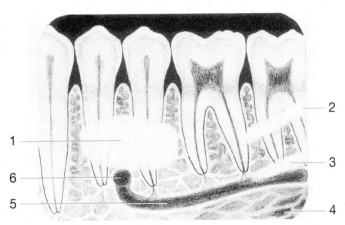

FIGURE 21–27 **Mandibular premolar view.** (**1**) Torus mandibularis, (**2**) oblique ridge, (**3**) mylohyoid ridge, (**4**) submandibular fossa, (**5**) mandibular canal, and (**6**) mental foramen.

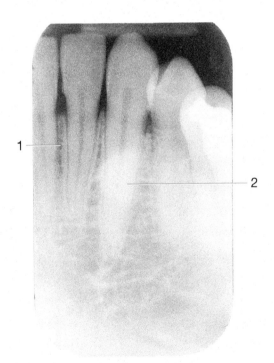

FIGURE 21–26 **Mandibular canine radiograph.** (**1**) Nutrient canal, and (**2**) torus mandibularis.

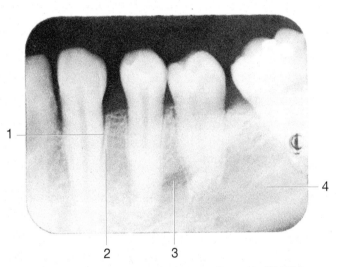

FIGURE 21–28 **Mandibular premolar radiograph.** (**1**) PDL space, (**2**) lamina dura, (**3**) mental foramen, and (**4**) submandibular fossa.

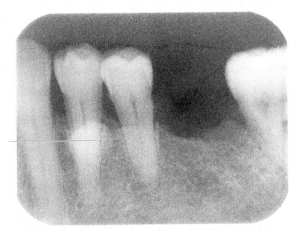

FIGURE 21–29 **Mandibular premolar radiograph.** Torus mandibularis.

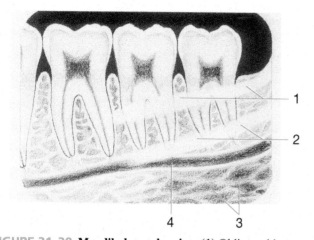

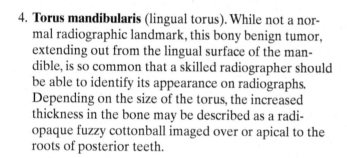

FIGURE 21–30 **Mandibular molar view.** (**1**) Oblique ridge, (**2**) mylohyoid ridge, (**3**) submandibular fossa, and (**4**) mandibular canal.

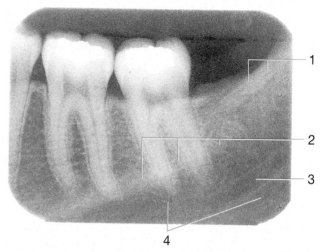

FIGURE 21–31 **Mandibular molar radiograph.** (**1**) Oblique ridge, (**2**) mylohyoid ridge, (**3**) mandibular canal, and (**4**) submandibular fossa.

4. **Torus mandibularis** (lingual torus). While not a normal radiographic landmark, this bony benign tumor, extending out from the lingual surface of the mandible, is so common that a skilled radiographer should be able to identify its appearance on radiographs. Depending on the size of the torus, the increased thickness in the bone may be described as a radiopaque fuzzy cottonball imaged over or apical to the roots of posterior teeth.

RADIOLUCENT FEATURES

1. **Mental foramen.** Small opening on the lateral side of the body of the mandible, often seen near the apices of the premolars; should not be mistaken for an abscess, cyst, or other pathological condition.
2. **Submandibular fossa.** Large irregular-shaped diffuse radiolucency inferior to the mylohyoid ridge and the roots of the mandibular molars. A decreased bone density in this region allows more x-rays to penetrate and reach the image receptor. Should not be mistaken for pathology.
3. **Mandibular canal.** Canal for the passage of the mandibular nerve and blood vessels, outlined by two paired, thin, barely visible, parallel radiopaque lines, which represent thin layers of cortical bone; often imaged in the premolar–molar areas inferior to the apices of the teeth.

REVIEW—Chapter summary

Radiographs represent two-dimensional images of three-dimensional structures. Different appearances of the same anatomical landmark on dental radiographs results from differing positions of the image receptor in the oral cavity, alterations in the position of the patient in relation to the angle of the x-ray beam, and when multiple structures may be recorded superimposed on top of each other.

A radiographer should be able to identify cranial and facial bones as well as specific landmarks and features of the maxilla and mandible. Dense, compact cortical bone appears radiopaque. Cancellous or spongy bone, formed by interconnected trabeculae, is described radiographically as having a honeycomb appearance with varying degrees of radiopacity. Bone may sometimes appear almost radiolucent if trabeculae spaces are large or the bone is thin. The supporting cancellous bone of the maxilla and the

mandible that supports the teeth is the alveolar process. The lamina dura is the hard cortical bone that lines the alveolus. The lamina dura appears radiographically as a thin radiopaque border that outlines a tooth root. The PDL space appears radiographically as a thin radiolucent border between the lamina dura and the root of a tooth. Thin radiolucent nutrient canals are sometimes recorded on mandibular anterior radiographs, on radiographs of edentulous areas, and within the maxillary sinus wall.

Radiographs may record primary teeth in various stages of resorption in response to the developing permanent dentition which may appear in various stages of development with incomplete crown and root formation. Tooth enamel, dentin, and cementum appear radiopaque; the pulp chamber and root canal appear radiolucent. Cementum and dentin are indistinguishable radiographically.

An organized and systematic approach to radiographic interpretation will assist a beginning radiographer in developing skills. An organization flow chart suggests the following steps to interpretation of bony landmarks: determine if the radiograph is a maxillary or mandibular view; determine if the radiograph is an anterior or posterior view; determine if the structure in question is radiopaque or radiolucent; determine if the structure in question has the characteristics of a border, process, ridge, spine, tubercle, tuberosity, canal, foramen, fossa, meatus, sinus, space, or suture.

RECALL—Study questions

1. The angle of the x-ray beam may distort the appearance of an anatomical structure *because* some landmarks may take on a different appearance on the right and on the left sides.
   a. Both the statement and reason are correct and related.
   b. Both the statement and reason are correct but NOT related.
   c. The statement is correct, but the reason is NOT.
   d. The statement is NOT correct, but the reason is correct.
   e. NEITHER the statement NOR the reason is correct.

2. Which of the following facial bones could appear on a periapical radiograph?
   a. Occipital
   b. Parietal
   c. Frontal
   d. Zygoma

3. Bone sometimes has a mixed radiopaque-radiolucent appearance due to the nature of the
   a. cortical plates.
   b. trabeculae patterns.
   c. alveolar process.
   d. lamina dura.

4. Which of the following will most likely appear as a radiopacity outlining the tooth root?
   a. PDL space
   b. Lamina dura
   c. Nutrient canal
   d. Cementum

5. When nutrient canals open at the surface of the bone, they often appear radiographically as
   a. small radiolucent dots.
   b. large radiopaque lines.
   c. small radiolucent lines.
   d. small radiopaque dots.

6. Which of these structures appears radiolucent?
   a. Enamel
   b. Cementum
   c. Dentin
   d. Pulp

7. Which of the following is the best recommended sequence for identifying a normal radiographic anatomical landmark?
   a. 1. Determine if radiograph is maxilla or mandible view.
      2. Determine if radiograph is anterior or posterior view.
      3. Determine if structure is radiopaque or radiolucent.
   b. 1. Determine if radiograph is anterior or posterior view.
      2. Determine if structure is radiopaque or radiolucent.
      3. Determine if radiograph is maxilla or mandible view.
   c. 1. Determine if structure is radiopaque or radiolucent.
      2. Determine if radiograph is maxilla or mandible view.
      3. Determine if radiograph is anterior or posterior view.
   d. 1. Determine if radiograph is maxilla or mandible view.
      2. Determine if structure is radiopaque or radiolucent.
      3. Determine if radiograph is anterior or posterior view.

8. Which of the following structures may be recorded radiographically superimposed over the roots of the maxillary molars?
   a. Mastoid process
   b. Maxillary tuberosity
   c. Zygomatic process
   d. Mylohyoid ridge

9. Each of these features will appear radiolucent EXCEPT one. Which one is the EXCEPTION?
   a. Foramen
   b. Suture
   c. Canal
   d. Spine

10. Each of these features will appear radiopaque EXCEPT one. Which one is the EXCEPTION?
    a. Ridge
    b. Sinus
    c. Tubercles
    d. Process

11. Each of the following may appear on a periapical radiograph of the maxillary anterior region EXCEPT one. Which one is the EXCEPTION?
    a. Nasal septum
    b. Median palatine suture
    c. Maxillary tuberosity
    d. Inverted Y

12. Each of the following may appear on a periapical radiograph of the maxillary posterior region EXCEPT one. Which one is the EXCEPTION?
    a. Maxillary sinus
    b. Incisive foramen
    c. Zygomatic arch
    d. Hamulus

13. Which of these mandibular anatomical features may be recorded on a periapical radiograph of the maxillary posterior region?
    a. Mandibular canal
    b. Submandibular fossa
    c. Inferior border of the mandible
    d. Coronoid process

14. Each of the following may appear on a periapical radiograph of the mandibular anterior region EXCEPT one. Which one is the EXCEPTION?
    a. Genial tubercles
    b. Mental ridge
    c. Coronoid process
    d. Lingual foramen

15. Each of the following may appear on a periapical radiograph of the mandibular posterior region EXCEPT one. Which one is the EXCEPTION?
    a. Mental foramen
    b. Pterygoid plate
    c. Mandibular canal
    d. Mylohyoid ridge

16. The inverted Y landmark is composed of the intersection of what two structures?
    a. Lateral wall of the nasal cavity and anterior border of the maxillary sinus.
    b. Anterior border of the maxillary sinus and inferior border of the mandible.
    c. Lateral wall of the nasal cavity and soft tissue shadow of the nose.
    d. Inferior border of the zygomatic process and the anterior nasal spine.

REFLECT—Case study

Your colleague is viewing a full mouth series of radiographs and describing the following features. Can you name each of the anatomic landmarks?

1. A dense, vertical radiopacity separating two paired oval radiolucencies observed in the maxillary anterior region

2. Large, paired oval radiolucencies separated by a dense, vertical radiopacity observed in the maxillary anterior region

3. A thin radiolucent line resembling a fracture observed between the maxillary central incisors

4. A round or pear-shaped radiolucency observed between the maxillary central incisors

5. A broad, U-shaped radiopacity observed superimposed over the maxillary posterior teeth roots

6. A radiopaque downward projection of bone that appears pointed or hook-like observed in the far posterior region of the maxilla

7. A large triangular radiopacity observed superimposed over the maxillary tuberosity region

8. A large radiolucency outlined by a thin radiopaque border that is observed in almost all periapical radiographs of the maxilla, from the canine posteriorly

9. A very small, round radiolucency observed in the midline inferior to the mandibular incisors

10. A horizontal radiopaque line extending from the premolar region to the symphysis

11. A round radiolucency that resembles an abscess observed near the apex of the mandibular second premolar

12. A horizontal radiopaque line observed in the mandibular posterior region, superimposed across the molar roots

13. A horizontal radiopaque line observed in the mandibular posterior region, inferior to the line described in #12 and inferior to the molar roots

14. A large, irregularly shaped, diffuse radiolucency observed inferior to the line described in #13.

RELATE—Laboratory application

Developing the ability to recognize, identify, and describe radiographic anatomy of the head and neck region takes practice. Using the illustrations in this chapter, compare the appearance of the structures labeled with how they appear on a skull, pointing out each of the landmarks in the figures.

To make it easier to locate these bones or structures, turn the skull so that it is oriented in the same direction as the illustration at which you are looking. Many structures can be seen readily; others may only be seen from one specific direction.

RESOURCES

White, S. C., & Pharoah, M. J. (2014). Intraoral anatomy. *Oral radiology: Principles and interpretation* (7th ed.). St. Louis, MO: Elsevier.

Visit www.pearsonhighered.com/healthprofessionsresources to access the student resources that accompany this book. Simply select Dental Hygiene from the choice of disciplines. Find this book and you will find the complementary study tools created for this specific title.

Recognizing Normal Radiographic Anatomy—Panoramic Radiographs

CHAPTER OUTLINE

OBJECTIVES

Following successful completion of this chapter, you should be able to:

1. Define the key terms.
2. Describe the unique appearance of normal anatomy as recorded by a panoramic radiograph.
3. Explain why panoramic radiographs present with streaked and blurred images.
4. List the types of tissues and artifacts that will be recorded on panoramic radiographs.
5. Describe the appearance of air spaces on a panoramic radiograph.
6. Explain how the panoramic technique produces ghost images.
7. Identify maxillofacial bony anatomic landmarks of the maxilla and surrounding tissues as viewed on a panoramic radiograph.
8. Identify maxillofacial bony anatomic landmarks of the mandible as viewed on a panoramic radiograph.
9. Identify the hyoid bone and cervical vertebra as viewed on a panoramic radiograph.
10. Identify maxillofacial soft tissues as viewed on a panoramic radiograph.
11. Identify maxillofacial air spaces as viewed on a panoramic radiograph.
12. Identify positioning guide artifacts as viewed on a panoramic radiograph.
13. Identify ghost image artifacts as viewed on a panoramic radiograph.

KEY TERMS

Artifacts
Ghost image
Glossopharyngeal air space
Maxillofacial
Nasopharyngeal air space
Palatoglossal air space
Torus palatinus (palatal torus)

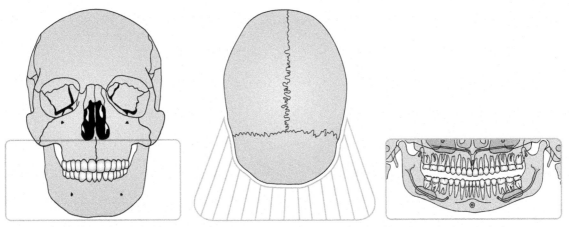

FIGURE 22–1 **Broad, wide view.** Panoramic radiographic image flattens and broadens the anatomical structures of the skull.

Introduction

Panoramic radiography produces a unique maxillofacial image. The principles of tomography, based on a moving x-ray source and corresponding moving image receptor, allow panoramic radiographs to record anatomic tissues a section at a time, producing an image a slice at a time that are then put together side by side on an image receptor. The wide panoramic broadening of the dental arches combined with superimposition of structures that lie along the same x-ray beam path produce unusual anatomical relationships not seen on intraoral radiographs. This chapter demonstrates how the skills developed for interpretation of intraoral radiographs can be expanded and adapted for successful interpretation of panoramic images.

Interpretation Fundamentals

Anatomical structures recorded by intraoral radiographs are also recorded on panoramic radiographs. To understand why anatomy imaged on intraoral radiographs takes on a unique appearance on a panoramic radiograph, consider the panoramic technique's ability to separate structures to make it possible to focus on a narrow slice of tissue at a time. Three-dimensional anatomical structures of the head and neck appear broadened and wider in the same way that a map of the world flattens and broadens the images of a globe. On a panoramic radiograph, the maxilla, mandible, and other bones of the skull are imaged as if these structures were split vertically in half at the midsagittal plane, and each half is folded outward (Figure 22–1 ■). In addition to the bones of the skull, a panoramic radiograph records the cervical vertebra of the spine and the hyoid bone, located in the neck inferior to the mandible. These structures often appear twice, beyond or superimposed over the mandibular rami at the extreme right and left edges of the radiograph (Figure 22–2 ■). It is important to understand this broadening and duplicate structure appearance to be able to correctly identify anatomical landmarks.

A significant point to remember regarding the panoramic technique is that structures located at increasingly greater distances from the center of the focal trough will be increasingly blurred out of the image. The goal of panoramic technology is to isolate and produce a relatively sharp image of the dental arches, while attempting to blur out structures that are not of interest for a dental diagnosis. However,

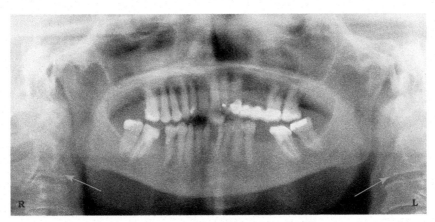

FIGURE 22–2 **Appearance of cervical vertebra imaged twice.**

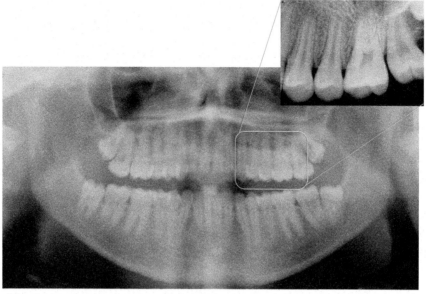

FIGURE 22–3 Comparison of intraoral and panoramic radiographs. Apply knowledge of landmarks that would be recorded on a periapical radiograph to aid in interpretation of a panoramic radiograph.

these other structures are not completely eliminated from the image. Panoramic images present with significant radiopaque and radiolucent blurring and streaking of the structures that are located just outside the focal trough. So, an understanding of how to read panoramic radiographs must be based on normal anatomy identification, and needs to address the presence of **artifacts**, or nonanatomical images that are typically recorded by panoramic radiographs.

To develop the skills needed to recognize normal anatomic structures viewed on a panoramic radiograph, build on the knowledge of how normal anatomy appears on intraoral radiographs and transfer this knowledge to the panoramic image. For example, when viewing the maxillary posterior region on a panoramic image, visualize a periapical radiograph taken in this same area (Figure 22–3 ■). The structures identified on the periapical radiograph will most likely be observed on the panoramic radiograph as well. Skills developed to identify anatomical landmarks on an intraoral radiograph can assist with developing the skills needed to identify these same landmarks on a panoramic radiograph.

All of the anatomical features of the maxilla and mandible and the dentition that are recorded on intraoral radiographs will be recorded on panoramic radiographs. It is important to remember that a panoramic radiograph will image additional bones and structures of the oral facial or **maxillofacial** region including the maxillary sinus, the temporomandibular joint (TMJ), and possibly cartilage and calcifications of ligaments located in the neck. It may be helpful to review dental and head and neck anatomy prior to practice of locating and identifying these structures on a panoramic radiograph. A working knowledge of the skull and facial bones and their landmarks will assist with identifying these structures on a panoramic image. The cranial and facial bones that may be recorded on dental radiographs are illustrated in Figures 22–4 ■ and 22–5 ■ and summarized in Box 22–1.

Soft Tissues

In addition to the dentition and bony structures, panoramic radiographs are likely to record soft tissues. When recorded, these tissues are usually superimposed over other structures and sometimes are only faintly or partially visible.

Box 22–1 Bones of the Skull

- Frontal
- Mandible
- Maxilla
- Nasal
- Occipital
- Parietal
- Sphenoid
- Temporal
- Zygoma

Practice Point

A panoramic radiograph records more structures of the maxillofacial region than the dentition and the surrounding supporting bone. Although an oral health care professional is primarily concerned with the oral cavity, panoramic radiographs must be interpreted by a dentist for all deviations from normal anatomy. Research has indicated that it is possible to identify carotid arterial plaques on some panoramic radiographs. This serious medical condition known as carotid artery stenosis can lead to a stroke, and other vascular events. When suspected carotid artery calcifications are recorded on a panoramic radiograph, the dentist must immediately refer the patient to a physician for further evaluation.

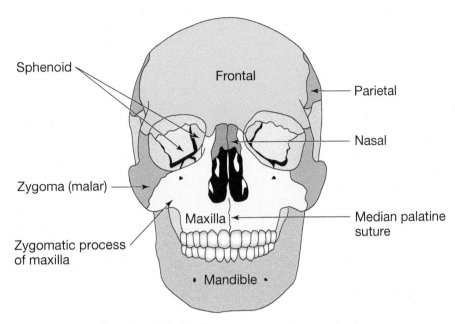

FIGURE 22–4 **Front view of the skull.**

An outline of a soft tissue landmark may be superimposed over bony tissue where it can mimic the appearance of a fracture. It is important to understand the location and typical appearance of these soft tissue structures to avoid mistaking them for other diagnoses.

The neck region, apical to the mandible, has additional soft tissue structures that can be recorded on a panoramic radiograph. These include cartilage, calcified ligaments, and lymph nodes. While not of interest in dental diagnoses these structures should be examined and identified. There is evidence that panoramic radiographs provide opportunistic screening for calcified carotid artery plaques. It is important that the radiographic appearance of the normal and calcified anatomic structures be identified to avoid mistaking these for a serious condition that would require a medical referral (see Chapter 26).

Air Spaces

Adding to the superimposition of anatomical structures is the appearance of air spaces, or regions of the skull where there is less bone or thin bony structures. Air does not attenuate the x-ray beam as much as hard or soft tissue. For this reason, air spaces appear with varying degrees of radiolucency on a panoramic radiograph. The radiolucencies produced by air spaces can be so dark that they may obscure other structures, compromising the diagnostic ability of the panoramic radiograph. Whereas bony tissue and sometimes soft tissue may be desirable to capture on a panoramic

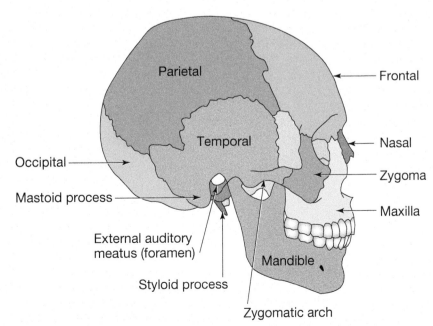

FIGURE 22–5 **Lateral view of the skull.**

radiograph, radiolucencies produced by air spaces do not add diagnostic information to the image. Careful positioning of a patient into the focal trough will help minimize the appearance of air spaces (see Chapter 17).

Positioning Guides

Panoramic machine positioning guides, such as a chin rest and biteblock, used to place the dental arches into the focal trough may be recorded on the panoramic image. Manufacturers of panoramic machines try to minimize this occurrence; however, because these positioning guides are within the path of the x-ray beam they are sometimes recorded. Care should be taken to identify these artifacts so that they are not confused with normal anatomical landmarks or the presence of disease.

Ghost Images

The rotation of the panoramic x-ray tube head and the use of a focal trough to isolate slices of an image create ghost images. **Ghost images** are mirror or second images of structures that are penetrated by the x-ray beam twice. Consider that when the panoramic process begins, if the x-ray tube head is on the patient's right side, the x-ray beam will penetrate the patient's tissues on the right side first. However, at this moment in time, the x-ray beam is calibrated to focus on recording the anatomical structures on the left side. At any given moment during the panoramic procedure structures are either in focus or being blurred out of focus; essentially the goal of tomography is to eliminate one side to more clearly view the other side (see Chapter 17). As the panoramic x-ray tube head and image receptor rotate, the x-ray beam is refocused to record the next section of anatomy, while blurring out the previously in-focus section. In principle when a structure is outside the focal trough it will not be imaged on the radiograph. However, a magnified, unsharp ghost image often appears.

For example, when viewing a panoramic image of a clearly recorded right side mandible, a ghost image of the left side mandible can be observed superimposed over the right, as a mirror image. Being able to identify typical ghost images will assist in interpreting panoramic radiographs.

Radiographic Appearance of Bony Landmarks of the Maxilla and Surrounding Tissues

A thorough knowledge of the anatomy of the skull, combined with the skills developed for identifying the appearance of these structures on intraoral radiographs, will provide the framework upon which to learn how these anatomical landmarks appear on a panoramic radiograph. The following landmarks may be recorded on panoramic radiographs. Note that some landmarks are more readily observed than others. Additionally, each bilateral landmark should be observed on both sides for symmetry. To assist with learning how to identify these structures, they are organized by region, and for ease of study, an alphabetical listing is presented. Note: an asterisk (*) denotes structures that are also recorded on intraoral radiographs (Figures 22–6 ■ and 22–7 ■).

ANTERIOR REGION

Anterior nasal spine*—V-shaped radiopacity representing pointed bony projection of maxilla located at most anterior point of floor of nasal cavity at base of nasal septum

Incisive canal—Not often visible; bilateral tunnel-like radiolucency with radiopaque borders observed extending from floor of nasal cavity inferior toward alveolar ridge between maxillary incisors

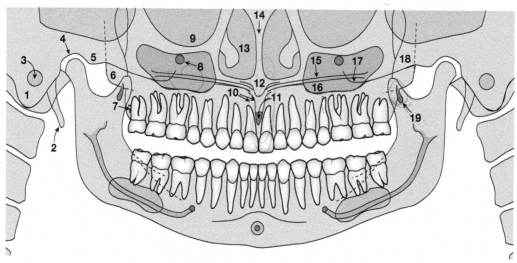

FIGURE 22–6 **Bony landmarks of maxilla and surrounding region.** (**1**) Mastoid process, (**2**) styloid process, (**3**) external auditory meatus, (**4**) glenoid fossa, (**5**) articular eminence, (**6**) lateral pterygoid plate, (**7**) maxillary tuberosity, (**8**) infra-orbital foramen, (**9**) orbit of the eye, (**10**) incisive canal, (**11**) incisive foramen, (**12**) anterior nasal spine, (**13**) nasal cavity, (**14**) nasal septum, (**15**) hard palate, (**16**) maxillary sinus, (**17**) zygomatic process of the maxilla, (**18**) zygoma, and (**19**) hamulus.

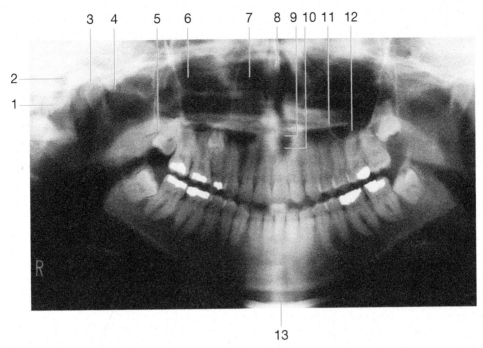

FIGURE 22–7 **Bony landmarks of maxilla and surrounding region.** (**1**) Mastoid process, (**2**) external auditory meatus, (**3**) glenoid fossa, (**4**) articular eminence, (**5**) maxillary tuberosity, (**6**) orbit of the eye, (**7**) nasal cavity, (**8**) nasal septum, (**9**) incisive canal, (**10**) incisive foramen, (**11**) hard palate, (**12**) maxillary sinus, and (**13**) chin rest (artifact).

Incisive foramen* — Not as distinctly recorded as it is on a periapical radiograph; round or oval radiolucency between roots of maxillary central incisors representing an opening in bone

Infraorbital foramen — Bilateral, small round radiolucent opening in bone inferior to border of orbit

Nasal cavity (nasal fossa)* — Bilateral, pear-shaped radiolucency located superior to maxilla incisor roots

- Nasal septum* — Radiopaque, vertical bony wall that separates right and left nasal fossae

- Nasal conchae* — Bilateral, slightly radiopaque, thin bony extensions of nasal wall often superimposed over radiolucent cavity; do not mistake these normal landmarks for pathology

Orbit — Bilateral, large round radiolucent bony cavity of eye socket, outlined by radiopaque border located superior to, or superimposed over, part of maxillary sinuses; usually only one-third to one-half of each orbit is visible

- Infraorbital ridge — Bilateral, thin radiopaque line inferior to radiolucent orbit

- Infraorbital canal — Bilateral, faint radiolucent tube outlined by faint parallel radiopaque lines extending vertically from inferior border of orbit inferiorly toward maxillary sinus

- Infraorbital foramen — Bilateral, faint radiolucent oval at end of infraorbital canal

POSTERIOR REGION

External auditory meatus — Bilateral, round radiolucent opening in temporal bone located anterior and superior to mastoid process

Hamulus* — Bilateral, tiny radiopaque hooklike process of bone that extends downward and slightly backward from medial pterygoid plate of sphenoid bone

Lateral pterygoid plate* — Bilateral, radiopaque winglike bony projection of sphenoid bone located posterior to maxillary tuberosity

Mastoid process — Bilateral, prominent rounded protrusion of temporal bone located posterior and inferior to TMJ; appears as rounded radiopacity at extreme far edge of radiograph

Maxillary sinus* — Bilateral, radiolucent cavity located within maxilla apical to maxillary posterior teeth; anterior wall begins near root of canine and extends posterior to third molar region

Maxillary tuberosity* — Bilateral, rounded bony prominence of varied radiopacity distal to third molar

Middle cranial fossa — Bilateral, large diffuse mixed radiopaque and radiolucent appearance at far upper corners of radiograph

Pterygomaxillary fissure — Bilateral, large elongated teardrop-shaped radiolucency representing space between posterior border of maxilla and lateral pterygoid plate of sphenoid bone

Styloid process—Bilateral, long narrow radiopaque spine extending downward from inferior surface of temporal bone, just anterior to mastoid process

Zygomatic process of the maxilla*—Bilateral bony process of maxilla, forming cheek bone, extends laterally to articulate with zygoma, which continues to extend laterally to articulate with temporal bone; thick, bulky radiopaque process, resembling a J or U shape located apical to, or superimposed over, roots of maxillary first molar

- Zygoma*—Bilateral, thick horizontal radiopaque band that extends posterior from zygomatic process of maxilla to connect with zygomatic process of temporal bone

- Articular eminence—Bilateral, slight convex protrusion extending inferior from zygomatic process of temporal bone; located anterior to glenoid fossa

- Glenoid fossa—Bilateral, slight concave depression in zygomatic process of temporal bone posterior to articular eminence; head of mandibular condyle recorded resting in glenoid fossa

- Zygomatico-temporal suture—Bilateral, distinct radiolucent suture that joins zygomatic process of temporal bone with temporal process of zygoma; do not mistake this normal landmark for a fracture

OBSERVED IN BOTH ANTERIOR AND POSTERIOR REGIONS

Hard palate—Horizontal, thick radiopaque band superior to maxillary teeth representing bony wall that separates oral cavity from nasal cavity; appears to traverse across both anterior and posterior regions

- **Torus palatinus (palatal torus)**—Common benign tumor that manifests as dense bony extension from inferior surface of palate; depending on size, torus will appear as a radiopaque thickening of palate superior to or superimposed over roots of maxillary teeth

Radiographic Appearance of Bony Landmarks of the Mandible (Figures 22–8 ■ and 22–9 ■)

ANTERIOR REGION

Genial tubercles*—Tiny, round radiopacity surrounding tiny, round radiolucent lingual foramen inferior to apices of mandibular incisor teeth

Lingual foramen*—Tiny, round radiolucent opening located in center of radiopaque genial tubercles

Mental fossa*—Radiolucent depressed area of bone in region of roots of mandibular incisor teeth

Mental ridge*—Bilateral, thick radiopaque band representing prominence of bone located on external surface of mandible; extends anteriorly from premolar area to midline

POSTERIOR REGION

Angle of the mandible—Bilateral corner where body of mandible meets and joins ascending ramus of mandible

Condyle—Bilateral, dense, radiopaque rounded head and neck extension of ramus of mandible; observed articulating in glenoid fossa of zygomatic process of temporal bone; due to its important role as part of TMJ, examine both condyles for symmetry

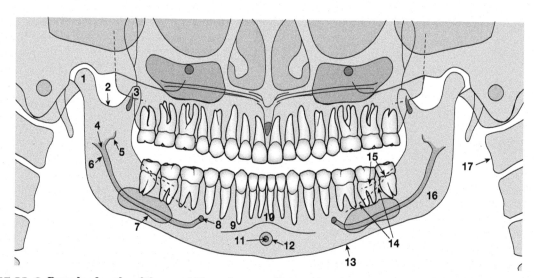

FIGURE 22–8 Bony landmarks of the mandible and surrounding region. (1) Mandibular condyle, **(2)** mandibular notch, **(3)** coronoid process, **(4)** mandibular foramen, **(5)** lingula, **(6)** mandibular canal, **(7)** submandibular fossa, **(8)** mental foramen, **(9)** mental ridge, **(10)** mental fossa, **(11)** lingual foramen, **(12)** genial tubercles, **(13)** inferior border of the mandible, **(14)** mylohyoid ridge, **(15)** oblique ridge, **(16)** angle of the mandible, and **(17)** cervical vertebrae.

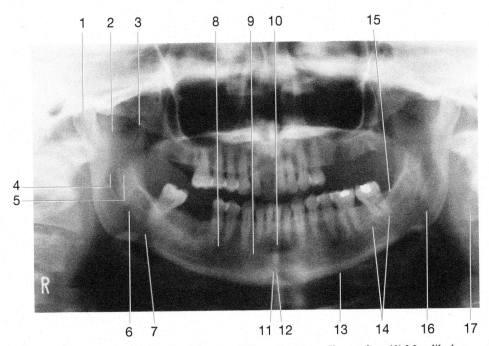

FIGURE 22–9 **Bony landmarks of the mandible and surrounding region.** (**1**) Mandibular condyle, (**2**) mandibular notch, (**3**) coronoid process, (**4**) mandibular foramen, (**5**) lingula, (**6**) mandibular canal, (**7**) submandibular fossa, (**8**) mental foramen, (**9**) mental ridge, (**10**) mental fossa, (**11**) lingual foramen, (**12**) genial tubercles, (**13**) inferior border of the mandible, (**14**) mylohyoid ridge, (**15**) oblique ridge, (**16**) angle of the mandible, and (**17**) cervical vertebrae.

Coronoid process*—Bilateral, large, radiopaque triangular prominence of bone located on anterior superior ramus of mandible

Lingula—Bilateral, small radiopaque projection of bone located anterior and adjacent to mandibular foramen

Mandibular canal*—Bilateral, radiolucent, long tunnel-like passageway outlined by parallel radiopaque lines representing canal walls; extends from mandibular foramen on medial aspect of ramus of mandible to mental foramen on lateral aspect of body of mandible

Mandibular foramen—Bilateral, radiolucent round or oval opening in bone on lingual aspect of ramus

Mandibular notch—Bilateral concavity of bone posterior to coronoid process on superior border of ramus

Mental foramen*—Bilateral, small, round radiolucent opening near roots of mandibular premolars

Mylohyoid ridge*—Bilateral, dense radiopaque bony ridge extending diagonally inferior on lingual aspect of ramus; continuing anterior to apices of teeth roots

Oblique ridge*—Bilateral, dense, radiopaque bony ridge extending inferior on lateral aspect of mandible; continuing anterior along cervical portion of molar and premolar roots

Submandibular fossa*—Bilateral, diffuse radiolucent concavity observed inferior to mylohyoid ridge and roots of mandible molars

OBSERVED IN BOTH ANTERIOR AND POSTERIOR REGIONS

Inferior border of the mandible*—Dense radiopaque band of thick cortical bone that outlines lower border of mandible

Radiographic Appearance of Other Bony Landmarks

Cervical spine—Radiopaque vertebrae appear on both sides of extreme right and left edges of radiograph

Hyoid bone—Radiopaque horseshoe-shaped bone located in neck region inferior to mandible; may be recorded superimposed over inferior border of mandible and often takes on varied appearance and shape (Figure 22–10 ■)

Radiographic Appearance of Soft Tissues

A panoramic radiograph is unique in that some soft tissue structures attenuate the beam of radiation enough to become visible on the radiograph. A panoramic radiograph is not used to diagnose diseases of these soft tissues. Instead these structures should be identified to distinguish them as normal and not mistake them for pathology or problems requiring further investigation (Figures 22–11 ■ and 22–12 ■).

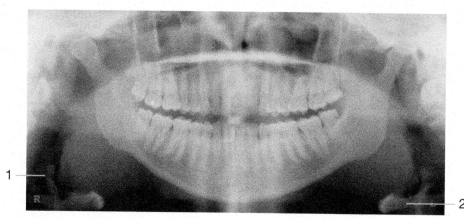

FIGURE 22–10 **(1) Cartilage**, and **(2) hyoid bone**.

Cartilage—At lower corners of radiograph inferior to mandible, various faintly radiopaque cartilage tissues (thyroid cartilage, tritial) may be observed (see Figure 22-10)

Ear—Observed at edges of radiograph as faint radiopaque outline, often of ear lobe, superimposed over styloid process, anterior and inferior to mastoid process

Epiglottis—Faint radiopaque slightly pointed or elongated triangular flap of cartilage can be observed extending out from lower corners of radiographic image

Lipline—Horizontal radiopaque line superimposed over anterior teeth that can mimic fractures; instructing patient to close lips together around bite guide helps avoid recording lip (see Figure 17–18)

Soft palate—Faint diagonal radiopaque structure above and posterior to maxillary tuberosity and posterior to hard palate, separating oral cavity from nasal cavity

Tongue—Correctly positioned, resting flat against palate, minimizes appearance of tongue and of palatoglossal airspace; when visible, radiopaque dorsal surface of tongue appears superimposed over ramus; recall that panoramic view of tongue will be broadened and much wider than it appears clinically

Radiographic Appearance of Air Spaces

The principle of tomography and the panoramic process produces images that present with an overall faint radiopaque streaking characteristic. However, upon close examination many radiolucencies and the subsequent streaking associated with these will be noted. The maxillofacial region contains many cavities and sinuses collectively called air spaces. A panoramic image that presents with an evenly distributed radiopaque streaking is preferred for ease of diagnoses. When radiolucent air spaces are pronounced, interpretation of normal radiographic landmarks becomes increasingly difficult. Correct patient positioning within the focal trough of the panoramic machine will help to minimize the appearance of these air spaces. The following represent the most common air spaces that may be recorded on panoramic radiographs (Figures 22–13 ■ and 22–14 ■).

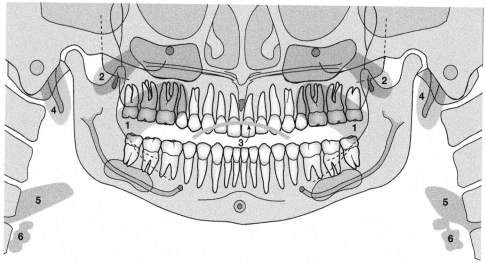

FIGURE 22–11 **Soft tissue images.** (**1**) Tongue, (**2**) soft palate, (**3**) lipline, (**4**) ear, (**5**) epiglottis, and (**6**) cartilage.

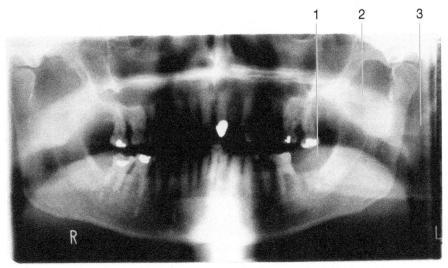

FIGURE 22–12 **Soft tissue images.** (**1**) Tongue, (**2**) soft palate, and (**3**) ear.

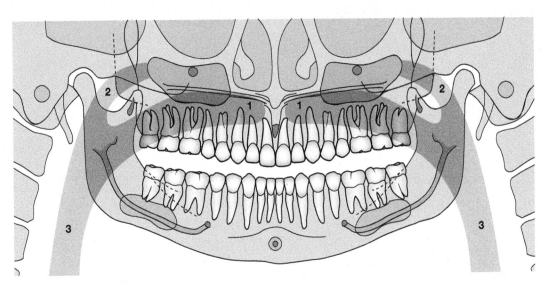

FIGURE 22–13 **Air space images.** (**1**) Palatoglossal, (**2**) nasopharyngeal, and (**3**) glossopharyngeal.

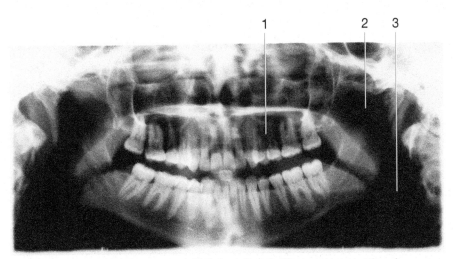

FIGURE 22–14 **Air space images.** (**1**) Palatoglossal, (**2**) nasopharyngeal, and (**3**) glossopharyngeal.

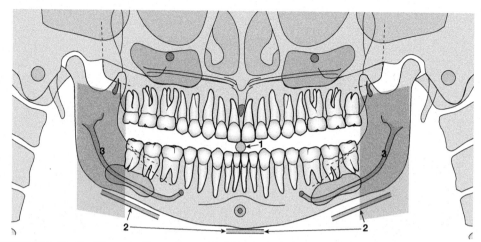

FIGURE 22–15 **Positioner guide artifacts.** (**1**) Biteblock, (**2**) chin rest, and (**3**) side positioner guides.

Palatoglossal air space—Radiolucency between palate and tongue that presents if tongue is not correctly positioned against palate during exposure; radiolucency appears superimposed on or above apices of maxillary teeth.

Nasopharyngeal air space—Bilateral, diagonal radiolucent streak superior to radiopaque soft palate; emphasized when patient's chin is incorrectly tipped down

Glossopharyngeal air space—Bilateral, vertical radiolucent band superimposed over ramus of mandible representing portion of pharynx located posterior to tongue and oral cavity

Radiographic Appearance of Positioning Guides

Because they are in the path of the primary x-ray beam during exposure, the following panoramic x-ray machine head positioner guides may be recorded on the radiograph (Figures 22–15 ■ and 22–16 ■). Panoramic machines that utilize light beams as guides help to eliminate machine part artifacts (see Figure 17-20).

Biteblock—Round or square, depending on shape of biteblock or bite pin, radiopacity observed between occluding anterior teeth; if biteblock has indented groove where patient is instructed to occlude, incisal edges of these teeth may be partially obscured by presence of biteblock

Chin rest—Radiopaque horizontal line or band, depending on thickness of material, appearing inferior to inferior border of mandible; depending on height dimension of panoramic radiograph's recording area, chin rest may or may not be recorded; additionally, some panoramic machines use a forehead rest instead of a chin rest, eliminating this artifact

Lateral (side) positioner guides—Faint radiopaque vertical lines representing outline of guides may be visible superimposed over left and right side posterior teeth; panoramic machines utilizing beams of light to position patient within focal trough eliminate this artifact

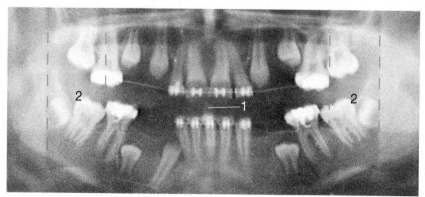

FIGURE 22–16 **Positioner guide artifacts.** (**1**) Biteblock, and (**2**) side positioner guides.

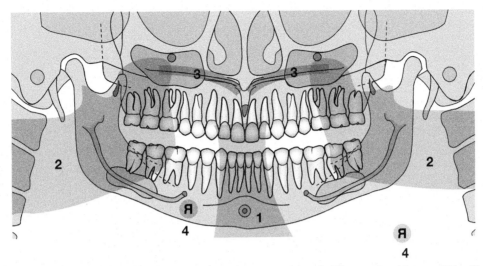

FIGURE 22–17 **Ghost images.** (**1**) Spinal column (cervical vertebrae), (**2**) opposite side mandible, (**3**) palate, and (**4**) "R" (right side) identification marker.

Right "R" or left "L" identification marker—Film-based panoramic machines will have identifying markers placed purposefully in path of x-ray beam to label right or left side of radiograph; while image of "R" or "L" is desirable, it is important to note that these markers may record a ghost image

Radiographic Appearance of Ghost Images

Ghost images enlarge and magnify structures; most to the extreme that they are not recognizable and do not interfere with diagnoses. However, there are some pronounced ghost images that require identification to avoid misinterpreting them. Ghost images will present on the opposite side of the radiograph than where the structure is located. Due to the fixed slight negative vertical angle of the x-ray beam, ghost images present superior to where the actual structure is located. In general, if trying to identify a blurred and faintly visible structure, try looking at the opposite side, slightly lower to determine if the blurred object in question is a ghost image (Figures 22–17 ■ and 22–18 ■).

Cervical vertebra of the spinal column—While the spinal column is often recorded twice, on each side of the radiograph, its ghost image will appear in the center of the image as a radiopacity superimposed over the anterior teeth.

Hard palate—The palate and the ghost image of the palate often present as a *double* image; a vertical ghost image appears superior to the location of the palate, resembling the presence of two structures.

Mandible—The ghost image of the right side mandible appears superimposed over the left side and the ghost image of the left side mandible appears superimposed over the right side. These ghost images will be recorded as mirror images of each other, in a slightly higher position.

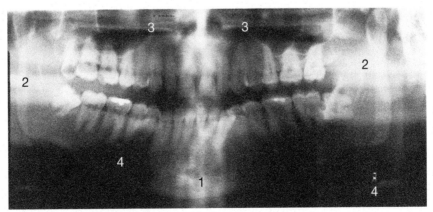

FIGURE 22–18 **Ghost images.** (**1**) Spinal column (cervical vertebrae), (**2**) opposite side mandible, (**3**) palate, and (**4**) "R" identification marker.

REVIEW—Chapter summary

Panoramic radiographs present with a broad, widened image of the maxillofacial anatomy. Based on tomography, panoramic radiographs focus on recording one section of tissue at a time, while blurring out other sections, resulting in images with significant radiopaque and radiolucent streaking. All anatomic landmarks recorded on intraoral radiographs will be recorded on panoramic radiographs. Panoramic radiographs record bony and soft tissue landmarks, air spaces, and parts of the panoramic machine used as positioning guides. Because every structure of the maxillofacial region is penetrated by the x-ray beam twice during exposure, panoramic radiographs will present with ghost images. Ghost images represent a mirror, or second image of a structure located in a higher position on the opposite side of the radiograph. Interpretation skills learned for reading intraoral radiographs can be applied to panoramic interpretation. The ability to identify the following anatomical landmarks and artifacts is required for successful interpretation of panoramic radiographs: bony landmarks of the maxilla, mandible, cervical spine, hyoid bone; soft tissues and air spaces of the maxillofacial region; positioning guide artifacts and ghost images.

RECALL—Study questions

1. Panoramic radiographs present a broad, widened view of maxillofacial structures, *because* the panoramic technique is based on tomography.
   a. Both the statement and reason are correct and related.
   b. Both the statement and reason are correct but NOT related.
   c. The statement is correct, but the reason is NOT.
   d. The statement is NOT correct, but the reason is correct.
   e. NEITHER the statement NOR the reason is correct.

2. Anatomy positioned _____ the dimensions of the focal trough will _____ on a panoramic image.
   a. within, not appear
   b. within, appear relatively sharp
   c. outside, appear relatively sharp
   d. outside, not appear

3. Which of the following would NOT be considered a radiographic artifact?
   a. Glossopharyngeal air space
   b. Chin rest positioning guide
   c. Ghost image of the mandible
   d. Cervical vertebra

4. Which of the following maxillofacial bones imaged on a panoramic radiograph would NOT be recorded by an intraoral radiograph?
   a. Hyoid
   b. Nasal
   c. Sphenoid
   d. Zygoma

5. Panoramic radiographs are sometimes prescribed to diagnose diseases of soft tissues.
   Superimposed images of soft tissues over bone can mimic the appearance of a fracture.
   a. The first statement is true. The second statement is false.
   b. The first statement is false. The second statement is true.
   c. Both statements are true.
   d. Both statements are false.

6. Positioning the tongue flat against the hard palate for the duration of the panoramic exposure will minimize the appearance of which of the following air spaces?
   a. Glossopharyngeal
   b. Nasopharyngeal
   c. Palatoglossal

7. What is the term given to an image of a structure that is recorded a second time, opposite of its location and with less sharpness?
   a. Air space
   b. Ghost image
   c. Panorama
   d. Tomograph

8. Each of the following is likely to be observed in the maxillary anterior region on a panoramic radiograph EXCEPT one. Which one is the EXCEPTION?
   a. Incisive canal
   b. Nasal conchae
   c. Infraorbital ridge
   d. Middle cranial fossa

9. Each of the following is likely to be observed in the maxillary posterior region on a panoramic radiograph EXCEPT one. Which one is the EXCEPTION?
   a. External auditory meatus
   b. Hamulus
   c. Infraorbital foreman
   d. Mastoid process

10. Each of the following is likely to be observed in the mandibular anterior region on a panoramic radiograph EXCEPT one. Which one is the EXCEPTION?
    a. Angle of the mandible
    b. Genial tubercles
    c. Lingual foramen
    d. Mental fossa

11. Each of the following is likely to be observed in the posterior region on a panoramic radiograph EXCEPT one. Which one is the EXCEPTION?
    a. Condyle
    b. Lingula
    c. Mental ridge
    d. Oblique ridge

12. Which of the following is the most likely interpretation that fits this description: large bilateral circular radiolucency observed superior to or superimposed over the maxillary sinus, in the anterior region?
    a. Glenoid fossa
    b. Orbit
    c. Nasal fossa
    d. Zygomatico-temporal suture

13. Which of the following is the most likely interpretation that fits this description: long, narrow radiopaque spine extending downward from the inferior surface of the temporal bone, observed in the posterior maxillary region?
    a. Styloid process
    b. Pterygomaxillary fissure
    c. Maxillary tuberosity
    d. Zygomatic process of the maxilla

14. Which of the following is the most likely interpretation that fits this description: radiolucent depressed area of bone observed inferior to the roots of the mandibular anterior teeth?
    a. Genial tubercles
    b. Mandibular foramen
    c. Mental foramen
    d. Mental fossa

15. Which of the following is the most likely interpretation that fits this description: faint radiopaque, slightly pointed or elongated triangular structure observed extending out from the lower corners of a panoramic radiograph?
    a. Ear lobe
    b. Epiglottis
    c. Soft palate
    d. Tongue

16. Which of the following panoramic machine positioning guides would not be likely to be recorded on the radiograph as an artifact?
    a. Bite pin
    b. Chin rest
    c. Forehead stop
    d. Lateral positioners

REFLECT—Case study

A colleague is viewing a panoramic radiograph and questions why the image appears streaked and slightly blurry. He is asking you what caused this appearance, so that he can recommend that the radiograph be retaken with the appropriate corrective action. Based on your knowledge of panoramic technology provide your colleague with an explanation for the appearance of the panoramic image; include an explanation of ghost imaging and the creation of artifacts.

RELATE—Laboratory application

To assist with developing the ability to recognize, identify, and describe the unique presentation of anatomy observed on a panoramic radiograph, it can be helpful to build on interpretation skills developed for reading intraoral radiographs. Obtain samples of full mouth series of radiographs and panoramic radiographs. Compare the radiographic anatomy recorded by the intraoral radiographs with the appearance of these structures as recorded by the panoramic radiograph.

RESOURCES

Ludlow, J. B., & Tyndall, D. A. (1999) *Panoramic radiographic anatomy*. Retrieved from University of North Carolina School of Dentistry website: http://www.dentistry.unc.edu/resources/NRA/PanAnatomy/pananat.html

White, S. C., & Pharoah, M. J. (2014). Panoramic imaging. *Oral radiology: Principles and interpretation* (7th ed.). St. Louis, MO: Elsevier.

Visit www.pearsonhighered.com/healthprofessionsresources to access the student resources that accompany this book. Simply select Dental Hygiene from the choice of disciplines. Find this book and you will find the complementary study tools created for this specific title.

Radiographic Appearance of Dental Materials and Foreign Objects

CHAPTER OUTLINE

OBJECTIVES

Following successful completion of this chapter, you should be able to:

1. Define the key terms.
2. Explain the need for a clinical examination in conjunction with radiographic interpretation.
3. Explain the effect two-dimensional radiographs have on the identification of dental materials.
4. Rank dental materials according to degree of radiopacity.
5. Describe the role radiographs play in evaluating dental restorations.
6. Identify the radiographic appearance of amalgam.
7. Identify the radiographic appearance of composite resin and glass ionomer.
8. Identify the radiographic appearance of full metal, PFM, and stainless steel crowns.
9. Identify the radiographic appearance of a fixed bridge.
10. Identify the radiographic appearance of retention pin and post and core restorative materials.
11. Identify the radiographic appearance of dental liners, bases, and cements.
12. Identify the radiographic appearance of endodontic fillers.
13. Identify the radiographic appearance of implants, orthodontic, and surgical materials.
14. Identify the radiographic appearance of an amalgam fragment.

KEY TERMS

Amalgam
Amalgam tattoo
Base material
Composite resin
Crown
Foreign object
Gutta-percha
Maryland bridge
Overhang
Post and core
Retention pin
Silver point

Introduction

An important dental radiographic interpretation skill is the ability to recognize deviations from normal radiographic anatomy. The most common anomalies or alterations to normal oral maxillofacial anatomy recorded by dental radiographic images will most likely be the presence of materials used in dental restorative treatments. These materials are considered **foreign objects**, or foreign bodies, as they do not represent normal physiologic structures. Foreign objects recorded by dental radiographs include those placed iatrogenically (purposefully for the treatment of pathology or a condition needing correcting), accidentally, or as a result of trauma. This chapter presents an overview of the radiographic appearance of common dental restorative materials and objects whose presence in the oral cavity is categorized as foreign.

Interpretation Fundamentals

Interpretation of radiographic findings is enhanced when a patient is present, facilitating a comparison of radiographic findings with a clinical examination. Attempting to determine what a particular finding is from a radiograph alone may be difficult. For example, a radiolucency observed within radiopaque enamel of a maxillary central incisor may suggest caries. However, a clinical examination may reveal the presence of a **composite resin** restoration, which can mimic decay radiographically (Figure 23–1 ■).

Remember that radiographs represent a two-dimensional image of three-dimensional objects. The superimposition of tooth surfaces can make it difficult to definitively identify the type, size, number, and location of restorations. For example, a facial surface restoration may be recorded superimposed with a lingual surface restoration, appearing as one restoration radiographically. Often, there is more than one type of material superimposed. For example, the appearance of a **base material** may be observed apical to a metallic or composite restoration, or the presence of metallic retention pins may be detected apical to a crown (Figure 23–2 ■). The radiographic appearance of restorative materials can vary depending on the angulation of the x-ray beam. For example, the horizontal direction of the x-ray beam may blend the appearance of two small restorations in such a manner that they appear as one large restoration.

Restorative materials may appear radiopaque or radiolucent (Box 23–1). Some restorations can be differentiated by relative degree of radiopacity; others are better identified by size and contour or by location on a tooth. For example, metal crowns will most often appear to have smooth margins, whereas the margins of amalgam restorations are irregular (Figure 23–3 ■). Metallic restorations of approximate equal density appear radiopaque. Therefore, it is impossible to determine whether a particular metal restoration is a gold or silver alloy. Looking at the size and contour of a restoration, it may be possible to make an educated guess as to what materials are generally used in such circumstances.

Aesthetic restorative materials, such as composite resin, glass ionomer, porcelain and ceramic, and intermediate and provisional restorative materials such as acrylic resin may appear radiopaque or radiolucent and may be barely visible or not detected at all. Some aesthetic dental materials, without added metal alloys, have a tendency to mimic decay radiographically; others exhibit about the same degree of radiopacity as dentin making these materials barely detectable radiographically (see Figures 23–1 and 23–2).

Evaluation of dental restorative materials is more likely to be conducted in conjunction with a clinical examination.

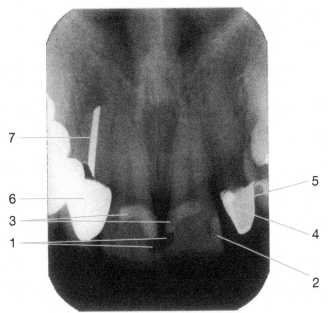

FIGURE 23–1 Dental materials. (**1**) Radiolucent composite resin. Do not mistake for caries. Note the prepared look. (**2**) Radiolucent dental base. Do not mistake for recurrent decay. (**3**) Radiopaque glass ionomer. Facial or lingual location cannot be definitively determined from two-dimensional image. (**4**) Radiopaque cement under crown. (**5**) Porcelain crown. (**6**) PFM crown. (**7**) Silver point endodontic filler.

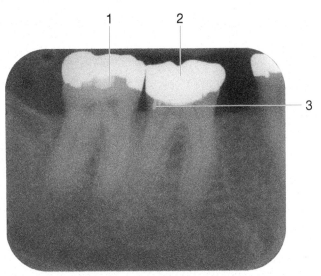

FIGURE 23–2 Dental materials. (**1**) Dental base, (**2**) amalgam, and (**3**) retention pin.

Box 23–1: Metallic and Nonmetallic Restorations

METALLIC DENTAL MATERIALS	NONMETALLIC DENTAL MATERIALS
MORE RADIOPAQUE	LESS RADIOPAQUE
Amalgam	Composite resin
Gold alloy	Glass ionomer
Stainless steel	Ceramic-porcelain
Fixed bridge clasp	Dental liner
Retention pin	Dental base
Silver point	Dental cement
Post and core	Gutta-percha
Implant	
Orthodontic band, wire, bracket	

However, because these materials can be recorded on radiographic images, it is important that they be identified and assessed. Radiographs can reveal the presence of recurrent decay, defective restoration margins that contribute to periodontal disease, and other potential problems that a clinical examination alone may not detect. It is equally important not to mistake foreign objects for pathology or other conditions requiring treatment intervention.

Identification of Common Dental Restorative Materials

- **Amalgam**

  Description: Combination of silver and other metal alloys (such as copper, tin, and zinc) used to restore

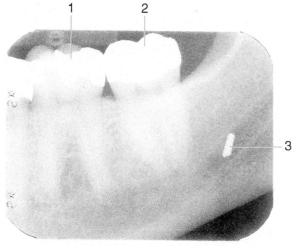

FIGURE 23–3 **Foreign objects.** (**1**) Irregular margins of amalgam, (**2**) smooth margins of full metal crown, (**3**) broken dental bur; accidentally lodged here during removal of third molar.

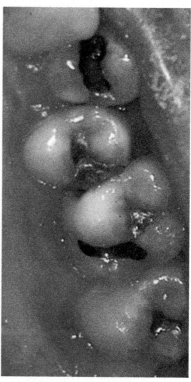

FIGURE 23–4 **Amalgam restorations.** Vary in size and shape.

function to decayed or damaged teeth. Varies in size and shape from a small pit and fissure, one-surface restoration to large expansive coverage of multiple surfaces (Figure 23–4 ■). **Amalgam** can be used to replace and build up extensive tooth destruction (core buildup) in preparation for placement of a crown.

Radiographic appearance: Most common and most easily recognized restorative material. Dense metal appears radiopaque with irregular margins and varies in size and shape and number of tooth surfaces affected. To differentiate from other metallic restorations, note that the radiopacity observed will most likely not cover the entire crown of a tooth; the less radiopaque enamel cusps will usually be visible superior to the restoration. Radiographs assist with evaluating amalgam restorations for recurrent decay and can reveal poorly contoured margins called **overhangs** (Figure 23–5 ■).

- **Composite resin**

  Description: Tooth-colored restorative material of an organic resin, usually bisphenol A-glycidyl methacrylate (BIS-GMA), with inorganic fillers such as quartz or silica that provide strength. When first introduced in the 1960s and 1970s composite resins were used mainly for esthetic restoration of anterior teeth. Composite resin is still used to provide esthetic solutions; for example, to repair a chipped anterior tooth surface or build out the mesial surfaces of central incisors to close a diastema (space). The improved strength of composite resin available today allow its

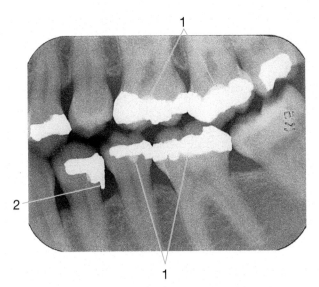

FIGURE 23–5 Irregular margins denoting amalgam restorations. Note the many shapes and sizes. (**1**) Dental base, (**2**) overhang.

use in all classifications of restorations, both anterior and posterior, and on one or multiple tooth surfaces (Figure 23–6 ■). Composite resin is also used as a bonding agent or cement in the attachment of crowns, fixed bridges, orthodontic bands, and other casting restorations (on-lays and in-lays) and as a pit and fissure sealant.

Radiographic appearance: Varies from radiolucent to slightly radiopaque. Composite resin used in older restorations or as a cement may appear radiolucent. When radiolucent, a composite resin restoration can mimic caries (see Figure 23–1). To help distinguish a composite resin restoration from caries, look for the restoration to appear to have straight margins and a prepared look, whereas the caries appears diffuse (see Figure 24–17). This radiolucent appearance can be observed apical to or under a crown or other type of dental material when composite resin is used as a dental liner or cement. A clinical examination may be needed to determine definitively whether

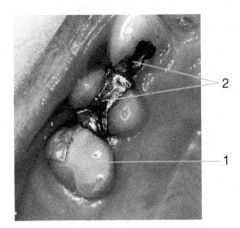

FIGURE 23–6 Composite resin (**1**) and amalgam (**2**) restorations.

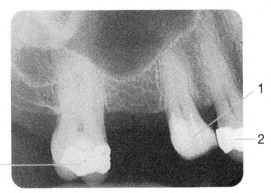

FIGURE 23–7 Composite resin restoration. (**1**) Appears slightly more radiopaque than dentin. Note the retention pins. (**2**) Amalgam restorations.

caries or composite is present. Composite resin in use today contains radiopaque fillers, aiding radiographic identification. Composite resin does not appear as radiopaque as amalgam (Figure 23–7 ■). Small restorations and small amounts of material used in pit and fissure sealants may not be recorded radiographically.

- **Glass ionomer**

Description: Tooth-colored restorative material made up of glass and ceramic particles and a polyacrylic acid, commonly used in dental cement (Figure 23–8 ■). Glass ionomer is used as a dental liner (applied to a cavity preparation to protect the pulp), as a dental cement, and as a pit and fissure sealant. The incorporation of a small amount of resin or a metal alloy has improved the strength of glass ionomer allowing its use as a dental restoration and in place of amalgam as a core buildup prior to the attachment of a crown.

Radiographic appearance: Can appear more distinctly radiopaque than composite resin due to an addition of a metal alloy used to reinforce the material; however, composite resin and glass ionomer are more often indistinguishable from one another radiographically. Glass ionomer is observed radiographically as a restoration on a tooth surface, and when used as a dental liner or cement, appearing as a distinct radiopacity under another restorative material such as an amalgam or crown (see Figures 23–1 and 23–5).

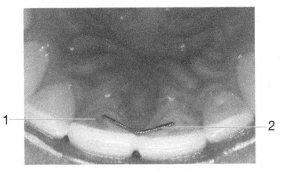

FIGURE 23–8 Cement and orthodontic materials. (**1**) Glass ionomer bonding, and (**2**) orthodontic wire.

- **Crown (full metal)**

  Description: A metal **crown** is the recommended restorative treatment when natural tooth structure is severely broken down and/or when a restoration with significant strength is needed. Depending on the metal alloy used, a full metal crown will appear gold or silver in color, making its use more common for the restoration of posterior teeth where esthetics are not a concern (Figure 23–9 ■). Occasionally a full metal crown is placed on an anterior tooth when a patient desires this appearance.

  Radiographic appearance: Appears radiopaque and is distinguished from amalgam by smooth margins. Whereas the natural tooth cusps will be observed in the presence of a large, multisurface amalgam restoration, a full metal crown replaces or covers the entire crown of a tooth and will be contoured to resemble the shape of the cusps (see Figure 23–3).

- **Crown (porcelain-fused-to-metal: PFM)**

  Description: A layer of tooth-colored ceramic-porcelain combination material is applied to a metal shell to achieve an esthetically pleasing restoration while retaining strength (see Figure 23–9). While desirable for use in restoring anterior teeth, PFM crowns work equally well at restoring posterior teeth.

  Radiographic appearance: The metal core of a PFM crown appears radiopaque, whereas the porcelain appears less radiopaque. The radiopaque shape of the metal shell will appear more rounded than a full metal crown and will not appear to be contoured to resemble the anatomic shape of the cusps of a tooth. The less radiopaque porcelain will outline the shape of the cusps (Figure 23–10 ■).

- **Crown (ceramic-porcelain)**

  Description: A full or three-quarter coverage crown fabricated entirely from a ceramic or porcelain material without a metal shell.

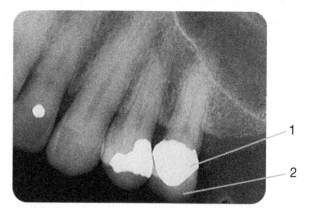

FIGURE 23–10 **PFM crown.** (**1**) Radiopaque metal shell, (**2**) less radiopaque ceramic porcelain outlining shape of anatomic crown.

  Radiographic appearance: Appears less radiopaque than a crown fabricated with a metal shell. The porcelain material will appear to be about the same radiopacity as dentin. An outline of the prepared tooth may be detected under the slightly see-through ceramic-porcelain material (see Figure 23–1).

- **Crown (stainless steel)**

  Description: A provisional, prefabricated metal shell used as a temporary restoration for a tooth that has been prepared to receive a permanent casting (fabricated outside the mouth by a dental laboratory) if esthetics is not a concern. May be used to restore a primary tooth until it is exfoliated.

  Radiographic appearance: As a temporary restoration, this metal is less dense and will allow the passage of more x-rays, giving the material a "see-through" appearance. These crowns are prefabricated and intended to be temporary, so they do not appear to fit the tooth very well (Figure 23–11 ■).

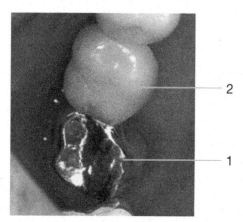

FIGURE 23–9 **Crown restorations.** (**1**) Full metal crown, and (**2**) PFM crown.

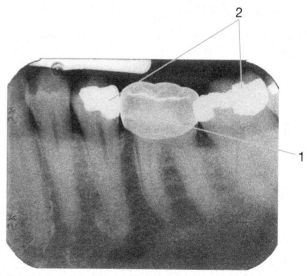

FIGURE 23–11 **Stainless steel crown.** (**1**) Note the "see-through" appearance. (**2**) Amalgam restorations.

- **Fixed bridge**

  Description: A combination of crowns and pontic(s) that when joined provide functional replacement for a lost or missing tooth or multiple teeth; may be constructed entirely of metal or a combination of porcelain fused to metal (Figure 23–12 ■). A **Maryland bridge** consists of a pontic with one or two metal clasps or wings on one or both sides that are cemented or bonded to adjacent natural teeth.

  Radiographic appearance: Full metal and PFM crowns on the abutment teeth will appear as previously described. The size and shape of the pontic(s) may vary depending on the functional needs of the space to be restored. For example, a three-unit bridge consisting of two abutments and one pontic may be used to replace not one, but two missing teeth. In this example the size of the pontic is fashioned to fit the space, and may not necessarily be an exact replication of the missing natural tooth (see Figure 23–12). A resin-bonded Maryland fixed bridge can be identified by the presence of radiopaque metal clasps or wings; a bonding agent used to cement the bridge in place may be recorded.

- **Retention pin**

  Description: A metal pin used to support a restoration; especially useful when tooth destruction is extensive or decay has undermined, or weakened a posterior tooth cusp or an anterior tooth incisal edge. A **retention pin** is partially inserted into the dentin. A restoration is then placed over the extension of the retention pin. Retention pins come in various sizes and diameters.

  Radiographic appearance: Retention pins appear radiopaque in an easily identified shape (Figure 23–13 ■; also see Figure 23–2). Because another restorative

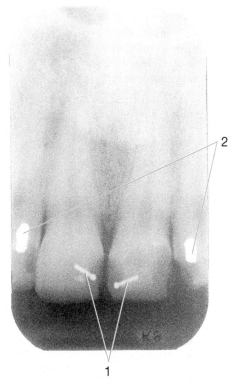

FIGURE 23–13 Retention pins. (1) Radiopaque pins help retain radiolucent composite resin restorations. **(2)** Radiopaque amalgam restorations.

material such as amalgam, composite resin, or a crown will be placed over the retention pin, it may be only partially recorded on a radiograph. Depending on the angle of the x-ray beam, a retention pin may be recorded on one radiograph and not on an adjacent image. It should be noted that retention pins will only be located in dentin and will not be observed penetrating the pulp. A retention pin should not be confused with a post and core restoration, which penetrates the pulp chamber and is only observed in conjunction with an endodontic filling material. These materials are described later.

- **Dental liners, bases, and cements**

  Description: In addition to composite resin and glass ionomer, other materials such as calcium hydroxide and zinc oxide-eugenol are utilized as intermediate restorations, cavity liners, bases, and cements. These materials are placed into a cavity preparation, when needed, to help limit sensitivity and to insulate and protect a tooth's pulp; and can be used to adhere crowns and orthodontic wires to a prepared tooth surface.

  Radiographic appearance: Because another restorative material such as an amalgam or composite will be placed over the dental liner, base, or cement, it may not be recorded on the radiograph. When recorded, these materials will appear slightly more radiopaque than the surrounding dentin (see Figures 23–1 and 23–5).

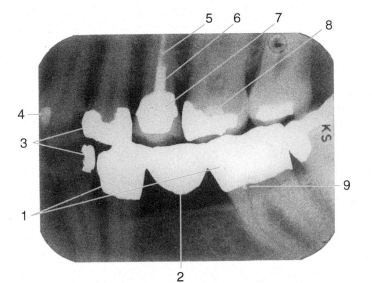

FIGURE 23–12 Fixed bridge. (1) Full metal crowns form bridge abutments, **(2)** metal pontic, **(3)** amalgam, **(4)** composite resin, **(5)** gutta-percha, **(6)** post and core, **(7)** PFM crown, **(8)** base material, **(9)** retention pin.

- **Endodontic filling material**

  Description: Gutta-percha, an organic material, is used to fill root canals following a pulpectomy (root canal therapy) in which the entire pulp structure is removed from a tooth. Root canals are further sealed with the use of a glass ionomer or zinc-oxide eugenol sealer. Occasionally a root canal will need a filling placed at the apex. Gutta-percha, or other restorative materials including amalgam and composite resins, can be used to seal the root canal.

  Radiographic appearance: A gutta-percha filled root canal will appear radiopaque (Figure 23–14 ■). A pulpal radiopacity resembling that of a metallic material indicates the root canal filling material is a **silver point** (see Figure 23–1). Silver points are no longer recommended as an endodontic filler, but may be observed in teeth treated prior to its discontinuation. A small radiopacity at the root apex indicates the use of amalgam or a composite resin that was placed as a retrograde restoration in response to an incomplete gutta-percha seal.

- **Post and core**

  Description: An amalgam or glass ionomer core buildup of an extensively damaged tooth may not be able to provide sufficient strength to support placement of a crown. If a tooth has undergone successful endodontic therapy, then a prefabricated or custom-made post may be used to supplement the buildup. The metal post is partially inserted and cemented into an endodontically treated root canal. The core buildup is placed on that portion of the core that extends beyond the height of the canal.

  Radiographic appearance: Prefabricated and custom-made posts appear radiopaque. The post is inserted and cemented into a pulp chamber, so the presence of endodontic filler will be observed. An important distinction when determining the difference between a **post and core** and a retention pin is location; a post penetrates a pulp root canal whereas a retention pin penetrates dentin only. Additionally, a post and core restoration can be distinguished from a retention pin by its significantly larger size (Figure 23–15 ■; also see Figure 23–2).

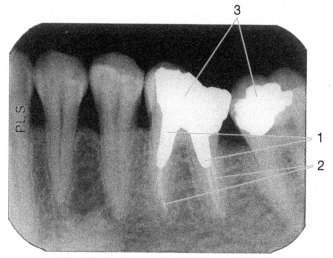

FIGURE 23–15 **Post and core.** (**1**) Post and core within the root canals, (**2**) gutta percha, and (**3**) amalgam restorations.

- **Implant**

  Description: Titanium screw or post surgically inserted into the dental arches for the purpose of providing a base upon which to secure a restorative treatment such as a crown or fixed bridge to replace missing or lost dentition.

  Radiographic appearance: Appears as a distinct radiopacity. To distinguish an implant from all other dental restorative materials, note its presence within the bone in an area of a missing tooth (Figure 23–16 ■).

- **Orthodontic and surgical materials**

  Description: Most orthodontic and surgical materials are fabricated using stainless steel, titanium, ceramic, or a composite material. Bonding agents used include previously listed cements and glass ionomers.

  Radiographic appearance: Metal orthodontic bands, wires, and brackets; and surgical wires, pins, and screws all appear as distinctly shaped radiopacities (Figures 23–17 ■ and 23–18 ■).

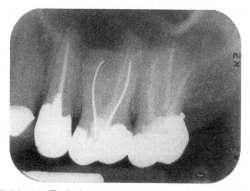

FIGURE 23–14 **Endodontic treatment.** Gutta-percha filled root canals.

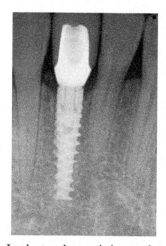

FIGURE 23–16 Implant replaces missing tooth root structure.

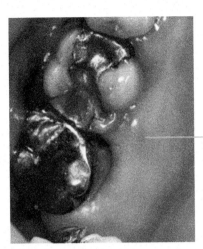

FIGURE 23–19 **Amalgam tattoo.**

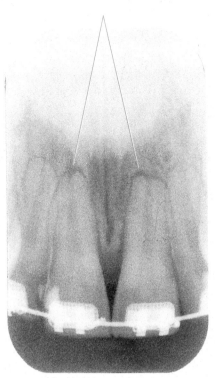

FIGURE 23–17 **Orthodontic appliance.** Note the root-end external resorption likely in response to orthodontic intervention.

Identification of Foreign Objects

- **Amalgam fragments**

  Description: Amalgam fragments may become harmlessly imbedded in soft tissue during placement or removal of a restoration, or during an extraction of a

tooth with an amalgam restoration present. Depending on the size of the fragment and where it becomes imbedded, an **amalgam tattoo** may result. An amalgam tattoo is the name given to the bluish-purple color of the soft tissue that covers the fragment (Figure 23–19 ■).

Radiographic appearance: Often found in edentulous areas of the mandible, fragments of amalgam appear radiopaque (Figure 23–20 ■).

- **Other foreign objects**

  Description: Foreign objects detected by radiographs should be differentiated from radiographic artifacts. A recording of a patient's eyeglasses that were accidentally positioned within the path of the x-ray beam during exposure is an artifact, an image that does not contribute to a diagnosis of a condition. Radiographic examination of dental materials can assist with detecting recurrent decay, periodontal disease, failure and the need for replacement or repair of the restorative treatment, among other conditions that a clinical

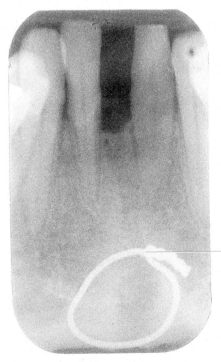

FIGURE 23–18 **Surgical wire.** Used to treat a fractured mandible.

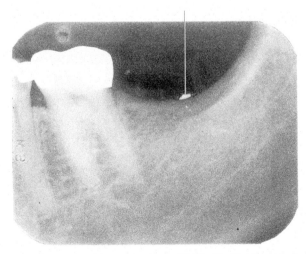

FIGURE 23–20 **Amalgam fragment.** Embedded in the soft tissue during extraction.

examination alone may miss. Radiographs also reveal the presence of other foreign objects that result from accidental or intentional trauma. Consider the following examples: a broken root tip that migrates into the maxillary sinus; a metal object that penetrates a tooth during mastication; dental material that becomes entrapped in an extraction site.

Radiographic appearance: The radiopacity of the foreign object will depend on its density. Note the radiopaque broken dental instrument in Figure 23–3.

REVIEW—Chapter summary

A dental assistant and dental hygienist should develop interpretation skills to recognize deviations from normal radiographic anatomy. The most common foreign objects recorded by dental radiographic images will most likely be dental restorative materials. Interpretation of radiographic findings is enhanced when a patient is present. Radiographs represent a two-dimensional image of three-dimensional objects resulting in superimposition that can make it difficult to definitively identify the type, size, number, and location of restorations. Some restorations can be differentiated by relative degree of radiopacity or radiolucency; others are better identified by size and contour or by location on a tooth. Aesthetic restorative materials may appear radiopaque or radiolucent.

Amalgam is easily recognized radiographically, appearing radiopaque with irregular margins. Radiographs assist with evaluating amalgam restorations for recurrent decay and overhangs. Composite resin and glass ionomer do not appear as radiopaque as amalgam and can vary in degree of radiopacity. Composite resin used in older restorations or as a cement may appear radiolucent. To help distinguish from caries, look for the restoration to appear to have straight margins and a prepared look, whereas caries appears diffuse.

Full metal crowns appear radiopaque and are distinguished from amalgam by smooth margins. The radiopaque metal shell of a PFM crown appears more rounded than a full metal crown with the less radiopaque porcelain outlining the shape of cusps. A ceramic-porcelain crown lacks the metal shell of full and PFM crowns, and will appear the same radiopacity as dentin. Prefabricated stainless steel crowns present with a "see-through" appearance and do not appear to fit the tooth very well. A fixed bridge consists of abutment teeth restored with crowns attached to one or more pontics. The size and shape of the pontic(s) varies depending on the functional needs of the space to be restored. A resin-bonded Maryland fixed bridge can be identified by the presence of radiopaque metal clasps or wings; a bonding agent used to cement the bridge in place may be recorded.

Retention pins, inserted into dentin, appear radiopaque in an easily identified shape. A retention pin should not be confused with a post and core restoration, which penetrates the pulp chamber and is only observed in conjunction with an endodontic filling material. Dental liners, bases, and cements appear slightly more radiopaque than the surrounding dentin. A gutta-percha filled root canal will appear less radiopaque than a root canal filled with a silver point. Implants, orthodontic, and surgical materials appear as distinct radiopacities based on shape.

Amalgam fragments imbedded in soft tissue appear radiopaque. Depending on the size of the fragment and where it becomes imbedded, an amalgam tattoo may result. Radiographs also reveal the presence of other foreign objects that result from accidental or intentional trauma.

RECALL—Study questions

1. Recurrent decay detected on a radiograph is classified as a foreign body *because* a foreign body represents alterations to normal oral maxillofacial anatomy.
   a. Both the statement and reason are correct and related.
   b. Both the statement and reason are correct but NOT related.
   c. The statement is correct, but the reason is NOT.
   d. The statement is NOT correct, but the reason is correct.
   e. NEITHER the statement NOR the reason is correct.

2. A radiographic image of a dental restoration aids in each of the following EXCEPT one. Which is the EXCEPTION?
   a. evaluating margins for defects.
   b. determining presence of recurrent decay.
   c. identifying tooth surface location.
   d. detecting an overhang.

3. It can be difficult to definitively identify type and size of a restoration recorded on a radiograph *because* radiographs represent a two-dimensional image of three-dimensional objects.
   a. Both the statement and reason are correct and related.
   b. Both the statement and reason are correct but NOT related.
   c. The statement is correct, but the reason is NOT.
   d. The statement is NOT correct, but the reason is correct.
   e. NEITHER the statement NOR the reason is correct.

4. Which of these appears the least radiopaque?
   a. Full metal crown
   b. Composite resin
   c. Post and core
   d. Implant

5. Which of these foreign objects recorded by dental radiographs would NOT have been placed iatrogenically?
   a. Amalgam tattoo
   b. Composite resin
   c. PFM crown
   d. Fixed bridge

6. Amalgam and a full metal crown can be distinguished from each other radiographically by
   a. degree of radiopacity.
   b. shape and margins.
   c. location in the mouth.
   d. use of retention pins.

7. Which of these dental restorative materials is most likely to mimic decay radiographically?
   a. Gold alloy
   b. Stainless steel
   c. Amalgam
   d. Composite resin

8. Glass ionomer and composite resin restorations can be distinguished from each other radiographically by margin shape.
   Composite resin restorations appear to have irregular margins.
   a. The first statement is true. The second statement is false.
   b. The first statement is false. The second statement is true.
   c. Both statements are true.
   d. Both statements are false.

9. Which of the following is least likely to be detected radiographically?
   a. Gutta-percha endodontic filling
   b. Ceramic-porcelain crown
   c. Glass ionomer sealant
   d. Composite resin restoration

10. A full metal crown appears radiographically as a rounded radiopacity that does not outline the anatomic shape of tooth cusps.
    A PFM crown presents a "see-through" radiopacity and does not appear to fit the tooth very well.
    a. The first statement is true. The second statement is false.
    b. The first statement is false. The second statement is true.
    c. Both statements are true.
    d. Both statements are false.

11. Each of these uses of dental materials will appear about the same radiopacity as dentin EXCEPT one. Which one is the EXCEPTION?
    a. Post
    b. Cement
    c. Liner
    d. Base

12. Which of the following would NOT be observed within the pulp?
    a. Retention pin
    b. Post and core
    c. Gutta-percha
    d. Silver point

13. Radiographs can detect amalgam fragments in oral soft tissue *because* the soft tissue in the location of the fragment may exhibit an amalgam tattoo.
    a. Both the statement and reason are correct and related.
    b. Both the statement and reason are correct but NOT related.
    c. The statement is correct, but the reason is NOT.
    d. The statement is NOT correct, but the reason is correct.
    e. NEITHER the statement NOR the reason is correct.

REFLECT—Case study

As technology and science advance, dental materials will continue to improve, providing oral health care professionals with a myriad of options for treating patients. Developments in composition and chemical properties are increasing the versatility of many dental materials, making radiographic detection and identification of these materials challenging. To improve radiographic interpretation skills, obtain a dental materials book for an in-depth study of the types of materials available, and how and where these materials are most likely to be used.

RELATE—Laboratory application

For a comprehensive laboratory practice exercise on this topic, see Thomson, E. M., & Bruhn, A. M. (2018). *Exercises in oral radiography techniques: A laboratory manual* (4th ed.). Hoboken, NJ: Pearson. Chapter 14, "Radiographic interpretation."

RESOURCES

American Association of Endodontists. (2013, April). AAE Position Statement. *Use of Silver Points.* Accessed from AAE website: https://www.aae.org/uploadedfiles/publications_and_research/guidelines_and_position_statements/silverpointsstatement.pdf.

Bird, D. L., & Robinson, D. S. (2015). Dental materials. *Modern Dental Assisting* (11th ed.). St. Louis, MO: Elsevier.

Hatrick, C. D., Eakle, W. S., & Bird, W. F. (2010). *Dental materials: Clinical applications for dental assistants and dental hygienists* (2nd ed.). St. Louis, MO: Elsevier.

Langlais, R. P. (2003). *Exercises in oral radiology and interpretation* (4th ed.). Philadelphia: Saunders.

Visit www.pearsonhighered.com/healthprofessionsresources to access the student resources that accompany this book. Simply select Dental Hygiene from the choice of disciplines. Find this book and you will find the complementary study tools created for this specific title.

24

The Use of Radiographs in the Detection of Dental Caries

CHAPTER OUTLINE

OBJECTIVES

Following successful completion of this chapter, you should be able to:

1. Define the key terms.
2. Explain why caries appear radiolucent on radiographs.
3. Define the role radiographs play in detecting caries.
4. Identify the ideal type of projection and technique factors that enhance a radiograph's ability to image caries.
5. List and describe the four categories of the caries depth grading system.
6. Describe the radiographic appearance of proximal surface caries.
7. Describe the radiographic appearance of occlusal surface caries.
8. Describe the radiographic appearance of buccal/lingual surface caries.
9. Describe the radiographic appearance of cemental/root surface caries.
10. Describe the radiographic appearance of recurrent and rampant caries.
11. Explain the importance of radiographically monitoring arrested caries.
12. Identify conditions that resemble dental caries radiographically and discuss how to distinguish these from caries.

KEY TERMS

Cementoenamel junction (CEJ)
Cervical burnout
Dentinoenamel junction (DEJ)
Mach band effect

Introduction

The detection of caries is probably the most common reason for exposing dental radiographs, especially bitewings. Dental hygienists and dental assistants who are skilled in identifying normal radiographic anatomy should be able to differentiate between the appearance of normal tooth structures and dental caries on a radiograph. This chapter describes the radiographic appearance of dental caries, presents a caries depth grading system, and offers tips for developing interpretation skills needed to identify the various stages of the caries process.

Detection of Dental Caries

Dental caries, or tooth decay, refers to a pathological process consisting of localized destruction of dental hard tissues by organic acids produced by microorganisms. The caries process is one of demineralization of tooth structure (enamel, dentin, cementum). This demineralization of tooth density allows more x-rays to pass through the tooth and darken the image. It is because of this that caries appear radiolucent on a radiograph (Figure 24–1 ■). The decalcification process requires 40 to 50 percent loss of calcium and phosphorus before the decreased density can be recorded by a radiograph. For this reason, the depth of penetration of a carious lesion is deeper clinically than it appears on a radiograph. Also, because the proximal surfaces of posterior teeth are broad, the loss of small amounts of mineral from incipient lesions may be difficult to detect on a radiograph (Figure 24–2 ■).

Even with these limitations, radiographs reveal carious lesions that may go undetected clinically, especially caries on the proximal surfaces, where teeth contact each other. To maximize their diagnostic ability, precisely expose and meticulously process all radiographs. Incorrect vertical or horizontal angulation will prevent a radiograph from imaging caries (Figure 24–3 ■). Achieving correct horizontal angulation is particularly important. Overlapping of the contact areas between the teeth will make it impossible to detect caries in these areas (Figure 24–4 ■).

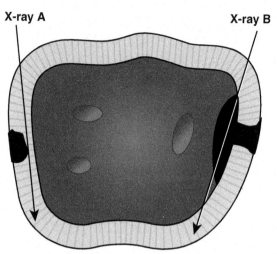

FIGURE 24–2 Ratio of caries to enamel. X-ray **(A)** passes through a small ratio of caries to enamel, making caries difficult to detect. X-ray **(B)** passes through a large ratio of caries to enamel, making caries detection easier.

Although bitewing radiographs are those of choice for the evaluation of caries due to the precise parallelism established between the tooth and the plane of the image receptor, a precisely placed periapical radiograph exposed using the paralleling technique will adequately image dental caries (Figure 24–5 ■). Although exposure factors (mA, kV, and exposure time) used will depend on the patient and the area to be recorded, some practitioners prefer to use a lower kV setting to image caries. A low kV setting produces a high-contrast image: black and white with few shades of gray in between. Because caries appear radiolucent against a radiopaque enamel (or lesser radiopaque dentin), in theory, a high-contrast image might be preferred for caries detection. However, research indicates that both low- and high-contrast images allow for adequate caries detection. More important than the kV setting is to produce radiographs that are free of angulation errors.

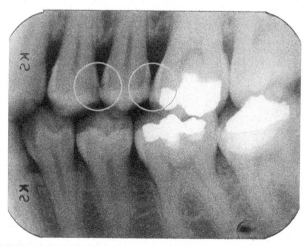

FIGURE 24–1 Proximal surface caries. Detected at the contact areas between adjacent teeth.

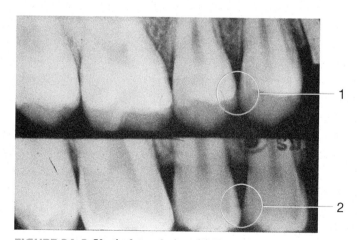

FIGURE 24–3 Vertical angulation. (1) Excessive vertical angulation prevents viewing these proximal surface carious lesions. **(2)** Correct vertical angulation reveals the proximal surface caries. Note the difference in alveolar bone crest heights between the two radiographs indicating a change in the vertical angulation.

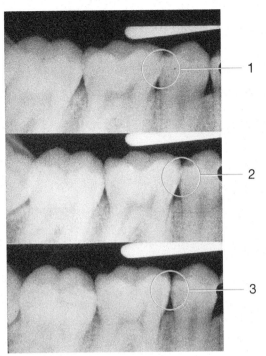

FIGURE 24–4 **Horizontal angulation.** (**1**) Incorrect horizontal angulation causes overlapping between adjacent teeth, which prevents viewing for interproximal caries. (**2**) Improved horizontal angulation, but caries difficult to view. (**3**) Correct horizontal angulation clearly images caries.

Classification of the Radiographic Appearance of Caries

To provide a framework upon which to build skills necessary for caries interpretation it is helpful to organize the caries process. Several systems are used to grade the depth of penetration of caries. A grading system suggested by Haugejorden and Slack is presented here (Figure 24–6 ▪). The advantage of this system is that it allows for accurate grading of the penetration of caries (establishes a baseline) and tracking of the progression and/or remineralization of

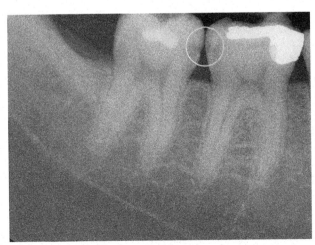

FIGURE 24–5 **Periapical radiograph records proximal surface caries.**

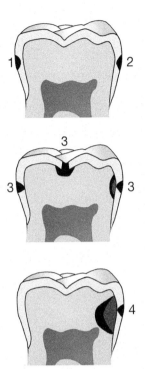

FIGURE 24–6 **Classification of dental caries recommended by Haugejorden and Slack.** (**1**) **C-1 Incipient Caries.** Penetrates less than halfway through enamel. (**2**) **C-2 Moderate Caries.** Penetrates more than halfway through enamel. (**3**) **C-3 Advanced Caries.** Penetrates DEJ, but less than halfway through dentin toward pulp. (**4**) **C-4 Severe Caries.** Penetrates more than halfway through dentin toward pulp.

the carious lesions at future appointments. These grades may also be called incipient, moderate, advanced, and severe.

- **C-1: Enamel caries**, also called incipient caries (meaning the first stage of existence), penetrates less than halfway through the enamel of the tooth toward the **dentinoenamel junction (DEJ)** (see Figure 24–6[1]).
- **C-2: Moderate caries** penetrates over halfway through the enamel toward the DEJ, but does not reach the DEJ. Moderate caries involves the enamel only (see Figure 24–6[2]).
- **C-3: Advanced caries** penetrates through the DEJ, but less than halfway through the dentin toward the pulp (see Figure 24–6[3]). Advanced caries invades both enamel and dentin.
- **C-4: Severe caries** penetrates over halfway through the dentin toward the pulp (see Figure 24–6[4]).

Caries can be further organized according to affected tooth surface: proximal (mesial and distal), occlusal, buccal or lingual, cemental (root surface); and may be categorized as recurrent, rampant, or arrested. Radiographs are most useful in detecting proximal surface caries. Occlusal, buccal/lingual, and cemental caries are more readily detected clinically. In fact, incipient and moderate occlusal, buccal/lingual, and cemental caries often do not show up on radiographs, even though these may be detected clinically. Advanced and severe occlusal, buccal/lingual, and cemental caries will appear radiographically, so it is important to recognize these (Table 24–1 ■).

Proximal Caries

Proximal surface caries, sometimes referred to as interproximal caries, are located on the mesial and distal tooth surfaces that contact adjacent teeth. Proximal surfaces are almost impossible to examine clinically, making radiographs vitally important in detecting caries in these areas. When examining a radiograph, check the mesial and distal tooth surfaces for caries at the points of contact between the teeth. Expand the examination of these points of contact apical to the estimated height of the gingival margin (Figure 24–7 ■). The location of the height of the gingival margin, which is soft tissue, is not recorded on a radiograph so estimate the gingival margin location based on where the alveolar bone crest height is recorded. Assume that the gingival margin will be located at least 1 mm above the level of bone imaged on a radiograph.

The shape of proximal caries begins as a radiolucent notch on the enamel (see Figure 24–6[1]). As demineralization of enamel progresses, caries take on a triangular shape (like a pyramid) with the apex pointing toward the DEJ and the base toward the outer surface of the tooth (see Figure 24–6[2]). At the DEJ the caries spread, undermining normal enamel, and again taking on a triangular shape as penetration continues toward the pulp (see Figure 24–6[3]). The base of this second triangle spreads along the DEJ and the apex points toward the pulp (see Figure 24–6[4]).

Occlusal Caries

Occlusal caries are located on the chewing surface of the posterior teeth. Because of the superimposition of the buccal and lingual cusps, incipient and moderate occlusal caries that are detected clinically may not be recorded on a radiograph (Figure 24–8 ■; also see Figure 24–6[3]).

Once penetration reaches the DEJ, advanced occlusal caries may be recorded on a radiograph (Figures 24–9 ■ and 24–10 ■). At the DEJ, occlusal caries will appear as a flat radiolucent line. Often no or little change is detected

Table 24–1 Radiographic Appearance of Caries

Grade	Severity	Proximal	Occlusal	Buccal/Lingual	Cemental
C-1	Incipient	Radiolucent notch less than halfway through enamel	Not evident radiographically	Not evident radiographically	Not applicable
C-2	Moderate	Radiolucent triangle, apex pointing toward DEJ, more than halfway through enamel, but does not invade DEJ	Not evident radiographically	Not evident radiographically	Not applicable
C-3	Advanced	Radiolucent double triangle, first triangle through enamel apex pointing toward DEJ; second triangle base spreading along DEJ, apex pointing toward pulp; radiolucency is less than halfway through dentin toward pulp	Flat radiolucent line, often with no or little change detected in enamel; radiolucency is less than halfway through dentin toward pulp	Not possible to distinguish advanced from severe; both appear as round radiolucency in middle of tooth with well-defined borders	Ill-defined, cresent-shaped radiolucency below CEJ; bone loss must be evident
C-4	Severe	Radiolucency may retain double triangle shape, or be so severe as to appear as large diffuse radiolucency more than halfway through dentin toward pulp	Large radiolucency detected in dentin below occlusal enamel; depending on extent of destruction, radiolucent breaks in occlusal enamel may be recorded; radiolucency is more than halfway through dentin toward pulp	Not possible to distinguish advanced from severe; both appear as round radiolucency in middle of tooth with well-defined borders	Ill-defined, crescent-shaped radiolucency below CEJ; bone loss must be evident

DEJ: dentinoenamel junction; CEJ: cementoenamel junction

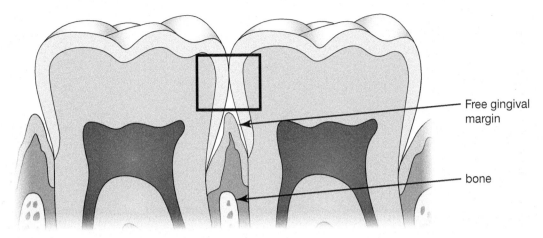

FIGURE 24–7 Area to examine for interproximal caries. View the area where two adjacent teeth contact, and apical down to where the gingival margin would most likely be (boxed area). Avoid mistaking caries in the region apical to the gingival margin, where the optical illusion cervical burnout is most likely to appear.

in the enamel radiographically at this stage. As demineralization progresses, the size of the radiolucency increases. It is important to note that when examining radiographs for occlusal caries, the area of interest is below the occlusal enamel, in the area of the dentin, and not from the top of the tooth. Changes (radiolucencies) in the dentin below the

occlusal enamel are indicative of occlusal caries. The irregularity of the cusps and occlusal surface pits and fissures do not usually indicate the presence of caries radiographically. As advanced caries progress to a severe stage, changes in the occlusal enamel are more likely to be recorded as the crown of the tooth breaks down.

Buccal and Lingual Caries

Buccal caries involves the buccal or facial surface of a tooth, and lingual caries involves the lingual surface (Figure 24–11 ■). Buccal and lingual caries are best detected clinically; early buccal and lingual carious lesions are almost impossible to detect radiographically. This is due to the superimposition of the normal tooth structures over the caries. As the demineralization becomes severe, caries appears as a radiolucency characterized by well-defined borders, often described as looking into a hole on

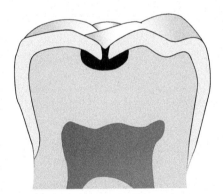

FIGURE 24–8 Early stages of occlusal caries. Early occlusal caries extend along the DEJ and may not be recorded on a radiograph, even though the lesion may be detected clinically.

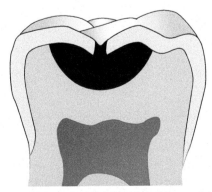

FIGURE 24–9 Advanced occlusal caries. Advanced (up to halfway toward the pulp) or severe occlusal caries (more than halfway toward the pulp) will most likely be recorded on a radiograph.

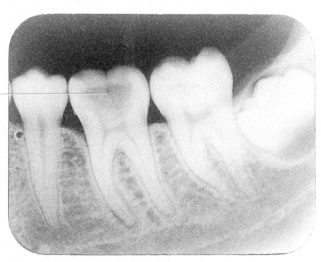

FIGURE 24–10 Severe occlusal caries. Large radiolucent lesion indicating caries of the first molar.

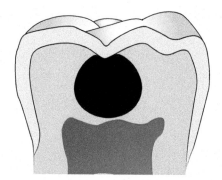

FIGURE 24–11 **Buccal or lingual caries.** Advanced buccal or lingual caries have well-defined borders.

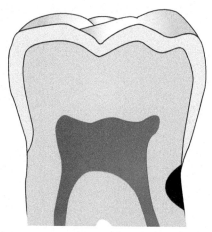

FIGURE 24–13 **Cemental (root) caries.** Gingival recession and bone loss precede the demineraliztion process to expose the root surfaces.

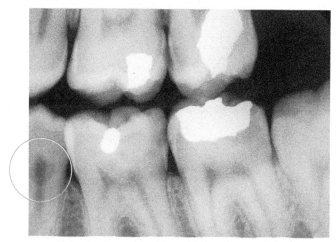

FIGURE 24–12 **Buccal or lingual caries.** Round radiolucency superimposed over the pulp chamber indicating caries of the second premolar.

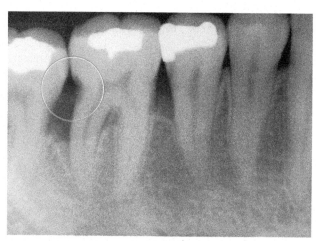

FIGURE 24–14 **Cemental (root) caries.** Large radiolucency indicating caries on the distal surface of the first molar. Note the bone loss exposing the root surface.

the radiograph (Figure 24–12 ■). It is impossible to tell the depth of buccal or lingual caries or the relationship to the pulpal tissue, because a radiograph is a two-dimensional image of three-dimensional structures.

Cemental (Root) Caries

Cemental caries (also known as root caries) develop between the enamel border and the free gingival margin on the cemental surface (Figure 24–13 ■). Bone loss and recession of the gingival tissue are necessary for the caries process to start on the root surfaces. Cemental caries may appear on the buccal, lingual, mesial, or distal surface of the tooth.

Radiographically, cemental caries appear as ill-defined, crescent-shaped radiolucencies just below the **cemento-enamel junction (CEJ)** (Figure 24–14 ■). Cemental caries may at times be misinterpreted as cervical burnout (discussed later in this chapter), an optical illusion of the radiographic image. Cemental caries are more easily detected clinically than radiographically.

Recurrent (Secondary) Caries

Recurrent or secondary caries is decay that occurs under a restoration or around its margins. Recurrent caries often occur because of poor cavity preparation, defective margins

of the restoration, or incomplete removal of caries prior to placement of a restoration. Recurrent caries appear radiographically as radiolucencies at the margins of restorations (Figure 24–15 ■).

Rampant Caries

Rampant caries are severe, unchecked, rapidly progressing caries that affect multiple teeth (Figure 24–16 ■).

Arrested Caries

Arrested caries are those caries that are no longer active. Carious lesions may become arrested if there is a significant shift in the oral environment from factors that cause caries to those that slow the caries process. Additionally, incipient enamel caries can remain dormant for long periods of time. Some carious lesions may even be reversed by remineralization. It is important that radiographic exams continue to monitor arrested caries to watch for changes.

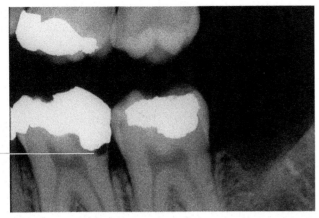

FIGURE 24–15 Recurrent caries. Radiolucency indicating caries adjacent to a metallic restoration.

Conditions Resembling Caries

A systematic approach to interpreting radiographs for caries should include an awareness of conditions that may mimic the appearance of caries (Procedure 24–1). Three conditions that resemble caries radiographically are the presence of nonmetallic restorations, cervical burnout, and the mach band effect.

Nonmetallic Restorations

Nonmetallic esthetic restorations may mimic decay radiographically (Figure 24–17 ■). Due to their radiolucent appearance, nonmetallic restorations such as composite, silicate, and acrylic resins may mimic decay (see Chapter 23). To aid in distinguishing a restoration from caries, look for

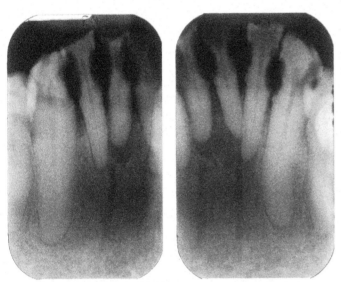

FIGURE 24–16 Rampant caries. Multiple radiolucencies indicating severe cemental caries.

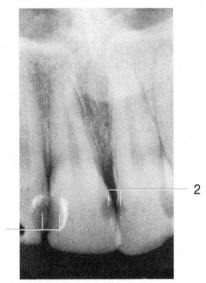

FIGURE 24–17 Nonmetalic restorations and caries. (1) Radiolucent nonmetallic restorations. Note radiopaque base or cavity liner. **(2)** Radiolucencies indicating caries.

Procedure 24–1

Radiographic interpretation for caries

See Procedure 20–1, Suggested sequence for viewing a full mouth series of radiographic images.

1. View all surfaces of each tooth.
2. Examine the contact points and the area just apical to the estimated gingival margin for radiolucencies indicating proximal caries.
3. Examine the dentin just apical to the occlusal enamel for radiolucencies indicating occlusal caries.
4. Examine the dentin in the middle of the tooth for a round radiolucency indicating buccal/facial or lingual caries.
5. If there is bone loss and evidence that cementum is exposed in the oral cavity, examine the cervical region of the tooth for an ill-defined, radiolucent crescent shape below the CEJ indicating cemental caries.
6. Examine existing restorations for recurrent decay.
7. Confirm findings and/or clarify uncertain interpretations with a clinical examination of the patient.
8. Consult the patient's chart for confirmation or clarification of findings as needed.
9. Present a preliminary interpretation for dentist's review.
10. Following confirmation by dentist, document findings on the patient's permanent record.

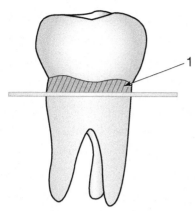

FIGURE 24–18 **Cervical burnout.** (**1**) Thin cervical root surface between dense crown and alveolar bone crest allows more x-rays to pass and reach the image receptor, producing an increased radiolucency.

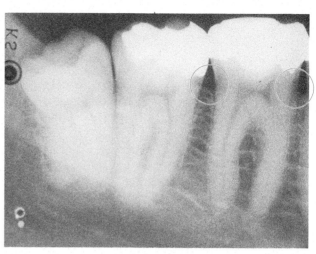

FIGURE 24–19 **Cervical burnout.** Note the radiolucent optical illusion of cervical burnout on the mesials and distals between the enamel and restorations and the alveolar crest of bone.

a restoration to have straight borders, or a prepared look, with an overall even radiolucency. A radiopaque base material may also be present under a radiolucent nonmetallic restoration. Caries tend to have more diffuse borders and uneven radiolucencies that take on a triangular shape, with the apex pointing toward the DEJ or pulp. A clinical examination may be required to make a final determination.

Cervical Burnout

Cervical burnout is an optical illusion created when the eye must distinguish between a very light (white) area and a very dark (black) area on the radiograph. The area of the tooth most likely to produce this optical illusion is the cervical root, or neck of the tooth. In this region, the concavity of the root surfaces allows greater penetration by x-rays (Figure 24–18 ◼). This area will appear especially dark next to radiopaque structures. When the radiopaque enamel on one side and the radiopaque lamina dura on the other side sandwich the radiolucent cervical of the tooth in between, the effect is an increased darkness called cervical burnout. Cervical burnout often appears as an irregularly shaped radiolucent area with a fuzzy outline seen on the mesial and/or distal surfaces of a tooth along the cervical line (Figure 24–19 ◼). To assist in distinguishing cervical burnout from caries, remember to focus caries detection only in the area of the contact points of adjacent teeth and apical to the estimated gingival margin (see Figure 24–7). Cervical burnout appears more apical, placing it in a position estimated to be under the gingival margin.

Mach Band Effect

Another optical illusion is a radiolucency caused by overlapping of the proximal surfaces of the teeth. When two proximal surfaces overlap (caused either by natural overlap

of misaligned teeth or by incorrect horizontal angulation of the x-ray beam), the result is a dense radiopacity outlined by radiolucent lines. These radiolucent lines represent an optical illusion called the **mach band effect**, resulting from the high contrast between the normal enamel and the dense overlapped enamel (Figure 24–20 ◼). The ability of these overlapped structures to produce this optical illusion illustrates how important it is to produce radiographs that do not have angulation errors.

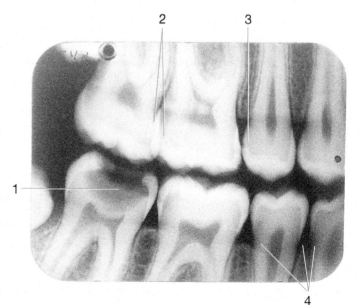

FIGURE 24–20 **Caries and optical illusions that mimic decay.** (**1**) Severe occlusal caries. (**2**) Radiolucent lines creating a mach band effect caused by overlapped enamel. (**3**) Incipient distal surface caries. (**4**) Cervical burnout.

REVIEW—Chapter summary

The detection of caries is often the most common reason for exposing dental radiographs. Caries appear radiolucent because demineralization of tooth structure allows more x-rays to pass through to reach the image receptor. Approximately 40 to 50 percent loss of hard tooth structure must occur before a decreased density can be recorded by a radiograph. Carious lesions are usually more advanced clinically than they appear on radiographs. Only precisely exposed and meticulously processed radiographs are useful in detecting caries.

Detecting proximal surface caries is the main purpose of bitewing radiographs. Carefully positioned periapical radiographs, exposed using the paralleling technique, are also valuable in detecting proximal surface caries. Radiographs detect proximal surface caries better than a clinical examination alone. A clinical examination is better at detecting early occlusal, buccal/lingual, and cemental caries.

An example of a caries depth grading system organizes the demineralization process into the following categories: incipient, moderate, advanced, and severe. The radiographic appearance of caries may also be classified according to location: proximal, occlusal, buccal/lingual, and cemental (root) surfaces. To best detect proximal surface caries, examine tooth surfaces at the point of contact and just apical to this point of contact to the estimated height of the gingival margin.

Incipient caries appears as a radiolucent notch extending less than halfway through the enamel; moderate caries appears as a radiolucent triangle extending more than halfway through the enamel; advanced caries appears as a radiolucent double triangle spreading along the DEJ, extending less than halfway toward the pulp; severe caries appears as a radiolucency extending through the dentin, more than halfway toward the pulp. Incipient and moderate buccal/lingual and cemental/root caries are not likely to be recorded radiographically even though these can be detected clinically. Once they reach the advanced and severe stages, buccal/lingual caries appears as a round radiolucency with well-defined borders; cemental/root caries appears as an ill-defined, crescent-shaped radiolucency. Significant bone loss must be evident before cemental/root caries occur. Cemental caries should not be misinterpreted as cervical burnout. Radiographic interpretation includes an understanding of recurrent, rampant, and arrested caries.

The following distinctions help to avoid mistaking nonmetallic restorations, cervical burnout, and mach band effect for caries. Nonmetallic restorations tend to have defined, prepared borders; cervical burnout appears so far apical as to position the radiolucency under the gingival margin; and mach band effect occurs adjacent to overlapped proximal surfaces.

RECALL—Study questions

1. Caries appears radiopaque, *because* more radiation passes through demineralization than through sound hard enamel.
   a. Both the statement and reason are correct and related.
   b. Both the statement and reason are correct but NOT related.
   c. The statement is correct, but the reason is NOT.
   d. The statement is NOT correct, but the reason is correct.
   e. NEITHER the statement NOR the reason is correct.

2. Each of the following will produce an ideal radiographic image for detecting caries EXCEPT one. Which one is the EXCEPTION?
   a. Bitewing radiographs
   b. Periapical radiographs
   c. Horizontal angulation that avoids overlapping
   d. Excessive vertical angulation

3. Caries in the earliest stage is called
   a. incipient.
   b. moderate.
   c. advanced.
   d. severe.

4. Radiographs are key to detecting incipient caries of which of these tooth surfaces?
   a. Occlusal
   b. Proximal
   c. Buccal/lingual
   d. Cemental

5. The key to successfully interpretating radiographs for proximal surface caries is to examine the contact point between adjacent teeth and just apical to the
   a. DEJ.
   b. CEJ.
   c. estimated gingival margin.
   d. alveolar bone crest.

6. What typical shape will an advanced proximal surface carious lesion most likely exhibit?
   a. Triangular
   b. Square
   c. Round
   d. Crescent

7. Which of the following proximal surface caries appears radiographically as a radiolucent notch that extends less than halfway through the enamel?
   a. Incipient
   b. Moderate
   c. Advanced
   d. Severe

8. Which of the following proximal surface caries appears radiographically as a radiolucent double triangle that extends less than halfway through the dentin toward the pulp?
   a. Incipient
   b. Moderate
   c. Advanced
   d. Severe

9. The key to successfully interpretating radiographs for occlusal caries is to examine
   a. the occlusal surface for changes in the pits and fissures.
   b. under the occlusal surface for changes in the dentin.
   c. the contact point between adjacent teeth for changes in the enamel.
   d. just apical to the contact point for changes in the DEJ.

10. Caries on which of the following surfaces appears radiographically as a round radiolucency in the middle of the tooth with well-defined borders?
    a. Proximal
    b. Occlusal
    c. Cemental
    d. Buccal/lingual

11. Caries on which of the following surfaces appears radiographically as an ill-defined crescent-shaped radiolucency below the CEJ?
    a. Proximal
    b. Occlusal
    c. Cemental
    d. Buccal/lingual

12. Caries that occurs under a restoration or around its margins is called
    a. recurrent.
    b. cemental.
    c. root.
    d. buccal.

13. Each of the following may mimic caries radiographically EXCEPT one. Which one is the EXCEPTION?
    a. Composite restorations
    b. Stainless stain crowns
    c. Cervical burnout
    d. Mach banding

14. An optical illusion created by an increased radiolucency observed at the cervical area of the tooth is called mach banding.
    The mach banding effect increases when overlap error occurs.
    a. The first statement is true. The second statement is false.
    b. The first statement is false. The second statement is true.
    c. Both statements are true.
    d. Both statements are false.

REFLECT—Case study

You are interpreting a full mouth series of radiographs on a patient who had dental hygiene services at your facility this morning. The completed patient's dental examination chart is available, but the patient has been dismissed. As you examine the radiographs, you notice the following:

1. Suspected incipient caries on the distal surface of the maxillary right first molar
   a. Describe the radiographic appearance of this suspect radiolucency.
   b. Indicate why you classified this suspect radiolucency as incipient.

2. Suspected moderate caries on the mesial surface of the maxillary left first premolar
   a. Describe the radiographic appearance of this suspect radiolucency.
   b. Indicate why you classified this suspect radiolucency as moderate.

3. Suspected advanced caries on the mesial surface of the mandibular left second premolar
   a. Describe the radiographic appearance of this suspect radiolucency.
   b. Indicate why you classified this suspect radiolucency as advanced.

4. Suspected severe caries on the distal surface of the mandibular right first molar
   a. Describe the radiographic appearance of this suspect radiolucency.
   b. Indicate why you classified this suspect radiolucency as severe.

5. Suspected advanced occlusal caries on the maxillary right second molar
   a. Describe the radiographic appearance of this suspect radiolucency.
   b. Indicate why you classified this suspect radiolucency as advanced.

6. Suspected cemental caries on the mesial surface of the mandibular right first premolar
    a. Describe the radiographic appearance of this suspect radiolucency.
    b. Indicate why you classified this suspect radiolucency as cemental.

7. The patient's chart indicates incipient occlusal caries detected clinically on the maxillary left first and second molars; however, these do not seem to be evident radiographically.
    a. Explain why these caries are not observed on the radiographs.

8. The patient's chart indicates incipient buccal caries detected clinically on the mandibular left first molar; however, this lesion does not seem to be evident radiographically.
    a. Explain why the buccal caries is not observed on the radiographs.

9. The radiographs reveal radiolucencies resembling cemental (root) caries on the mesial and distal surfaces of the mandibular right first and second premolars; however, the patient's chart does not indicate bone loss and no cemental caries were detected clinically.
    a. Explain the possible cause of these radiolucencies.

10. The periapical radiograph of the maxillary left molar region is overlapped between the maxillary first and second molars.
    a. Explain why detecting caries in this area will be compromised.
    b. What optical illusion will most likely present in this area?
    c. Describe the appearance of this optical illusion.

RELATE—Laboratory application

For a comprehensive laboratory practice exercise on this topic, see Thomson, E. M., & Bruhn, A. M. (2018). *Exercises in oral radiography techniques: A laboratory manual* (4th ed.). Hoboken, NJ: Pearson. Chapter 14, "Radiographic interpretation."

RESOURCES

Berry, H. (1983). Cervical burnout and mach band: Two shadows of doubt in radiologic interpretation of carious lesions. *Journal of the American Dental Association, 106*, 622.

Langlais, R. P. (2003). *Exercises in oral radiology and interpretation* (4th ed.). Philadelphia: Saunders.

White, S. C., & Pharoah, M. J. (2014). Dental caries. *Oral radiology: Principles and interpretation* (7th ed.). St. Louis, MO: Elsevier.

25

The Use of Radiographs in the Evaluation of Periodontal Diseases

CHAPTER OUTLINE

OBJECTIVES

Following successful completion of this chapter, you should be able to:

1. Define the key terms.
2. List the uses of radiographs in the assessment of periodontal diseases.
3. Differentiate between horizontal and vertical bone loss.
4. Identify three local contributing factors for periodontal disease that radiographs can help detect.
5. Explain the purpose of using radiographs to image root morphology.
6. List the limitations of radiographs in the assessment of periodontal diseases.
7. Explain the parameters for using vertical and horizontal bitewing, and periapical radiographs to record periodontal disease.
8. Recognize the roles vertical and horizontal angulations play in imaging periodontal diseases.
9. Describe the radiographic appearance of the normal periodontium.
10. Describe the radiographic appearance of gingivitis.
11. Describe the radiographic appearance mild periodontitis.
12. Describe the radiographic appearance of moderate periodontitis.
13. Describe the radiographic appearance of severe periodontitis.

KEY TERMS

Calculus
Furcation involvement
Gingivitis

Horizontal bone loss
Interdental septa
Local contributing factor
Localized bone loss
Occlusal trauma

Periodontitis
Periodontium
Triangulation
Vertical (angular) bone loss

Introduction

Dental radiographs, when used to supplement a clinical examination, play a key role in the diagnosis, prognosis, management, and evaluation of periodontal diseases. Radiographic images can confirm bone loss and may assist with identifying local periodontal disease–contributing factors not detected clinically. To be of maximum benefit, radiographic images must be correctly exposed and meticulously processed. This chapter describes the radiographic appearance of periodontal diseases, presents a periodontal diseases classification framework upon which to base radiographic interpretation, and outlines radiographic techniques best suited for producing quality radiographs for the purpose of evaluating periodontal diseases.

Radiographic Appearance of Periodontal Diseases

Periodontal diseases are those that affect both soft tissues (gingiva) and hard tissues (bone) surrounding and supporting the teeth. The severity of periodontal disease may range from early inflammation of the gingiva to the destruction of periodontal ligaments (PDL) and supporting bone. The most common periodontal diseases are gingivitis and periodontitis. **Gingivitis** is inflammation of the gingiva and limited to soft tissues. **Periodontitis** also results from infection, but involves loss of alveolar bone.

Radiographs, in combination with a thorough clinical examination, allow an oral health care professional to evaluate and document periodontal diseases (Box 25–1). The uses of radiographic images in the assessment of periodontal diseases include the following:

- **Evaluate supporting bone.** Radiographs allow for the evaluation of crestal bone irregularities and **interdental septa** changes (alveolar bone between the teeth), and document the amount of bone remaining rather than the amount lost. The amount of bone loss is estimated as the difference between the physiologic bone level and the height of the remaining bone (Figure 25–1 ■).

Radiographs can be used to determine the pattern of bone loss: horizontal or vertical.

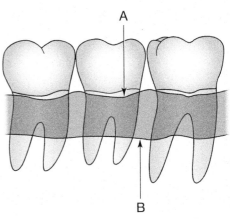

FIGURE 25–1 **Horizontal bone loss. (A)** Normal (physiologic) level of alveolar bone parallel to the CEJ. **(B)** Bone level associated with severe periodontal disease. Horizontal bone loss is the estimated difference between (A) and (B) (shaded area).

Horizontal bone loss describes bone height loss in which both buccal and lingual bony plates, as well as the intervening interdental bone, resorb simultaneously and at the same rate. Horizontal bone loss occurs along a plane which is said to be parallel to an imaginary line connecting the cementoenamel junctions (CEJs) of adjacent teeth (Figure 25–2 ■). **Vertical (angular) bone loss** occurs in an uneven manner where the resorption of bone between teeth sharing an interdental septum creates angular defects in the crestal bone along the adjacent teeth (Figures 25–3 ■ through 25–5 ■). Buccal and lingual plates of bone resorb at different rates and will appear to be at differing heights on the radiograph.

Radiographs also assist with determining the distribution of bone loss—localized or generalized. **Localized bone loss** is defined as a pattern of bone loss that is confined to less than 30 percent of all teeth. When bone loss involves more than 30 percent of all teeth, generalized bone loss is more descriptive

Box 25–1: Periodontal Bone Changes Recorded by Radiographs

- Crestal irregularities
- Interdental alveolar bone changes
- Pattern of bone loss (horizontal or vertical)
- Distribution of bone loss (localized or generalized)
- Severity of bone loss (mild, moderate, severe)
- Furcation involvement

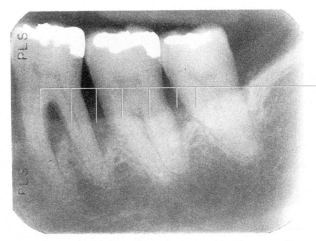

FIGURE 25–2 **Horizontal bone loss.** Level of bone loss is parallel to an imaginary line connecting the CEJ of the adjacent teeth.

Vertical bone loss

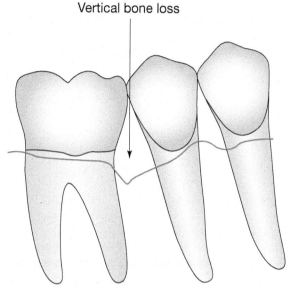

FIGURE 25–3 **Vertical bone loss.** Vertical bone loss appears angular where the resorption is greater on the side of one tooth than on the side of the adjacent tooth.

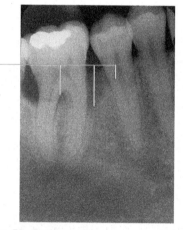

FIGURE 25–4 **Vertical bone loss.**

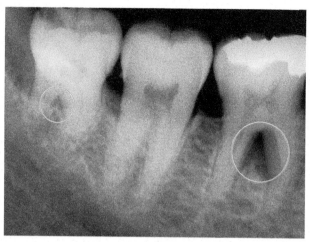

FIGURE 25–6 **Furcation involvement.** Note the radiolucencies in between the roots of these multirooted teeth.

of the condition. Following specific parameters suggested by various periodontal disease classification systems, radiographs can be used to determine the severity of bone loss—mild, moderate, or severe—and can detect **furcation involvement** (bone loss between the roots) of multirooted teeth (Figure 25–6 ■).

- **Reveal local contributing factors** Radiographs can detect conditions such as amalgam overhangs, poorly contoured crown margins, and calculus deposits, each of which attract and can lead to a buildup of bacterial pathogens that cause periodontal diseases (Figure 25–7 ■). **Calculus**, essentially hardened plaque, appears slightly radiopaque (about the radiopacity of dentin) and must be significantly calcified to be recorded on radiographs. Depending on the density and the amount of a deposit, calculus may appear as pointed or irregular projections on the proximal tooth surfaces, or as a ringlike radiopacity around the cervical neck of a tooth (Figure 25–8 ■).

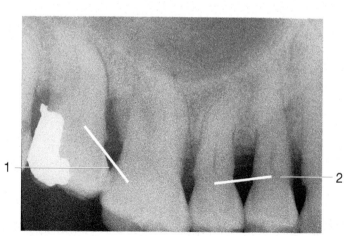

FIGURE 25–5 **Use the CEJ of adjacent teeth as a guideline.** (1) Vertical bone loss. (2) Horizontal bone loss.

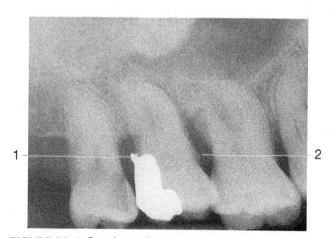

FIGURE 25–7 **Local contributing factors.** (1) Amalgam overhang and (2) calculus are likely to collect bacterial pathogens that can contribute to the progression of periodontal diseases.

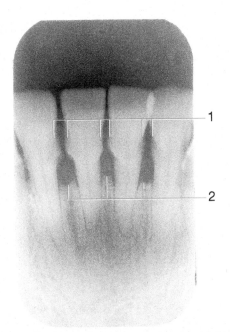

FIGURE 25–8 **Calculus. (1)** Large deposits around the cervical region of the teeth. **(2)** Height of alveolar bone remaining as a result of periodontal disease.

Radiographs often reveal the effects of traumatic occlusion, another contributing factor for periodontal disease. **Occlusal trauma** does not cause periodontal disease, but has been shown to hinder the body's response to the disease. The effects of excessive occlusal forces are detected on radiographs as a widening of the PDL space (Figure 25–9 ■), called **triangulation**. Triangulation appears to form a radiolucent angular gap, with its base toward the tooth crown and its point toward the root apex, between the radiopaque lamina dura and the root surface of the tooth.

- **Assess anatomical configurations.** Radiographs reveal information about tooth root morphology. Determining tooth root length, shape, and width, and evaluating bone support between multirooted

teeth and between adjacent teeth roots, can aid in planning disease interventions and help predict treatment outcomes. Detecting the presence of dilacerations (see Chapter 26) and evaluating bone support between multirooted teeth and along narrow, close, or fused roots provides additional data for determining treatment protocols based on expected outcomes. For example, bone loss involving a tooth with a short root may predict a poor prognosis, whereas a tooth with a long root may be predicted to have a better treatment outcome (Figure 25–10 ■). Additionally, bone loss is likely to have an increased adverse effect on teeth with roots that are in close proximity. Roots that closely share an interdental septum will more likely share a loss of bone.

- **Document the prognosis and treatment intervention.** Providing information on the tooth root-to-crown ratio, and adjacent tooth root proximity, allows radiographs to help guide treatment plans and predict outcomes.
- **Serve as a baseline and a means for evaluating the results of treatment.** Radiographs provide documentation on the progression of disease and provide a permanent record of the condition of the bone throughout the course of the disease and treatment.

Although radiographs provide a valuable adjunct to a clinical examination, they have the following limitations:

- **Radiographs are a two-dimensional image of three-dimensional objects.** Radiographs lack the third dimension of depth, which results in bone and tooth structures being superimposed over each other. This superimposed image often hides bone loss on the buccal and lingual surfaces and in furcation areas, especially in the posterior region of the oral cavity.

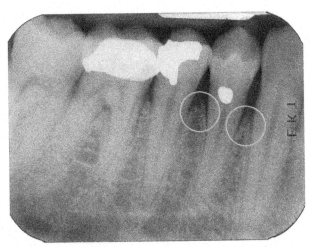

FIGURE 25–9 **Triangulation.** Widening of the PDL space indicative of occlusal trauma.

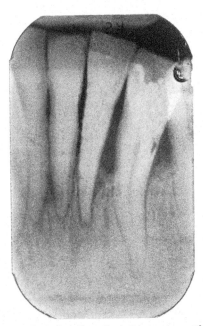

FIGURE 25–10 **Root length and root-to-crown ratio.** Although the bone loss observed on this radiograph is significant, the long, dilacerated root improves the prognosis for the canine.

- **Changes in soft tissue not imaged.** Because soft tissue is not recorded on radiographs, gingivitis cannot be detected radiographically. Radiographs do not add information regarding the location and/or depth of periodontal pockets.
- **Cannot distinguish treated versus untreated disease.** Radiographs do not indicate the presence or absence of active disease. For example, a reduction in crestal bone height remaining after a patient has undergone treatment and is now on periodontal maintenance therapy would be considered stabilized and categorized as a state of health. Without a clinical examination to determine the presence of inflammation or increased probing depths, the radiographic finding of bone loss alone cannot be used to distinguish between treated and untreated disease.
- **Actual destruction more advanced clinically.** Radiographs cannot detect early signs of periodontal diseases. A significant loss of bone density must occur before radiographic changes are detected.

Radiographic Techniques for Imaging Periodontal Diseases

Bitewings, especially a vertical bitewing series of both anterior and posterior radiographs, are most useful for examining the **periodontium** (Figure 25–11 ■; also see Chapter 15). Vertical bitewing radiographs, with the longer dimension of the image receptor positioned vertically, offer a gain in recording height over horizontal bitewing radiographs. The precise parallelism established between the tooth and the plane of the image receptor when taking bitewing radiographs makes it possible to image the alveolar crestal bone accurately. To achieve this same degree of accuracy with periapical radiographs, use the paralleling technique. Place the image receptor parallel to the long axis of the teeth to ensure that the images of the bone and teeth on the radiograph are not distorted.

To be a useful diagnostic aid, a radiograph must be positioned precisely and exposed with accurate vertical and horizontal angulations of the x-ray beam. Incorrect angulation can render a radiograph worthless for evaluating periodontal disease. Excessive vertical angulation may not reveal bone loss, whereas inadequate vertical angulation may result in a radiographic image that falsely indicates bone loss when there is none (Figures 25–12 ■ and 25–13 ■). Horizontal angulation actually plays two important roles in evaluating periodontal disease. First, accidental incorrect horizontal angulation results in overlapping of the contact areas between the teeth, making it impossible to determine the condition of interdental bone. Second, purposefully varying the horizontal angulation slightly may actually increase the chances of identifying interdental defects and furcation involvement. For example, a bitewing series of seven radiographs (see Chapter 15) and a full mouth series of multiple periapical and bitewing radiographs (see

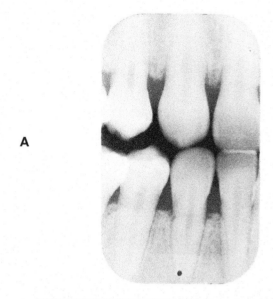

A

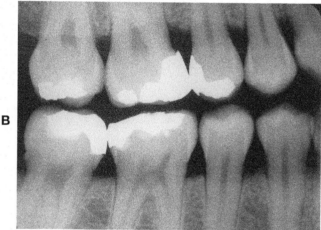

B

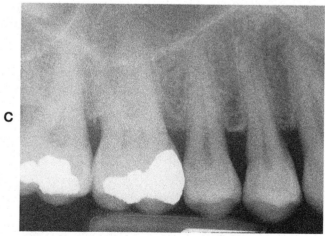

C

FIGURE 25–11 **Comparison of bitewing and periapcial radiographs imaging the periodontium. (A)** Vertical bitewing. **(B)** Horizontal bitewing. **(C)** Periapical.

Chapter 13) will contain images that were produced with different horizontal angles. The varying angulations used allow for valuable comparisons among multiple views of the condition of the periodontium (Figure 25–14 ■).

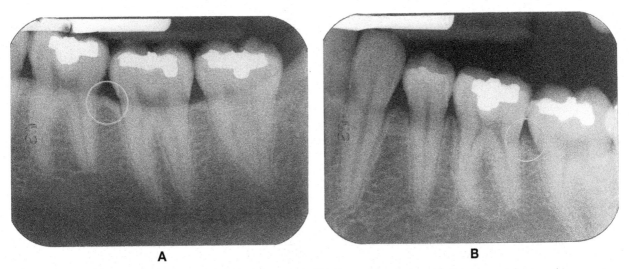

FIGURE 25-12 Correct and incorrect vertical angulation. (A) Correct vertical angulation accurately records crestal bone indicating no bone loss between the mandibular first and second molars. **(B)** Incorrect vertical angulation produces a radiolucent, cupping-out appearance of the lamina dura falsely indicating bone loss between these same teeth.

Although exposure factors (mA, kV, and exposure time) will depend on the patient and the area to be recorded, some practitioners prefer to use a higher kV setting to image alveolar bone conditions. A high kV setting produces a low-contrast image: black and white with many shades of gray in between. Because bone changes that accompany periodontal diseases will begin to produce radiolucencies in the radiopaque alveolar crest, in theory, a low-contrast image might be preferred as a way to detect early signs of bone destruction. However, research indicates that both low- and high-contrast images allow for adequate periodontal disease

evaluation. More important than the kV setting is to produce radiographs that are free of angulation errors.

Radiographic Interpretation of Periodontal Diseases

A dental radiographer should be familiar with the radiographic appearance of the normal periodontium to be able to identify deviations from normal that may indicate possible periodontal diseases (Procedure 25–1). When noted radiographically, these deviations can be quantified along

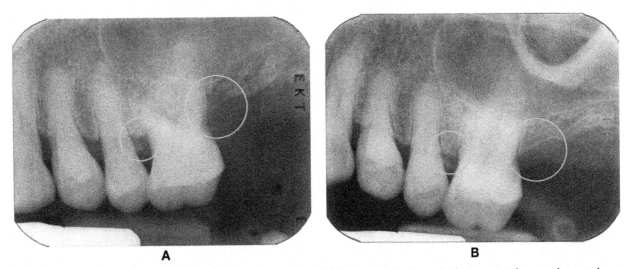

FIGURE 25-13 Correct and incorrect vertical angulation. (A) Correct vertical angulation accurately records crestal bone indicating bone loss mesial and distal to the maxillary first molar. **(B)** Incorrect vertical angulation produces a false appearance to the level of bone in these same areas.

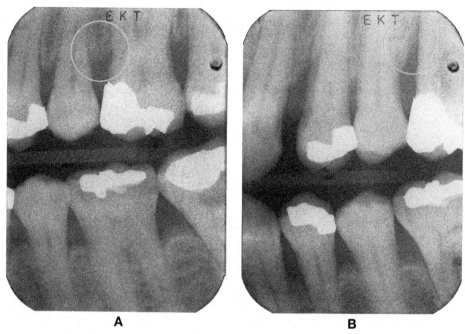

FIGURE 25–14 Example of varying horizontal angulation. (A) Correct horizontal angulation, but image does not reveal the vertical (angular) defect on the mesial of the maxillary first molar. **(B)**. Slightly varied horizontal angulation of the same region now reveals the vertical bony defect.

a continuum from early to advanced changes. When interpreting these changes, it is helpful to have guidelines. There have been several classification systems developed for categorizing periodontal diseases; most are based on etiologic factors of the disease and tissue response to treatment. Many of these systems continue to be revised and updated based on ongoing research. All classification systems use both clinical and radiographic data to determine a diagnosis and quantifiers for periodontal diseases. Because the focus of this chapter is on the radiographic interpretation of periodontal diseases, the following four classifications of periodontal disease are used (Table 25–1 ■).

Health or Gingivitis

Radiographs do not image soft tissue, and therefore the radiographic appearance of the periodontium in all types and severities of gingivitis appears the same as normal bone. The lamina dura (dense cortical plate of the bony tooth socket) appears as an unbroken, dense radiopaque line around the roots of the teeth. The alveolar crest is located 1 to 2 mm apical to the CEJ of the teeth (Figure 25–15 ■). In the posterior region of the oral cavity, normal alveolar bone is flat, smooth, and parallel to an imaginary line drawn between adjacent CEJ (Figure 25–16 ■). In the anterior region of the oral cavity, normal alveolar bone appears pointed (Figure 25–17 ■).

Procedure 25–1

Radiographic interpretation for periodontal disease

See Procedure 20–1, Suggested sequence for viewing a full mouth series of radiographic images.

1. View all surfaces of each tooth.
2. Note the alveolar bone height. Use the CEJ as a reference point. Measure with a probe as needed (see Figure 20–9).
3. Examine the PDL space, following it around the entire tooth. Note widening, triangulation.
4. Examine the furcation area of multirooted teeth for radiolucencies.
5. Identify local contributing factors such as restoration overhangs and calculus.
6. Confirm findings and/or clarify uncertain interpretations with a clinical examination of the patient.
7. Consult the patient's chart for confirmation or clarification of findings as needed.
8. Present a preliminary interpretation for dentist's review.
9. Following confirmation by dentist, document findings on the patient's permanent record.

Table 25–1 Radiographic Periodontal Disease Classification

Classification	Radiographic Appearance
Health or Gingivitis	*Alveolar crest:* Unbroken, radiopaque; bone level 1–2 mm below and parallel to CEJ *Anterior:* Pointed *Posterior:* Flat, smooth
Mild Periodontitis	*Alveolar crest:* Loss of density with slight radiolucency evident; bone level ≥2 mm and ≤3 mm below CEJ, indicating up to 15% bone loss *Anterior:* Blunted *Posterior:* Fuzzy, cupping-out appearance
Moderate Periodontitis	*Alveolar crest:* Bone level ≥3 mm and ≤5 mm below CEJ, indicating 16–30% bone loss *Anterior and posterior:* Horizontal and/or vertical patterns of bone loss observed *Posterior:* Furcation radiolucencies evident
Severe Periodontitis	*Alveolar crest:* Bone level >5 mm below CEJ, indicating greater than 30% bone loss *Anterior and posterior:* Evidence of tooth position changes, drifting

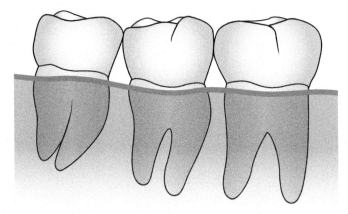

FIGURE 25–15 **Health or Gingivitis.** Alveolar crest located 1 to 2 mm apical to the CEJ of the teeth.

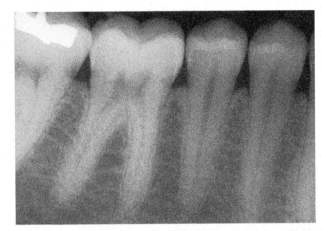

FIGURE 25–16 **Health or Gingivitis—posterior region.** Flat radiopaque appearance of the lamina dura and thin radiolucent line of the PDL space.

The PDL space appears as a thin radiolucent line between the lamina dura and the root of the tooth.

Mild Periodontitis

The alveolar crest is located 2 to 3 mm apical to the CEJ of the teeth indicating up to a 15 percent bone loss (Figure 25–18 ■). Loss of crestal bone density that often appears as a fuzzy cupping-out of the alveolar crest is the first radiographic indication of periodontal disease (Figure 25–19 ■). The alveolar crest appears blunted in the anterior region of the oral cavity (Figure 25–20 ■). In the posterior region of the oral cavity triangulation, a widening of the PDL space becomes evident at the mesial or distal surfaces of the teeth.

Moderate Periodontitis

Moderate bone loss (16 to 30 percent) may appear in both the horizontal and vertical planes as indicated by bone levels between 3 and 5 mm below the CEJ of the teeth (Figures 25–21 ■ and 25–22 ■). As the bone levels continue to resorb, radiolucencies may appear in the furcations of multirooted teeth (Figure 25–23 ■).

Severe Periodontitis

The advanced stage of periodontal disease (greater than 30 percent bone loss) is characterized radiographically by severe horizontal and/or vertical bone loss of greater than 5 mm below the CEJ of the teeth, evidence of furcation involvement, widened PDL spaces, and indications of changes in tooth position (Figures 25–24 ■ through 25–26 ■).

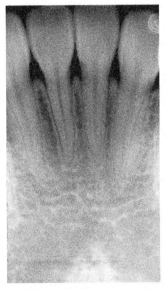

FIGURE 25–17 **Health or Gingivitis—anterior region.** Pointed radiopaque appearance of the lamina dura and thin radiolucent line of the PDL space.

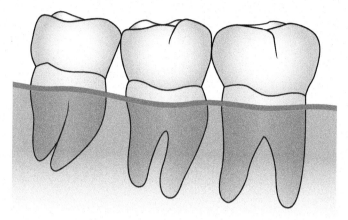

FIGURE 25–18 **Mild Periodontitis.** Alveolar crest located 2 to 3 mm apical to the CEJ of the teeth.

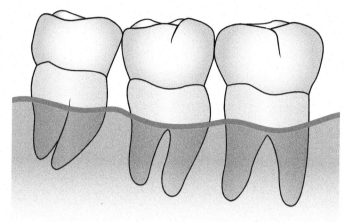

FIGURE 25–21 **Moderate Periodontitis.** Alveolar crest located 3 to 5 mm apical to the CEJ of the teeth.

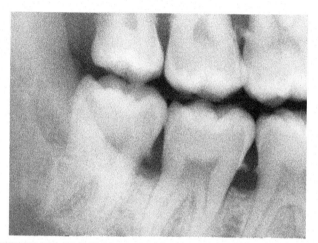

FIGURE 25–19 **Mild Periodontitis—posterior region.** Radiolucent cupping-out of the lamina dura, especially visible between the mandibular first and second molars. Radiopaque calculus visible on the proximal surfaces of the teeth.

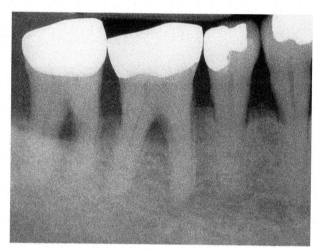

FIGURE 25–22 **Moderate Periodontitis—posterior region.** Horizontal and vertical patterns of bone loss observed. Radiolucency in the furca of the mandibular molars. Radiopaque calculus visible on the proximal surfaces of the teeth.

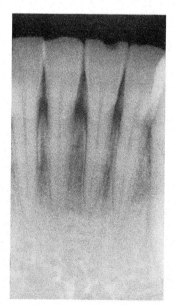

FIGURE 25–20 **Mild Periodontitis—anterior region.** Blunting of the lamina dura and radiolucent widening of the PDL space. Radiopaque calculus visible on the proximal surfaces and across the cervical necks of the teeth.

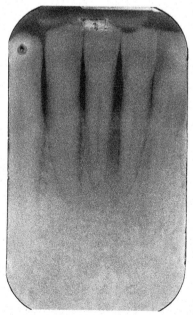

FIGURE 25–23 **Moderate Periodontitis—anterior region.** Bone level 3 to 5 mm apical to the CEJ, indicating 16–30% bone loss.

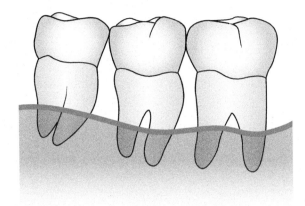

FIGURE 25–24 Severe Periodontitis. Bone level greater than 5 mm apical to the CEJ, indicating greater than 30% bone loss.

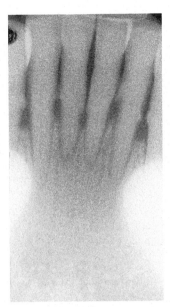

FIGURE 25–26 Severe Periodontitis—anterior region. Bone level greater than 5 mm apical to the CEJ, indicating greater than 30% bone loss. Radiopaque calculus visible on the proximal surfaces of the teeth.

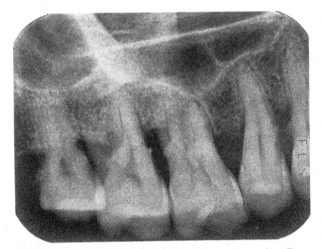

FIGURE 25–25 Severe Periodontitis—posterior region. Bone level greater than 5 mm apical to the CEJ. Radiolucencies indicating furcation involvement. Radiopaque calculus visible on the proximal surfaces of the teeth.

REVIEW—Chapter summary

Periodontal diseases affect both soft tissues (gingivitis) and bone around the teeth (periodontitis). To be of maximum benefit, radiographs must be positioned precisely and exposed with accurate vertical and horizontal angulations of the x-ray beam. The uses of radiographs in the diagnosis, prognosis, management, and evaluation of periodontal diseases include imaging supporting bone, locating local contributing factors, recording anatomical configurations, evaluating prognosis and treatment intervention needs, and serving as a baseline for identifying and documenting the progression of the disease and the results of treatment.

Horizontal bone loss occurs along a plane parallel to an imaginary line connecting the CEJ of adjacent teeth. Vertical bone loss occurs in an uneven manner creating angular defects in the crestal bone along the affected teeth. Localized bone loss involves less than 30 percent of all teeth; generalized bone loss involves more than 30 percent of all teeth. Local factors that contribute to periodontal diseases

that radiographs play a role in detecting include amalgam overhangs, poorly contoured crown margins, and calculus deposits. Radiographs reveal information about tooth root morphology that can aid in planning disease interventions and help predict treatment outcomes.

Two-dimensional radiographs are limited in their ability to record three-dimensional teeth and supporting bone. Radiographs do not contribute diagnostic information on changes in soft tissue. Treated disease cannot be distinguished from untreated disease, and the actual destruction of bone is more clinically advanced than what is revealed on radiographs.

The ideal radiographs for imaging periodontal diseases are bitewings, particularly vertical bitewings, or periapical radiographs exposed with the paralleling technique. Radiographs are important aids in identifying changes in the periodontium and can assist in classifying various stages of periodontal disease: mild, moderate, and severe.

RECALL—Study questions

1. Each of the following may be determined from a dental radiograph EXCEPT one. Which one is the EXCEPTION?
   a. Bone loss
   b. Pocket depth
   c. Furcation involvement
   d. Local contributing factors

2. List four uses of radiographs in the assessment of periodontal diseases.
   a. _____
   b. _____
   c. _____
   d. _____

3. Which of the following terms describes bone loss that occurs in a plane parallel to the CEJ of adjacent teeth?
   a. Irregular
   b. Vertical
   c. Horizontal
   d. Periapical

4. Significant bone loss that results in a radiolucency observed in the area between the roots of multirooted teeth is called
   a. localized bone loss.
   b. interdental septa.
   c. local contributing factor.
   d. furcation involvement.

5. Radiographs may help to locate each of the following local contributing factors for periodontal diseases EXCEPT one. Which one is the EXCEPTION?
   a. Calculus
   b. Poorly contoured crown margin
   c. Deep pocket
   d. Amalgam overhang

6. Excessive occlusal force may result in a widening of the periodontal ligament space.
   Widening of the periodontal ligament space is called furcation involvement.
   a. The first statement is true. The second statement is false.
   b. The first statement is false. The second statement is true.
   c. Both statements are true.
   d. Both statements are false.

7. Dental radiographs play a key role in documenting the location and depths of periodontal pockets.
   Dental radiographs may serve as a baseline and as a means for evaluating the outcomes of periodontal treatments.
   a. The first statement is true. The second statement is false.
   b. The first statement is false. The second statement is true.
   c. Both statements are true.
   d. Both statements are false.

8. List four limitations of dental radiographs in the assessment of periodontal diseases.
   a. _____
   b. _____
   c. _____
   d. _____

9. Which of the following would be best for imaging a mild, generalized periodontal status?
   a. Select periapical radiographs using the bisecting technique.
   b. Select periapical radiographs using the paralleling technique.
   c. Posterior horizontal bitewing radiographs.
   d. Posterior and anterior vertical bitewing radiographs.

10. Correct horizontal angulation is needed to accurately image interdental bone levels.
    Altering the horizontal angulation can reveal additional information regarding interdental bone levels.
    a. The first statement is true. The second statement is false.
    b. The first statement is false. The second statement is true.
    c. Both statements are true.
    d. Both statements are false.

11. Alveolar crests pointed in the anterior region and a radiopaque flat, smooth lamina dura 1 to 2 mm apical to the CEJ in the posterior region describes
    a. Health or Gingivitis
    b. Mild Periodontitis
    c. Moderate Periodontitis
    d. Severe Periodontitis

12. Radiolucent changes observed on a radiograph such as a fuzzy, cupping-out of crestal bone, and a blunted appearance of the lamina dura in the anterior region describes
    a. Health or Gingivitis
    b. Mild Periodontitis
    c. Moderate Periodontitis
    d. Severe Periodontitis

REFLECT—Case study

Describe what radiographic changes in the periodontium you would expect to observe when interpreting a seven-image series of vertical bitewing radiographs based on the following:

1. Health or Gingivitis

2. Mild Periodontitis

3. Moderate Periodontitis

4. Severe Periodontitis

RELATE—Laboratory application

For a comprehensive laboratory practice exercise on this topic, see Thomson, E. M., & Bruhn, A. M. (2018). *Exercises in oral radiography techniques: A laboratory manual* (4th ed.). Hoboken, NJ: Pearson. Chapter 14, "Radiographic interpretation."

RESOURCES

American Academy of Periodontology. (2015). Task force report on the update to the 1999 classification of periodontal diseases and conditions. *Journal of Periodontology, 86,* 835–838.

Langlais, R. P. (2003). *Exercises in oral radiology and interpretation* (4th ed.). Philadelphia: Saunders.

White, S. C., & Pharoah, M. J. (2014). Periodontal diseases. *Oral radiology: Principles and interpretation* (7th ed.). St. Louis, MO: Elsevier.

Visit www.pearsonhighered.com/healthprofessionsresources to access the student resources that accompany this book. Simply select Dental Hygiene from the choice of disciplines. Find this book and you will find the complementary study tools created for this specific title.

Describing Radiographic Anomalies, Lesions, and Opportunistic Screening

OBJECTIVES

Following successful completion of this chapter, you should be able to:

1. Define the key terms.
2. Use correct terminology to describe the radiographic appearance of dental anomalies.
3. Describe anomalies and pathologic lesions by density, size, shape, border, architecture, location, and affect on surrounding tissues.
4. Differential between radiolucent, radiopaque, and lucent-opaque lesions.
5. Explain how to document the size of a lesion detected on a radiographic image.
6. Differentiate between regular- and irregular-shaped lesions detected on a radiographic image.
7. Differentiate between a well-defined and a poorly-defined border of a lesion detected on a radiographic image.
8. Explain the difference between lesion architecture that is unilocular, multilocular, focal opacity, multifocal, or a target lesion.
9. Explain the importance of documenting location of anomalies and lesions detected on a radiographic image.
10. Explain the importance of examining adjacent structures and surrounding tissues for changes caused by an anomaly or lesion.
11. List and describe the radiographic appearance of common developmental anomalies.
12. List and describe the radiographic appearance of common radiolucent lesions.
13. List and describe the radiographic appearance of common radiopaque lesions.
14. Differentiate between external and internal resorption.
15. List and describe the radiographic appearance of common lucent-opaque lesions.
16. Explain the significance of opportunistic screening.

Introduction

Radiographs play a valuable role in the detection of diseases and conditions that might not be discovered by a clinical examination alone. A patient may present with signs and symptoms that require the exposure of dental radiographs to determine a diagnosis. Other times radiographs exposed for one condition may reveal other conditions or problems that need treatment intervention. Although a dentist is responsible for determining the diagnosis and treatment of conditions revealed on dental radiographic images, it is important that all members of the oral health care team develop the skills required to recognize deviations from normal anatomic landmarks. Equally important is the ability to describe radiographic findings using terms familiar to other health care professionals. This chapter introduces radiographic descriptive terminology and provides an overview of the radiographic appearance of some of the more commonly occurring developmental anomalies, lesions, and other conditions of the teeth and jaws.

Descriptive Terminology

Radiographic interpretive findings must be described and documented in a patient's dental record using terminology understood by other professionals. The use of standard terminology aids in communication between oral health care practitioners, other medical professionals, and health insurers for the purpose of third-party payment. *Radiopaque* and *radiolucent* are familiar terms used to describe the appearance of radiographic findings. Anomalies and pathologic lesions and conditions must also be described by size, shape, border, architecture, location, and affect on surrounding tissues. Many pathologic lesions have a characteristic or unique appearance that assists with determining a diagnosis, underlining the importance of using correct descriptive terminology. A dentist or specialist will use the descriptors to assist with a **differential diagnosis**, distinguishing the type of lesion from other possibilities.

DENSITY. Describing the density of an object is relative, and depends on the appearance of adjacent tissues. Comparing a finding to the density of normal supporting bone can be used as guidance. In general, describe a suspicious finding as radiolucent if it appears darker than normal bony trabeculae; radiopaque if it appears lighter. An **anomaly** may be distinctly radiolucent or radiopaque, or present a mixed appearance. A mixed radiolucent and radiopaque (**lucent-opaque**) lesion may take on a wispy appearance, referred to as ground-glass or cotton-wool.

Determining density assists with identifying a lesion. A radiolucent appearance usually is indicative of tissue breakdown or destruction that allows more radiation to penetrate the tissue and reach the image receptor. A radiopaque appearance indicates the growth or penetration of a lesion by more calcified or denser tissue that blocks radiation from reaching the image receptor. A lucent-opaque lesion may indicate a simultaneous buildup of denser or calcified tissues that are replacing tissues undergoing destruction.

SIZE. Documenting the size of a lesion is important not only as an aid to differential diagnosis, but to record changes over time or treatment outcomes. Radiographic images record structures at their approximate size allowing for a reasonably accurate measurement. As is the case in medical documentation, oral and maxillofacial lesions are measured in millimeters, or, if large enough, centimeters. Depending on the shape of the anomaly or lesion, two measurements should be taken: height and width. If interpreting film-based radiographs, use a periodontal probe to more precisely determine an accurate measurement; use digital software rulers when interpreting digital images (Figure 26–1 ■).

SHAPE. When a lesion shape can be distinguished, for example, as round, oval, scalloped, or linier, the descriptor *regular* is applied. Regular-shaped lesions are most often associated with an even growth of the lesion, which expands outward from a center as the lesion grows in size. An irregular shape is often indicative of growth or expansion that occurs in different directions from multiple centers at differing rates.

BORDER. A lesion will have a well-defined or a poorly-defined border. A well-defined border separates the lesion from the surrounding structures. Bone will appear normal up to the edge of the lesion. A **corticated** border appears as a radiopaque outline that encapsulates the lesion, and may appear thin or thick. A poorly-defined border will not distinctly separate a lesion from the surrounding normal tissue. A lesion with a poorly-defined border will appear diffuse, making it difficult to determine the boundaries of the lesion.

A well-defined border is often indicative of a slow-growing lesion. Slow growth and even expansion of

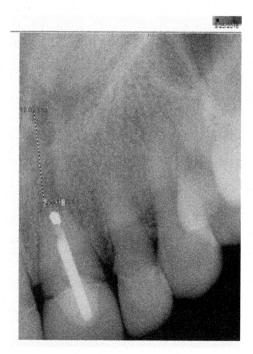

FIGURE 26–1 Document measurement. Digital software used to measure height and width of a radiolucent lesion.

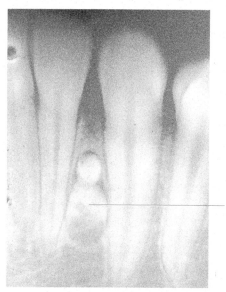

FIGURE 26–2 Odontoma. Consisting of small, misshaped teeth located within a radiolucent fibrous capsule.

a lesion gives surrounding healthy bone time to generate a defense in the form of a thickened cortex against the expanding pathologic lesion. Many benign pathologic lesions fit this description. A poorly-defined border usually indicates that a lesion is invading surrounding tissues rather than pushing against them. A more rapidly growing and expanding lesion may not give surrounding bone time to generate a defense wall. Infection and malignant lesions usually have poorly-defined borders.

ARCHITECTURE. The makeup or internal architecture of a lesion should be described using terminology specific to radiolucent and radiopaque pathology. A close examination of a lesion will determine if it is made up of one or more internal compartments. Radiolucent compartments are called loculations. A **unilocular** lesion is not compartmentalized, but appears as a single radiolucent part. **Multilocular** refers to a lesion with more than one radiolucent compartment, appearing to be separated by radiopaque walls or septa. Radiopaque lesions use the term **focal opacity** to describe the architecture of a lesion that appears as a single entity. When multiple radiopaque lesions appear to be joined or in an overlapping relationship, the term **multifocal** is applied. A focal opacity that presents with a radiolucent, ringlike outline is called a **target lesion**.

In addition to selecting correct terminology to document architectural makeup, a lesion should be examined for the presence of multiple types of tissues within its borders. This is especially important when evaluating lucent-opaque lesions. A characteristic unique to a specific type of odontogenic tumor is the presence of a fibrous capsule containing enamel, dentin, and cementum that would normally be combined to form a tooth (Figure 26–2 ■).

LOCATION. Examine radiographic images for the possibility that an abnormal condition is detected bilaterally or unilaterally. Specifically describe the location of the anomaly or lesion. The location may be categorized as localized or generalized. The detection of multiple separate, but characteristically similar lesions in different locations throughout the maxillofacial region would be documented as a generalized condition. The documentation for a single lesion is localized. If multiple lesions are close enough to be considered in the same location, and/or appear to overlap or otherwise give the appearance of being connected, the condition will most likely be categorized as localized. Use specific tooth locations, if applicable, to document location, even if the tooth is not present. For example, a dental record entry that reads—a round radiolucency adjacent to the distal root of the mandibular right first molar—or—a linear radiopacity in the edentulous region of the mandibular left third molar—would clearly convey to another professional where the finding is located.

Document location of anomalies and lesions in relation to adjacent normal anatomic structures. Use the same terminology learned to describe surfaces and positions of teeth—mesial, distal, posterior, anterior, etc. Periapical, pericoronal, and interradicular also describe specific locations. Whereas the familiar term *periapical* describes a position around a root tip, **pericoronal** refers to a location around a tooth crown. This description would apply to an unerupted tooth, where a radiographic image may detect abnormalities associated with a tooth crown. A lesion located between teeth roots is termed **interradicular**. As with other descriptors used to document the appearance, certain lesions and conditions occur only in specific locations, further assisting with a differential diagnosis.

Additionally, tissues located in specific oral maxillofacial regions give rise to specific pathoses and abnormalities, making documentation of location important to differential diagnosis. A lesion noted near the temporomandibular joint must be considered to be cartilaginous in nature, while a lesion located above the mandibular canal will probably be **odontogenic** (pertaining to the development of teeth) in nature.

EFFECT ON SURROUNDING TISSUES. Examine adjacent structures and surrounding tissues for changes caused by an anomaly or lesion. The effect a lesion has on surrounding tissues such as cortical bone and lamina dura plays an important role in differential diagnosis. An expanding lesion may push adjacent structures out of normal position. An invasive lesion may damage or cause an adjacent structure to resorb.

Radiographic Appearance of Developmental Anomalies

Begin the interpretation process with an examination to determine the presence or absence of teeth—followed by an assessment of tooth morphology and eruption patterns—before determining if deviations from normal and/or suspected pathology is detected (see Procedure 20–1). Dental anomalies are relatively common, so it is important to develop skills at identifying normal structures to be better prepared to notice when a deviation presents. The following represent a few of the more common development anomalies detected by dental radiographs.

- **Hypodontia.** The failure of a tooth or multiple teeth to develop. Third molars are the most common congenitally missing teeth, followed by second premolars and maxillary lateral incisors (Figure 26–3 ■). Radiographs play a valuable role in assessing dentition eruption patterns for children and adolescents.
- **Hyperdontia.** It is equally important that the presence of **supernumerary** (extra) teeth be detected (Figure 26–4 ■). Supernumerary teeth can form in any region of the oral cavity and are likely to be misshaped or oddly formed. Supernumerary fourth molars are called distomolars due to their location

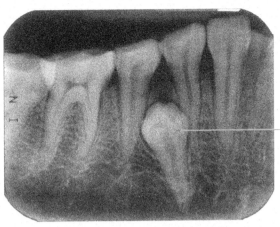

FIGURE 26–4 **Supernumerary tooth.** Impacted supernumerary premolar.

distal to the third molars (Figure 26–5 ■). Mesiodens is the name given to a supernumerary tooth that forms near the maxillary midline. Often there is not a space for these extra teeth to erupt into, leading to additional problems. Complications associated with supernumerary teeth that can be detected by a radiographic examination include impaction, cyst formation, and the malposition, blocked eruption, or resorption of adjacent teeth (Figure 26–6 ■).
- **Dens in dente.** Literally, a tooth within a tooth, dens invaginatus presents as an invagination of enamel within the body of the tooth; radiographically, it is detected as a teardrop shape within the pulp. This anomaly occurs most frequently in the maxillary lateral incisor (Figure 26–7 ■).
- **Dilaceration.** Describes a tooth root with a sharp bend or abnormal curvature. **Dilaceration** may occur on any tooth. Due to two-dimensional recording, radiographic detection is more likely when the abnormal bend curves toward the mesial or distal than toward the facial or lingual (see Figures 26–6 and 26–8 ■).
- **Supernumerary root.** A tooth may abnormally form an extra root (see Figure 30–6). A supernumerary root is more likely to occur with third molars, mandibular premolars, and canines.

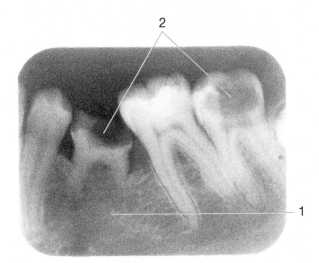

FIGURE 26–3 **Congenitally missing tooth. (1)** Second premolar did not develop under this primary molar. **(2)** Note severe caries.

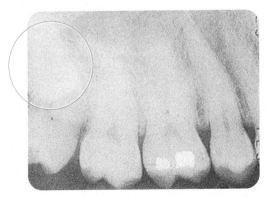

FIGURE 26–5 **Distomolar.** Impacted supernumerary fourth molar.

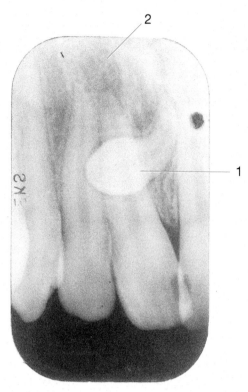

FIGURE 26–6 **Mesiodens.** (**1**) Supernumerary tooth with dilacerated root structure located near midline between central incisors. Note the well-defined corticated radiopaque border. (**2**) Periapical radiolucency with poorly-defined diffuse border.

- **Fusion.** A developmental disturbance that results when two adjacent teeth fuse together during growth, forming one large tooth. Fusion occurs in enamel and dentin, and sometimes the pulp chambers of adjacent

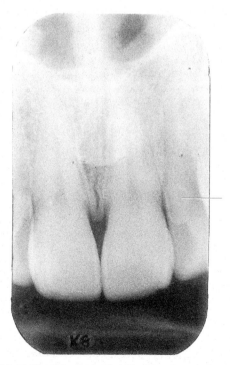

FIGURE 26–7 **Dens in dente.** An invagination of the enamel within the body of the lateral incisor.

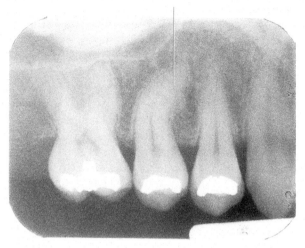

FIGURE 26–8 **Dilaceration.** Sharp bend in root of second premolar.

teeth. A radiographic examination will usually detect two separate pulp chambers (Figure 26–9 ■). Size and shape, and the degree to which two adjacent teeth fuse will vary. Fusion is more likely to affect anterior teeth.

- **Gemination.** Results when a single tooth germ divides and forms two joined teeth. Similar to fusion, the size and shape of the joined teeth will vary. A radiographic examination will usually detect one large shared pulp chamber rather than two smaller joined pulp chambers observed in fusion. Gemination is more likely to occur in primary dentition. The presence of adjacent teeth distinguishes this anomaly from fusion.

Appearance of Radiolucent Lesions

PERIAPICAL RADIOLUCENCY. A radiolucency surrounding the apices or root tips of a tooth is indicative of pathological changes. Periapical infections usually result from

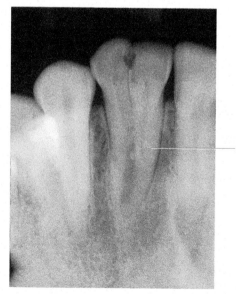

FIGURE 26–9 **Fusion** of mandibular lateral and central incisors.

pulpal inflammation. Bacteria from caries infect the pulp and gain access to periapical bone by way of tooth root canals. As a rule, in the early stages a pulpal or periapical infection is barely discernible radiographically as a break, or loss of radiopacity, in the lamina dura. As infection becomes chronic, a circular radiolucency develops around the root apices. The three most common periapical lesions observed on radiographs are abscess, granuloma, and cyst. These lesions cannot be definitively diagnosed based on a radiographic examination alone. Detection of an apical lesion on a radiograph must be carefully correlated with other assessment information before a diagnosis can be made (Figure 26–10 ■).

DENTIGEROUS CYST. A dentigerous or follicular cyst is observed as a radiolucency surrounding the crown only of an unerupted tooth—most often third molars and supernumerary teeth (Figure 26–11 ■). If the involved tooth is able to erupt, the cyst will be destroyed by natural means (Figure 26–12 ■).

NONODONTOGENIC CYSTS. Periapical and dentigerous cysts are categorized as odontogenic, of tooth origin. Nonodontogenic cysts arise from epithelium other than that associated with tooth formation. Two nonodontogenic cysts that can be detected by a radiographic examination are the incisive canal (nasopalatine) cyst located within the incisive canal, and the rare globulomaxillary cyst which arises between the maxillary lateral incisor and the canine (Figures 26–13 ■ and 26–14 ■).

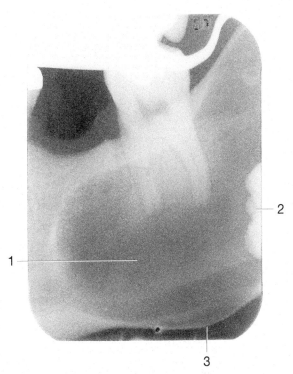

FIGURE 26–11 **Dentigerous cyst (1)** involving (**2**) impacted third molar. (**3**) Note expansion and thinning of cortical bone in response to lesion. (Purposeful vertical positioning of image receptor was used to better record lesion.)

Appearance of Radiopaque Lesions

PERIAPICAL RADIOPACITIES. Two forms of **ossification** (conversion of structures into hardened bone) are often recorded by radiographs. Condensing osteitis occurs when sclerotic (hardened) bone is formed as a result of infection or chronic irritation caused by pulpal necrosis from an adjacent tooth. Therefore, condensing osteitis is always associated with a nonvital tooth, a condition that cannot be determined radiographically. Osteosclerosis occurs when regions of abnormally dense bone form, but not as a

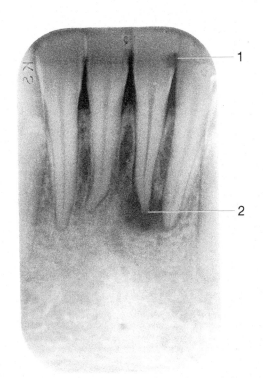

FIGURE 26–10 **Periapical pathology.** (**1**) Caries. (**2**) Round radiolucent lesion may be periapical abscess, granuloma, or cyst.

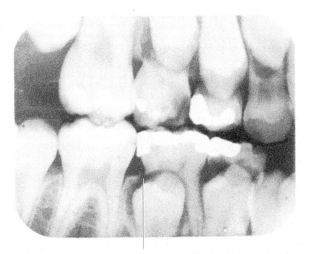

FIGURE 26–12 **Follicular cyst** surrounding crown of unerupted second premolar. Note the physiologic external resorption of the primary teeth roots in response to erupting permanent teeth.

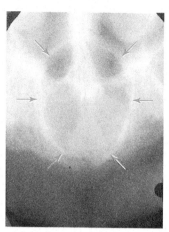

FIGURE 26–13 **Incisive canal cyst.** Arrows outline an incisive canal (nasopalatine) cyst in an edentulous maxilla. Note the well-defined corticated border.

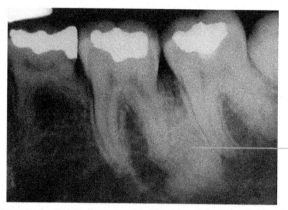

FIGURE 26–15 **Radiopaque lesion.** Irregular-shaped diffuse radiopaque lesion. A clinical examination to determine tooth vitality is needed to distinguish between condensing osteitis and osteosclerosis. Note the radiolucent PDL spaces indicating this lesion is separate from the teeth.

direct result of infection or irritation. Although the cause is unknown, osteosclerosis commonly occurs in the interseptal premolar region; it is also often associated with fragments of retained primary roots. Differentiating between condensing osteitis and osteosclerosis observed on a radiographic examination requires a clinical examination to determine tooth vitality (Figures 26–15 ■ and 26–16 ■).

HYPERCEMENTOSIS. Seen radiographically as an excessive formation of cementum along a tooth root, this enlargement will usually take on a bulbous appearance toward the root apex (Figure 26–17 ■). Hypercementosis is distinguished from other radiopacities surrounding or near the tooth roots by the radiolucent and radiopaque outlines of the periodontal ligament (PDL) space and lamina dura, respectively. When observing hypercementosis, the PDL space contains the radiopacity and separates it from bone. This distinction will help to avoid mistaking hypercementosis for sclerotic bone.

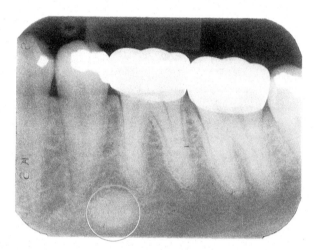

FIGURE 26–16 **Radiopaque lesion.** Focal opacity representing sclerosed bone. A clinical examination to determine tooth vitality is needed to distinguish between condensing osteitis and osteosclerosis.

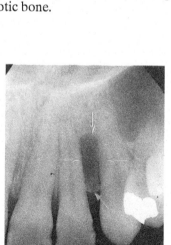

FIGURE 26–14 **Globulomaxillary cyst.** Interradicular globulomaxillary cyst.

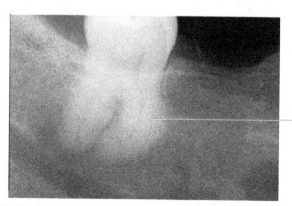

FIGURE 26–17 **Hypercementosis.** Overgrowth of cementum on the roots of the molar. Note that the PDL space and lamina dura surround this lesion indicating that it is attached to the tooth.

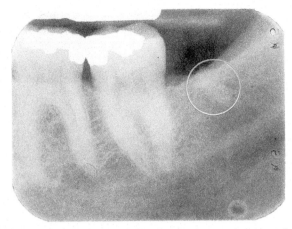

FIGURE 26–18 **Retained root fragment** in an extraction site.

PULP STONES. Calcifications in the dental pulp occur in the form of small radiopaque nodules of varied size. Pulp stones are common but of little significance, unless root canal therapy is needed on the affected tooth.

RETAINED ROOT FRAGMENT. Radiographs may detect pieces of tooth structures embedded in the bone of the dental arches, particularly evident in an edentulous area. A root tip or other piece of tooth structure may break off and be inadvertently left behind following extraction; or remain behind as a result of severe decay or trauma that broke off the crown of the tooth (Figure 26–18 ■). Retained root tips may be clearly visible radiographically or less so, depending on their size and degree of resorption.

Radiographic Appearance of Tooth Resorption

Evidence of tooth resorption is a common finding on dental radiographs. Natural physiologic resorption, such as when the roots of primary teeth resorb in response to erupting permanent teeth, is considered normal (see Figure 26–12). Other resorptive processes, however, are the result of infection, trauma, or some unusual condition. Tooth resorption may be external or internal. External resorption is most often characterized by root-end resorption, where teeth roots appear shorter than normal as the resorption progresses (Figure 26–19 ■). External resorption is not limited to the root apex, but can occur anywhere along a tooth root or crown. Other examples of external resorption include resorption caused by pressure from an adjacent impacted or unerupted tooth; resorption caused by slow-growing tumors; or trauma, such as when teeth are moved too rapidly during orthodontic treatment(see Figure 23-17). When the cause is unknown, it is called **idiopathic** resorption.

Internal resorption typically appears as a radiolucent widening of a tooth root canal, indicating that the resorption process is taking place within the dentin. Typically this, *from the inside out*, resorption widens the appearance of the pulp chamber or root canal, sometimes taking on a radiolucent oval or round shape as the resorption progresses (Figure 26–20 ■).

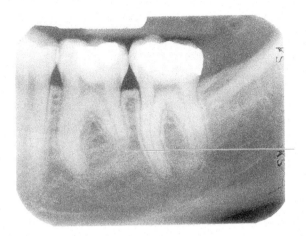

FIGURE 26–19 **External resorption.** Idiopathic resorption of distal root of first molar.

Appearance of Lucent-Opaque Lesions

ODONTOMA. One of the most common ondontogenic tumors detected by a dental radiographic examination is the odontoma. Odontogenic tumors result from abnormal proliferation of cells and tissues involved in odontogenesis (the formation of the teeth). An odontoma forms when enamel, dentin, and cementum form irregular shapes resembling small misshaped teeth whose number varies widely. These toothlike structures appear radiopaque and are located within a radiolucent fibrous capsule that can resemble a cyst (see Figure 26–2).

PERIAPICAL CEMENTAL DYSPLASIA. Sometimes called cementoma, periapical cemental dysplasia (PCD) is a bone dysplasia derived from periodontal ligaments of fully developed and erupted teeth. Early PCD is radiolucent and

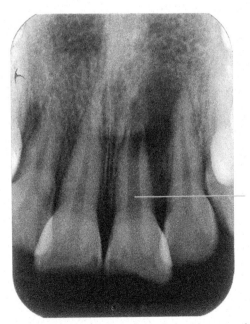

FIGURE 26–20 **Internal resorption.** Idiopathic resorption noted as a widening of the pulp chamber.

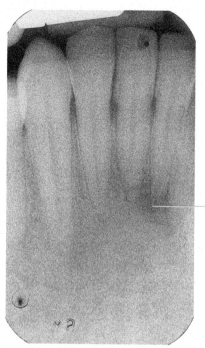

FIGURE 26–21 Periapical cemental dysplasia (PCD). Lucent-opaque lesion.

appears identical to pathological cysts. In later stages of development, PCD appears as radiopaque masses encompassed by a radiolucent line or halo (Figure 26–21 ■). Due to its changing radiolucent to radiopaque appearance, PCD may be difficult to diagnose without knowledge of other clinical data.

Opportunistic Screening

Radiographs should be thoroughly interpreted with the patient present so that a clinical examination can contribute to a diagnosis. A series of radiographs may need to be more thoroughly evaluated at a time set aside for this purpose. Radiographs must be evaluated for all possible findings. A dentist will not only examine a specific area of interest, but will thoroughly evaluate adjacent teeth, supporting bone, and all tissues of the maxillofacial region for other possible anomalies and pathoses. For example, a panoramic radiograph prescribed to assess unerupted third molars must be evaluated for incidental findings including developmental anomalies, caries, periodontal disease, and pathologic manifestations of the entire maxillofacial structures—not just the oral cavity. A radiograph may be prescribed to address one condition, but detect another. A radiographic examination that detects anomalies and/or lesions different from which the examination was prescribed is called an opportunistic screening.

Two possible opportunistic screening uses of dental panoramic radiographs currently being researched are the detection of carotid stenosis and osteoporosis. While it is not currently recommended that panoramic radiographs be prescribed for the evaluation of these conditions, in the

future they may possibly play a role in preliminary detection. Additionally, research is not conclusive regarding predictive ability or treatment recommendations of incidental findings recorded on a dental panoramic radiograph. The static two-dimensional property and the inherent image distortion make a panoramic radiograph an unreliable tool at determining the extent and progression of these conditions. Nevertheless, research continues to show correlations between dental radiographs and the detection of these conditions, so dentists are being advised to examine panoramic radiographs thoroughly and to refer patients for a medical examination when needed. To accurately interpret a dental radiograph for these conditions, an oral health care practitioner will most likely need special training. The following interpretation guidelines are offered to help increase awareness of opportunistic screening and are not meant to be instructional.

CAROTID STENOSIS. Stenosis, a constriction of the carotid arteries by the accumulation of atherosclerotic plaque, is a risk factor for a vascular event such as stroke. Panoramic radiographs have been shown to record plaques that are significantly calcified. These radiopaque calcifications vary widely in shape (e.g., round, linear, or clustered in nodular masses) and are observed in the region of the carotid bifurcation into the internal and external branches of the artery. To estimate the location of the bifurcation, draw an imaginary line at a 45-degree angle from the angle of the mandible, extending posterior and inferior approximately 0.5 to 0.75 inch (1.5 to 2 cm) to a region adjacent but not attached to the cervical vertebrae at about the level of C-3 and C-4 (Figure 26–22 ■). Before determining the presence of a carotid artery calcification, a thorough interpretation must identify all radiopaque normal anatomy most likely to be recorded in this region (Box 26–1).

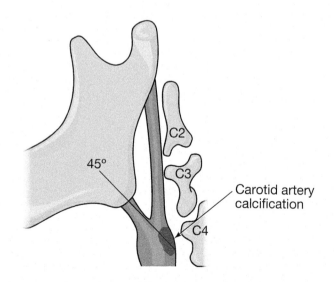

FIGURE 26–22 Estimated location of carotid bifurcation on a panoramic radiograph; a 45-degree angle from the angle of mandible to cervical vertebrae C-3 and C-4.

Box 26–1: Anatomy to Be Distinguished from Carotid Artery Calcification

- Auricle (ear lobe)
- Calcified acne
- Calcified lymph nodes
- Epiglottis
- Hyoid bone
- Phleboliths (calcified thrombi in soft tissues of cheeks)
- Sialoliths (salivary gland calcifications)
- Soft palate
- Styloid ligaments (Figure 26–23 ■)
- Styloid process
- Thyroid cartilage
- Tongue
- Tonsillothis (calcification formed in crevice of tonsillar tissues)
- Triticeous cartilage (nodule on thyrohyoid ligament)
- Vertebrae

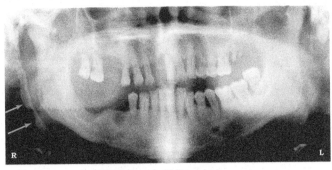

FIGURE 26–23 **Calcified styloid ligament.**

these models continue to provide research data, they do not yet have a role in general practice.

These diseases and other conditions often progress without signs and symptoms making it unlikely that a patient would pursue diagnostic medical testing. Compared to other medical testing, dental radiographs are more frequently performed. A large percentage of the population is likely to have undergone a dental radiographic examination. The opportunity to screen for potentially serious medical conditions as an incidental finding will add to the benefits of dental radiography.

OSTEOPOROSIS. A disease characterized by the loss of skeletal bone density, osteoporosis results in fragility that increases risk of fracture. Dental radiographs have the ability to record altered bone trabeculae patterns and changes in the width of cortical bone of the inferior border of the mandible. Interpreting these bone changes for a possible correlation with osteoporosis requires the use of special mathematical formulas and digital analyses not practical for use in general practice. Researchers continue to develop mathematical models to design indexes used to study the feasibility of dental radiographs to measure bone density (Figure 26–24 ■). Some models measure thickness of cortical bone outlining the inferior border of the mandible; others analyze density of trabecular microstructure. Although

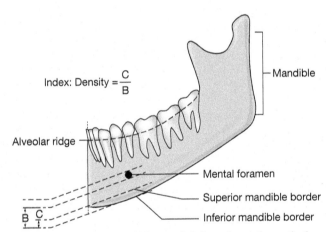

Index: Density $= \dfrac{C}{B}$

FIGURE 26–24 **Sample index model.** Sample mathematical index measures thickness of cortical bone of the mandible.

REVIEW—Chapter summary

Oral health care professionals must develop skills required to recognize deviations from normal anatomic landmarks and be able to describe radiographic findings using terms familiar to other health care professionals. Correct descriptive terminology aids in determining a differential diagnosis. Anomalies and pathologic lesions and conditions must be described according to density, size, shape, border, architecture, location, and effect on surrounding tissues. Density is described as radiolucent if it appears darker than normal bony trabeculae, radiopaque if it appears lighter, and lucent-opaque if a mixed appearance is evident. Lesions may be regular or irregular in shape, and are measured in millimeters or centimeters. Radiolucent lesions are unilocular or multilocular; radiopaque lesions are focal opacity or multifocal; and have a well-defined or poorly-defined border. Lesions may occur in a single or generalized location, and may be unilateral or bilateral. Use specific tooth locations, if applicable, to document lesion location, even if the tooth is not present. Mesial, distal, posterior, anterior, periapical, pericoronal, interradicular also describe specific locations. An expanding lesion may push adjacent structures out of normal position; an invasive lesion may damage or cause an adjacent structure to resorb.

Common dental anomalies recorded by dental radiographs include hypodontia, the failure of a tooth or multiple teeth to develop; hyperdontia, the development of supernumerary teeth; mesiodens, a supernumerary tooth formed at the maxillary midline; dens in dente, an invagination of enamel within the body of the tooth; dilaceration, an abnormal bend or curve of a tooth root; a supernumerary tooth root; fusion of two adjacent teeth; and gemination, a tooth germ that divides and forms two joined teeth.

Periapical radiolucencies can indicate pathological changes. Although a definitive diagnosis cannot be based on a radiographic examination alone, three common periapical radiolucent lesions are abscess, granuloma, and cyst. Dentigerous or follicular cyst is detected as a radiolucency-associated with the crown only of impacted or unerupted teeth. Odontogenic cysts originate from a tooth origin; nonodontogenic cysts arise from epithelium other than that associated with tooth formation.

Two forms of ossification seen as periapical radiopacities are condensing osteitis, associated with a nonvital tooth, resulting from infection or chronic irritation; and osteosclerosis, abnormally dense bone formed but not as a direct result of infection or irritation. Hypercementosis is an excessive formation of cementum along a tooth root and a bulbous enlargement near the root apex, separated from surrounding bone by the radiolucent outline of the PDL space. Pulp stones appear as calcified nodules of various sizes within the dental pulp. Depending on the degree to which it has resorbed, a radiopaque root tip or piece of tooth structure may be observed embedded in bone.

Tooth structure resorption may be external or internal. External resorption may occur at any point along the surface of the tooth; most common occurrence begins at root end. Internal resorption appears as a radiolucent widening of a tooth root canal, as the resorption begins within the dentin.

A common odontogenic tumor detected by radiographs is the odontoma, an irregular formation of enamel, dentin, and cementum resembling small misshaped teeth surrounded by a radiolucent fibrous capsule. An example of a lucent-opaque lesion is the bone dysplasia PCD, derived from periodontal ligaments of fully developed and erupted teeth. Early PCD is radiolucent, changing to radiopaque in later stages.

A radiograph may be prescribed to address one condition, but detect something else. Dental radiographs are not prescribed to detect carotid stenosis and osteoporosis, but may possibly fulfil a role of opportunistic screening.

RECALL—Study questions

1. Each of the following should be used to describe anomalies and pathologic lesions detected by radiographs EXCEPT one. Which one is the EXCEPTION?
   a. Shape
   b. Border
   c. Color
   d. Size

2. Describing the density of an object is relative, *because* density depends on the appearance of adjacent tissues.
   a. Both the statement and reason are correct and related.
   b. Both the statement and reason are correct but NOT related.
   c. The statement is correct, but the reason is NOT.
   d. The statement is NOT correct, but the reason is correct.
   e. NEITHER the statement NOR the reason is correct.

3. Which of the following does NOT describe object density?
   a. Lucent-opaque
   b. Radicular
   c. Radiolucent
   d. Radiopaque

4. Lesions detected by radiographs may appear round, oval, scalloped, or linear.
   Lesions with these shapes are expanding in different directions at differing rates.
   a. The first statement is true. The second statement is false.
   b. The first statement is false. The second statement is true.
   c. Both statements are true.
   d. Both statements are false.

5. What term describes a radiopaque border that outlines and encapsulates a lesion detected on a radiograph?
   a. Lucent-opaque
   b. Focal
   c. Corticated
   d. Idiopathic

6. What term describes the architecture of a lesion with radiolucent compartments?
   a. Focal opacity
   b. Multilocular
   c. Target lesion
   d. Unilocular

7. What term describes a lesion located around an unerupted tooth crown?
   a. Interproximal
   b. Periapical
   c. Pericoronal
   d. Interradicular

8. The failure of a tooth or multiple teeth to develop is called
   a. hyperdontia.
   b. hypodontia.
   c. supernumerary.
   d. dens in dente.

9. Which of the following is the best preliminary documentation for a radiolucency surrounding the root tips of a tooth?
   a. Periapical abscess
   b. Granuloma
   c. Cyst
   d. Periapical radiolucency

10. Which of the following radiographic findings is associated with a nonvital tooth?
    a. Condensing osteitis
    b. Pulp stones
    c. Osteosclerosis
    d. Hypercementosis

11. Radiographic evidence of resorption that appears to shorten a tooth root is called
    a. internal.
    b. primary.
    c. external.
    d. secondary.

12. What is the most likely interpretation of a radiographic lesion that resembles misshaped teeth?
    a. Dens in dente
    b. Odontoma
    c. Mesidens
    d. Germination

13. Which of the following appears radiolucent in its early stages and as a radiopaque mass in later stages?
    a. Globulomaxillary cyst
    b. Carotid stenosis
    c. Osteoporosis
    d. Periapical cemental dysplasia (PCD)

14. Dental radiographs should be prescribed as an opportunistic screening tool for carotid stenosis *because* a radiographic examination can be used to predict a vascular event.
    a. Both the statement and reason are correct and related.
    b. Both the statement and reason are correct but NOT related.
    c. The statement is correct, but the reason is NOT.
    d. The statement is NOT correct, but the reason is correct.
    e. NEITHER the statement NOR the reason is correct.

REFLECT—Case study

With permission to access archived patient records, search for records with panoramic radiographs. Using the information presented on opportunistic screening for carotid stenosis, locate the region of interest. Identify the angle of the mandible. Identify the cervical vertebrae. Direct your attention to locating radiopaque structures in this region. Using a head and neck anatomy and/or pathology textbook, match as many of these structures as possible with the list presented in Box 26–1. Note: If you cannot name a structure and suspect pathology, check the record to be sure that it was documented during a previous interpretation of the radiographs. If not, present your findings to your instructor for follow-up.

RELATE—Laboratory application

Obtain a pathology textbook and study the chapters and images for the developmental anomalies and lesions introduced in this chapter. With permission to access archived patient records, search for records with full mouth series radiographs. Interpret the radiographs for these anomalies and lesions. Check the record to be sure that findings were documented during a previous interpretation of the radiographs. If not, present your findings to your instructor for follow-up.

RESOURCES

Damaskos, S., Griniatsos, J., Tsekouras, N., et al. (2008). Reliability of panoramic radiograph for carotid atheroma detection: A study in patients who fulfill the criteria for carotid endarterectomy. *Oral Surgery Oral Medicine Oral Pathology Oral Radiology, 106,* 736–742.

Garoff, M., Johansson, E., Ahlqvist, J., et al. (2015). Calcium quantity in carotid plaques: Detection in panoramic radiographs and association with degree of stenosis. *Oral Surgery Oral Medicine Oral Pathology Oral Radiology, 120,* 269–274.

Horowitz, H. (2015). Identify tooth anomalies. *Dimensions of Dental Hygiene, 13*(6), 16, 18, 20–21.

Iannucci, J. M., & Howerton, L. J. (2017). Descriptive terminology, interpretation of trauma, pulpal lesions, and periapical lesions. *Dental radiography. Principles and techniques* (5th ed.). St. Louis, MO: Elsevier.

Torres, S. R., Chen, C. S. K., Lerouz, B. G., et al. (2015). Mandibular inferior cortical bone thickness on panoramic radiographs in patients using bisphosphonates. *Oral Surgery Oral Medicine Oral Pathology Oral Radiology, 119,* 584–592.

Virginia Commonwealth University School of Dentistry Department of Oral and Diagnostic Sciences. (2014, August 7). Oral radiology. Basic diagnostic skills modules. Describing a radiograph and interpreting what you see. Retrieved from VCU Web site: http://www.oraldiagnosticsciences.vcu.edu/courses/diagnostic/

Weiskircher, M. A., Gonzalez, S. M., & Palazzolo, M. (2015). Detect developmental tooth anomalies. *Dimensions of Dental Hygiene, 13*(8), 24–27.

White, S. C., & Pharoah, M. J. (2014). Soft tissue calcifications and ossifications. *Oral radiology: Principles and interpretation* (7th ed.). St. Louis, MO: Elsevier.

Visit www.pearsonhighered.com/healthprofessionsresources to access the student resources that accompany this book. Simply select Dental Hygiene from the choice of disciplines. Find this book and you will find the complementary study tools created for this specific title.

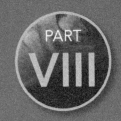

PART

VIII

Radiographic Techniques for Specific Needs

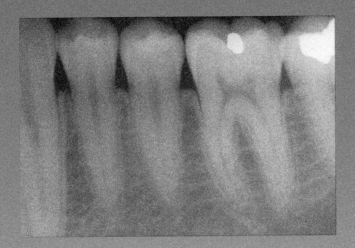

OUTLINE

Pediatric Radiographic Techniques

OBJECTIVES

Following successful completion of this chapter, you should be able to:

1. Define the key terms.
2. List signs and symptoms that would indicate a pediatric radiographic need.
3. List conditions a pediatric patient might present with that would prompt a need to adapt a standard radiographic procedure.
4. Identify factors that influence the number of radiographs, and size of image receptors to be exposed on a pediatric patient.
5. Explain the reasoning behind the recommendation to use the largest size image receptor that can be tolerated by a pediatric patient.
6. Determine the type and number of radiographs, and size of image receptor to use to image primary dentition.
7. Determine the type and number of radiographs, and size of image receptor to use to image transitional mixed dentition.
8. Identify extraoral radiographic examinations that may benefit a pediatric patient.
9. Demonstrate adaptations and modifications to standard paralleling and bisecting techniques that aid in obtaining a pediatric radiographic examination.
10. Adjust standard adult exposure settings to those settings considered appropriate for pediatric radiographs.
11. Commit to Image Gently® campaign goals.
12. Demonstrate a radiographic examination use of Show-Tell-Do.
13. Demonstrate a radiographic examination use of modeling.
14. Interpret a set of pediatric radiographic images.

KEY TERMS

Exfoliation
Image Gently®
Modeling
Pediatric dentistry
Permanent teeth
Primary teeth
Transitional mixed dentition

Introduction

Preventive oral health care is especially important during childhood. Dental radiographs play a valuable role in assessing growth and development, and in early detection of caries, which is of significant importance because children are at a higher risk for caries that progress more rapidly as compared with adults. Dental radiographic techniques and the types of projections used to image the oral cavity of children do not differ significantly from those used for adult patients. However, children usually present with physical characteristics such as a smaller, and sometimes more sensitive, oral cavity and behavioral considerations that may require adaptations to standard procedures. This chapter presents radiographic technique alterations, and behavior modification strategies to assist with obtaining diagnostic quality radiographs with minimal radiation exposure for a pediatric patient.

Assessment of Radiographic Need

Pediatric dentistry (*pedia* is Greek for "child") is the branch of dentistry that specializes in providing comprehensive preventive and therapeutic oral health care for children. The organization American Academy of Pediatric Dentistry, and other oral health and medical organizations, recommend that a child's first professional oral examination occur within 12 months following eruption of the first primary tooth, usually between 6 and 12 months of age. Early prevention is key to preventing tooth loss and developing good oral self-care habits. At this early age, teeth can usually be visually inspected clinically without a need for radiographs.

As with adult patients, an indication to expose dental radiographs on a child is based on unique signs, symptoms, and circumstances with which a patient presents. Evidence-based selection criteria provide guidelines for assessing radiographic needs of children and adolescents as well as adults (see Table 6–1). Children may present with a need for a radiographic examination for detection of caries and periodontal diseases; assessment of growth and development and orthodontic intervention; detection of congenital dental abnormalities, such as hypodontia and supernumerary teeth; evaluation of third molars; diagnosis of pathologic conditions such as an abscess or other infection; and assessment of the effect of trauma, such as a fall or accident, not only for **primary teeth,** but for the developing, unerupted **permanent teeth** as well.

Unless an accident, unexplained dental pain, or other unusual circumstance causes a need for radiographs, the selection criteria guidelines suggest a radiographic survey may not be necessary until all primary teeth have erupted, and prevent a visual inspection of proximal surfaces via a clinical examination. Patients without evidence of disease and with open interproximal contacts may not require a radiographic exam. Once teeth have erupted in such a manner that the proximal surfaces can no longer be viewed clinically, and caries are suspected, or a patient presents with high risk factors for caries, such as poor oral self-care or inadequate fluoride protection, radiographs may be indicated.

Image Receptor Size, Number, and Type of Projection

Once it has been determined that a radiographic examination is needed, a child's age, oral cavity size, and cooperation level must be considered to determine size and number of radiographs to expose (Box 27–1). Although a size 0 or 1 intraoral image receptor is often used for radiographic images of a child with primary teeth, the preferred size for **transitional mixed dentition,** the presence of both primary and permanent teeth, is a standard size 2 image receptor. Use the largest size image receptor that a pediatric patient can tolerate. The amount of radiation required does not change with different sizes of intraoral image receptors. Using a size 2 image receptor whenever possible instead of a size 0 or 1 will record a larger area, providing more information. It is important to record developing permanent teeth that are not visible clinically. Choice of image receptor size should be individualized based on anatomical limitations and tissue sensitivity. Select a smaller-size image receptor to aid with accurate and comfortable positioning rather than bending a large film or photostimulable phosphor (PSP) plate to make it fit. Additionally, a smaller-size digital sensor would more likely be retained correctly in position for the duration of the exposure.

The number of image receptors required depends on needs of the individual (see Table 15–1). When exposing bitewing radiographs prior to the eruption of the permanent second molar, two horizontal posterior bitewings, one on each side, is recommended. Following eruption of the permanent second molar, four horizontal (or vertical if

Box 27–1: Pediatric Radiographic Considerations

- Oral health needs
- Willingness to cooperate
- Attention span and emotional state
- Ability to understand and follow directions
- Ability to hold still throughout exposure
- Size of opening to oral cavity
- Size and shape of teeth and dental arches
- Sensitivity of oral mucosa
- Operator's ability to gain patient's trust
- Operator's ability to position image receptor
- Operator's knowledge of and ability to adapt standard techniques

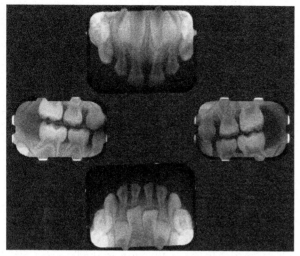

FIGURE 27–1 Radiographic survey of primary dentition.
One anterior occlusal radiographic image in each arch and one
posterior bitewing radiographic image on each side. (Courtesy
DP Gutz, DDS, University Nebraska Medical Center, College of
Dentistry, Lincoln, NE.)

periodontal disease is suspected) posterior bitewings must
be taken to image all proximal contacts without overlap.

If conditions exist that require additional exposures, the
following radiographic full mouth surveys are offered as
suggestions.

Primary Dentition

Small oral cavity size, tongue resistance, and a hypersensitive gag reflex can be barriers to obtaining quality
radiographic images for small children ages 3 to 6 years.
To overcome these challenges, the recommendation is to
expose four radiographic images, one anterior occlusal of
each arch (maxilla and mandible) and one posterior bitewing on each side (Figure 27–1 ■).

Transitional Mixed Dentition

At 6 years of age, the first permanent teeth usually
begin to erupt. The recommendation is to expose a minimum of 12 radiographic images. Ten periapical radiographs
should include one exposure in each of the four molar
regions, four canine exposures, and two incisor exposures.
Two bitewing radiographs should be exposed, one on each
side (Figure 27–2 ■).

Between ages 12 and 14 years, all permanent teeth
except third molars will have erupted. It is during this adolescent period that growth is rapid and metabolic changes
occur that heighten the possibility of dental caries and
increase the need for preventive oral hygiene care. At this
stage of dental development, the recommendation is to
expose the same number of radiographs as a full mouth
series for an adult patient (i.e., 14 periapical and 4 bitewing
radiographic images; see Figure 12–3).

Extraoral Radiographs

Evidence-based selection criteria guidelines indicate the
value of a panoramic radiograph for assessing growth and
development for pediatric patients. Panoramic radiographs
do not image structures with the detail and clarity of intraoral radiographs and, therefore, are limited in the ability
to reveal early carious lesions. However, these large radiographic images are ideal for viewing overall development
of the dental arches and other oral and maxillofacial structures (Figure 27–3 ■). Panoramic radiographs are often prescribed to supplement intraoral exposures, especially when
evaluating dentition eruption patterns and for assessing

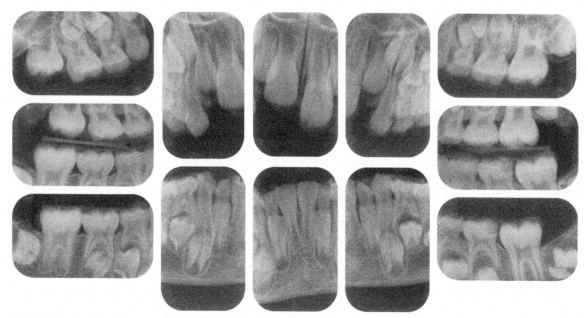

FIGURE 27–2 Radiographic survey of transitional dentition. Six anterior periapical radiographic images (three
on the maxilla and three on the mandible), one posterior periapical radiographic image in each quadrant, and one
posterior bitewing radiographic image on each side.

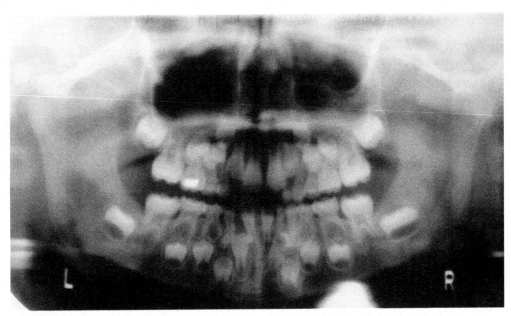

FIGURE 27–3 **Panoramic radiograph of transitional dentition.** Note eruption pattern.

development of third molars. A panoramic radiograph can sometimes be an acceptable substitute if an intraoral radiographic image receptor placement cannot be achieved. The panoramic radiographic procedure is usually well tolerated by a pediatric patient. A child must be able to hold still for the duration of the exposure cycle, usually 15 to 20 seconds, and be able to understand and cooperate with the positioning requirements necessary for producing a diagnostic image.

Other extraoral imaging examinations such as a lateral cephalometric radiograph and three-dimensional cone beam computed tomography (CBCT) used to assess adult patients can be used to provide valuable diagnostic information for pediatric patients as well. In fact, technological advancements in digital imaging is making CBCT a valuable tool in orthodontic assessment for pediatric patients (see Chapter 31).

Suggested Radiographic Techniques

Methods for exposing radiographic images on children are essentially the same as for those on adults. Although either the paralleling or bisecting technique can be used, the physical characteristics children present with usually require a slight variation in vertical angulation with either technique. A smaller oral cavity and lower palatal vault, a tendency toward a hypersensitive gag reflex and reduced tongue and muscle control, and sensitive oral mucosa due to growth and **exfoliation** (shedding) of primary teeth and eruption of permanent teeth require creative improvising on standard techniques to produce diagnostic-quality images in the presence of these challenges.

The paralleling technique is preferred for use on all patients because of its ability to produce accurate images with minimal distortion. The greatest challenge of using the paralleling technique with children is placing an image receptor parallel to the long axes of the teeth of interest. Switching to a smaller-sized image receptor may help with

this placement. Often, it is the size and weight of an image receptor holding device that children have difficulty tolerating. Switching to a smaller, lighter-weight image receptor holder, modifying an adult holder, or designing a custom holder may increase a pediatric patient's ability to tolerate placement (Figure 27–4 ■).

Once an image receptor is in position, the vertical angulation may still need to be increased slightly over the setting used for adult patients. The increase should be no more than 10 degrees to avoid dimensional distortion that can compromise image quality. Due to a shallow palatal vault, an image receptor will most likely lay flatter in position. Slightly increasing vertical angulation, 10 degrees or less, over perpendicular will help to record root apices and

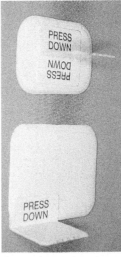

FIGURE 27–4 **Adapting an image receptor holder for pediatric use.** Bitewing bitetab positioned for use as a periapical image receptor holder. (Thomson, E. M. (1993). Dental radiographs for the child patient. *Dental Hygiene News,* 6(4), 24, with permission from Procter & Gamble Company.)

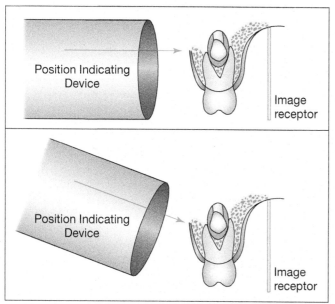

FIGURE 27–5 Slight increase in vertical angulation records more of the unerupted developing permanent teeth and will compensate for a shallow palatal vault.

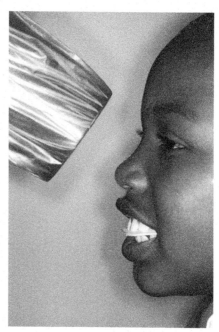

FIGURE 27–6 **Occlusal technique.** Use a size 2 image receptor to expose a maxillary occlusal radiograph.

reveal more information regarding unerupted developing permanent teeth (Figure 27–5 ■).

The bisecting technique inherently produces images with more distortion and magnification than the paralleling technique, but its greatest advantage is the ability to produce reasonably acceptable images when parallel image receptor positioning is not possible. The bisecting technique with its image receptor placement close to the teeth is usually well tolerated by a pediatric patient.

If a child cannot tolerate image receptor placement with either the paralleling or bisecting method, use an occlusal radiographic technique to achieve reasonably acceptable images. Whereas a size 4 image receptor is utilized for occlusal radiographs for adults, a size 2 image receptor will better fit a child's oral cavity (Figure 27–6 ■). The flat image receptor placement required for the occlusal technique is usually readily accepted by a pediatric patient. As with adults, use of a slight modification of vertical angulation is required for obtaining occlusal radiographs (Table 27–1 ■).

Practice Point

Children can easily understand the directive to bite on the image receptor as if it were a familiar flat-shaped item, such as a graham cracker. Occluding in this manner on the flat position of an image receptor placed for an occlusal radiograph is usually readily accepted. Once the image receptor is in position, align the central rays of the x-ray beam to produce an acceptable quality radiographic image.

ALARA Radiation Protection

It is important that all patients, children and adults, be protected from excess radiation exposure. The first step in reducing radiation exposure is the use of radiographic selection criteria to determine when radiographs are necessary. As outlined in Chapter 6, the "as low as reasonably achievable" (ALARA) practices apply to adults and children. Additional concerns regarding radiation exposure for a pediatric patient include a possible increase in sensitivity of immature, rapidly growing cells and tissues; smaller stature and overall size placing radiation-sensitive tissues closer to the path of the primary beam of radiation; and smaller, less dense bone structure requiring less radiation to produce an acceptable image. The amount of radiation required to expose an intraoral radiograph on a child of average size is less than that required for the same exposure on an average-sized adult patient. The reduction amount depends on size, body mass, and bone density of a patient. Generally, a reduction by one-half for children under 10 years of age and by one-fourth for children between the ages of 10 and 15 years is acceptable. Once a child reaches adolescence, 15 or 16 years of age, the exposure settings should be the same as for an adult patient.

An increase in the availability and prescription of CBCT examinations, especially for children, has prompted a need for strategies that bring a heightened awareness for radiation protection of pediatric patients. In 2007, the Alliance for Radiation Safety in Pediatric Imaging, a committee within the Society for Pediatric Radiology, along with several other professional radiologic and medical organizations formed the **Image Gently®** campaign to raise awareness for radiation safety and ALARA protocols for radiographic imaging of children. Dental organizations

Table 27–1 Pediatric Radiographic Techniques

Dentition Category	Type and Region	Image Receptor Size	Number of Image Receptors	Image Receptor Placement	Vertical Angulation	Horizontal Angulation	Point of Entry	Exposure
Primary dentition (ages 3 to 6 years)	Bitewing posterior	0 or 1	1 on each side	Line up behind distal half of mesially located primary maxillary or mandibular canine	+5 to +10 degrees	Perpendicular through primary first and second molar embrasure	A spot on occlusal plane between primary maxillary and mandibular first molars	Reduce adult exposure by 1/2
Primary dentition (ages 3 to 6 years)	Occlusal anterior	2	1 on each arch	Place long dimension across mouth (buccal to buccal; Figures 27–7 ▪ and 27–8 ▪)	*Maxilla:* Perpendicular to imaginary bisector +60 degrees *Mandible:* Perpendicular to imaginary bisector −30 degrees	Perpendicular to midsagittal plane	*Maxilla:* At tip of nose *Mandible:* At middle of chin	Reduce adult exposure by 1/2
Transitional dentition (ages 7 to 12 years)	Bitewing posterior	*Prior to eruption of permanent second molar:* 1 or 2	*Prior to eruption of permanent second molar:* 1 on each side	*Prior to eruption of permanent second molar:* Line up behind distal half of mesially located primary or permanent maxillary or mandibular canine (Figure 27–9 ▪)	*Prior to eruption of permanent second molar:* +5 to +10 degrees	*Prior to eruption of permanent second molar:* Perpendicular through primary first and second molar embrasure or, if erupted, first and second premolar embrasure	*Prior to eruption of permanent second molar:* A spot on occlusal plane between primary maxillary and mandibular first molars or, if erupted, first and second premolars	*Prior to eruption of permanent second molar:* Reduce adult exposure by 1/4 to 1/2

(continued)

Table 27–1 Pediatric Radiographic Techniques (continued)

Dentition Category	Type and Region	Image Receptor Size	Number of Image Receptors	Image Receptor Placement	Vertical Angulation	Horizontal Angulation	Point of Entry	Exposure
		After eruption of permanent second molar: 2	After eruption of permanent second molar: 2 on each side (1 premolar bitewing and 1 molar bitewing)	After eruption of permanent second molar: Use same criteria as for adult patient (see Table 15–3)	After eruption of permanent second molar: +10 degrees	After eruption of permanent second molar: Use same criteria as for adult patient (see Table 15–3)	After eruption of the permanent second molar: Use same criteria as adult patient (see Table 15–3)	After eruption of permanent second molar: Reduce adult exposure by 1/4 to 1/2
Transitional dentition (ages 7 to 12 years)	Anterior periapical	0 or 1	3 on each arch (1 central-lateral, 1 right canine, and 1 left canine)	Central-lateral incisors: Center behind primary or, if erupted, permanent central and lateral incisors (Figures 27–10 and 27–11)	Central-lateral incisors: Paralleling—Perpendicular to image receptor. Bisecting—Perpendicular to imaginary bisector Maxillary: +45 to +50 degrees Mandibular: −20 to −25 degrees	Central-lateral incisors: Perpendicular through left and right primary or, if erupted, permanent central incisor embrasure	Central-lateral incisors: At root tips of central incisors	Central-lateral incisors: Reduce adult exposure by 1/4 to 1/2
				Canine: Center behind primary or, if erupted, permanent canine (Figures 27–12 and 27–13)	Canine: Paralleling—Perpendicular to image receptor Bisecting—Perpendicular to imaginary bisector Maxillary: +55 to +60 degrees Mandibular: −25 to −30 degrees	Canine: Perpendicular at center of canine	Canine: At root tip of canine	Canine: Reduce adult exposure by 1/4 to 1/2

Transitional dentition (ages 7 to 12 years)	Posterior periapical	1 or 2	Prior to eruption of permanent second molars: 1 in each quadrant (4 molar periapicals)	Prior to eruption of permanent second molars: Line up behind distal half of primary or, if erupted, permanent maxillary canine (Figures 27–14 and 27–15)	Prior to eruption of permanent second molars: Paralleling—Perpendicular to image receptor Bisecting—Perpendicular to imaginary bisector Maxillary: +30 to +35 degrees Mandibular: −15 to −20 degrees	Prior to eruption of permanent second molars: Perpendicular through primary first and second molar embrasure or, if erupted, first and second premolar embrasure	Prior to eruption of permanent second molars: At root tip of primary first molar, or if erupted, root tip of first premolar	Prior to eruption of permanent second molars: Reduce adult exposure by 1/4 to 1/2
			After eruption of second permanent molar: 2 in each quadrant (4 premolar and 4 molar periapicals)	After eruption of second permanent molar: Same criteria as adult patient (see Table 13–2)	After eruption of second permanent molar: Paralleling—Perpendicular to image receptor Bisecting—Perpendicular to imaginary bisector Maxillary: +20 to +30 degrees Mandibular: -5 to -10 degrees	After eruption of second permanent molar: Same criteria as adult patient (see Table 13–2)	After eruption of second permanent molar: Same criteria as adult patient (see Table 13–2)	After eruption of second permanent molar: Reduce adult exposure by 1/4 to 1/2

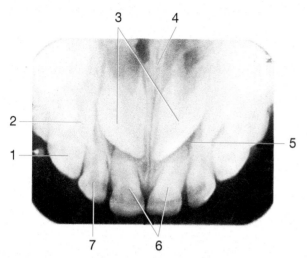

FIGURE 27–7 **Maxillary anterior occlusal radiograph exposed with size 2 film.** (**1**) Primary canine. (**2**) Unerupted permanent lateral incisor. (**3**) Unerupted permanent central incisors—note that root formation has not begun. (**4**) Median palatine suture. (**5**) Partially resorbed root of primary central incisor. (**6**) Primary central incisors. (**7**) Primary lateral incisor.

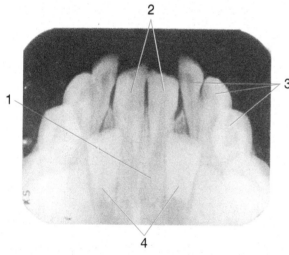

FIGURE 27–8 **Mandibular anterior occlusal radiograph exposed with size 2 film.** (**1**) Alveolar bone. (**2**) Partially erupted permanent central incisors. (**3**) Primary lateral incisor, canine, first molar. (**4**) Unerupted permanent lateral incisors.

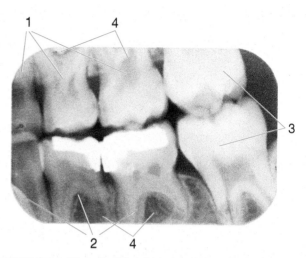

FIGURE 27–9 **Posterior bitewing radiograph.** (**1**) Primary maxillary canine, first, second molars. (**2**) Primary mandibular canine, first, second molars. (**3**) Permanent maxillary, mandibular first molars. (**4**) Note small image receptor size did not adequately record apical region to determine presence of premolars.

Patient Management

Obtaining quality radiographs on children may present challenges. A radiographer must be able to communicate and explain the procedure so that a child will understand what is expected. A patient must be able to follow directions and cooperate with the procedure requirements. The patient management skills of a radiographer should bring out a child's natural curiosity and eagerness to participate.

First impressions are important and lasting, and a child's first experience with the radiographic procedure should be pleasant and informative. The child should be a willing participant in the process. Only in an emergency

---

and specialty oral health care groups also support this alliance (Box 27–2). The Image Gently® campaign promotes ALARA recommendations that apply to both children and adult patients. These include the use of fast film and digital image receptors, x-ray beam filtration and collimating devices, appropriately reduced child exposure settings, following selection criteria guidelines for prescribing dental radiographs, and use of thyroid shielding (Figure 27–16 ■). Oral health care professionals are invited to sign an online pledge to Image Gently® committing to recognize campaign goals; to be open to suggestions on radiation safety changes; and agreeing to implement protocols and recommendations that help to reduce radiation exposure (Figure 27–17 ■).

Box 27–2: Oral Health Organizations in Support of Image Gently®

- American Academy of Oral and Maxillofacial Pathology
- American Academy of Oral and Maxillofacial Radiology
- American Academy of Oral and Maxillofacial Surgeons
- American Academy of Pediatric Dentistry
- American Academy of Periodontology
- American Association of Endodontists
- American Association of Orthodontists
- American Association of Public Health Dentistry
- American Dental Assistant Association
- American Dental Association
- American Dental Hygienists Association
- FDI World Dental Federation
- International Association of Dento-Maxillo-Facial Radiology

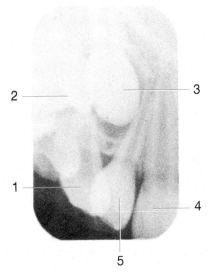

FIGURE 27–10 **Maxillary central-lateral incisors periapical radiograph.** (**1**) Primary lateral incisor. (**2**) Unerupted permanent central incisors. (**3**) Roots of primary central incisors showing signs of physiological resorption. (**4**) Primary central incisors.

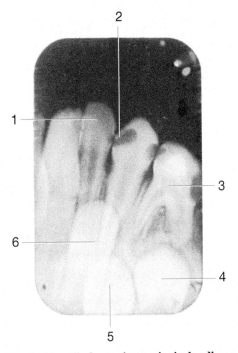

FIGURE 27–12 **Maxillary canine periapical radiograph.** (**1**) Primary canine. (**2**) Unerupted first premolar. (**3**) Unerupted permanent canine—note radiolucent dental follicle surrounding crown. (**4**) Permanent central incisor—note widened pulp chamber indicating root formation still in progress. (**5**) Permanent lateral incisor—appears to be tipped toward distal overlapping with primary canine.

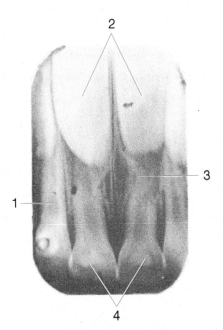

FIGURE 27–11 **Mandibular central-lateral incisors periapical radiograph.** (**1**) Unerupted permanent lateral incisor. (**2**) Caries on mesial surface of primary lateral incisor. (**3**) Permanent central incisors. (**4**) Large open apex on permanent teeth, indicating root formation still in progress.

or when a child's immediate health may be compromised should a radiographic examination continue under duress. If possible, it may be better to postpone a radiographic examination than to cause an unpleasant experience. Children can be told that they will "be bigger" next time and that the procedure will be easier now that they have "practiced" for it. Planting a positive thought is better than the risk of instilling a fear of the procedure.

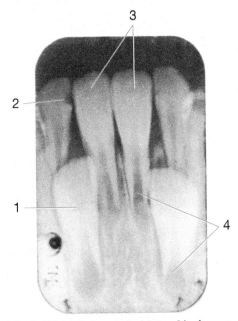

FIGURE 27–13 **Mandibular canine periapical radiograph.** (**1**) Primary lateral incisor. (**2**) Primary canine with radiolucencies indicative of caries. (**3**) Primary first molar. (**4**) Unerupted first premolar. (**5**) Unerupted permanent canine. (**6**) Unerupted permanent lateral incisor.

Most children react favorably to the authority of a confident, capable radiographer. Usually it is best to greet, and then take a child from the reception room to the examination room without the parent, to allow a radiographer to fully engage in communication with the child. Occasionally, if a child becomes difficult to manage, inviting a parent or older sibling

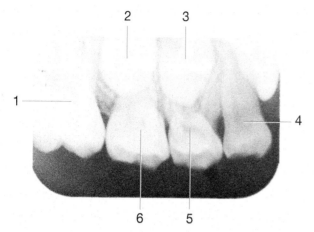

FIGURE 27–14 Maxillary molar periapical radiograph.
(**1**) Permanent first molar. (**2**) Unerupted second premolar.
(**3**) Unerupted first premolar. (**4**) Primary canine. (**5**) Primary
first molar—note almost total resorption of roots. (**6**) Primary
second molar.

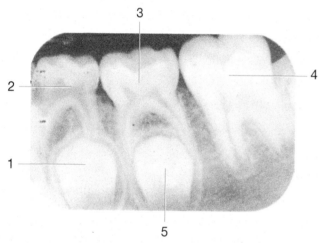

FIGURE 27–15 Mandibular molar periapical. (**1**) Unerupted
first premolar. (**2**) Primary first molar with partial resorption of
distal root. (**3**) Primary second molar. (**4**) Permanent first molar.
(**5**) Unerupted second premolar.

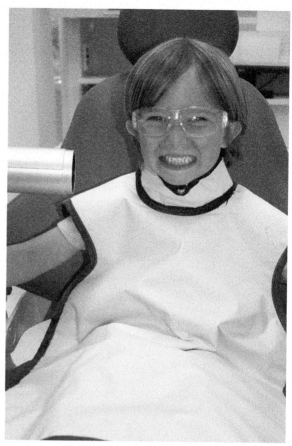

FIGURE 27–16 Child-size lead apron with thyroid collar.

Show-Tell-Do

The use of Show-Tell-Do is especially useful with pediatric
patients. Children, and adults, can be naturally fearful of
the unknown. Orienting a pediatric patient to radiographic
equipment will help to alleviate fear and will often pique
curiosity. Digital radiographic equipment can be especially
interesting and engaging for a pediatric patient. Demonstrate how a radiographic image is displayed on a computer
monitor. A child can be given a digital sensor to examine
and feel. Show a child different image receptor sizes and
then explain that the size that is "just right" will be chosen.
If an image receptor holder is to be used, allow it to be
handled and examined by the child. Carefully explain and
rehearse radiographic procedures. Use words and terminology to describe radiographic equipment on a level that a

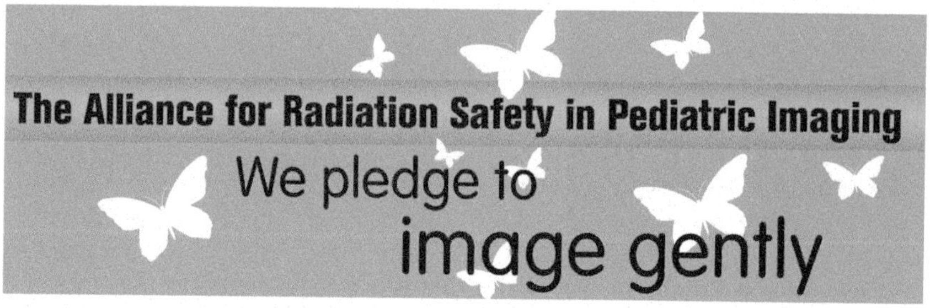

to accompany the child into the examination room may help
elicit cooperation. If a child is having trouble understanding
instructions or is unable to hold the image receptor in place,
a parent or accompanying adult may have to put on a protective lead/lead equivalent barrier and assist during exposure.

The Alliance for Radiation Safety in Pediatric Imaging
We pledge to
image gently

FIGURE 27–17 Image Gently® pledge logo. Pledge confirmation certificate and
logo for public display helps reassure patients of a practice commitment to reducing radiation exposure. (Courtesy of Alliance for Radiation Safety in Pediatric Imaging.)

child understands. Young children can be told that the x-ray tube head is a "camera" that takes special x-ray pictures of teeth; and that they can watch the computer monitor to see the pictures appear on the screen.

Modeling

Modeling, giving a patient an opportunity to observe a procedure being performed on another patient, can be a successful tool for alleviating fear of the unknown and gaining cooperation. A child may observe a cooperative older sibling or a parent undergoing the procedure. After image receptor placement, the child can accompany the radiographer out of the area, to the protected location of the control panel and assist in the exposure by watching for, and confirming, the illumination of the red exposure indicator light. Observation of, and participation in, obtaining a radiographic examination on another patient can help prepare a pediatric patient for the experience.

Communication

Use clear communication and good interpersonal skills to gain procedure acceptance and cooperation from children as would be done with adults. Praising a child for his or her cooperation and successful completion of each step of the procedure will encourage more of the same behavior. If a child's attention span is short, repeat praise and instructions with each exposure as often as necessary. Perform the examination quickly, but accurately.

Giving a pediatric patient a job to do and a sense of control, such as listening for the "beep" sound to be sure that the x-ray machine worked, will allow him or her to be a willing participant in the process and can lead to enhanced and active cooperation. However, be mindful over which procedures to maintain authority. Allowing a patient to hold and examine an image receptor is reasonable. Do not allow a child to place the holder into his or her own mouth. It is important to communicate that correct image receptor placement requires the expertise of a radiographer. Allowing a pediatric patient to try to place an image receptor and holder intraorally where he or she wants it to go may lead to less cooperation.

Many strategies that apply to managing adult patients and patients with special needs or specific oral conditions work well with pediatric patients (see Chapters 28 and 29). Whenever possible begin an examination with the potentially easier or more comfortable image receptor placement positions to gain acceptance, usually in the anterior region of the oral cavity. Tell a story that lasts throughout the examination procedure (distraction technique); count backwards from 5 to 0 while the patient holds his or her breath, to allow time to make the exposure (breathing exercise for hypersensitive gag reflex); and palpate tissues with an index finger to massage and desensitize sensitive mucosa and to simulate image receptor placement (Figure 27–18 ■). Additional patient management strategies will be presented in Chapters 28 and 29.

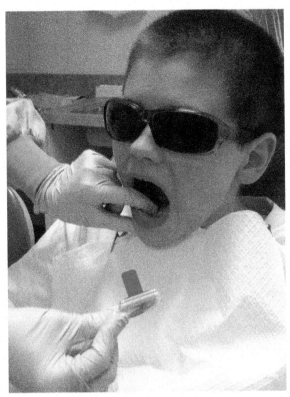

FIGURE 27–18 **Digital palpation** desensitizes sensitive mucosa prior to image receptor placement.

Radiographic Interpretation

Radiographs play an especially important role in detecting diseases and conditions that impact growth and development. Early detection can advantageously affect treatment outcomes. Interpret radiographs prescribed for pediatric patients in the same manner as those obtained for adults. An accurate interpretation of pediatric radiographs requires a working knowledge of dentition eruption patterns, primary and permanent tooth crown and root morphology, and the appearance of normal growth and development conditions.

Begin the interpretation process by identifying the presence or absence of teeth. This requires knowing which permanent tooth develops apical to, and then erupts into, the space occupied by a primary tooth. Determine any deviation from a normal eruption pattern, such as the presence of a supernumerary tooth, or a congenitally missing tooth. Next, examine the morphology of each primary tooth, noting normal physiologic root resorption that occurs in response to an erupting permanent tooth. Examine morphology of each unerupted permanent tooth noting the appearance of a dental follicle or sac. In early development stages, a tooth crown appears completely encircled within a radiolucent dental follicle; in later stages a thinning radiolucent outline surrounds the crown and elongates as the root takes shape. Examine partially and fully erupted permanent teeth and note the widened pulp chambers and large open apices indicating that normal root formation is still in progress. This appearance may be observed radiographically until about two or three years following tooth eruption as root formation continues after

eruption. Continue the interpretation process to determine deviations from normal development that would need a referral to determine a pathologic condition (see Figures 27–7 through 27–15).

REVIEW—Chapter summary

Pediatric radiographic techniques and the types of projections used to image oral and maxillofacial regions do not differ significantly from those used for adult patients. However, children present with unique characteristics that may require adaptation to standard procedures. Evidence-based selection criteria guidelines are used to prescribe radiographs for children and adolescents. A radiographic examination may be prescribed for detection of caries, oral diseases, dental abnormalities; and to assess growth and development and trauma. Radiographs record the condition of primary teeth and developing, unerupted permanent teeth. Once teeth have erupted preventing visual inspection of proximal surfaces for caries, radiographs may be prescribed.

The number of radiographs and size of image receptor selected will depend on age, oral cavity size, and cooperation level. Size 0 or 1 is appropriate for bitewing radiographs of primary dentition, prior to eruption of first permanent molars; size 2 is appropriate for transitional mixed dentition. Use the largest size image receptor that a child can tolerate. If necessary, an occlusal radiograph may be substituted for a periapical radiograph. Following eruption of permanent second molars, bitewing and full mouth surveys for children follow the adult guidelines.

If an image receptor cannot be held securely in place for the duration of the exposure, intraoral occlusal, panoramic, and other extraoral radiographs may be an acceptable substitute. Extraoral radiographs and cone beam computed tomography (CBCT) provide information regarding development of dental arches and other oral and maxillofacial structures.

Adjust standard radiographic techniques to meet the needs of a pediatric patient's smaller oral cavity, potential hypersensitive gag reflex, and soft tissue sensitivity due to the eruption process. The paralleling method is the technique of choice; however, image receptor placement may be easier with the bisecting method. Use a small, lighter-weight image receptor holder or design a custom holder to increase

tolerance to placement. Due to a shallow palatal vault, an image receptor may lay flatter in position. Slightly increase vertical angulation, 10 degrees or less, over perpendicular to assist with recording root apices and unerupted developing permanent teeth.

Pediatric radiographs require less radiation to produce an acceptable quality image due to decreased size, body mass, and bone density. Reduce adult exposure settings for children under 10 years of age by one-half, and by one-fourth for children 10 to 15 years of age. Adolescents 15 to 16 years of age and older require the same exposure settings as an adult. The Image Gently® campaign was organized to promote and advocate the need for increased radiation safety specifically for children. Oral health care professionals are invited to pledge commitment to implementing radiation safety protocols and following suggestions and recommendations that help to reduce radiation exposure.

A pediatric patient's first experience with a radiographic procedure should produce acceptable diagnostic quality radiographs under pleasant circumstances. A successful outcome is more likely when good communication elicits cooperation. Most children react favorably to the authority of a confident, capable radiographer. Show-Tell-Do and modeling are valuable patient management tools. Orient a pediatric patient to radiographic equipment to alleviate fear of the unknown. Provide a way to give a pediatric patient a sense of control that can lead to enhanced cooperation, but be mindful about maintaining authority.

Interpret pediatric radiographs in the same manner as those obtained for adults. Develop a working knowledge of dentition eruption patterns and primary and permanent tooth morphology to accurately interpret pediatric radiographs. Interpretation should include an observation of the appearance of normal growth and development conditions including physiologic external resorption, dental sac or follicle, widened pulp chambers, and large open apices.

RECALL—Study questions

1. List five conditions that might indicate a need to expose dental radiographs on a child.
   a. _____
   b. _____
   c. _____
   d. _____
   e. _____

2. Which of the following conditions noted during a clinical examination of a pediatric patient would most likely prompt a need for an adaptation to standard radiographic procedures?
   a. Proximal surfaces visible clinically
   b. Shallow palatal vault
   c. Inadequate self-care
   d. Child > 15 years of age

3. What size image receptor is recommended for imaging transitional mixed dentition?
   a. Size 0
   b. Size 1
   c. Size 2
   d. Size 4

4. Each of the following need to be considered when deciding what size image receptor to use for a pediatric radiograph EXCEPT one. Which one is the EXCEPTION?
   a. Cooperation level
   b. Size of dental arches
   c. Size of mouth opening
   d. Amount of plaque present

5. Which image receptor size would be easiest to position for a bitewing radiograph on a 5-year-old patient?
   a. Size 0
   b. Size 1
   c. Size 2
   d. Size 4

6. Which of the following is the best reason to use the largest size intraoral image receptor that a child will tolerate?
   a. So that a decreased number of image receptors will have to be exposed
   b. To enable compatible use with the paralleling technique
   c. To record more information about a larger area
   d. So that the radiation exposure time can be reduced

7. Which of the following is the suggested number and type of radiographs to expose if a 3-year-old patient required a full mouth examination?
   a. 2 bitewing and 2 occlusal
   b. 2 bitewing and 2 periapical
   c. 2 bitewing and 4 periapical
   d. 4 bitewing and 10 periapical

8. Which of the following is the suggested number and type of radiographs to expose if a 10-year-old patient required a full mouth examination?
   a. 2 bitewing and 8 periapical
   b. 2 bitewing and 10 periapical
   c. 4 bitewing and 10 periapical
   d. 4 bitewing and 14 periapical

9. Which of the following is the suggested number and type of radiographs to expose if a 15-year-old patient required a full mouth examination?
   a. 2 bitewing and 6 periapical
   b. 4 bitewing and 8 periapical
   c. 4 bitewing and 10 periapical
   d. 4 bitewing and 14 periapical

10. If a child cannot tolerate placement of an image receptor for exposure of a periapical radiograph, which of the following can be an acceptable substitute?
    a. Bitewing
    b. Panoramic
    c. Occlusal
    d. Both b and c

11. What slight change in angulation is usually required when using the bisecting technique to obtain pediatric radiographs?
    a. Increase vertical angulation
    b. Decrease vertical angulation
    c. Direct horizontal angulation mesiodistally
    d. Direct horizontal angulation distomesially

12. Exposure setting for a child under 10 years of age should be
    a. reduced by one-half the exposure used for adults.
    b. reduced by one-third the exposure used for adults.
    c. reduced by one-fourth the exposure used for adults.
    d. the same exposure as used for adults.

13. Exposure setting for a child between 10 and 15 years of age should be
    a. reduced by one-half the exposure used for adults.
    b. reduced by one-third the exposure used for adults.
    c. reduced by one-fourth the exposure used for adults.
    d. the same exposure as used for adults.

14. Exposure setting for a child over 16 years of age should be
    a. reduced by one-half the exposure used for adults.
    b. reduced by one-third the exposure used for adults.
    c. reduced by one-fourth the exposure used for adults.
    d. the same exposure as used for adults.

15. The Image Gently® campaign was formed to
    a. develop state-of-the-art pediatric imaging systems.
    b. raise awareness of radiation safety for children.
    c. review regulations governing the use of ionizing radiation on children.
    d. study the effects of changing pediatric exposure times.

16. The management strategy known as modeling can alleviate fear of a radiographic procedure *because* modeling allows a child to observe, prior to undergoing, the procedure.
    a. Both the statement and reason are correct and related.
    b. Both the statement and reason are correct but NOT related.
    c. The statement is correct, but the reason is NOT.
    d. The statement is NOT correct, but the reason is correct.
    e. NEITHER the statement NOR the reason is correct.

17. A radiolucent widening of the pulp chamber of a maxillary central incisor observed on a radiographic image of a pediatric patient is most likely
    a. external resorption.
    b. internal resorption.
    c. incomplete root formation.
    d. dental follicle.

REFLECT—Case study

Consider the following chart that lists sample exposure settings for an adult patient. Complete the chart to reflect the recommendations presented in this chapter regarding exposure settings for a pediatric patient.

Film
speed: F

PID
length: 12 in. (30.5 cm)

mA: 7

kVp: 70

| | Impulses | | |
Bitewings	Adult	Child (under 10 yrs)	Child (10–15 yrs)
Posterior	20	—	—
Anterior	16	—	—
Periapicals			
Maxillary anterior	18	—	—
Maxillary premolar	22	—	—
Maxillary molar	24	—	—
Mandibular anterior	16	—	—
Mandibular premolar	18	—	—
Mandibular molar	20	—	—

RELATE—Laboratory application

Visit the Alliance for Radiation Safety in Pediatric Imaging Image Gently® Web site at: www.imagegently.org. Prepare a presentation to share with your class on how oral health care professionals can participate in increasing awareness of the need for radiation protection of pediatric patients and in adopting radiation safety best practices.

RESOURCES

Alliance for Radiation Safety in Pediatric Imaging. (2014). Image Gently® Campaign. Retrieved from Alliance for Radiation Safety in Pediatric Imaging Web site: http://www.imagegently.org

American Academy of Pediatric Dentistry. (2015). Guidelines on prescribing dental radiographs for infants, children, adolescents, and persons with special health care needs. *Journal of Pediatric Dentistry, 37*(reference manual), 319–321.

Carestream Dental. (2015). *Successful intraoral radiography.* Retrieved from Carestream Dental Web site: http://www.carestreamdental.com/ImagesFileShare/.sitecore.media_library.Files.Film_and_Anesthetics.8665_Successful_Intraoral_Brochure.pdf

Pinkham, J., Casamassimo, P., Fields, H. W., McTigue, D. J., & Nowak, A. J. (2013). *Pediatric dentistry: Infancy through adolescence* (5th ed.). St. Louis, MO: Elsevier Saunders.

Thomson, E. M. (2008). Panoramic radiographs and the pediatric patient. Part 1. *Dimensions of Dental Hygiene, 6*(2), 26–29.

White, S. C., & Pharoah, M. J. (2014). Prescribing diagnostic imaging. *Oral radiology: Principles and interpretation* (7th ed.). St. Louis, MO: Elsevier.

Visit www.pearsonhighered.com/healthprofessionsresources to access the student resources that accompany this book. Simply select Dental Hygiene from the choice of disciplines. Find this book and you will find the complementary study tools created for this specific title.

Radiographic Techniques for Patients with Special Needs

OBJECTIVES

Following successful completion of this chapter, you should be able to:

1. Define key terms.
2. Discuss strategies for managing apprehension during a radiographic examination.
3. Discuss strategies for managing patients with autism spectrum disorder (ASD).
4. Explain ways to manage a patient with disabilities.
5. Identify opportunities to develop cultural sensitivity and cultural competence.
6. Discuss strategies for managing radiographic procedures for a patient with age-related changes.
7. Use evidence-based guidelines to educate patients who may be reluctant to accept radiographic assessment of need.

KEY TERMS

Autism spectrum disorder (ASD)
Cultural competence

Disability

Speech reading

Introduction

Radiographic examinations are prescribed based on signs and symptoms with which a patient presents. The procedures used to obtain a radiograph examination require this same careful individualized attention to meet unique patient needs. Radiographic techniques should be selected and performed based on oral maxillofacial, medical, physical, psychological, emotional, and cultural considerations with which a patient exhibits. Skills necessary to meet these challenges must be developed to successfully produce diagnostic quality radiographic images while practicing ALARA (as low as reasonably achievable). This chapter presents radiographic techniques that can assist with producing quality radiographic images for patients with special needs (Table 28–1 ■).

Patient with Apprehension

If a patient perceives radiographic procedures as unpleasant, apprehension may manifest. A patient may have had a negative experience with a past radiographic procedure, causing him or her to project those negative feelings onto the current situation. It is important to show an apprehensive patient empathy, concern, and a pleasant and reassuring attitude.

It is equally important that a radiographer not project his or her own negative feelings or experiences regarding the procedure into the current situation. If a radiographer has personal views regarding the experience as uncomfortable or not necessary, he or she must not assume that the patient shares those views. Most patients are not apprehensive about radiographic procedures, and nothing should be said or done that would prompt a patient to become anxious.

To prevent or reduce apprehension, the following are suggested:

- **Develop a rapport.** Take time to explain radiographic procedures and allow the patient to ask questions. A conversation that demonstrates attentive listening and empathy can help relax an apprehensive patient.
- **Project confidence.** A skilled radiographer who demonstrates confidence will gain trust and

Table 28–1 Radiographic Management of Special Needs

Special Need	Anticipated Challenge	Management Strategy
Apprehension	Cooperation with procedure	Develop rapport Project confidence Maintain authority Be organized Reassure patient
Wheelchair-bound	Access to radiographic equipment	Transfer to examination chair
Visual impairment	Communication	Explain procedure in detail Use touch to help describe equipment and procedures Announce when exiting and entering the area Explain need to remove personal eyewear
Hearing impairment	Communication	Establish alternative methods of communication
Culturally diverse	Communication	Be aware of communication styles, zones of territory, meanings of gestures
Age-related changes	Tolerance of image receptor	Use smaller, lighter-weight image receptor and holder, and comfort-designed products Supplement with extraoral radiographs
Radiation therapy	Reluctance to radiographic examination	Demonstrate empathy with shared concern Educate patient on use of evidence-based criteria for assessment of radiographic need Explain radiation safety protocol
Pregnancy	Reluctance to radiographic examination	Demonstrate empathy with shared concern Educate patient on use of evidence-based criteria for assessment of radiographic need Explain radiation safety protocol

cooperation. Apprehension may be increased when it is perceived that an operator is unsure of oneself.

- **Maintain authority.** Maintain control over the radiographic procedure. Be gentle, but firm. A patient who trusts a radiographer's ability may have less cause to become anxious. Consider this example: A patient is allowed to take control of the procedure by dictating how an image receptor should be placed. Letting go of control of how and where an image receptor is placed may add to the creation of stress or patient apprehension. The patient may now feel responsible for directing the procedure and may become increasingly anxious that the radiographer is not performing the technique correctly or that the radiographs may not come out right and will have to be retaken.
- **Be organized.** Progress through the procedure rapidly and accurately. For example, expose the easier maxillary anterior projections first, gaining patient confidence, prior to progressing to the potentially more difficult posterior areas.
- **Provide reassurance.** Compliment apprehensive patients on their ability to cooperate with the procedure. Continually provide reassuring feedback throughout the examination.

Extreme Cases of Apprehension

Occasionally, a patient with an extreme case of anxiety can be difficult to manage. This may occur with **autism spectrum disorder (ASD)**. The prevalence of ASD is on the rise, with 1 in 68 children age 8 years diagnosed more recently compared with 1 in 150 children in the year 2000, increasing the likelihood that these patients will be encountered in practice. ASD is a complex disorder characterized as deficits with communication, leading to social situations and behaviors that create anxiety. ASD ranges from a mild form of the disorder where an individual may exhibit slight social impairments to a severe form denoted by speech impediments, unexpected or repetitive behaviors, severe emotional outbursts, and hypersensitivity to new places, situations, and stimuli. A dental radiographic examination, especially when unfamiliar to an individual with ASD, may elicit anxiety.

Dental radiographers should be trained in intervention strategies and specific social and communication techniques in advance of performing radiographic examinations for a patient with ASD. Avoiding a severe anxiety reaction to dental radiography procedures is best accomplished through preventive measures. Helpful tools that can prepare an individual with ASD for a radiographic examination include video technologies, mobile applications, and picture cards that help familiarize a patient with the dental environment and radiographic equipment, reducing anxiety that results when encountering the unknown (Figure 28–1 ■). Media tools can demonstrate and familiarize a patient with procedures, and provide a radiographer with guidelines for communication that can be reinforced during the examination. Individuals with ASD can view mobile application images or video clips repetitively prior to an appointment to alleviate anxiety and feel more comfortable once in the oral health care environment. During the examination use videos or picture cards as a prompt for what will happen next and to aid verbal and nonverbal communication.

In rare cases conscious sedation, general anesthesia, and/or medical restraint may be necessary for patients with ASD unable to be managed with any of the above strategies. Consider the risks and complications of these alternatives, and use only as a last resort.

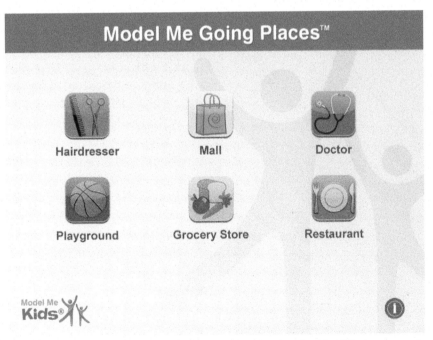

FIGURE 28–1 Technology for reducing anxiety associated with ASD. (Courtesy of Model Me Kids, LLC.)

Patient with Disabilities

A **disability** is defined as a physical or mental impairment that substantially limits one or more of an individual's major life activities. Be prepared to accommodate patients with disabilities.

- **Talk directly to the patient.** Do not ask a patient's caregiver questions that should be directed to the patient. For example, do not say to the caregiver, "Can he (or she) stand up?" Instead, speak directly to the patient and say, "Can you stand up?"
- **Offer assistance to disabled patients.** Ask the patient how you can best be of assistance.
- **Do not ask personal questions about the patient's disability.**

Individual Who Uses a Wheelchair

It can sometimes be difficult to maneuver a patient who uses a wheelchair into a position close enough to the dental x-ray machine to obtain prescribed radiographs (Figure 28–2 ■). Take care to ensure that the dental x-ray machine extension arm can support the x-ray tube head in the correct position without drifting. Unless using a total-support wheelchair, it may be best to transfer a patient to the dental examination chair to complete the radiographic examination. Patients can be transferred from wheelchair to dental chair by use of the following techniques:

- **Patient who can temporarily support weight** can be transferred by placing the wheelchair alongside the examination chair. Set the brakes of the wheelchair and elevate the examination chair to the height of the wheelchair. Move or remove both the wheelchair and the examination chair arms from between the chairs.

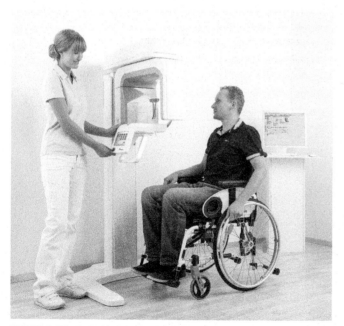

FIGURE 28–2 Panoramic machine that can accommodate wheelchair-bound patient. (Courtesy of Air Techniques, Inc.)

Place one end of a transfer sliding board, designed for this purpose, under the patient and the other end across the dental chair. Have the patient move or slide sideways from the chair, onto the board and onto the examination chair with the caregiver and radiographer assisting as needed.

- **If a patient is unable to support weight,** the caregiver and radiographer together must assist with the transfer. Follow the patient's and the caregiver's directions on how to proceed. Working together, one person should take a position behind the patient and the other person should be in front of and facing the patient, to facilitate lifting the patient from the wheelchair into the examination chair. Use a transfer belt that wraps around the patient's waist to hold the patient steady during this movement.

Individual with a Visual Impairment

A visually impaired or blind patient requires special consideration during radiographic procedures. Communicate using clear verbal explanations of each step of the procedure before it is performed. When exposing multiple radiographic images, it is important to maintain verbal contact to reorient the patient each time an image receptor is placed and removed from the oral cavity. Use touch to demonstrate placement of the image receptor and the feel of the receptor holder prior to its placement to help eliminate the feeling of anxiety when facing the unknown.

Personal eyewear worn by a patient with a visual impairment may have to be temporarily removed if it is determined that the eyewear will be positioned within the path of the primary x-ray beam. Explain the need for this, and allow a patient to remove his or her own glasses. Immediately following the procedure, allow the patient to resume wearing personal eyewear.

Maintain communication. Announce when leaving the examination room during radiation exposure, and let the patient know how long he or she will be left alone in the examination room during radiographic film processing or while scanning photostimulable (PSP) plates. Immediately announce your return to the operatory by speaking directly to the patient.

Individual with a Hearing Impairment

Communication is important to the success of all radiographic procedures. A patient must receive explicit detailed instructions before, during, and at the end of each image

Practice Point

Never gesture to another person in the presence of a patient with a visual impairment. Blind persons are sensitive to gesture communication and may feel you are "talking behind their back."

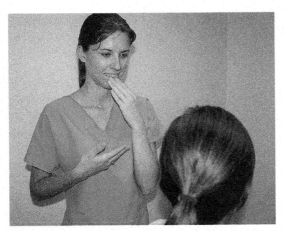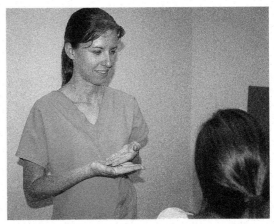

FIGURE 28–3 **Radiographer using American Sign Language (ASL)** to communicate that the radiographic examination is going well.

receptor placement and radiographic exposure. The production of quality radiographs depends on a patient's ability to understand and follow these instructions. Communication with a hearing-impaired patient requires knowledge of what method of communication works best for the patient. Always ask a hearing-impaired or deaf patient how he or she prefers to communicate. Options for communication are:

- Written instructions
- Relative or caregiver as interpreter
- Gestures

If a patient uses **speech reading** (reading lips), face the patient and speak slowly and clearly, allowing the patient to read facial expressions and gestures. Because a face mask is recommended as personal protective equipment (PPE; see Chapter 9) during radiographic procedures, it is important that the patient and radiographer agree on the meaning of certain gestures before putting on a face mask. A hearing-impaired patient will appreciate a radiographer who has learned a few sign language gestures to facilitate communication (Figure 28–3 ∎).

If a patient uses a hearing aid device, it may have to be removed prior to exposing a panoramic radiograph (see Chapter 17). Explain the procedure and ensure patient understanding of required cooperation needed prior to asking a patient to remove the device. Immediately following the procedure, allow the patient to resume wearing his or her hearing aid device.

Cultural Competency

Cultural competence can be defined as the level of knowledge-based skills required to provide effective clinical care to patients from a particular ethnic or racial group. The wide range of cultural beliefs and values in today's global society means that a radiographer is increasingly likely to find oneself performing radiographic examinations on patients of a variety of racial, ethnic, and cultural backgrounds. Educating patients from a variety of cultural backgrounds regarding

the role radiographs play in the diagnosis and treatment of oral diseases requires an awareness of possible cross-cultural barriers, such as language, beliefs, traditions, and familial influences. Dental radiographers who are sterotypical, prejudiced, and/or unsure of how to treat patients with cultural diversity contribute to the growing access to care barriers.

Because good communication is the foundation on which quality radiographs are produced, strive to develop a better understanding of cultures most likely to be encountered in the community where an oral health care practice is located. To assist in developing cultural sensitivity take into consideration a patient's:

- **Communication style.** Is eye contact considered respectful or a sign of rudeness? Is discussion of the oral cavity personal and private? Is a patient comfortable having a family member translate personal or sensitive information? Does the culture perceive or value oral wellness?
- **Comfortable zones of territory.** Does touch convey acceptance, or is it offensive? Is a patient uncomfortable being treated by a professional of the opposite gender? Are certain articles of clothing or jewelry worn that a patient would be uncomfortable removing for a radiographic procedure?
- **Nonverbal gestures.** Does the meaning of a hand gesture carry over to the same thing to the patient in his or her culture? Are there hand gestures needed to convey instructions regarding the radiographic procedure that might be considered impolite in another culture?

Being aware of other value systems and incorporating other cultural perspectives into practice is likely to gain trust and cooperation necessary for successful radiographic examinations (Figure 28–4 ∎). Being aware of attitudes toward, gaining knowledge in, and developing skills for interacting with diverse cultures can help reduce barriers to oral health care and gain acceptance of preventive procedures, including radiographic examinations (Box 28–1).

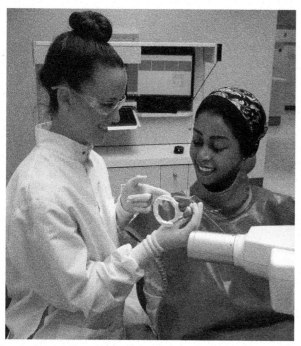

FIGURE 28–4 **Culturally competent radiographer** communicates to gain trust and cooperation necessary for a successful radiographic examination.

Other Special Needs Considerations

Age-Related Changes

Normal, age-related changes affecting the health of an individual do not necessarily mean that older adult patients

---

Box 28–1: Developing Cultural Awareness

Attitude

Become aware of one's own cultural background.

Identify and eliminate personal bias toward diverse cultures.

Acknowledge the role cultural influences play on patient oral health care decisions.

Knowledge

Learn about cultural differences, traditions, and beliefs.

Discover personal values of individual culturally diverse patients.

Engage patients in collaborative discussions regarding cultural influences.

Skill Development

Participate in multicultural experiences.

Develop respect for cultures different than one's own.

Demonstrate professionalism and kindness toward diverse cultures.

---

will present with unique conditions requiring special radiographic procedures. However, it is important to be aware of an increased incidence of conditions that may require adjustments or alterations in standard radiographic techniques. Soft tissue changes noted in an aging population may affect oral mucosa and lips. Reduced salivary flow can lead to an increase in sensitivity and reduction in pliability of soft tissues, hindering or preventing accurate image receptor placement. Muscle function that diminishes with age can affect an individual's ability to maintain firm pressure on an image receptor positioner for the duration of an exposure. Residual effects of stroke, such as paralysis, may reduce the ability to move or control the tongue, or result in unsteadiness and tremors that present a challenge to holding still during exposures. Alzheimer's disease—which often results in inattentiveness to instructions, loss of coordination, and other motor abnormalities, including exaggerated reflexes—should be taken into consideration when planning to expose radiographs.

It is important to communicate with older adult patients to ensure that they can follow instructions for a successful outcome to the radiographic procedure. Most of the suggestions presented for managing other special needs patients can be applied to aid in obtaining quality radiographic images for an older adult patient. These include using a smaller image receptor with a lighter-weight image receptor holder and applying a commercial product that reduces image receptor edge sharpness (Figure 28–5 ■).

Radiation Therapy

A patient who is currently receiving or has recently undergone radiation therapy for the treatment of cancer may have questions regarding the radiation dose needed to expose dental radiographs. A patient may be reluctant to receive additional radiation, no matter how small. An informative discussion with the patient should include an opportunity to

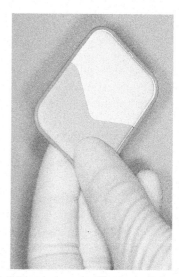

FIGURE 28–5 **Edge protectors.** Film is available with commercially applied edge softeners.

ask questions and to make clear that concerns for radiation safety are shared by the oral health care team. A prescription to expose dental radiographs is based on an assessment of need, carefully weighing benefits and risks. Although an oncology patient may have received large therapeutic doses of radiation, this is not a contraindication to exposing dental radiographs necessary for an oral diagnosis. The radiation dose required to expose dental radiographs is minimal, and its use is justified to gain potential benefits to oral and overall health.

Pregnancy

In the past there has been controversy regarding the exposure of diagnostic radiographs, including dental radiographs, during pregnancy. Modern radiation producing equipment and image receptors that require minimal radiation exposure continue to significantly reduce the radiation dose of a dental radiographic examination. Additionally, research continues to link poor oral health with other diseases that affect overall health, making oral care an important requirement during pregnancy. The American Dental Association (ADA) and the American College of Obstetricians and Gynecologists (ACOG) recommend prophylactic oral health assessments, including necessary dental radiographs during pregnancy. The ACOG has deemed routine oral health care, including dental radiographic examinations, safe during pregnancy; and that pregnancy is not a reason to delay necessary radiographic examinations and subsequent treatment, especially when a delay has the potential to lead to a worsening problem or future complications.

REVIEW—Chapter summary

Radiographic techniques should be selected and performed based on oral maxillofacial, medical, physical, psychological, emotional, and cultural considerations with which a patient presents. Basic radiographic procedures may need to be altered to manage patients with special needs. Radiographic procedures involving an apprehensive patient may be managed by developing a rapport with the patient, projecting confidence, maintaining authority, being organized, and reassuring the patient throughout the procedure.

A dental radiographic examination can elicit anxiety in an individual with autism spectrum disorder (ASD), especially if the procedure is new or unfamiliar. Extreme anxiety may be difficult to manage. Avoid a severe anxiety reaction to dental radiography procedures through preventive measures. Media tools can assist with familiarizing and preparing an individual with ASD for a radiographic examination; and they can be used repetitively prior to and during the examination as a prompt for what will happen next and to aid verbal and nonverbal communication.

A disability is a physical or mental impairment that substantially limits one or more of an individual's major life activities. Be prepared to accommodate patients with disabilities: talk directly to the patient; ask the patient how best to offer assistance; and do not ask personal questions regarding the patient's disability. A wheelchair-bound patient may need to be transferred to an examination chair to accommodate placement of the x-ray tube head.

Establish clear communication to facilitate radiographic examinations for visual- and hearing-impaired patients. A patient's personal eyewear may need to be removed if in the path of the primary x-ray beam during exposure. Establish an alternative communication method with a hearing-impaired patient who uses speech reading prior to putting on a personal protective mask.

Cultural competence requires knowledge-based skills, and an accepting and respectful attitude to provide effective care to patients from different cultures. Cultural competency is expressed as a nonjudgmental attitude when presented with diverse cultures. To assist in developing cultural sensitivity take into consideration a patient's communication style, comfortable zones of territory, and possible dual meanings to nonverbal gestures. Be aware of a patient's value systems to gain trust and cooperation necessary for successful radiographic examinations.

Normal age-related changes may prompt alteration in radiographic techniques. Soft tissue changes affecting sensitivity of oral mucosa and lips, reduced salivary flow, reduced muscle function, and reduction in pliability of soft tissues noted in an aging population may hinder or prevent accurate image receptor placement.

Some patients, especially those who have received radiation therapy, and patients who are pregnant may be reluctant to consent to necessary dental radiographs. It should be explained to all patients that radiographs are prescribed according to evidence-based criteria, and recommended only when a beneficial diagnosis can result.

RECALL—Study questions

1. List five actions for managing an apprehensive patient.
   a. _____
   b. _____
   c. _____
   d. _____
   e. _____

2. A dental radiographic examination can produce severe anxiety in a patient with autism spectrum disorder (ASD) *because* patients with extreme anxiety are often hypersensitive to new and unfamilar situations.
   a. Both the statement and reason are correct and related.
   b. Both the statement and reason are correct but NOT related.
   c. The statement is correct, but the reason is NOT.
   d. The statement is NOT correct, but the reason is correct.
   e. NEITHER the statement NOR the reason is correct.

3. Use of each of the following can assist in reducing anxiety for patients with autism spectrum disorder (ASD) EXCEPT one. Which one is the EXCEPTION?
   a. Video clips
   b. Mobile applications
   c. Picture cards
   d. Safety glasses

4. When performing radiographic services for a patient with a disability
   a. remove the patient's eyewear for him or her prior to exposures.
   b. offer to assist the patient in the manner that he or she wants.
   c. communicate with the caregiver instead of talking directly to the patient.
   d. ask personal questions about the patient's disability.

5. A sliding board during a wheelchair transfer is used for patients who can temporarily support their own weight. Patients who cannot temporarily support their own weight must remain in the wheelchair during a radiographic examination.
   a. The first statement is true. The second statement is false.
   b. The first statement is false. The second statement is true.
   c. Both statements are true.
   d. Both statements are false.

6. To assist a patient with a visual impairment during a radiographic examination
   a. avoid discussing patient's disability.
   b. use gestures to communicate with a caregiver.
   c. announce when entering and leaving the area.
   d. speak louder to make patient aware of your presence.

7. Take each of the following into consideration when interacting with a patient from a different culture EXCEPT one. Which one is the EXCEPTION?
   a. Lowered intellectual capacity
   b. Personal territory zone
   c. Communication style
   d. Multiple meanings to hand gestures

8. Which of the following is NOT helpful to developing cultural competence?
   a. Learn about cultural differences, traditions, and beliefs.
   b. Acknowledge that cultural values are more important than individual values.
   c. Engage patients in collaborate discussions regarding cultural influences.
   d. Identify and eliminate personal bias toward diverse cultures.

9. Older adults who present with soft tissue degeneration that makes placement of an image receptor uncomfortable may benefit from each of the following EXCEPT one. Which one is the EXCEPTION?
   a. Applying an edge protector to the image receptor
   b. Using a smaller-sized image receptor
   c. Using a lighter-weight image receptor holder
   d. Rinsing with an antimicrobial product prior to image receptor placement

10. Which of the following is correct protocol for dental radiographic assessment of a pregnant patient?
    a. Expose necessary radiographs as per assessment.
    b. Expose necessary radiographs only if an emergency.
    c. Postpone necessary radiographs until the third trimester of pregnancy.
    d. Postpone necessary radiographs until after delivery.

REFLECT—Case study

Select one of the special needs listed in Table 28–1. Assume that you will need to perform a full mouth series radiographic examination for this patient. Research the special need to learn all you can to best prepare to communicate with the patient and successfully perform the procedure. Share challenges and tips and technique alterations you learn or develop with your class.

RELATE—Laboratory application

For a comprehensive laboratory practice exercise on this topic, see Thomson, E. M., & Bruhn, A. M. (2018). *Exercises in oral radiography techniques: A laboratory manual* (4th ed.). Hoboken, NJ: Pearson. Chapter 10, "Patient Management Skill Development."

RESOURCES

American College of Obstetricians and Gynecologists. (2013, July 26). Dental x-rays, teeth cleanings. Safe during pregnancy. Retrieved from ACOG Web site: http://www.acog.org /About-ACOG/News-Room/News-Releases/2013 /Dental-X-Rays-Teeth-Cleanings-Safe-During-Pregnancy

American Dental Association. (2012, November 28). ADA updates dental radiograph recommendations. Retrieved from ADA Web site: http://www.ada.org/en/publications/ada-news/2012-archive /november/ada-updates-dental-radiograph-recommendations

Charbonneau, C. J., Neufeld M. J., Craig B. J., & Donnelly, L. R. (2009). Increasing cultural competence in the dental hygiene profession. *Canadian Journal of Dental Hygiene*, *43*, 297–305.

Darby, M. L., & Walsh, M. M. (2015). Cultural competence. *Dental hygiene theory and practice* (4th ed.). St. Louis, MO: Elsevier.

Elmore, J., Bruhn, A., & Bobzien, J. (2016). Research: Interventions for the reduction of dental anxiety and corresponding behavioral deficits in children with autism spectrum disorder (ASD). *Journal of Dental Hygiene*, *90*, 111–120.

Khan, F. M. (2014). *The physics of radiation therapy* (5th ed.). Philadelphia: Lippincott Williams & Wilkins.

White, S. C., & Pharoah, M. J. (2014). Prescribing diagnostic imaging. *Oral radiology: Principles and interpretation* (7th ed.). St. Louis, MO: Elsevier.

Wilkins, E. M. (2015). Patients with special needs. *Clinical practice of the dental hygienist* (12th ed.). Philadelphia: Lippincott Williams & Wilkins.

Visit www.pearsonhighered.com/healthprofessionsresources to access the student resources that accompany this book. Simply select Dental Hygiene from the choice of disciplines. Find this book and you will find the complementary study tools created for this specific title.

Radiographic Techniques for Specific Oral Conditions

OBJECTIVES

Following successful completion of this chapter, you should be able to:

1. Define the key terms.
2. Demonstrate ability to appropriately adapt standard radiographic techniques to meet specific oral condition challenges.
3. List and define gag reflex stimuli.
4. Describe methods to prevent and manage a gag reflex during a radiographic examination.
5. Demonstrate recommended image receptor placement when challenged with large, sensitive tori.
6. Demonstrate image receptor placement for use with the paralleling and the bisecting techniques in edentulous regions.
7. Explain the need to expose multiple radiographs of malaligned teeth.
8. Explain how to avoid canine-premolar and molar overlap.
9. Describe the difference between a standard and a disto-oblique periapical radiograph.
10. List steps to obtain a maxillary and a mandibular disto-oblique periapical radiograph.
11. Explain the need to alter an image receptor positioner to prevent unequal distribution of the arches.
12. Explain how to overcome the challenge of not imaging distal of canines on a bitewing radiograph.
13. Explain how to overcome the challenge of not imaging root apices on a periapical radiograph.

KEY TERMS

Disto-oblique periapical radiographs

Edentulous

Hypersensitive gag reflex

Psychogenic stimuli

Tactile stimuli

Introduction

Oral conditions may present that challenge the ability to obtain quality radiographs. Unique oral characteristics may require modifications and adaptations of basic techniques in order to produce desired diagnostic results. Anatomical limitations such as rotation or misalignment of teeth, variations in the size of the oral cavity, height or sensitivity of the palate, and unique anatomic structures and tooth morphology may present obstacles to obtaining diagnostic quality radiographs unless an acceptable variation on standard technique is applied. Additionally, specific problems not encountered when using film may arise with the use of a digital sensor. What sets a skilled radiographer apart from the average is the ability to alter techniques to meet challenging conditions, and still produce diagnostic quality images. This chapter outlines acceptable alterations of standard techniques to help meet special oral conditions.

Hypersensitive Gag Reflex

A gag reflex is a protective mechanism that serves to clear the airway of obstruction. The receptors for a gag reflex are located in the soft palate and lateral posterior third of the tongue. Two reactions occur prior to initiation of a gagging reaction. The first is a cessation of respiration, and the second is a contraction of the muscles of the abdomen and the throat.

All individuals have gag reflexes, but some are more sensitive than others. A **hypersensitive gag reflex** is probably the most troublesome problem for accurate image receptor placement. Two stimuli that must be diminished or eliminated to reduce the occurrence of a hypersensitive gag reflex are:

1. **Psychogenic stimuli**, which originates in the mind; it may result from a suggestion of gagging or as a result of a past experience of gagging.
2. **Tactile stimuli**, which originates from touch; it is a physical reaction to a feeling of the airway being blocked.

Reducing Psychogenic Stimuli

To help avoid stimulating a gag reflex that originates in the mind, it may be helpful to apply strategies for alleviating apprehension (see Chapter 28). If a patient reports a past experience with gagging during the radiographic procedure, or a gag reflex is likely to occur, try the following preventive measures:

- **Do not suggest gagging.** Do not ask the question, "Are you a gagger?" The power of suggestion is a strong psychogenic stimulus and can initiate a gag reflex. Unless a patient brings it up first, do not mention it.
- **Empathize.** If a patient brings up the subject of gagging, do not dismiss the concern as "all in the mind." Instead, show empathy and explain that there are tricks and techniques that have been shown to help avoid stimulating a gagging reaction to image receptor placement, and that you are trained in how to apply these techniques to help the patient control his or her gag reflex.
- **Use the power of suggestion.** Prior to applying a technique that can assist in avoiding a gag reflex, explain it to the patient. Letting a patient know that a technique will be altered to help him or her manage a gag reflex will increase the likelihood of its success. A patient will often be embarrassed by an involuntary gagging reaction and will be eager to accept methods to help regain control. Just as the suggestion of gagging can bring forth the reflex, the suggestion of easing the reflex can help avoid it from presenting.
- **Apply distraction techniques.** There are many ways to divert a patient's attention away from the oral cavity. This can be done by maintaining an engaging dialogue or telling the patient to think of something pleasant, such as a favorite vacation. However, if a gag reflex presents at the onset of the procedure, it may be better to tell a patient that you are going to give him or her a distraction task to perform. For example, a patient may be instructed to bite hard and concentrate on maintaining firm and constant pressure on the image receptor holder's biteblock; concentrate on raising an arm or maintain a clenched fist; or forcibly press the head back against the head rest of the examination chair. Anything that helps to divert the patient's attention from the oral cavity may lessen the likelihood of initiating a gag reflex (Figure 29–1 ■).
- **Explain controlled breathing.** A gag reflex is often stimulated by a sense of not being able to breathe. Explain this to a patient and together, plan a breathing exercise that the patient can concentrate on while the image receptor is placed intraorally and in position for the duration of the exposure. For example, a patient may be coached to breathe deeply through the nose or the mouth, to hum a familiar song, or to hold the breath while silently counting to 10 slowly, by which time the exposure can be completed and the image receptor removed from the oral cavity.

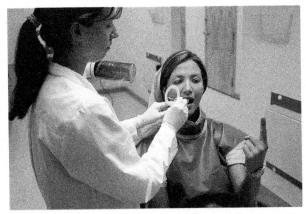

FIGURE 29–1 Distraction techniques. Patient is concentrating on keeping a steady and rhythmic bending and straightening of index finger to help manage a gag reflex.

Reducing Tactile Stimuli

Some patients have an accentuated gag reflex because of hypersensitive pharyngeal tissues. Chronic sinus problems and postnasal drip can contribute to gagging as mucus and saliva accumulate into the nasopharyngeal area. Reduce tactile stimuli when placing the image receptor by use of the following techniques:

- **Begin exposures in the anterior regions first.** Anterior image receptor placements are less likely to initiate a gag reflex, as opposed to those in the maxillary molar region which are more likely to initiate a gagging response. When exposing a series of bitewing radiographs, place and expose the premolar radiograph before placing and exposing the molar image. It is often easier to prevent a gag reflex than to subdue it once excited. Placing an image receptor in the anterior regions first allows a patient to get used to the procedure, builds acceptance, and will usually permit the potentially more difficult posterior placements without incident. Additionally, fears from psychogenic stimuli are more likely to have been forgotten by the time the maxillary molar exposure is made.
- **Place the image receptor firmly and expertly.** For all projections, insert the image receptor into the mouth parallel with the plane of occlusion. When in proper position, rotate into place against the appropriate structures (see Figure 15–10). Retain in position without movement and avoid sliding the image receptor across sensitive oral mucosa.
- **Use the bisecting technique** (see Chapter 14). The manner in which an image receptor is positioned when utilizing the bisecting technique may be less likely to initiate a gag reflex for some patients. Placing the image receptor close to the lingual surface of the teeth may help to avoid sensitive areas of the oral cavity such as the region near the soft palate, and avoids the need to significantly alter a resting tongue position, both of which may be less likely to stimulate a gag reflex for some patients.
- **Confuse the senses.** Stimulating the oral mucosa with digital palpation (rubbing with the finger) serves two purposes. Using touch sensation to simulate where the image receptor will be placed, a patient can experience and prepare for placement of the image receptor. Second, palpation helps to massage and desensitize soft tissue to make placement of the image receptor feel less foreign. Another technique that helps confuse the senses and lower the risk of gagging is to instruct a patient to rinse with cold water, ice cubes, or an antimicrobial oral rinse product just prior to image receptor placement. Placing table salt on the middle or tip of the tongue has also been shown to be effective at reducing the occurrence of a gag reflex. When introducing any of these agents, care must be

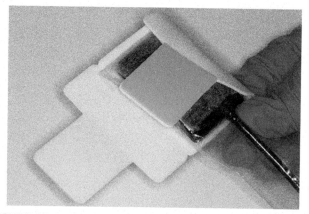

FIGURE 29–2 Edge protectors. Applying a commercial product to reduce feeling of image receptor edge sharpness.

taken to be sure that there are no contraindications for their use. For example, teeth may be sensitive to cold; and a patient may be on a salt-restricted diet.
- **Use special products.** A different image receptor holding device may be successful at avoiding stimulation of, or managing a patient with a hypersensitive gag reflex. Patients may find different image receptor holders more comfortable than others. Additionally, there are products on the market, such as edge protectors and soft plastic barriers, that may reduce the feeling of edge sharpness that some patients report as stimulating a gag reflex. While these products may work for some patients, others find that the addition of bulk or thickness to the image receptor makes it less tolerable (Figure 29–2 ■).

Extreme Hypersensitive Gag Reflex

Occasionally, a patient will present with a hypersensitive gag reflex that cannot be managed by the previously discussed suggestions. It may be necessary to substitute a smaller-sized image receptor, such as a size 1 or 0 for the standard 2 size. Take as many intraoral radiographs as possible and then supplement these with extraoral radiographs. In rare cases a dentist may prescribe a topical anesthetic to numb the areas causing a gag reflex. The risks and contraindications of topical anesthetic must be considered. It should be noted that some patients experience increased anxiety as the result of the numbing sensation produced by topical anesthetic, especially in the soft palate and oral pharyngeal area, so its use must be prescribed judiciously and with caution.

Large Sensitive Tori

Torus palatinus or palatal torus is a benign outgrowth of bone along the midline of the hard palate. Torus mandibularis or lingual torus is a benign outgrowth of bone along the lingual aspect of the mandible in the canine-premolar area. These bony outgrowths on the palate and the lingual surfaces of the mandible present in various sizes.

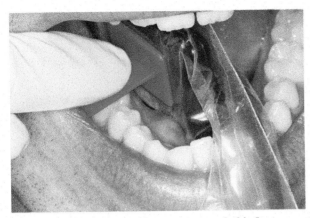

FIGURE 29–3 **Placement of image receptor behind mandibular torus.**

Large tori may interfere with precise image receptor placement. In addition to intrusion into the oral cavity, the oral mucosa covering tori can be thin and sensitive. Placing the edge of an image receptor directly on top of tori will not only increase patient discomfort, but will most likely result in cutting the root apices off the resultant image. Instead, place the image receptor on the far side of a torus. When placing an image receptor in the presence of mandibular tori, position between the torus and tongue (Figure 29–3 ■). This recommended placement may prove difficult when bitewing stick-on tab holders are used. Positioning the image receptor away from the teeth requires that a patient bite on the very end of the bitewing tab. To aid with proper placement in such cases, a bite tab would need to be lengthened (see Figure 15–8).

Edentulous Arches

Radiographs provide valuable information when prescribed to image fully and partially **edentulous** (without teeth) dental arches. A radiographic examination can reveal conditions not detected by a clinical examination alone, such as the presence of retained roots, impacted teeth, foreign bodies, cysts, and other pathological lesions. Radiographs can also be used to determine the condition and extent of remaining bone, especially useful in an assessment for the placement of implants.

The absence of teeth to serve as landmarks to guide positioning of the image receptor requires an ability to estimate best positions. Visualizing and establishing horizontal and vertical planes is more difficult without the presence of teeth as guides. However, because the teeth are not the focus of the examination, and overlapping error is not a concern, a fair amount of leeway in horizontal angulation is permissible; although take care to minimize distortion. Achieving accurate vertical angulation is important, especially when the focus is an examination of alveolar bone.

Periapical radiographs may be taken of edentulous areas using either the paralleling or the bisecting technique. The paralleling technique is preferred because radiographic detail is improved and dimensional distortion is minimized. When utilizing the paralleling technique to image an edentulous region, place the image receptor parallel to the long axis of the edentulous ridge using a sterile cotton roll or polystyrene bite block to support the image receptor holder (Figure 29–4 ■). A sterile cotton roll or polystyrene bite block is used as a substitute for a missing tooth, allowing the arches to occlude together to stabilize the image receptor and holder into the correct parallel position. Once the image receptor is stabilized into a position parallel to the long axis of the edentulous ridge, use the external aiming device of the image receptor holder to determine the vertical and horizontal angulation, and centering of the x-ray beam.

If parallel placement of an image receptor into an edentulous region is difficult to stabilize correctly, apply the bisecting technique instead. Position the image receptor against the lingual surface of the edentulous ridge, where it will not be parallel. Determine the vertical angulation

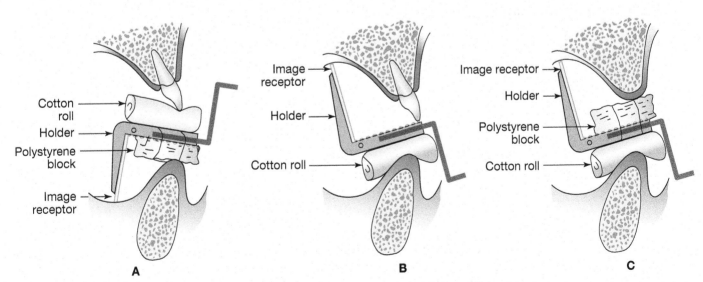

FIGURE 29–4 **Stabilization of image receptor.** (**A** and **B**) Partially edentulous. (**C**) Completely edentulous.

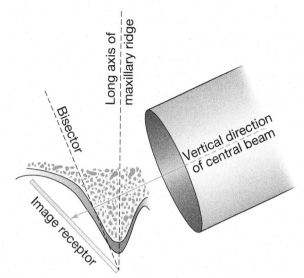

FIGURE 29–5 **Bisecting technique.** Direct central rays of x-ray beam perpendicular to bisector, halfway between plane of image receptor and an imaginary line drawn vertically through edentulous ridge which substitutes for the long axis of a tooth.

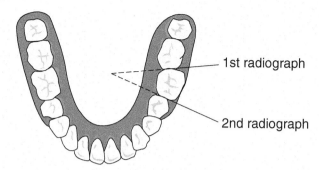

FIGURE 29–6 **Different horizontal angulation is required when teeth are malaligned.**

by bisecting the angle formed between the recording plane of the image receptor and an imaginary line through the ridge that substitutes for the long axes of the teeth (Figure 29–5 ■). This position often results in some dimensional distortion; however, acceptable radiographic images can still be produced. The horizontal angle and centering of the x-ray beam is determined in the same manner as that used for the paralleling technique. Take note that exposure settings for edentulous regions can usually be set at slightly less than those required for an area where teeth are present.

Teeth Alignment and Malalignment

When teeth are malaligned or crowded, it may be necessary to take additional radiographs at various horizontal angles to image every proximal surface and interproximal space clearly, with no overlap. Position each image receptor perpendicular to the embrasures of each tooth as necessary (Figure 29–6 ■).

CANINE-PREMOLAR Standard periapical and bitewing radiographs for imaging the canine will almost always produce overlap between the distal surface of the canine and the mesial surface of the premolar. This overlap occurs because the curve of the dental arches in this region superimposes the lingual cusp of the premolar onto the distal edge of the canine. Due to this expected outcome it is important to take steps to clearly record the distal portion of the canine on a standard premolar periapical or bitewing image when taking a series of radiographs. If a series of images will not be taken and/or to help minimize this overlap recorded by a standard canine radiograph, adjust the horizontal angulation slightly to direct the central rays of the x-ray beam to

intersect the image receptor from the distal. Shifting the position indicating device (PID) slightly toward the posterior will help separate these two teeth on the resultant image and avoid anatomic overlap (Figure 29–7 ■).

MOLAR Because the proximal surfaces of molars are in a mesiodistal relationship to the midsagittal plane, conventional image receptor placement parallel to the buccal surfaces may result in overlapping of the contact areas and closure of the embrasure spaces. To assist with avoiding the occurrence of molar overlap error, an image receptor should be positioned perpendicularly to the embrasures. To achieve this position, place the image receptor slightly diagonal, with the front edge at a greater distance from the lingual surfaces of the teeth than the back edge (Figure 29–8 ■).

Disto-oblique Periapical Radiographs

Disto-oblique periapical radiographs utilize an alteration in a standard direction of the x-ray beam to image posterior structures such as impacted third molars, when posterior image receptor placement cannot be tolerated. Standard vertical and horizontal angulation utilized when exposing periapical radiographs may be altered slightly (no more than 15 degrees) to project posterior objects forward or anteriorly onto an image receptor (Procedure 29–1).

For example, if an impacted third molar is positioned so far posterior in the oral cavity that the standard image receptor placement is not likely to record it, the PID and tube head can be moved to direct the central rays of the x-ray beam to project the impacted tooth forward onto the image receptor (Figure 29–9 ■). By directing the x-ray beam mesially, the posterior object will be projected anteriorly. Because the central rays will intersect the plane of the image receptor at an oblique angle, there will be slight overlap and distortion of the image (Figure 29–10 ■). However, the goal of a disto-oblique periapical radiograph is to record a posteriorly located object or structure that could not be imaged with standard techniques, so this distortion is tolerated.

Maxillary disto-oblique periapical radiographs require three changes to standard maxillary molar periapical radiograph techniques. The first and most important step is to

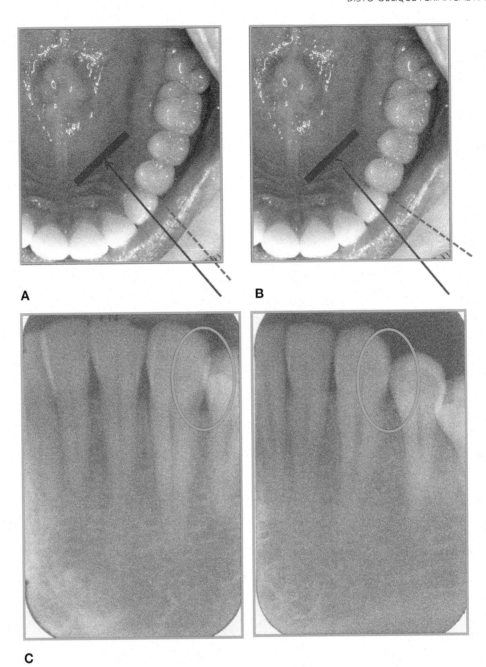

A

B

C

FIGURE 29–7 **Minimize canine and premolar overlap.** (**A**) Curve of arches in this region superimposes premolar lingual cusp onto distal edge of canine. (**B**) Shift horizontal angle slightly to direct x-ray beam to intersect image receptor from the distal to help avoid overlap. (**C**) Note elimination of overlap error in the radiograph on the right.

shift the horizontal angulation of the x-ray beam to project posterior objects anteriorly. Second is to increase the vertical angulation. Most impactions, or foreign objects in the posterior region of the maxilla, are located in a superior position to erupted teeth. Increasing vertical angulation of the x-ray beam will record more of the periapical region. And third, increase exposure to the next higher timer setting. The oblique horizontal and vertical angles cause the x-ray beam to take a longer passage through the oral tissues,

including the dense bone of the zygomatic arch, necessitating a slight increase in radiation to produce adequate image density.

The mandibular disto-oblique periapical radiograph requires only a change to the horizontal angulation, to project the anatomic structure or foreign object of interest forward. Most impactions and foreign objects of the posterior mandible will be located at the level of, or higher than, the erupted teeth so no change is required in the direction of

Procedure 29–1

Disto-oblique periapical radiographs

Maxillary Disto-oblique Periapical Radiograph

1. Place image receptor as close as allowable into the ideal posterior position.
2. Align horizontal and vertical angulations for a standard maxillary molar periapical radiograph.
3. From this standard alignment, shift the tube head and PID 10 degrees to direct the central rays of the x-ray beam to intersect the image receptor obliquely from the distal.
4. Increase the vertical angulation 5 degrees to direct the central rays of the x-ray beam to intersect the image receptor obliquely from a superior angle.
5. Check that the image receptor is centered in the middle of the x-ray beam.
6. Increase the recommended exposure setting to the next higher exposure setting.

Mandibular Periapical Radiograph*

1. Place image receptor as close as allowable into the ideal posterior position.
2. Align horizontal and vertical angulations for a standard mandibular molar periapical radiograph.
3. From this standard alignment, shift the tube head and PID 10 degrees to direct the central rays of the x-ray beam to intersect the image receptor obliquely from the distal.
4. Check that the image receptor is centered in the middle of the x-ray beam.

*No change is made to the standard vertical angulation or to the exposure setting.

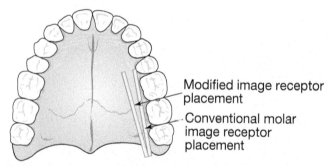

Modified image receptor placement

Conventional molar image receptor placement

FIGURE 29–8 Minimize molar overlap. Position anterior portion of image receptor a greater distance away from lingual surfaces of the teeth.

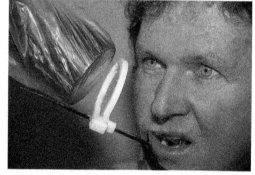

FIGURE 29–9 Disto-oblique periapical technique. Shift horizontal angulation so central rays of x-ray beam are directed 10 degrees from distal; increase vertical angulation 5 degrees. Note the PID and external aiming ring are no longer aligned.

the vertical angulation. There are no thick bony structures, like the zygoma, to penetrate, so the exposure time does not have to be increased.

Image Receptor and Positioner Challenges

Evaluating image receptor placement for correctness is critical to obtaining diagnostic quality images and avoiding errors. Determining the accuracy of and responding appropriately to less than ideal placement of an image receptor are necessary skills.

Image receptor positioners with an external aiming device are invaluable in assisting with correct alignment of the x-ray beam. If an image receptor positioner cannot be

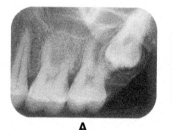
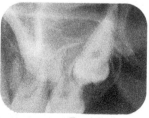

A B

FIGURE 29–10 Comparison of standard and disto-oblique periapical radiographs. (A) Standard periapical radiograph records a portion of an unerupted third molar. **(B)** Disto-oblique periapical radiograph records a larger portion of the unerupted tooth. Note overlap caused by horizontal angle shift; and crowns cut off image caused by vertical angle shift.

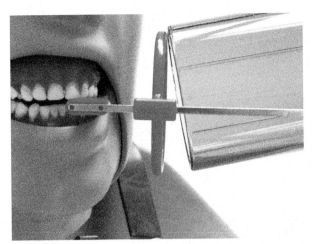

FIGURE 29–11 **Indicator ring is not a dictator.** PID at +10 degrees vertical angle for bitewing exposure instead of aligning with aiming ring.

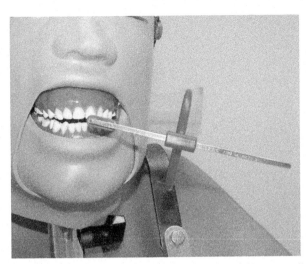

FIGURE 29–13 **Unequal recording of dental arches.** Naturally long facial cusps on the maxillary arch force image receptor positioner into drooping position.

placed precisely, the x-ray beam may be directed incorrectly. A radiographer may choose to align the x-ray beam to the image receptor itself, instead of relying on the external aiming device alone (Figure 29–11 ■). This is a means of using the aiming device as an "indicator," and not the absolute "dictator" on where to line up the x-ray beam. Although image receptor positioners with external aiming devices assist in producing diagnostic radiographs, some conditions hinder ideal placement of these holders.

Bitewing Radiograph Challenge: Unequal Recording of Dental Arches

Unequal recording of the dental arches by bitewing radiographs results in an image that does not record enough information on one or the other arch, either maxilla or mandible, usually prompting a retake. The most common occurrence is a recording of more mandibular structures, or cutting off maxillary structures (Figure 29–12 ■). This results when naturally long facial cusps of maxillary posterior teeth force the image receptor and holding device into a downward position. The hard plastic bite block of an image receptor positioner is forced into a downward drooping position by the extended facial cusps on the maxillary arch (Figure 29–13 ■).

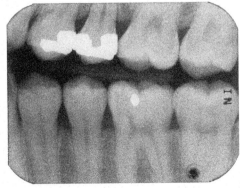

FIGURE 29–12 **Unequal recording of dental arches.** Note that less maxillary anatomy is recorded, indicating inadequate vertical angulation.

To overcome this anatomic challenge, reassemble the image receptor positioner to allow for occlusion on the opposite side of the arch (Figure 29–14 ■). Occluding on the side opposite the image receptor positioner will allow the facial cusps of the maxillary posterior teeth on the opposite side to affect the holder by propping it upward to achieve an accurate 10-degree vertical angulation.

Bitewing Radiograph Challenge: Not Imaging Distal of Canines

Rigid, inflexible direct digital sensors may make it difficult to produce a premolar bitewing radiograph that meets image standards, which require recording the distal edges of both the maxillary and mandibular canines (see Table 15–3). This may occur when using a film packet as well, but the inflexibility of a digital sensor and the presence of the universal serial bus (USB) sensor cable, combined with potentially sensitive mandibular lingual mucosa, make it particularly difficult to position a sensor sufficiently forward in the oral cavity. To overcome this obstacle, when using either a digital sensor or a film packet, position the image receptor farther away from the lingual surface, while simultaneously moving it anteriorly toward the mandibular canine on the opposite side (see Figure 18–1). To reduce the chance that overlap error occurs in this altered position, ensure that the entire length of the image receptor is moved farther away from the lingual surfaces of the teeth; avoid moving only the anterior section and not the posterior section of the image receptor away from the lingual surfaces. Once in position, align the PID to direct the central rays of the x-ray beam to intersect the image receptor perpendicularly.

Periapical Radiograph Challenge: Not Recording Teeth Apices

Shallow palate, tori, naturally long roots of canine teeth, and smaller overall recording dimensions of digital sensors all contribute to not adequately recording all teeth

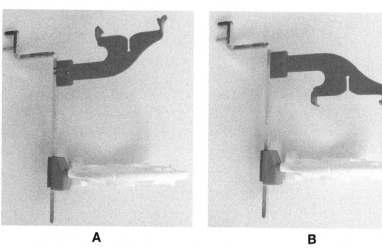

A   **B**

FIGURE 29–14 Minimize unequal recording of dental arches. (A) Standard assembly of an image receptor holding device with extension arm and external aiming ring. **(B)** Alternate assembly to assist with minimizing unequal recording of dental arches.

apices. Moving the image receptor in toward the center of the oral cavity and increasing vertical angulation of the x-ray beam by up to 15 degrees over what is indicated will facilitate in recording more of the apical region (Figure 29–15 ■). Do not vary vertical angulation by more than 15 degrees, or noticeable distortion and error will result. Altering an image receptor holding device may also provide enough recording area to image root apices (Figure 29–16 ■).

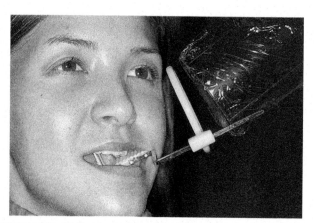

FIGURE 29–15 Increasing vertical angulation to assist with recording root apices. Note the PID and external aiming ring are no longer aligned.

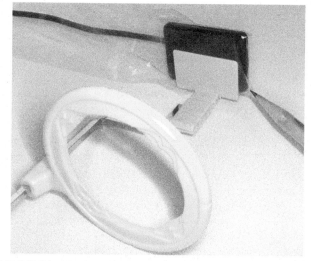

FIGURE 29–16 Alteration of image receptor positioner to assist with recording root apices. This stick-on biteblock is placed to increase the apical position of the sensor in the oral cavity.

REVIEW—Chapter summary

Anatomical limitations may present obstacles in obtaining diagnostic quality radiographs unless an acceptable variation on standard technique is applied. Specific challenges not encountered when using film may arise with the use of a digital sensor. A hypersensitive psychogenic or tactile stimulated gag reflex is probably the most troublesome problem for accurate image receptor placement. A hypersensitive gag reflex may be prevented or managed by establishing patient rapport and demonstrating empathy; explaining techniques and procedures; employing distraction and breathing exercises; beginning examination in the anterior region; placing image receptor and positioner expertly; using the bisecting technique; using a smaller-sized image receptor; applying pressure sensation to desensitize mucosa; and/or using products that confuse the senses and increase comfort. Extreme cases of a hypersensitive gag reflex may require supplementing an intraoral examination with extraoral radiographs or judicious prescribing of topical anesthesia.

Large or sensitive tori may interfere with image receptor placement. Correct placement of an image receptor is between the torus and tongue; and not on top of a torus. Placement of an image receptor in edentulous regions may require the use of a sterilized cotton roll or polystyrene block to stabilize the image receptor holder in a secure position parallel to the long axis of the edentulous ridge. When utilizing the bisecting technique, position the image receptor against the lingual surface of the edentulous ridge; determine the vertical angulation by bisecting the angle formed between the recording plane of the image receptor and an imaginary line through the ridge that substitutes for the long axes of the teeth.

It may be necessary to take additional radiographs at various horizontal angles to image all interproximal spaces with no overlap when teeth are malaligned. Standard periapical and bitewing radiographs for imaging the canine will almost always produce overlap between the distal surface of the canine and the mesial surface of the premolar. To minimize canine-premolar overlap, adjust the horizontal angulation slightly to direct the central rays of the x-ray beam to intersect the image receptor from the distal. A mesiodistal relationship of molars to the midsagittal plane often results in overlap. To minimize molar overlap, position an image receptor slightly diagonal with the front edge at a greater distance from the lingual surfaces to line up perpendicular to the embrasures.

Disto-oblique periapical radiographs require an alteration in standard horizontal and/or vertical angulation to project posterior objects forward or anteriorly onto an image receptor. To obtain a maxillary disto-oblique periapical radiograph, shift the dental x-ray tube head and PID 10 degrees to direct the central rays of the x-ray beam to intersect the image receptor obliquely from the distal; increase vertical angulation 5 degrees to direct the central rays of the x-ray beam to intersect the image receptor obliquely from a superior angle; and increase the exposure to the next higher setting. To obtain a disto-oblique mandibular periapical radiograph, shift the dental x-ray tube head and PID 10 degrees to direct the central rays of the x-ray beam to intersect the image receptor obliquely from the distal; no change is needed in the vertical angulation or the exposure setting.

The external aiming device of an image receptor holder serves as an indicator and not a dictator for alignment of the x-ray beam. Experiment with an alternate image receptor positioner assembly to allow for occlusion on the opposite side of the arch from the location of the image receptor to avoid unequal recording of the dental arches on bitewing radiographs. Position an image receptor farther away from the lingual surface, while simultaneously moving anterior toward the mandibular canine on the opposite side to record the distal edge of canines. Move an image receptor in toward the center of the oral cavity and increase vertical angulation of the x-ray beam by up to 15 degrees or alter an image receptor holder to record more of the apical region.

RECALL—Study questions

1. A perception that the airway has become blocked is called a psychogenic stimulus for a gag reflex. Eliminating psychogenic stimuli will assist with managing a hypersensitive gag reflex.
   a. The first statement is true. The second statement is false.
   b. The first statement is false. The second statement is true.
   c. Both statements are true.
   d. Both statements are false.

2. A patient who is told that gagging is "all in the mind" will experience fewer gagging problems *because* all patients have a gag reflex that is psychogenic.
   a. Both the statement and reason are correct and related.
   b. Both the statement and reason are correct but NOT related.
   c. The statement is correct, but the reason is NOT.
   d. The statement is NOT correct, but the reason is correct.
   e. NEITHER the statement NOR the reason is correct.

3. Asking a patient to do each of the following can help avoid exciting a gag reflex during a radiographic examination procedure EXCEPT one. Which one is the EXCEPTION?
   a. Think about a past experience with gagging.
   b. Rinse with ice water prior to image receptor placement.
   c. Breathe through the nose.
   d. Press the head against the headrest during the procedure.

4. Placement of an image receptor into which of these regions is most likely to initiate a gag reflex?
   a. Maxillary premolar
   b. Maxillary molar
   c. Mandibular premolar
   d. Mandibular molar

5. A patient is more likely to have a gagging response to a radiographic examination
   a. when the bisecting technique is used.
   b. if he or she concentrates on image receptor placement.
   c. after stimulation of the oral mucosa with digital palpation.
   d. while performing a breathing exercise during image receptor placement.

6. The presence of a large mandibular torus may make which of these radiographic technique steps difficult?
   a. Aligning accurate horizontal angulation
   b. Determining correct vertical angulation
   c. Placing an image receptor precisely
   d. Directing central rays of the x-ray beam at the center of an image receptor

7. The best image receptor placement for a patient with a torus palatinus is
   a. between the torus and the tongue.
   b. on the top of the torus.
   c. near the front of the torus.
   d. behind the torus.

8. The paralleling technique is the best technique for imaging partially edentulous regions.
   The bisecting technique is the best technique for imaging completely edentulous regions.
   a. The first statement is true. The second statement is false.
   b. The first statement is false. The second statement is true.
   c. Both statements are true.
   d. Both statements are false.

9. Each of the following can help manage overlap error when challenged with malaligned teeth EXCEPT one. Which one is the EXCEPTION?
   a. Increase vertical angulation no more than 15 degrees.
   b. Position image receptor perpendicular to tooth embrasures.
   c. Vary the horizontal angle of exposure.
   d. Expose multiple radiographs.

10. To minimize canine-premolar overlap, direct the central rays of the x-ray beam toward the image receptor slightly oblique from the
    a. mesial.
    b. distal.
    c. occlusal.
    d. apical.

11. To help avoid molar overlap, place an image receptor
    a. parallel to the buccal surfaces of the molars.
    b. perpendicular to the buccal surfaces of the molars.
    c. parallel to the molar embrasures.
    d. perpendicular to the molar embrasures.

12. When exposing a disto-oblique periapical radiograph of the maxilla, which of the following changes should be made to a standard periapical radiograph?
    a. 5-degree shift in vertical angulation
    b. 10-degree shift in horizontal angulation
    c. Increase exposure time setting
    d. All of the above

13. When exposing a disto-oblique periapical radiograph of the mandible, which of the following changes should be made to a standard periapical radiograph?
    a. 5-degree shift in vertical angulation
    b. 10-degree shift in horizontal angulation
    c. Increase in exposure time setting
    d. All of the above

14. Assembling an image receptor holder so that a patient will occlude on the side opposite from where the image receptor is positioned will assist in avoiding which of these errors?
    a. Overlapping of molars
    b. Unequal recording of dental arches
    c. Cutting root apices off the image
    d. Not imaging the distal of the canines

15. The presence of a USB cable and the inflexibility of a digital sensor present a challenge for recording the distal surfaces of both maxillary and mandibular canines on a bitewing radiograph *because* these characteristics make it difficult to position a digital sensor sufficiently forward in the oral cavity.
    a. Both the statement and reason are correct and related.
    b. Both the statement and reason are correct but NOT related.
    c. The statement is correct, but the reason is NOT.
    d. The statement is NOT correct, but the reason is correct.
    e. NEITHER the statement NOR the reason is correct.

16. To assist with recording the entire root apex of a canine, place an image receptor
    a. at an angle to the distal edge of the canine.
    b. as close as possible to the lingual surface of the canine.
    c. away from the canine in toward center of the oral cavity.
    d. more toward the canine on the opposite side.

REFLECT—Case study

You will be taking a full mouth series of radiographs on a patient who appears apprehensive when she tells you that her last experience taking radiographs could not be completed because she experienced a gagging problem. She states that she was so embarrassed that she did not return to complete the examination.

1. Explain how you would respond to this patient. Include how you would develop a rapport, project confidence, and maintain authority.

2. Prepare a conversation that addresses your ability to perform the procedure; how the procedure today can be different than the past experience; and what techniques will be introduced to help the patient prevent and manage a gag reflex.

3. Answer the following questions:

   a. Why should you not tell this patient that gagging is all in her mind?

   b. What area of the oral cavity should you try placing the image receptor first, and why?

   c. What is the purpose of thanking and praising the patient for her cooperation with the procedure?

   d. What is the difference between psychogenic and tactile stimuli? Give an example of each.

   e. What is the purpose of asking the patient to do breathing exercises during radiographic exposures?

   f. What role could rinsing with ice water or placing salt on the tongue have prior to image receptor positioning?

   g. At what point during the procedure would you tell the patient that you were altering a technique, or using a strategy for controlling a gag reflex, and why?

RELATE—Laboratory application

For a comprehensive laboratory practice exercise on this topic, see Thomson, E. M., & Bruhn, A. M. (2018). *Exercises in oral radiography techniques: A laboratory manual* (4th ed.). Hoboken, NJ: Pearson. Chapter 12, "Supplemental Radiographic Techniques."

RESOURCES

American Dental Association: Council on Scientific Affairs. U.S. Department of Health and Human Services: Public Health Service. Food and Drug Administration. (2012). *Dental radiographic examinations: Recommendations for patient selection and limiting radiation exposure.* Washington, DC: Author.

Dentsply Sirona. (2014). *Intraoral radiography with Rinn XCP/XCP DS Instruments.* York, PA: Dentsply Int. Inc. Retrieved from Dentsply Sirona Web site: https://www.dentsply.com/content/dam/dentsply/pim/manufacturer/Preventive/X_ray/Arms__Rings/Comfortwand/XCP-Intraoral-Radiography-Education-Manual.pdf

Thomson, E. M., & Bruhn, A. M. (2018). Supplemental radiographic techniques. *Exercises in oral radiography techniques: A laboratory manual* (4th ed.). Hoboken, NJ: Pearson.

Visit www.pearsonhighered.com/healthprofessionsresources to access the student resources that accompany this book. Simply select Dental Hygiene from the choice of disciplines. Find this book and you will find the complementary study tools created for this specific title.

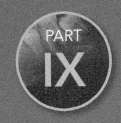

Alternate Imaging Modalities

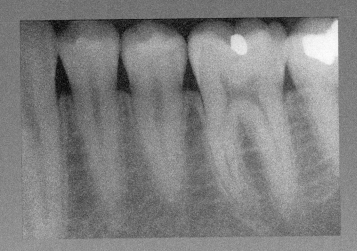

OUTLINE

Supplemental and Extraoral Radiographic Techniques

OBJECTIVES

Following successful completion of this chapter you should be able to:

1. Define the key terms.
2. Explain the need for multiple radiographs during endodontic procedures.
3. Describe the characteristics of an image receptor positioner used to expose working radiographs during endodontic procedures.
4. List three methods of localization.
5. Explain the relationship between shadow casting principles and the definitive method of localization.
6. Explain the role the tube shift method of localization plays in imaging root canals.
7. List the two radiographic images needed for the right angle method of localization.
8. Explain the S.L.O.B. rule.
9. Utilize the buccal-object rule to determine the buccal-lingual location of a foreign object.
10. Explain the need for a specialized image receptor positioner when using a handheld x-ray device.
11. List possible uses for duplicate radiographs.
12. Describe the difference between duplicating and radiographic film.
13. List possible uses of extraoral radiographs.
14. Identify types of extraoral radiographs used to image the oral and maxillofacial regions.

KEY TERMS

Antemortem radiograph
Buccal-object rule
Cephalostat

Digitization
Duplicate radiograph
Film duplicator

Localization
Postmortem radiograph
S.L.O.B. rule

Introduction

Supplemental radiographic examinations address a variety of specific oral and maxillofacial diagnostic needs. Some techniques are readily available for use in general practice settings, while others are more likely to be performed in specialized practices and nontraditional settings. A skilled dental radiographer should have an understanding of available supplemental intraoral and extraoral imaging techniques. This chapter provides an overview of essential procedures and ancillary techniques that enable oral health care practitioners to provide specialized care.

Radiographic Techniques for Endodontics

Endodontic therapy is the treatment of a diseased tooth by removing infected nerves and tissues from the pulp cavity and replacing with therapeutic filling material, usually gutta-percha (see Figure 23–14). Successful endodontic therapy or root canal treatment depends on the exposure of multiple radiographs, some of which require a specialized image receptor positioner and an alteration in standard radiographic technique. An initial radiograph is exposed to determine preoperative condition and to make a diagnosis; a posttreatment radiograph is used to ensure the canal is filled and sealed satisfactorily. The paralleling technique and a standard image receptor positioner can be utilized to expose the pre- and posttreatment radiographs.

During the procedure, working radiographs are needed to determine the number, shape, and length of a root canal, possible calcification or obstructions such as the presence of pulp stones, position of endodontic instruments in the canal, and placement of filling material and sealer. Use the paralleling technique for these working radiographs due to its ability to produce accurate images. However, instruments and materials used during endodontic treatment (rubber dam, files, and gutta-percha points) hinder precise placement of an image receptor in a standard holder (Figure 30–1 ■). The presence of these instruments, which must be left in place, makes it impossible for a patient to

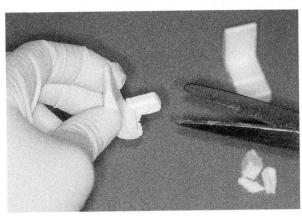

FIGURE 30–2 **Film holder modification** for use during endodontic treatment.

bite down on the biteblock of an image receptor positioner to hold it securely in place to ensure an accurate recording. Avoiding distortion and magnification of the image is a major concern because the length of each root canal must be accurately and precisely measured. Additionally, endodontic therapy requires that at least 4 to 5 mm below the root apex be recorded, making it imperative that an image receptor be positioned correctly. In the past, radiographers would sometimes improvise and modify a standard image receptor positioner for use during an endodontic procedure (Figures 30–2 ■ and 30–3 ■). The current availability of positioners designed specifically for use with endodontic treatment may provide better and more reliable results (Figure 30–4 ■).

Multirooted teeth and teeth with multiple root canals pose a challenge for the two-dimensional recording ability of intraoral radiographs. Superimposition and a static, one-angle perspective limit the ability to accurately image the number and length of a tooth's root canals. This is one of the reasons endodontic therapy requires the exposure of multiple radiographs. Exposing multiple radiographs at different horizontal or vertical angulation can assist with separating and bringing into view superimposed root canals (Figure 30–5 ■). The specific technique used to achieve this is the tube shift method of object localization.

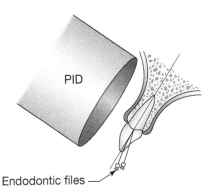

FIGURE 30–1 **Tooth undergoing endodontic treatment**. Files prevent occlusion on a standard image receptor bite block.

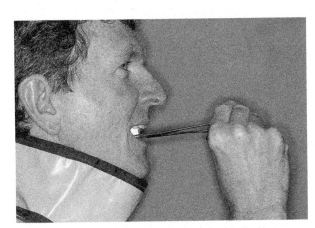

FIGURE 30–3 **Hemostat as film holder** for use during endodontic treatment.

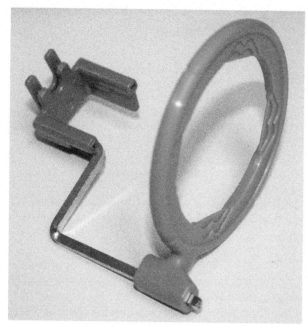

FIGURE 30–4 **Endodontic image receptor holder.**

Object Localization

Object **localization** is a supplemental technique that can be used to derive three-dimensional information from two-dimensional radiographic images; this is especially valuable during root canal therapy and for determining facial or lingual position of impacted teeth and foreign objects. There are three methods of localization.

Definitive Evaluation Method

The definitive method of localization is based on shadow casting principles explained in Chapter 4. The principle that an object positioned farther away from the image receptor will be magnified and less clearly imaged is the basis for the definitive method. Because intraoral image receptor placement positions the receptor close to the lingual surface of the teeth, those objects on the lingual are more likely to appear distinctly defined on the resultant radiograph. Those objects positioned more toward the facial or buccal will be farther away from the image receptor and therefore more likely to appear magnified and less clearly imaged on the resultant radiograph (Figure 30–6 ■). Although true in principle, the definitive method of localization is not consistently reliable.

Right-Angle Method

Once identified on a periapical radiograph, a better way to determine whether an impacted tooth or foreign object is located on the buccal or the lingual is to expose an occlusal radiograph. A cross-sectional occlusal radiograph, as described in Chapter 16, places an image receptor at a right angle to a tooth or dental arch. In this position the occlusal radiograph will image the object of interest clearly on the buccal or lingual (Figure 30–7 ■).

Tube Shift Method (Buccal-Object Rule)

The tube shift method, also called the **buccal-object rule,** is the most versatile method of localization. To apply the tube shift method two radiographs are needed. The two radiographic images must have been exposed using either a different horizontal or a different vertical angulation. If a full mouth series of periapical, or a complete set of bitewing radiographs, or a combination of both are available and the object in question is imaged in more than one radiograph, it is possible to apply the tube shift method when reading the radiographs to determine the buccal or lingual location of the object.

The principle behind the tube shift method is that if the structure or object in question appears to have moved

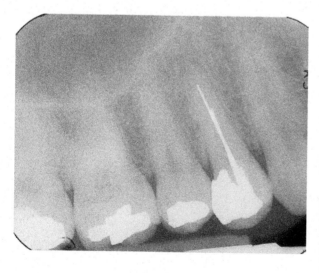
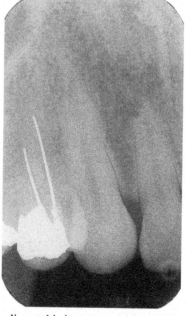

FIGURE 30–5 **Horizontal angle change** between these two radiographic images provides additional information regarding the number and length of root canals.

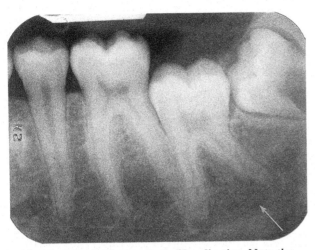

FIGURE 30–6 **Definitive method of localization.** Note the barely visible supernumerary root on this first molar. Applying the definitive method of localization, it is most likely a buccal root. The buccal position would place this root a greater distance away from the image receptor, resulting in its magnified and less distinctly defined appearance.

in the same direction as the horizontal- or vertical shift of the dental x-ray tube, then the structure or object is located on the lingual. Conversely, if the move is in the opposite direction of the shift of the tube, the structure or object is located on the buccal or facial. The tube shift method is summarized as the **S.L.O.B. Rule,** which stands for "same on lingual–opposite on buccal" (Figures 30–8 ■ and 30–9 ■).

Handheld X-ray Devices

Portable, handheld x-ray generating equipment plays a valuable role in obtaining a radiographic examination when a wall-mounted dental x-ray machine is not accessible or feasible. Handheld devices are often used in nontraditional settings such as mobile clinics, and have a role in dental

forensics. Prior to using a handheld device, be thoroughly familiar with the manufacturer's operating instructions, and be prepared to appropriately adapt or alter techniques used with a wall-mounted dental x-ray machine. Of particular importance is the need to use an image receptor positioner that is compatible with the handheld backscatter ring shield.

The metal positioning arm of a standard image receptor positioner with an external aiming attachment can interfere with the handheld backscatter ring shield in such a way as to prevent proper alignment, and possibly create a wider than necessary x-ray beam diameter exposure for a patient. This occurs when attempting to maneuver the open end of the position indicating device (PID) of the handheld appropriately close to the aiming ring, only to be blocked by the extension of the metal arm (Figure 30–10 ■). Not being able to position the PID close to the aiming ring increases risk of alignment errors, and increases the target-skin surface distance the x-ray beam must travel resulting in a wider diameter

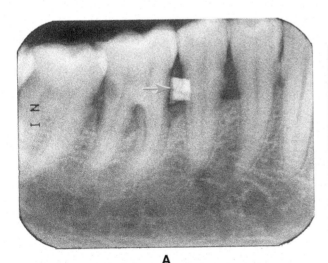

A

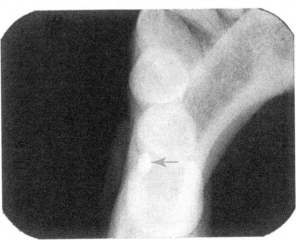

B

FIGURE 30–7 **Right-angle method of localization. (A)** A foreign object appears in the periodontal pocket between the second premolar and the first molar. It is impossible to tell from this periapical radiograph whether the object is located toward the buccal or the lingual. **(B)** The occlusal radiograph, placed at a right angle position to the tooth, clearly images the object on the buccal side of the pocket.

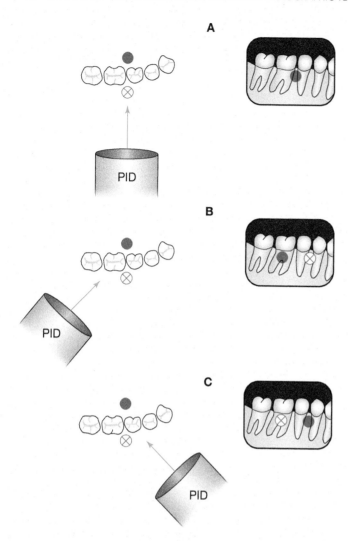

FIGURE 30–8 **Horizontal tube shift. (A)** Original radiograph records buccal and lingual objects superimposed. **(B)** When tube head is moved to distal, buccal object appears to shift to mesial and lingual object appears to shift to distal. **(C)** When tube head is moved to mesial, buccal object appears to shift to distal and lingual object appears to shift to mesial.

beam of radiation than is necessary for exposure of the image receptor. Using a positioning biteblock only, without the metal arm and aiming ring attachment will allow the PID to be positioned close to the skin surface, but will eliminate the alignment guideline needed to determine correct angles.

It is imperative that an image receptor positioner with an alignment guide be used with handheld x-ray devices. When using a wall-mounted dental x-ray machine, a skilled radiographer can be reasonably accurate at determining correct angles and centering the x-ray beam without relying on an image receptor positioner with an external aiming device. However, when using a handheld x-ray device, the operator must take a position behind the unit, which prohibits the front or side view a radiographer would need to determine accurate and precise angulations. Manufacturers of image receptor holding devices are producing equipment with a shortened metal extension arm specifically designed for use with handheld x-ray devices (Figure 30–11).

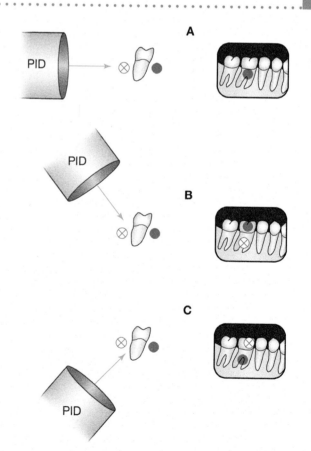

FIGURE 30–9 **Vertical tube shift. (A)** Original radiograph records buccal and lingual objects superimposed. **(B)** When tube head is moved to superior, buccal object appears to shift to inferior and lingual object appears to shift to superior. **(C)** When tube head is moved to inferior, the buccal object appears to shift to superior and lingual object appears to shift to inferior.

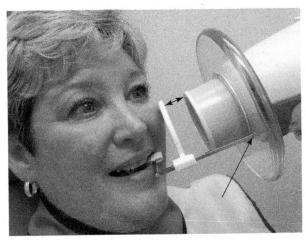

FIGURE 30–10 **Metal extension arm contacts backscatter ring shield prohibiting correct positioning of the PID.**

Film Duplication

Original film-based radiographs must remain with a patient's permanent record. Supplemental film duplication techniques can make copies available for other purposes (Box 30–1). A **duplicate radiograph,** an identical copy of the original, is produced with a film duplicator and duplicating film.

Duplicating film is available in a variety of sizes to accommodate the duplication of one or multiple intraoral films and extraoral panoramic radiographs (see Chapter 7). Duplicating film emulsion is specially formulated to work with a **film duplicator** that emits ultraviolet light. There are different sizes of film duplicator models available commercially (Figure 30–12 ■). The operation of a film duplicator must take place in a darkroom under safelight conditions. After exposure to ultraviolet light, duplicating film is time-temperature processed using developer and fixer in the same manner as radiographic film (Procedure 30–1).

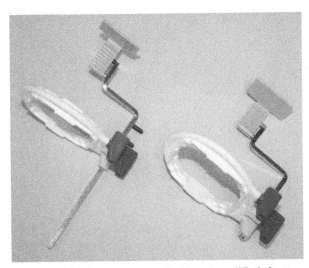

FIGURE 30–11 **Traditional long** (left) **and modified short** (right) **metal extension arms.**

Box 30–1: Possible Uses of Duplicate Radiographs

- Referral to a specialist
- Accompany a biopsy
- Patient moves or chooses another dentist
- Consultation with other professionals
- Third-party payment approval
- Adding to evidence-based practice through publication, professional study group discussion
- Legal cases

Extraoral Two-Dimensional Radiographs

While panoramic radiographic equipment is readily available in most general oral health care practice settings, other extraoral imaging techniques usually require special equipment often limited to specialty practices (Figure 30–13 ■). While radiographers employed in specialty practices will be specifically trained to perform these techniques, all radiographers should have a basic understanding of the types of extraoral radiographs prescribed to image the oral maxillofacial region. A working knowledge of standard extraoral examinations is required for patient education and to communicate with other health care professionals.

The purpose of extraoral radiographs is to examine structures of the oral cavity and the maxillofacial region that includes the maxilla and mandible, facial bones and sinuses, and the temporomandibular joint (TMJ). Extraoral radiographic images are used to:

- Examine large areas of the dental arches and skull
- Study growth and development of bone and teeth
- Detect fractures and evaluate trauma
- Detect pathological lesions and diseases
- Detect and evaluate impacted teeth
- Evaluate temporomandibular disorder (TMD)

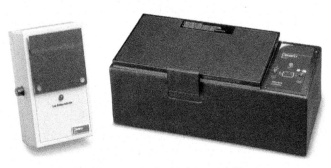

FIGURE 30–12 **Radiograph duplicating machines** accommodate duplication of one or multiple films at a time. Built-in ultraviolet fluorescent light source with timer permits variations in density. (Courtesy of Dentsply Sirona.)

Procedure 30–1

Film duplication

1. Remove original radiographs from mount and place on duplicator glass surface with the embossed dots concave to allow for close, tight contact between original radiographs and duplicating film.
2. Under safelight conditions, remove a sheet of duplicating film from the box. Use scissors if necessary to cut film to size.
3. Place duplicating film, emulsion-side down, on top of original radiographs.
4. Close duplicator cover, set desired exposure time, and depress exposure button. To produce a darker duplicate image, decrease exposure time; increase for a lighter duplicate. (Decreasing and increasing duplication exposure time has the opposite effect on the density of the image than increasing and decreasing x-ray exposure time has on radiographic film.)
5. Process duplicating film in the same time-temperature manner as radiographic film.

- Plan treatment for dental implants and prosthetic appliances
- Serve as a substitute when an intraoral examination is not possible

Orthodontic, prosthodontic, oral surgical practices, and practitioners who specialize in dental implants and treatment of TMD are increasingly relying on three-dimensional imaging (see Chapter 31). However, two-dimensional extraoral imaging modalities continue to be used to diagnose and treat conditions of the oral cavity and head and facial regions. For example:

- **Orthodontists** use facial profile radiographic images, produced with **cephalostat** headplates (*cephalometric* means "measuring the head") to record, measure, and compare changes in growth and development of maxillofacial bones and dentition.
- **Prosthodontists** use facial profile radiographs to record the contour of the lips and face and the relationship of the natural teeth before extraction to help in constructing prosthetic appliances that look natural (Figure 30–14 ■).
- **Oral surgeons** use extraoral radiographs to evaluate trauma; to determine the location and extent of fractures; to locate impacted teeth, abnormalities, and malignancies; and to evaluate injuries to the TMJ (Figure 30–15 ■).

There are many techniques for exposing radiographic images of the oral cavity and the maxillofacial region. It is not within the scope of this book to describe every available technique, so the examinations presented in Table 30–1 ■ are the most common extraoral images where the x-ray source and image receptor remain static, and do not rotate around the patient.

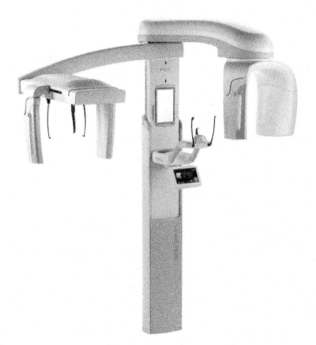

FIGURE 30–13 A combination panoramic and cephalometric dental x-ray machine. (Courtesy of Progeny, A Midmark Company.)

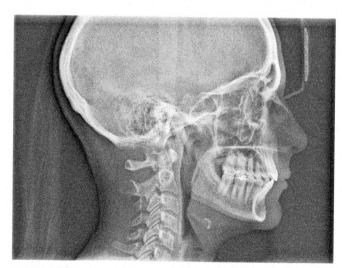

FIGURE 30–14 Cephalometric radiograph with outline of soft tissue profile. (Courtesy of Progeny, A Midmark Company.)

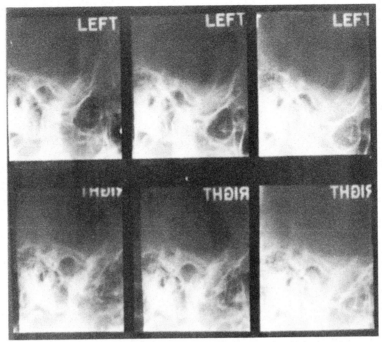

FIGURE 30–15 Serial radiographs of TMJ positions during occlusion, at rest, and with the mouth open. (Courtesy of McCormack Dental X-ray Laboratory.)

Table 30–1 Extraoral Radiographic Images of the Maxillofacial Region

Type of Radiograph	Area of Interest	Purpose	Positioning
Lateral cephalometric (lateral skull)	Entire skull from side (lateral); sinus cavities	Prior to orthodontic intervention, at various stages of treatment, upon completion of treatment; to evaluate growth/ development, trauma, pathology, developmental abnormalities; can reveal facial soft tissue profile with use of a filter; to establish pre-/ posttreatment records	Image receptor — Central ray — X-ray beam
Posteroanterior (PA) cephalometric (posterior skull)	Entire skull in posteroanterior plane; orbit; frontal sinus	To examine facial growth/ development, disease, trauma, developmental abnormalities; used to supplement lateral cephalometric because right and left sides of facial structures are not superimposed on each other	Image receptor — Central ray — X-ray beam

(continued)

Table 30–1 **Extraoral Radiographic Images of the Maxillofacial Region** *(continued)*

Type of Radiograph	Area of Interest	Purpose	Positioning
Waters	Middle third of face to include zygoma, coronoid process, sinuses	To evaluate maxillary, frontal, ethmoid sinuses	Tip of nose 0.75 inch from image receptor; X-ray beam; Central ray; Image receptor
Reverse Towne	Condyles	To examine fractures of condylar neck	X-ray beam; Central ray; Image receptor; Mouth open, head tipped down
Submentovertex	Base of skull; condyles; sphenoid sinus; zygoma	To evaluate position/orientation of condyles; fractures of zygomatic arch	Frankfort plane; X-ray beam; Central ray; Floor; Image receptor
Transcranial	Head of condyle; glenoid fossa; temporal bone; TMJ in open, closed, and at rest positions	Aids in diagnosing ankylosis (stiffening of TMJ); malignancies, fractures, and tissue changes caused by arthritis	Sagittal plane; Image receptor; Central ray; X-ray beam +25°

REVIEW—Chapter summary

While some supplemental radiographic examinations and ancillary techniques are more likely to be performed in specialized practices, others are readily available for use in general practice. Endodontic therapy requires exposure of standard initial preoperative and posttreatment radiographs, and exposure of working radiographs using a specialized image receptor positioner and an alteration in standard radiographic technique. Multiple radiographs exposed at different horizontal or vertical angulation can assist with separating and bringing into view superimposed root canals.

Object localization methods add a third dimension to two-dimensional radiographs. The definitive method is least reliable. The right angle method uses a periapical radiograph and a cross-sectional occlusal radiograph. The tube shift method is based on the S.L.O.B. (same on lingual–opposite on buccal) rule. The object in question is located on lingual if it moves in the same direction as a horizontal or vertical shift of the x-ray tube and on buccal if it moves in the opposite direction as a horizontal or vertical shift of the x-ray tube.

Operator position when using a handheld x-ray device is behind the unit blocking a front or side view needed to determine accurate and precise angulations. An image receptor positioner with a shortened metal extension arm must be used with a handheld x-ray device to avoid interference with the backscatter ring shield. Interference would likely prevent proper alignment and possibly create a wider than necessary x-ray beam diameter exposure for a patient.

Ancillary radiographic techniques include digitization and duplication of film-based radiographs. Film-based radiographs can be converted to a digital format by scanning or by using a digital camera to photograph the existing radiograph. Duplicate copies of film-based radiographs have many uses and are produced by a commercially made duplicator and special duplicating film. Duplicate film gets darker with less exposure to ultraviolet light, and lighter with longer exposure. The duplication process must take place under safelight conditions. Duplicating film is processed in the same manner as radiographic film.

Oral health care personnel properly trained in forensic identification may play a role in responding to a mass fatality incident. Postmortem and antemortem radiographs are compared for positive victim identification.

Extraoral radiographs are used to examine structures of the oral and maxillofacial region for the purpose of determining pathologic conditions, trauma and fractures, growth and development, assessment of impacted teeth, evaluation of TMD, and in treatment planning for dental implants and prosthetics. Orthodontic, prosthodontic, and oral surgical practices and practitioners specializing in dental implants and TMD are major users of extraoral imaging modalities. These professionals are likely to prescribe lateral and PA cephalometric, Waters, reverse Towne, submentovertex, and transcranial examinations.

RECALL—Study questions

1. Which of the following supplemental radiographic techniques is least likely to be performed in general practice?
   a. PA cephalometric radiographic examination
   b. Film-based radiograph duplication
   c. Endodontic radiographic examination
   d. Object localization radiographic interpretation

2. During endodontic treatment which of the following radiographs would require the use of a specialized image receptor positioner?
   a. Initial preoperative
   b. Working
   c. Posttreatment
   d. Recall

3. How many working radiographs are usually required during endodontic treatment?
   a. Three
   b. Four
   c. Five
   d. As many as needed to complete the procedure

4. Which object localization method best aids in identification of root canals?
   a. Definitive
   b. Right angle
   c. Tube shift

5. Object localization adds which of the following dimensions to two-dimensional radiographs?
   a. Buccal-lingual
   b. Anterior-posterior
   c. Mesial-distal
   d. Inferior-superior

6. Which of the following methods of object localization utilizes a cross-sectional occlusal radiograph?
   a. Definitive
   b. Right angle
   c. Tube shift

7. If the x-ray tube is shifted to the mesial and the object in question shifts to the distal, the object is located on the lingual.

This is an example of the definitive method of localization.
   a. The first statement is true. The second statement is false.
   b. The first statement is false. The second statement is true.
   c. Both statements are true.
   d. Both statements are false.

8. Which of the following is true regarding the metal extension arm of an image receptor positioner appropriate for use with a handheld dental x-ray device?
   a. Should be shorter than standard
   b. Should be longer than standard
   c. Should be replaced with a plastic arm
   d. Should be removed

9. A film duplicator emits
   a. x-ray energy.
   b. infrared light.
   c. white light.
   d. ultraviolet light.

10. A _____ exposure time produces a duplicate radiographic image with _____ density.
    a. short; decreased
    b. short; increased
    c. long; increased

11. For which of these purposes are extraoral radiographs least suitable?
    a. Detecting interproximal caries
    b. Locating an impacted tooth
    c. Viewing a sinus obstruction
    d. Determining the extent of a fracture

12. Which of these extraoral radiographic examinations is most likely to be performed in general practice?
    a. PA cephalometric
    b. Reverse Towne
    c. Panoramic
    d. Submentovertex

13. Which of these extraoral radiographic examinations is most likely to be performed in an orthodontic practice?
    a. Transcranial
    b. Lateral cephalometric
    c. Waters
    d. Reverse Towne

REFLECT—Case study

Consider the following patients and conditions. Which of the six extraoral radiographs described in this chapter might be the *best* recommendation for these cases? (*Note:* Radiographs of the skull are difficult to interpret due to the numerous structures that exist in a very small area. These structures often appear superimposed over each other, requiring multiple views to obtain a good diagnosis. Therefore, in some of these cases, although there is usually a *best* answer, there may be more than one correct answer.)

1. An adolescent presents for an orthodontic consultation. Occlusal and facial disharmonies need to be assessed prior to treatment intervention.

2. A difficult extraction case presents with a severely decayed maxillary molar. During the extraction procedure, a root tip fractures and is possibly impacted in a sinus cavity.

3. A medically compromised patient suffered a seizure and fell. A fractured mandibular condyle is suspected.

4. A patient presents with a history of degenerative joint disease that may be affecting the TMJ. An examination for the purpose of diagnosing TMD is prescribed.

5. A patient presents for extractions and construction of a maxillary full denture and a mandibular partial denture.

RELATE—Laboratory application

Using Procedure 30–1, produce a duplicate copy of a set of bitewing radiographs. Experiment with increasing and decreasing the exposure time and compare the results.

RESOURCES

Bird, D. L., & Robinson, D. S. (2015). Extraoral imaging. *Modern dental assisting in endodontics* (11th ed.). St. Louis, MO: Elsevier.

Bruhn, A., Newcomb, T., & Giles, B. (2016). Evaluating imaging techniques for intraoral forensic radiography with the dental hygienist as part of the forensic radiology team. *Journal of Forensic Identification, 66,* 22–36.

Farman, A. G., Nortje, C. J., & Wood, R. E. (1993). *Oral and maxillofacial diagnostic imaging.* St. Louis, MO: Mosby.

Horner, K., Drage, N., & Brettle, D. (2008). *21st century imaging.* London: Quintessence Publishing Co.

Newcomb, T., Bruhn, A., & Giles, B. (2015). Critical issues: Mass fatality incidents and the role of the dental hygienist, are we prepared? *Journal of Dental Hygiene, 89,* 143–151.

White, S. C., & Pharoah, M. J. (2014). Extraoral projections and anatomy. *Oral radiology: Principles and interpretation* (7th ed.). St. Louis, MO: Elsevier.

Visit www.pearsonhighered.com/healthprofessionsresources to access the student resources that accompany this book. Simply select Dental Hygiene from the choice of disciplines. Find this book and you will find the complementary study tools created for this specific title.

Three-dimensional Imaging

Ann M. Bruhn, BSDH, MS

CHAPTER OUTLINE

OBJECTIVES

Following successful completion of this chapter, you should be able to:

1. Define the key terms.
2. Describe the purpose and use of three-dimensional imaging.
3. Describe the three suggested categories of oral conditions for the prescription of a cone beam computed tomography (CBCT) examination.
4. Explain how CBCT differs from medical computed tomography (CT).
5. Explain the purpose of changing the field of view (FOV).
6. Explain the effect changing voxel size has on an image.
7. List the three anatomical planes of CBCT slice image data.
8. List oral conditions that would most benefit from a CBCT examination.
9. Discuss how CBCT settings can reduce radiation exposure.
10. Describe the appearance of artifacts that occur on CBCT images.
11. Explain the challenges to interpretation of image data produced by CBCT technology.

KEY TERMS

Anatomical planes
Axial plane
Computed tomography (CT; CT scan)
Cone beam computed tomography (CBCT)
Coronal plane
Cupping artifact
Field of view (FOV)
Flat panel detector (FPD)
Reconstruction
Sagittal plane
Scatter correction algorithm
Slice data
Streaking artifact
Trajectory
Voxel (volume element)

Introduction

Cone beam volumetric imaging (CBVI), more commonly known as **cone beam computed tomography (CBCT)**, is based on existing technology in the medical field known as **computed tomography (CT)** or **CT scan**. CBCT produces three-dimensional (3-D) radiographic images similar to those produced by a medical CT scan, but with a lower dose of radiation. The use of CBCT technology is rapidly growing, albeit while advantages and limitations are being identified and explored. Guidelines for CBCT use—including prescription criteria, administration and documentation requirements, and quality control for radiation safety standards—continue to evolve. CBCT does not replace two-dimensional (2-D) extraoral imaging modalities, including panoramic radiographs; and the benefits and risks of CBCT must be carefully considered prior to prescribing and using this technology. This chapter provides an overview of this cutting-edge technology.

Purpose and Use of Three-dimensional Imaging

CBCT was first developed in the 1990s for use in oral and maxillofacial imaging and has since become the most important advancement in oral radiographic imaging since the development of panoramic technology. CBCT is essentially medical CT technology that has been specifically adapted for oral health care applications. Its integration into oral health care has increased significantly in recent years. This is due in part to the accessibility of CBCT machines. A few years ago, a patient would most likely need to be referred to a medical imaging center to have an examination. Today, CBCT machines are being marketed for use in general and specialty oral health care practices (Figure 31–1 ■). Most CBCT machines currently available allow an operator to switch between 2-D and 3-D imaging options. These combination machines generate enhanced 2-D panoramic and other extroral radiographs in addition to CBCT images (Figure 31–2 ■).

A CBCT examination is prescribed when an increase in clarity and detail of anatomic structures and pathologic conditions is necessary for diagnosis. While a CBCT examination requires less radiation exposure than a medical CT, the radiation dose is significantly greater than 2-D extra- and intraoral imaging. A dentist will need to assess the use of CBCT carefully based on the needs of an individual patient. To assist with a decision to prescribe a CBCT examination, experts suggest that oral conditions be classified according to the benefits a CBCT examination is likely to produce. The suggested categories are called *Standard of Care*, *Preferred*, and *Not Necessary* (Table 31–1 ■). As research continues to add to the body of knowledge on this relatively new technology, these classifications may be modified. Currently, practitioners can use these guidelines to determine assessment of need.

- The *Standard of Care* category lists conditions and treatments for which the beneficial diagnostic

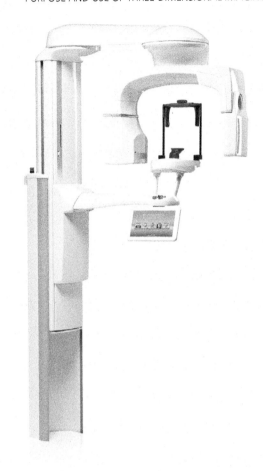

FIGURE 31–1 **CBCT imaging machine.** Designed for the oral health care practice. (Courtesy of Planmeca.)

information expected from CBCT significantly outweighs the risk of radiation exposure. Practitioners who prescribe CBCT for these conditions can be assured that they are in line with what experts agree are the standards of care for that condition.

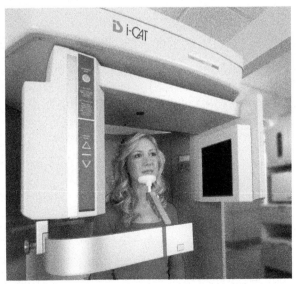

FIGURE 31–2 **Combination CBCT/panoramic imaging machine.** (Courtesy of Gendex Dental Systems/Imaging Sciences Intl.)

Table 31–1 Oral Conditions for the Prescription of CBCT

Standard of Care	Preferred	Not Necessary
Dental implant assessment	Location of inferior alveolar nerve prior to oral surgical procedures	Simple evaluation of TMJ before orthodontic treatment
Surgical tooth extraction and impaction evaluation	Endodontic therapy	Periodontal evaluation
Orthodontic assessment	Evaluation of sinus cavities	Caries detection
Surgical guide to reconstruction	Evaluation of bony defects (fenestration, dehiscence)	Determining location of impacted third molars
Challenging presurgical diagnostic situations	Evaluation of oral pathologic lesions	
	Temporomandibular joint (TMJ) evaluation for associated problems	

- Conditions classified under the *Preferred* category require more careful consideration as a practitioner must assess whether the risk versus benefit warrants a CBCT examination; or could extra- and/or intraoral 2-D radiographs provide enough information to make a diagnosis and appropriately treat the condition.
- Conditions listed under the *Not Necessary* category can usually be adequately interpreted and diagnosed using 2-D extra- and/or intraoral imaging.

Fundamentals of Cone Beam Computed Tomography

To understand the complex process of CBCT, review the principle of tomography used to produce panoramic dental images (see Chapter 17). Tomography uses a moving radiation source and image receptor to record layers or slices of structures located within a selected plane of tissue, while blurring structures outside the selected plane making them less visible. Unlike panoramic imaging, CT technology produces enhanced 3-D images out of the recorded slices of tissue with no superimposed blurring of the structures that lie outside the selected plane.

A patient undergoing a traditional CT examination of the maxillofacial region is placed into a supine position on a table with the head positioned inside a scanner (Figure 31–3 ∎). The scanner emits a narrow, fan-shaped x-ray beam that rotates 360 degrees around the head multiple times while up to 2,000 digital image receptors receive the data. The table supporting the patient moves as the x-rays focus on each new layer or slice of tissue during the rotations. Digital software then translates the data received by the image receptors into an image displayed on a computer monitor. CT is a highly regarded, accurate method for imaging both soft and hard bony tissues, but the large radiation dose only rarely justifies use in dental applications. The evolution of CBCT technology that reduces radiation dose provides new options for diagnosing and treating oral conditions.

Similar to CT, a CBCT examination provides accurate, multiplanar (multiple planes or slices) of images with no superimposed blurring. However, CBCT differs from medical CT technology in several ways. CBCT is more effective at imaging hard tissues, making this technology ideally suited to recording oral and maxillofacial structures; and patient positioning is usually seated or standing upright, similar to positioning used for a panoramic examination. The main difference between CBCT and CT is that instead of a narrow, fan-shaped x-ray beam that rotates multiple times 360 degrees around a patient, CBCT utilizes a cone-shaped x-ray beam collimated to limit radiation exposure to a region that corresponds to the dental arches; and rotates in one full or partial rotation around the head (180 to 360 degrees). It is this cone-shape collimation of the x-ray beam that significantly reduces radiation dose. The x-ray beam rotates around a full or partial **trajectory** or path, and travels through the anatomic structures to an image receptor that captures the scan data from the entire cone-shape area simultaneously and in a sequential manner to produce a planar, volumetric data set (Figure 31–4 ∎). This raw data, collectively called projection data, is then processed or reconstructed by computer software to produce enhanced 2-D and 3-D images (Figure 31–5 ∎). While CBCT examinations are prescribed for their ability to produce 3-D images, software settings also allow images to be displayed on a monitor as 2-D images that look similar to digital extraoral radiographs. Future technological development may

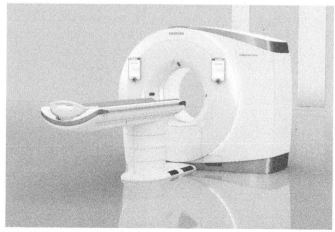

FIGURE 31–3 **CT scanner.** (Courtesy of Siemens Medical Solutions USA, Inc.)

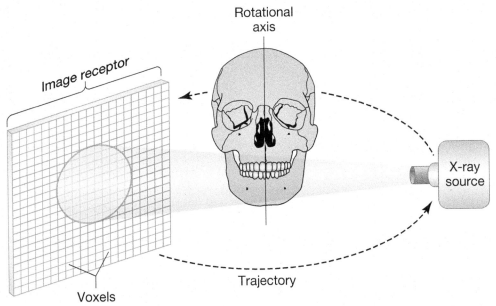

FIGURE 31–4 **Trajectory of exposure.** Cone-shaped x-ray beam passes through anatomy to image receptor while rotating 180 to 360 degrees in a single rotation around a rotational axis.

soon allow the display to resemble intraoral images of a full mouth series.

Another difference between CT and CBCT is the ability to reduce or enlarge the **field of view (FOV)**. FOV is the area of interest that will be exposed during the scanning process. Reducing or enlarging the FOV allows for a customized exposure based on the needs of a patient and on what data is needed from the examination. For example, a localized approximately 5-cm FOV may be selected to examine only the TMJ; a medium 10-cm FOV might be selected when the area of interest is both the mandible and maxilla (Table 31–2 ■; Figure 31–6 ■). Matching the size of the FOV with the area of interest can keep radiation exposure "as low as reasonably achievable" (ALARA). Using a smaller FOV is also linked to a higher resolution image and limiting the amount of scatter radiation produced.

Projection data captured by CBCT differs from data captured by standard 2-D digital imaging. Extra- and intra-oral digital sensors use pixels to capture a 2-D image; a CBCT sensor, called a **flat panel detector (FPD)**, utilizes

voxels to construct volumes of 3-D images. Recall that a pixel has two dimensions represented by an x-coordinate and a y-coordinate. A **voxel** (*vol*, short for volume; and *el*, short for element) adds a dimension, a z-coordinate, to form a cube that can capture more data that will then be used to produce a 3-D image (Figure 31–7 ■). Voxel size ranges between 0.076 and 0.125 mm and can be manually selected depending on the desired outcome. Voxel size influences image resolution, electronic image noise, and possibly the amount of radiation exposure required to produce an acceptable image. A larger voxel size setting can be expected to result in slightly decreased image detail and spatial resolution, but with reduced electronic noise; a smaller voxel size produces increased image detail and spatial resolution, but with a slightly greater appearance of electronic noise. The decision to use a larger or smaller voxel size setting is based on the image resolution and detail needed for an accurate diagnosis, balanced with an expected amount of electronic noise. Regarding radiation exposure, research suggests that a smaller voxel setting will require an increased radiation exposure to produce a diagnostic image. However, studies assessing the effective radiation dose when comparing large and small voxel size settings alone without other variables such as FOV are not currently conclusive.

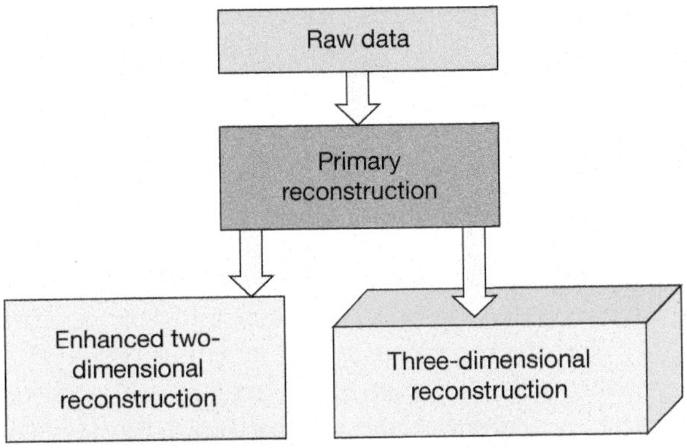

FIGURE 31–5 **Reconstruction of projection data.**

Raw data

↓

Primary reconstruction

↓   ↓

Enhanced two-dimensional reconstruction   Three-dimensional reconstruction

Table 31–2 Examples of FOV Sizes

Large	Medium	Focused
Entire oral and maxillofacial region	Maxillary arch, mandibular arch or both	Limited areas (e.g., one side of the arch)

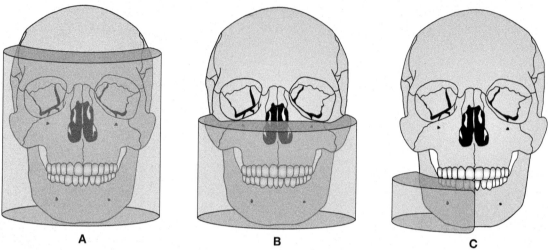

FIGURE 31–6 **FOV Sizes.** (**A**) Large. (**B**) Medium. (**C**) Focused.

Anatomical Planes

Once an image receptor receives raw data, **scatter correction algorithms**, built into CBCT computer software, reconstruct the digital signal into enhanced 2-D and 3-D images that are displayed on a monitor (Figure 31–8 ■). The reconstruction process is complex and can take the computer software between 5 and 30 minutes to complete. The resulting 3-D images are based on **anatomical planes**, imaginary lines that bisect the body and are used to describe locations of anatomy. CBCT images are displayed and can be interpreted and studied from thin **slice data** in three anatomical planes—axial, sagittal, and coronal. The **axial plane** (x-coordinate), sometimes referred to as the transverse plane, divides anatomy into an upper and lower section; the **coronal plane** (y-coordinate) divides anatomy vertically into a front and back section; and the **sagittal plane** (z-coordinate) divides anatomy vertically into a right and left side. All three anatomical planes when viewed together are known as image **reconstruction** (Figure 31–9 ■).

Images can be displayed in a variety of formats and, through use of computer software, can be viewed from various angles within the three anatomical planes. For example, a localized cross-sectional view is helpful when the area of interest is small and specific image detail is required for an accurate diagnosis. Structures displayed in the sagittal plane are similar to those recorded by 2-D extra- and intraoral radiographic images and are therefore not as challenging to interpret by experienced radiographers. The anatomy presented by slice data within the coronal, and especially within the axial planes is not as familiar to interpreters of 2-D radiographic images, who would most likely require specific training to accurately interpret CBCT images (Figure 31–10 ■).

Incorporating Three-dimensional Imaging in Oral Health Care

CBCT has improved diagnosing capabilities over 2-D radiographs for a variety of oral conditions and diseases. One of the most valuable uses of a CBCT examination is to diagnosis and plan treatment for dental implants. CBCT has the ability to demonstrate a 3-D representation of bone shape and contours of edentulous ridges. CBCT is able to accurately image the location of critical structures, such as the inferior alveolar nerve and maxillary sinus, prior to placement of dental implants. The ability to image a specific implant site in the axial plane, and with multiple cross-sectional views, allows for precise treatment planning prior to implant placement (Figure 31–11 ■).

Another important use of the diagnostic capabilities of CBCT is in determining and monitoring orthodontic intervention. Orthodontists have found that CBCT is more reliable than 2-D radiographs in determining location and position of unerupted, impacted, and supernumerary teeth, and other growth and developmental anomalies. Orthodontic diagnoses and pretreatment planning require the exposure of multiple types of 2-D radiographs, including panoramic and lateral and anterior-posterior cephalometric images (see Chapter 30). A

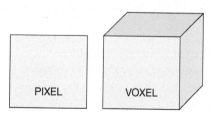

FIGURE 31–7 **Comparison of pixel and voxel.** Voxel captures a third dimension.

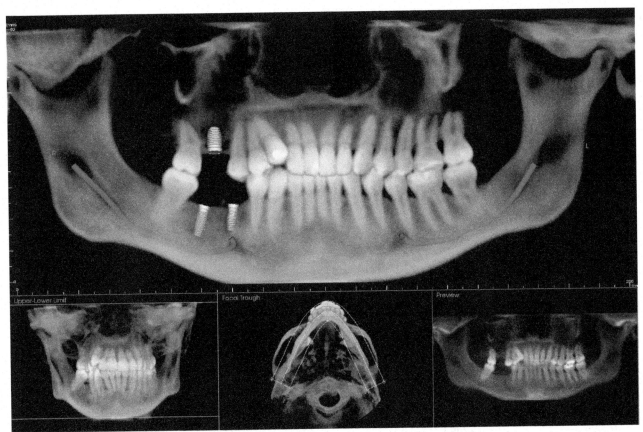

FIGURE 31–8 **Images produced by CBCT and reconstructed software viewed on a computer monitor.** (Courtesy of Kavo Kerr.)

CBCT examination may be a valuable substitute for these radiographic series, producing the additional benefit of more detailed 3-D images obtained with a comparable radiation dose.

CBCT may aid endodontists with diagnosing pathology for patients whose clinical symptoms do not present on intraoral or 2-D extraoral radiographs; particularly when symptoms are associated with a tooth previously treated with endodontic therapy. CBCT imaging has been shown to have the ability to detect periapical lesions at an earlier stage than 2-D radiographs, when treatment will have the best chance of a successful outcome. CBCT further assists during the course of endodontic treatment with an enhanced ability to precisely identify the presence of extra root canals, and when tooth root morphology presents a challenge for the imaging capabilities of 2-D radiographs. Although valuable, CBCT should not be used routinely pre- or posttreatment or during endodontic treatment, but rather assessed based on diagnostic need.

Technological advances that continue to reduce radiation exposure and improve the imaging capabilities of CBCT technology may see more recommended uses in the near future. The development of computers that can receive, manipulate, and store large data files, and monitors that can display complex images, will further the adoption of CBCT. The smaller size and footprint of the equipment used to obtain CBCT has increasingly allowed for its adoption in oral health practice settings outside of medical imaging centers. Since 2-D images can be extracted from CBCT image data (see Figure 31–5), more general practitioners may adopt the technology, further enlarging its potential application. As with any new technology, the potential for overuse exists, prompting a cautious examination of benefits and risks of radiation exposure.

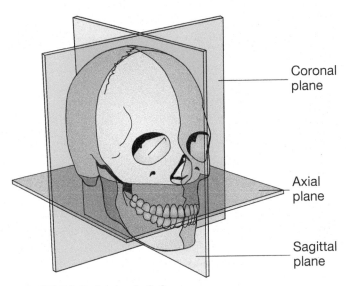

Coronal plane

Axial plane

Sagittal plane

FIGURE 31–9 **Anatomical planes.**

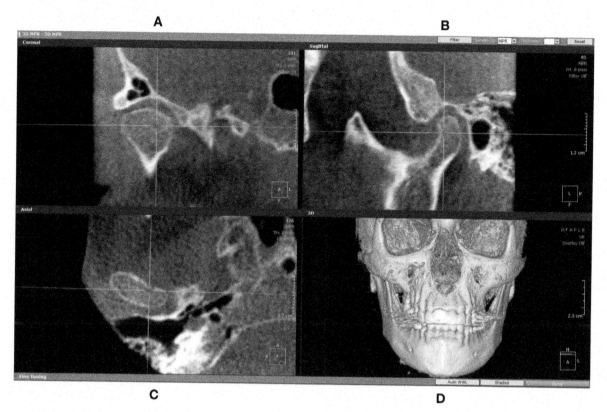

FIGURE 31–10 **Slice data.** (**A**) Coronal plane. (**B**) Sagittal plane. (**C**) Axial plane. (**D**) 3-D reconstruction. (Courtesy of Dale A. Miles, DDS, MS, FRCD(C), Diplomate, ABOM & ABOMR, CEO, Cone Beam Radiographic Services, LLC, President, EasyRiter, LLC.)

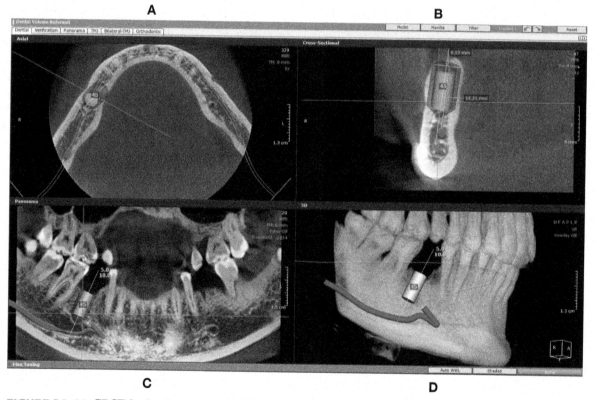

FIGURE 31–11 **CBCT for implant assessment.** (**A**) Axial plane. (**B**) Cross-sectional view. (**C**) Panoramic view. (**D**) Reconstructed 3-D view. Note location of inferior alveolar nerve highlighted in red by the computer program. (Courtesy of Dale A. Miles, DDS, MS, FRCD(C), Diplomate, ABOM & ABOMR, CEO, Cone Beam Radiographic Services, LLC, President, EasyRiter, LLC.)

ALARA

Radiation dose amounts from all types of diagnostic oral and maxillofacial examinations depend on many factors, and may be expressed using different quantifiers. It has been estimated that the effective dose from a CBCT examination using a large FOV ranges from 29 to 569 microseiverts (μSv). These estimates are generally lower than the estimated effective dose from a medical CT scan of the maxilla and mandible, between 240 and 1200 μSv and 480 and 3324 μSv, respectively. The advantage of prescribing CBCT over CT is a lowered radiation dose. However, the estimated effective dose from CBCT is still significantly higher than the dose expected from 2-D extra- and intraoral radiographic examinations. For comparison purposes, the estimated effective dose of a film-based panoramic radiograph is approximately 7 μSv.

CBCT is not meant to replace conventional 2-D oral and maxillofacial radiographic examinations for many conditions; and must not be utilized as a screening tool for occult disease. Because of the increased radiation dose, prescription of a CBCT examination must be based on a deliberate assessment of benefit and risks. CBCT should only be considered for use when it can be determined that other standard radiographic examinations will not contribute adequately to the diagnosis or treatment plan for the condition. Conversely, CBCT should be considered prior to exposing a series of extra- and/or intraoral radiographs to prevent duplication and overlap of exposures, negating the need for one or the other.

Depending on the type of equipment used, exposure factors can usually be adjusted to reduce or limit radiation in compliance with ALARA. Determine milamperage (mA), kilovoltage (kV), and collimated FOV settings based on patient characteristics and the needs of the examination. A lead/lead equivalent barrier including a thyroid collar should be used, unless it will interfere with acquisition of the image. Operators of CBCT must

be specifically trained in use of the equipment to safely administer an examination and perform regular equipment calibrations to ensure reliable output and proper exposure setting parameters.

Limitations

The presence of artifacts, images other than anatomy or pathology that do not contribute to a diagnosis, can be a significant problem affecting image quality. Artifacts and electronic noise are more likely to occur with CBCT technology than with medical CT scans. The cone-shape beam, and use of a lower radiation energy, can lead to the production of scatter radiation that negatively affects an image (Figure 31–12 ■). The increased scatter radiation produced by CBCT also contributes to decreased contrast

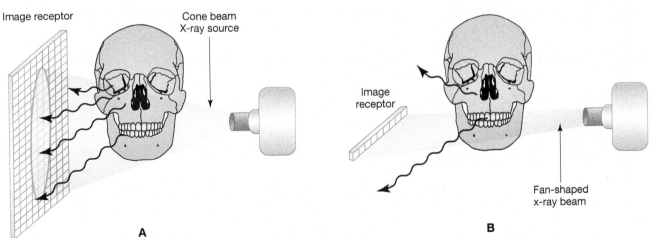

FIGURE 31–12 Scatter radiation. CBCT cone-shaped x-ray beam creates more scatter radiation that reaches the image receptor than CT fan-shaped x-ray beam resulting in increased occurrence of artifacts.

of soft tissue, making CT scans better at imaging conditions that require a comparison of hard and soft tissue structures. CBCT antiscatter or scatter correction algorithms software help to minimize artifacts and improve contrast.

Differential absorption of x-ray photons creates distortion in the form of streaking and cupping artifacts. **Streaking artifacts**, radiolucent lines observed across an image, are most likely to occur when the x-ray beam passes through two objects of equal high density that are close to one another, such as adjacent teeth with large metallic restorations (Figure 31–13 ■). The presence of a large metallic restoration can also create a **cupping artifact**, which presents as a radiolucent distortion surrounding the dense radiopaque appearance of the metal object (Figure 31–14 ■). The mechanism for these occurrences is the inherent tendency for lower energy x-ray photons to be absorbed by an image receptor instead of higher energy x-ray photons.

Artifacts can also occur due to patient movement during the scanning process. These artifacts present as a double, or duplicate, appearance of anatomical structures that appear to have been imaged twice. Patient movement may occur during a CBCT scan because of the time required for exposure; usually between 10 and 90 seconds depending on the FOV. To avoid movement artifacts, assess a patient's ability to cooperate with the procedure and/or utilize stabilizing aids such as a chin or head rest, and bite guides. The chance of artifacts occurring due to patient movement is usually reduced when using a smaller FOV, which requires a shorter exposure time.

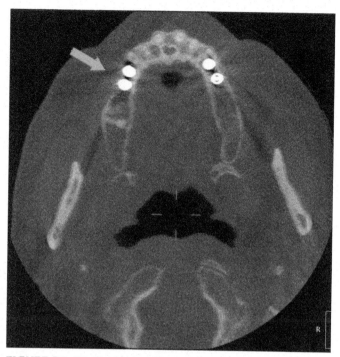

FIGURE 31–14 Cupping artifacts. (Courtesy of Dale A. Miles, DDS, MS, FRCD(C), Diplomate, ABOM & ABOMR, CEO, Cone Beam Radiographic Services, LLC, President, EasyRiter, LLC.)

Interpretation

The decision to prescribe a CBCT examination comes with the responsibility, both ethically and legally, for interpreting the images. Interpretation of a CBCT image is a daunting task. Unless specifically trained as an oral and maxillofacial radiologist, an oral health care practitioner is not likely to attempt a definitive interpretation without assistance. A CBCT examination produces as many as 500 image slices for each of the three anatomical planes, resulting in 1500 image slices available for interpretation.

A comprehensive interpretation must include detection of conditions affecting anatomy beyond the oral cavity such as diseases and abnormalities noted in the nasal airways, paranasal sinuses, craniofacial structures, cervical vertebrae, and other tissues outside the dentition and supporting structures. It is critical that the entire image data set be reviewed and interpreted. While an examination may have been prescribed for a specific dental need, the prescribing oral health care professional is responsible for detection and subsequent recommendations for treatment or referral of all conditions revealed by the examination (Figure 31–15 ■). A comprehensive interpretation may be obtained through collaboration with a maxillofacial radiologist consultant who would be responsible for interpreting the images and providing a report or summary to the referring dentist. A practitioner who plans to adopt CBCT as a standard of care would be expected to obtain these interpretation skills.

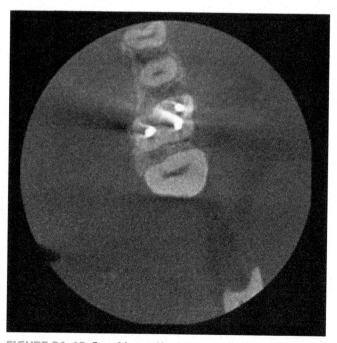

FIGURE 31–13 Streaking artifacts. (Courtesy of Planmeca.)

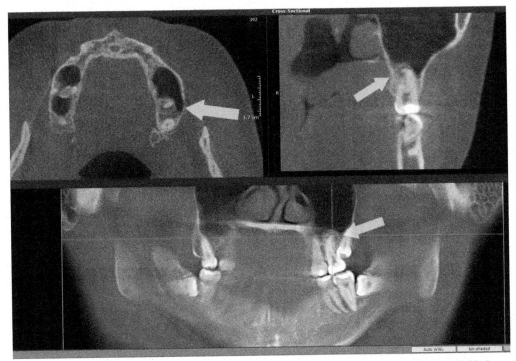

FIGURE 31–15 CBCT interpretation. CBCT examination prescribed to assess impacted third molar incidentally reveals unsuspected periapical pathology of an adjacent tooth (arrows). (Courtesy of Dale A. Miles, DDS, MS, FRCD(C), Diplomate, ABOM & ABOMR, CEO, Cone Beam Radiographic Services, LLC, President, EasyRiter, LLC.)

REVIEW—Chapter summary

Cone beam computed tomography (CBCT), also called cone beam volumetric imaging (CBVI), is essentially medical computed tomography (CT) that has been specifically designed to produce 3-D radiographic images of the oral and maxillofacial region. A CBCT examination is prescribed when detail of pathologic conditions is necessary for diagnosis. Due to the large radiation dose required, use of CBCT must be carefully assessed. Experts categorize specific oral conditions for prescribing CBCT examinations into the following categories: *Standard of Care*, *Preferred Use*, and *Not Necessary* to guide practitioners with its use. Examples of conditions categorized as *Standard of Care* include implant assessment, surgical tooth extraction, and orthodontic assessment. Examples of conditions categorized as *Preferred* include endodontic therapy and location of the inferior alveolar nerve prior to oral surgical procedures. CBCT is not recommended for noncomplex conditions that can be adequately assessed with 2-D images such as caries and periodontal diagnoses.

CT and CBCT examinations produce enhanced 3-D images from multiplanar recorded slices of tissue without superimposed blurring of structures that lie outside a selected plane. There are differences between CT and CBCT. Most importantly, CT uses a narrow, fan-shaped x-ray beam that rotates multiple times 360 degrees around a patient; conversely, CBCT uses a cone-shaped x-ray beam

collimated to limit radiation exposure to a region that corresponds to the area of interest, and rotates in one full or partial rotation around the head. CBCT is more effective than CT at imaging hard tissues of the oral and maxillofacial area, and allows for the adjustment of the size of the field of view (FOV) to customize exposure as needed.

A CBCT image receptor, usually a flat panel detector (FPD), utilizes voxels to capture raw data. A larger voxel size decreases spatial resolution, decreases electronic noise, and may possibly require less radiation exposure to produce an acceptable image. A smaller voxel size increases spatial resolution, increases electronic noise, and may possibly require more radiation exposure to produce an acceptable image. Digital software such as scatter correction algorithms reconstruct projection data into enhanced 2-D and 3-D images that are shown on a computer monitor. Images are displayed and can be interpreted and studied from thin slice data in three anatomical planes—axial, coronal, and sagittal.

CBCT is considered valuable in assessment and treatment related to dental implants, orthodontics, and endodontic therapy, and technological advances may lead to additional uses. Assess benefits to be gained from CBCT examination with risks of radiation exposure. CBCT should be considered prior to exposing a series of extra- and/or intraoral radiographs to prevent duplication and overlap of exposures, negating the need for one or the other.

Artifacts and electronic noise such as radiolucent streaking and cupping are more likely to occur with CBCT than CT technology. Reduce patient movement artifacts by assessing ability to cooperate with the procedure; utilizing stabilization aids; and reducing the FOV, which decreases the length of time a patient must hold still. Prescribing a CBCT examination comes with an ethical and legal responsibility to thoroughly interpret the images. A maxillofacial radiologist consultant may assist an untrained oral health care practitioner in obtaining a definitive interpretation.

RECALL—Study questions

1. Which of the following is true regarding cone beam computed tomography (CBCT)?
   a. Requires more radiation than computed tomography (CT)
   b. Produces 3-D radiographic images
   c. Replaces standard 2-D extraoral radiographs
   d. Records structures that lie outside a selected plane

2. CBCT is useful for each of the following EXCEPT one. Which one is the EXCEPTION?
   a. Orthodontic assessment
   b. Temporomandibular disease (TMD) evaluation
   c. Dental implant treatment planning
   d. Detecting proximal surface dental caries

3. Which of the following conditions would be categorized as *Preferred* for use of CBCT?
   a. Endodontic therapy
   b. Location of impacted third molar
   c. Surgical guide to reconstruction
   d. Temporomandibular joint (TMJ) assessment

4. CBCT significantly reduces radiation dose over a CT examination *because* CBCT uses a fan-shaped x-ray beam of exposure.
   a. Both the statement and reason are correct and related.
   b. Both the statement and reason are correct but NOT related.
   c. The statement is correct, but the reason is NOT.
   d. The statement is NOT correct, but the reason is correct.
   e. NEITHER the statement NOR the reason is correct.

5. Which of the following refers to the size of the area that will be exposed by a CBCT examination?
   a. Trajectory
   b. Anatomic plane
   c. Field of view (FOV)
   d. Cone-shaped collimation

6. Which of the following is used by CBCT to capture image data in three dimensions?
   a. Pixel
   b. Voxel
   c. Slice
   d. Plane

7. A larger voxel size setting _____ spatial resolution and _____ electronic noise.
   a. decreases, decreases
   b. increases, increases
   c. decreases, increases
   d. increases, decreases

8. A CBCT scan obtains image data in each of the following planes EXCEPT for one. Which one is the EXCEPTION?
   a. Sagittal
   b. Coronal
   c. Axial
   d. Apical

9. A CBCT examination plays a valuable role in endodontic therapy *because* CBCT can detect periapical lesions at an earlier stage than 2-D radiographs.
   a. Both the statement and reason are correct and related.
   b. Both the statement and reason are correct but NOT related.
   c. The statement is correct, but the reason is NOT.
   d. The statement is NOT correct, but the reason is correct.
   e. NEITHER the statement NOR the reason is correct.

10. Each of the following has led to the increased use of CBCT technology for oral and maxillofacial conditions EXCEPT one. Which one is the EXCEPTION?
    a. Development of computers that can receive, manipulate, and store large data files
    b. The availability of a flat-panel detector (FPD) digital image receptor
    c. Smaller size and footprint of equipment used to obtain CBCT
    d. Both 2-D and 3-D images can be extracted from image data

11. Which of the following examinations would require the least amount of radiation exposure?
    a. CBCT medium FOV
    b. CBCT focused FOV
    c. CT mandibular arch
    d. Lateral cephalometric radiograph

12. Each of the following may help avoid CBCT image artifacts EXCEPT one. Which one is the EXCEPTION?
    a. Decrease exposure time.
    b. Instruct patient to remain still.
    c. Increase FOV.
    d. Utilize head stabilizing aids.

13. Interpreting a CBCT image may be challenging for a practitioner not specifically trained for this task *because* CBCT records conditions affecting anatomy beyond the oral cavity.
    a. Both the statement and reason are correct and related.
    b. Both the statement and reason are correct but NOT related.
    c. The statement is correct, but the reason is NOT.
    d. The statement is NOT correct, but the reason is correct.
    e. NEITHER the statement NOR the reason is correct.

REFLECT—Case study

A CBCT examination has been prescribed for a pediatric orthodontic assessment. Consider how you would prepare for an informative discussion in response to the following questions a parent may ask.

1. What is CBCT?
2. Why has CBCT been prescribed?
3. What does the CBCT machine look like?
4. How will my child be prepared for the examination?
5. Will he or she have to do something during the exposure?
6. How long does the examination take?
7. What steps will be taken to protect my child from radiation exposure?
8. When will the dentist have the examination results?
9. Will additional dental radiographs have to be exposed?
10. Can I have a copy of the images?

RELATE—Laboratory application

Design a recordkeeping pamphlet that a patient could use to keep track of diagnostic radiographic examinations. Title your pamphlet: "My Dental Imaging History" or something similar. For ideas to include in your pamphlet, visit the U.S. Food and Drug Administration (FDA) website at: http://www.fda.gov/downloads/Radiation-EmittingProducts/RadiationSafety/RadiationDoseReduction/UCM235128.pdf

RESOURCES

American Academy of Endodontists and American Academy of Oral and Maxillofacial Radiology. (2015, May). AAE and AAOMR joint position statement. Use of cone beam computed tomography in endodontics 2015 update. Retrieved from AAE Web site: https://www.aae.org/uploadedfiles/clinical_resources/guidelines_and_position_statements/cbctstatement_2015update.pdf

American Academy of Oral and Maxillofacial Radiology. (2013, August). Clinical recommendations regarding use of cone beam computed tomography in orthodontics. Position statement by the American Academy of Oral and Maxillofacial Radiology. *Oral Surgery, Oral Medicine, Oral Pathology, Oral Radiology, 116*(2), 238–257.

American Dental Association Council on Scientific Affairs. (2012). The use of cone-beam computed tomography in dentistry. *Journal of the American Dental Association, 143,* 899–902.

Chau, A. C. M., & Fung, K. (2009). Comparison of radiation dose for implant imaging using conventional spiral tomography, computed tomography, and cone-beam computed tomography. *Oral Surgery, Oral Medicine, Oral Pathology, Oral Radiology, 107,* 559–565.

Ludlow, J. B., & Ivanovic, M. (2008). Comparative dosimetry of dental CBCT devices and 64-slice CT for oral and maxillofacial radiology. *Oral Surgery, Oral Medicine, Oral Pathology, Oral Radiology, 106,* 106–114.

Ludlow, J. B., Davies-Ludlow, L. E., Brooks, S. L., et al. (2006). Dosimetry of 3 CBCT devices for oral and maxillofacial radiology: CB Mercuray, NewTom 3G and i-CAT. *Dentomaxillofacial Radiology, 35,* 219–226.

Miles, D. A. (2013). *Color atlas of cone beam volumetric imaging for dental applications* (2nd ed.). Chicago: Quintessence Publishing Co.

Miles, D. A., & Danforth R. A. (2008). *A clinician's guide to understanding cone beam volumetric imaging (CBVI)*. The Academy of Dental Therapeutics and Stomatology, a division of PennWell, 1–15.

Spin-Neto, R., Gotfredsen, E., & Wenzel, A. (2013). Impact of voxel size variation on CBCT-based diagnostic outcome in dentistry: a systematic review. *Journal of Digital Imaging, 26*(4), 813–820.

Tyndall, D. A., Price, J. B., Tetradis, S., et al. (2012, June). Position statement of the American Academy of Oral and Maxillofacial Radiology on selection criteria for the use of radiology in dental implantology with emphasis on cone beam computed tomography. *Oral Surgery, Oral Medicine, Oral Pathology, Oral Radiology, 113*(6), 817–826.

White, S. C., & Pharoah, M. J. (2014). Cone beam computed tomography. *Oral radiology: Principles and interpretation* (7th ed.). St. Louis, MO: Elsevier.

Visit www.pearsonhighered.com/healthprofessionsresources to access the student resources that accompany this book. Simply select Dental Hygiene from the choice of disciplines. Find this book and you will find the complementary study tools created for this specific title.

ANSWERS
to Study Questions

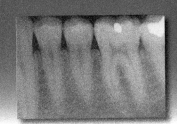

Chapter 1

1. c
2. a
3. d
4. e
5. b
6. d
7. c
8. b
9. c
10. d
11. a
12. b
13. d
14. Use Box 1-1 to list uses.

Chapter 2

1. a
2. Use chapter information and Figure 2-1 to draw diagram.
3. d
4. c
5. b
6. b
7. a
8. d
9. b
10. Use chapter information to list properties.
11. a
12. c
13. d
14. b
15. d
16. c
17. Use chapter information to list sources.
18. b

Chapter 3

1. d
2. c
3. a
4. b
5. c
6. b
7. a
8. a
9. c

10. Use chapter information to list conditions.
11. Use chapter information and Figure 3-8 to draw and label diagram.
12. c
13. d
14. b
15. a

Chapter 4

1. Use chapter information to list criteria.
2. d
3. c
4. b
5. d
6. a
7. d
8. c
9. a
10. d
11. b
12. c
13. d
14. a

Chapter 5

1. a
2. c
3. d
4. b
5. Use chapter information to list responses.
6. c
7. a
8. d
9. c
10. b
11. c
12. a
13. b
14. d
15. d
16. c

Chapter 6

1. d
2. d
3. b

4. c
5. b
6. c
7. d
8. c
9. d
10. a
11. b
12. d
13. c
14. c
15. b
16. Use Table 6-3 to list organizations.

Chapter 7

1. a
2. d
3. c
4. b
5. b
6. c
7. c
8. d
9. a
10. c
11. c
12. a
13. b
14. d
15. a

Chapter 8

1. d
2. e
3. b
4. a
5. c
6. c
7. b
8. e
9. d
10. c
11. b
12. a
13. c
14. c
15. d
16. a
17. a

Chapter 9
1. d
2. d
3. a
4. a
5. Use chapter information to list items.
6. c
7. b
8. b
9. c
10. b
11. d
12. b
13. a
14. c
15. b

Chapter 10
1. d
2. a
3. d
4. b
5. c
6. d
7. a
8. a
9. b
10. c
11. d
12. c
13. b
14. a
15. a
16. c

Chapter 11
1. d
2. a
3. b
4. c
5. a
6. d
7. b
8. a
9. a
10. d
11. c
12. b
13. Use chapter information to list responses.

Chapter 12
1. c
2. a
3. b
4. a

5. a
6. c
7. b
8. d
9. a
10. a
11. b
12. d
13. c
14. d
15. Use chapter information to list contraindications.
16. d
17. a
18. b

Chapter 13
1. d
2. a
3. c
4. d
5. c
6. b
7. a
8. c
9. a
10. c
11. b
12. d

Chapter 14
1. b
2. b
3. d
4. c
5. a
6. a
7. d
8. c
9. d
10. d
11. b
12. b
13. d
14. a
15. c
16. a
17. c

Chapter 15
1. c
2. b
3. b
4. d
5. a
6. c
7. b
8. c

9. d
10. c
11. a
12. d
13. c
14. d
15. d

Chapter 16
1. a
2. d
3. d
4. b
5. c
6. a
7. b
8. a
9. c
10. d

Chapter 17
1. c
2. a
3. c
4. d
5. a
6. c
7. c
8. a
9. c
10. b
11. b
12. d
13. c
14. d
15. c
16. d
17. b
18. a

Chapter 18
1. d
2. a
3. c
4. c
5. a
6. b
7. d
8. b
9. c
10. a
11. d
12. d
13. a
14. c
15. c
16. a
17. b

Chapter 19

1. b
2. d
3. d
4. c
5. a
6. d
7. b
8. b
9. a
10. a
11. d
12. c

Chapter 20

1. Use chapter information to list advantages.
2. d
3. b
4. d
5. b
6. d
7. a
8. d
9. c
10. b
11. c
12. a
13. d

Chapter 21

1. b
2. d
3. b
4. b
5. a
6. d
7. a
8. c
9. d
10. b
11. c
12. b
13. d
14. c
15. b
16. a

Chapter 22

1. a
2. b
3. d
4. a
5. b
6. c
7. b
8. d

9. c
10. a
11. c
12. b
13. a
14. d
15. b
16. c

Chapter 23

1. e
2. c
3. a
4. b
5. a
6. b
7. d
8. d
9. c
10. d
11. a
12. a
13. b

Chapter 24

1. d
2. d
3. a
4. b
5. c
6. a
7. a
8. c
9. b
10. d
11. c
12. a
13. b
14. b

Chapter 25

1. b
2. Use chapter information to list uses.
3. c
4. d
5. c
6. a
7. b
8. Use chapter information to list limitations.
9. d
10. c
11. a
12. b

Chapter 26

1. c
2. a

3. b
4. a
5. c
6. b
7. c
8. b
9. d
10. a
11. c
12. b
13. d
14. e

Chapter 27

1. Use chapter information to list conditions.
2. b
3. c
4. d
5. a
6. c
7. a
8. b
9. d
10. d
11. a
12. a
13. c
14. d
15. b
16. a
17. c

Chapter 28

1. Use chapter information to list actions.
2. a
3. d
4. b
5. a
6. c
7. a
8. b
9. d
10. a

Chapter 29

1. c
2. e
3. a
4. b
5. b
6. c
7. d
8. a
9. a
10. b

11. c
12. d
13. b
14. b
15. a
16. c

Chapter 30

1. a
2. b
3. d
4. c
5. a

6. b
7. d
8. a
9. d
10. b
11. a
12. c
13. b

Chapter 31

1. b
2. d
3. a

4. c
5. c
6. b
7. a
8. d
9. a
10. b
11. d
12. c
13. a

GLOSSARY

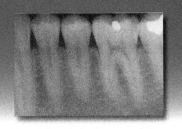

Absorbed dose: Amount of energy deposited in any form of matter, such as hard and soft tissues of the body, by any type of ionizing radiation. The units for measuring the absorbed dose are the gray (Gy) and the rad (radiation absorbed dose).

Absorption: The process through which radiation imparts some or all of its energy to any material through which it passes.

Active listening: Requires that a person pay attention to what is being said verbally, and observe nonverbal communication, to respond in a manner that demonstrates an understanding of what is being said.

Acute radiation syndrome (ARS): Symptoms of short-term radiation effects after a massive dose of ionizing radiation.

Added filtration: Added to the inherent filtration built into a dental x-ray machine, in the form of thin disks of aluminum, inserted between the x-ray tube and the lead collimator when inherent filtration is not sufficient to meet radiation safety requirements.

ALARA: "As low as reasonably achievable" concept that any radiation dose that can be lowered without major difficulty, great expense, or inconvenience should be reduced or eliminated. Adopted as a culture and attitude by professionals who work with ionizing radiation to minimize radiation exposure and risks.

Ala–tragus line: An imaginary plane or line from the ala of the nose (winglike projection at the side of the nose) to the tragus of the ear (cartilaginous projection in front of the acoustic meatus of the ear). Important in deciding the correct head position for determining angles and points of entry for radiographic techniques.

Alternating current (AC): A flow of electrons in one direction, followed by a flow in the opposite direction; important concept in the operation of a dental x-ray machine.

Aluminum equivalent: Thickness of a material affording the same degree of attenuation of the primary x-ray beam as aluminum, under specified conditions.

Alveolar process: The most coronal portion of the alveolar bone. Appears radiopaque.

Alveolus: A section of alveolar bone that forms a bony socket in which the roots of a tooth are held in position by periodontal ligaments. The outline of the socket is observed radiographically as the radiopaque lamina dura.

Amalgam: Metallic restorative material that appears radiopaque.

Amalgam tattoo: Bluish-purple color observed in gingiva caused by fragments of amalgam left under the tissue; appears radiopaque.

Analog: Relating to the mechanism in which data is represented by continuously variable physical quantities.

Anatomical planes: Imaginary lines bisecting the body or a specific anatomical area of interest into the coronal, axial, and sagittal planes. Used to identify location of anatomical structures and conditions.

Angulation: Referring to dental radiographic techniques, the direction in which the x-ray tube head and position indicating device (PID) and central rays of the x-ray beam are directed toward the oral structures and an image receptor. *See* Horizontal angulation, Negative angulation, Positive angulation, and Vertical angulation.

Anode: The positive electrode in the dental x-ray tube that serves to provide a target to stop or significantly slow high-velocity electrons, converting their kinetic energy into x-rays (electromagnetic energy).

Anomaly: A deviation from the normal.

Antemortem radiograph: Any image that was exposed before death that is used to compare with postmortem radiographs for identification of human remains.

Antihalation coating: A dye added to the nonemulsion side of duplicating film to prevent backscattered ultraviolet light from coming through the films and creating an unsharp image.

Artifacts: Images recorded on radiographs other than anatomy or pathology that do not contribute to a diagnosis of the patient's condition.

Artificial intelligence: Ability of a computer to perform decision making similar to a human being.

Aseptic: The absence of microorganisms that cause infection.

Atom: The smallest particle of an element that retains the properties of that element. Atoms are composed of a number of subatomic particles. *See* Electron, Neutron, and Proton.

Autism spectrum disorder (ASD): Developmental disorder affecting social and behavioral interactions and causing obsessive and repetitive behaviors.

Automatic processor: A machine that develops, fixes, washes, and dries radiographic film.

Axial plane: Anatomical plane that divides an area of interest into superior and inferior slices of data in a horizontal dimension.

Backscatter ring shield: A leaded acrylic circular ring surrounding the position indicating device (PID) of a handheld dental x-ray machine that serves to protect an operator from backscatter radiation when used appropriately.

Barrier envelope: Plastic sheaths used to seal intraoral film packets, phosphor plates, and digital sensors to protect from contact with fluids in the oral cavity during exposure.

Base material: A thick layer of cement used as a cavity preparation under a restoration. Base material often appears slightly more radiopaque than dentin.

Binding energy: The internal energy within an atom that holds its components together.

Biodegradable: Capable of being broken down into harmless products by living organisms such as those found in a wastewater treatment facility.

Bisecting technique: A dental radiographic technique in which the central rays of the x-ray beam are directed perpendicular to an imaginary bisector of the angle formed by the recording plane of the image receptor and the long axes of the teeth.

Bisector: An imaginary line that bisects the angle formed by an intraoral image receptor when placed against a tooth.

Biteblock: The portion of an image receptor holding device that a patient occludes on to hold an image receptor in position during exposure.

Bitetab: An extension attached at the center of an image receptor that a patient occludes on to stabilize the image receptor during a bitewing exposure.

Bitewing radiograph: An intraoral radiograph that records the crown portion of both the maxillary and mandibular teeth.

Buccal-object rule: Principle that structures portrayed in two or more radiographs exposed at different angles will appear to shift positions.

Calcium tungstate: Barium strontium sulfate salt crystals used in intensifying screens that fluoresce and emit energy in the form of blue light when x-rays are absorbed.

Calculus: Calcified microbial plaque.

Cancellous (trabecular) bone: Soft spongy bone that makes up the bulk of the inside portion of most bones; appears radiographically as mixed radiolucent-radiopaque honeycomb compartments.

Cassette: A rigid or flexible light-tight extraoral film or digital phosphor plate holder.

Cathode: The negative electrode in the x-ray tube that serves to supply the electrons necessary to produce x-rays.

CBCT: *See* Cone beam computed tomography.

CCD: *See* Charge-coupled device.

CEJ: *See* Cementoenamel junction.

Cementoenamel junction (CEJ): The area where the enamel covering of a tooth crown meets the cementum covering of a tooth root.

Cementum: Thin layer of dense tissue that covers a tooth root; radiographically indistinguishable from dentin. When hypercementosis presents, the overgrowth of cementum will appear radiopaque and bulbous.

Central rays: The central portion of the primary beam of radiation.

Cephalostat: A device used to stabilize the head during exposure of an extraoral lateral cephalometric radiograph.

Cervical burnout: A radiolucency often observed on the mesial and distal tooth root surfaces near the cementoenamel junction (CEJ) caused by a concave root shape at the cervical line; appearance mimics caries.

Chain of infection: The sequence of the transmission of infectious diseases made up of six links: a susceptible host, a pathogen, a reservoir, entrance and exit portals, and a mode of transmission.

Chairside manner: Refers to the conduct of a dental radiographer while working with a patient.

Charge-coupled device (CCD): A solid-state detector used as a digital image receptor that replaces dental radiographic film. Converts x-rays to an electronic signal that is sent to a computer via a universal serial bus (USB) cable; has a wider dynamic range than complementary metal oxide semiconductor (CMOS-APS) technology.

Cloud file sharing: Secure computer storage systems for transferring large data files between patients, insurance companies, and other medical professionals.

CMOS: *See* Complementary metal oxide semiconductor.

Code of ethics: A professional organization's principles to assist members in achieving a high standard of ethical practice.

Collimation: Restriction of the useful beam to an appropriate size. Beam diameter used to expose intraoral dental radiographs is collimated not to exceed 2.75 inches (7 cm) at the skin surface.

Collimator: A diaphragm, usually lead, designed to restrict dimensions of the useful beam.

Complementary metal oxide semiconductor (CMOS): A solid-state detector used as a digital image receptor that replaces dental radiographic film. Converts x-rays to an electronic signal that is sent to a computer via a universal serial bus (USB) cable or wirelessly via a radio signal. Requires less computer system power and has a narrower dynamic range than charge-coupled device (CCD) technology.

Composite resin: Tooth-colored restorative material made up of an organic resin, usually bisphenol A-glycidyl methacrylate (BIS-GMA), with inorganic fillers such as quartz or silica that provide strength; radiopacity is about the same as dentin.

Computed tomography (CT; CT scan): Medical radiographic imaging technique that uses a fan-shaped x-ray beam to record a "slice" of tissue producing a three-dimensional image.

Cone: Older term used to describe the positioning indicating device (PID).

Cone beam computed tomography (CBCT): Technology based on medical computed tomography (CT) that has been designed specifically for three-dimensional imaging of the oral and maxillofacial regions.

Conecut error: An intraoral radiographic technique error that results when the central rays of the x-ray beam are not directed toward the center of an image receptor, resulting in a blank area in that part of the radiograph that was not reached by the radiation.

Confidentiality: Private information, such as dental records, protected by law from being shared with nonprivileged individuals.

Contact point: Area on a tooth surface that touches an adjacent tooth; the mesial surface of one tooth makes contact with the distal surface of the tooth adjacent to it in the dental arch.

Contrast: The visual differences between shades ranging from black to white in adjacent areas of a radiographic image. *See* Long-scale contrast and Short-scale contrast.

Control panel: That portion of a dental x-ray machine that houses the controls: line switch, timer, milliamperage and kilovoltage selectors, and exposure button.

Coronal plane: Anatomical plane that divides an area of interest into anterior and posterior slices of data in the vertical dimension.

Cortical bone: The solid, dense, radiopaque outer portion of bone.

Corticated: Refers to a thin or thick border that appears as a radiopaque outline encapsulating a lesion.

Cough etiquette: Also called respiratory hygiene, consists of steps taken to prevent the transmission of respiratory pathogens that includes covering the mouth and nose when coughing and sneezing.

Coulombs per kilogram (C/kg): *Système Internationale* unit for measuring radiation exposure. A coulomb is a unit of electrical charge (equal to 6.25×10^8 electrons). The unit C/kg measures electrical charges (ion pairs) in a kilogram of air.

Cross-sectional technique: An occlusal radiographic technique in which the central rays of the x-ray beam are directed perpendicular to the image receptor.

Crown: (1) That portion of a tooth covered with enamel, and appears radiopaque. (2) A metallic, porcelain, or combination of metal and porcelain tooth restoration;

radiopacity varies depending on the density of the material.

CT: *See* Computed tomography.

Cultural competence: The level of knowledge-based skills required to provide effective clinical care to patients from a particular ethnic or racial group.

Cumulative effect: The theory that radiation-exposed tissues accrue damage and may function at a diminished capacity with each repeated exposure.

Cupping artifact: An artifact sometimes present on a cone beam computed tomography (CBCT) image that appears as a radiolucent distortion surrounding a dense radiopaque metal object, such as a large metallic restoration.

Darkroom: A light-tight room with special safelighting where x-ray film is handled and processed.

Daylight loader: A light-shielded compartment attached to an automatic processor allowing films to be unwrapped in a room with white light.

Dead pixel: Term given to a damaged pixel that does not respond to x-radiation exposure and therefore will not record radiographic information.

DEJ: *See* Dentinoenamel junction.

Density: The degree of darkening or blackening of a radiographic image. A radiographic image that appears light is said to have little density; a radiographic image that appears dark is said to have more density.

Dentin: Hard tissue that makes up a large portion of a tooth, surrounding the pulp and covered by enamel on the crown and by cementum on the root. Appears slightly less radiopaque than enamel.

Dentinoenamel junction (DEJ): The area where the dentin and enamel covering of a tooth crown meet.

Deterministic effect: Also called nonstochastic effect. Observable adverse biological effects caused by radiation exposure. The severity of change in tissues depends on the radiation dose.

Developer: The chemical solution used in film processing that reduces silver halide crystals within film emulsion to metallic silver making a latent image visible.

Diagnosis: The art of differentiating and determining the nature of a problem or disease. *See* Differential diagnosis.

DICOM: *See* Digital Imaging and Communication in Medicine.

Differential diagnosis: Form of diagnosis that distinguishes the type of lesion or condition from all other possibilities.

Digital imaging: A method of producing a filmless radiographic image using a sensor or phosphor plate that captures x-ray energy, and transmits electronic data to a computer, that processes and displays the radiographic image on a computer monitor. The terms *digital imaging* and *digital radiography* are often used interchangeably.

Digital Imaging and Communications in Medicine (DICOM): A joint committee formed in 1983 by the American College of Radiology and the National Electrical Manufacturers Association to create a standard method for electronic transmissions of digital images, the goal of which is to achieve compatibility and ease exchange of electronic information between digital image systems.

Digital subtraction: Computer software manipulation that merges two radiographic images of the same area, taken at different times allowing similar portions of the image to cancel each other out and reveal changes.

Digitization: Conversion of a film-based radiograph into a digital form that can be processed by a computer.

Dilaceration: Describes a tooth root with a sharp bend or abnormal curvature.

Direct current (DC): Electric current that flows continuously in one direction; similar to current produced in batteries. An important concept in the operation of a dental x-ray machine. Ideal for use with digital imaging systems.

Direct ion storage (DIS) monitor: A personnel radiation monitoring device that uses a miniature ion chamber to absorb radiation. Exposure is monitored through digital processing.

Direct supervision: Requires a dentist be present when a radiographer is performing a radiographic examination.

DIS: *See* Direct ion storage monitor.

Disability: A physical or mental impairment that substantially limits one or more of an individual's major life activities.

Disclosure: The process of informing a patient about the risks and benefits of a treatment procedure such as a radiographic examination.

Disinfection: Chemical applications that reduce disease-producing microorganisms to an acceptable level.

Distomesial overlap: When the projection angle of the x-ray beam is directed obliquely from distal to mesial, resulting in an overlapping error that appears more severe in the anterior region of the image.

Disto-oblique periapical radiographs: Images that utilize a dental x-ray machine tube shift to help record posterior objects such as impacted third molars. The tube head is shifted to the distal allowing the position indicating device (PID) to direct the central rays of the x-ray beam to intersect the image receptor obliquely from the distal, projecting the posterior object forward onto the image receptor.

Dose equivalent: Term used to measure radiation through an analytical comparison of the biological effects of various types of radiation. Defined as the product of the absorbed dose × a biological effect qualifying factor. Quantum physicists have determined that the qualifying factor for x-rays is "1" so absorbed dose and dose equivalent are numerically equal. The units for measuring dose equivalent are sievert (Sv) and rem.

Double exposure: Incorrectly using the same image receptor to expose two radiographs, which results in an over-exposed, double-image error.

Duplicate radiograph: An identical copy of an original radiograph obtained either through use of double intraoral film packets or with duplicating film and a duplicator made especially for this purpose.

Duplicating film: A photographic film used in conjunction with a film duplicator that uses infrared and ultraviolet light to make copies of intra- and extraoral film-based radiographs.

Dynamic range: Allowable amount of radiation that can be received by a digital image receptor and produce an acceptable, diagnostic quality radiographic image.

Edentulous: Without teeth; condition may present as partially edentulous, areas of the jaws with no teeth; or completely edentulous.

Effective dose equivalent: Term used to make more accurate comparisons between different radiographic exposures; measures the risk of the exposure producing a biological response; compensates for the differences in area exposed and the tissues that may be in the path of the x-ray beam. Measured in microsieverts (μSv).

Electromagnetic radiation: Forms of energy propelled by wave motion as photons; a combination of electric and magnetic energy. Has no charge, mass, or weight and travels at the speed of light in a vacuum. Differs in wavelength, frequency, and properties.

Electromagnetic spectrum: A convenience-based diagram where electromagnetic radiations are arranged according to wavelength. No clear-cut separation exists between various radiations; consequently, overlapping of wavelengths is common. Longer waves are measured in meters; shorter waves are measured in angstrom units.

Electron: A small, negatively charged particle of an atom.

Electron cloud: A mass of free electrons that hovers around a filament wire of the cathode when it is heated to incandescence. The number of free electrons increases as the milliamperage is increased.

Elon: Developer solution reducing agent that converts exposed silver halide crystals to black metallic silver. Builds up gray tones in a radiographic image.

Elongated image: Refers to a distortion of the radiographic image in which the tooth structures appear longer than the anatomical size. Often caused by insufficient vertical angulation of the central rays of the x-ray beam.

Elongation: A radiographic image that appears stretched out.

Embrasure: Space between the sloping proximal surfaces of the teeth. The space may diverge facially, lingually, occlusally, or apically; important to alignment of an intraoral image receptor to achieve correct horizontal angulation.

Empathy: The ability to share in another's emotions or feelings.

Emulsion: The gelatinous coating on radiographic film containing silver halide crystals.

Enamel: Dense, hard tissue of a tooth crown covering the dentin; appears radiopaque.

Encryption: A means to provide secure digital data transfer via mechanisms such as password protection.

Energy: The ability to do work and overcome resistance.

Energy levels: Term used in chemistry and physics to denote the spherical levels or electron shells that contain the electrons of an atom.

Ethics: A sense of moral obligation regarding right and wrong behavior.

Exfoliation: Shedding of primary teeth.

Exposure: A measure of ionization produced in air by x- or gamma radiation. The units of exposure are coulombs per kilogram (C/kg) and the roentgen (R).

Exposure button: Keypad or switch that activates an x-ray production process.

Exposure factors: Settings for milliamperage (mA), exposure time, and kilovoltage (kV).

Extension arm: (1) Flexible arm from which a dental x-ray tube head is suspended. (2) That part of an image receptor positioner that attaches a biteblock to an indicator ring.

External aiming device: An indicator ring or rectangle attached to an extension arm used to assist in locating correct angles and points of entry needed to expose intraoral radiographs, eliminating the need for precise patient head positioning.

Extraoral: Outside the oral cavity.

Extraoral film: Dental radiographic film designed for use in conjunction with intensifying screens to obtain extraoral (outside the oral cavity) radiographs.

Eyewash station: Sink with faucets designed for the purpose of flushing the eyes with copious amounts of water in response to an accidental chemical contamination.

Facilitation skills: Actions such as respectfulness, courtesy, empathy, patience, honesty, and tactful communication used to enhance and ease the way to good working relationships with others.

Field of view (FOV): The area of interest that will be exposed and recorded during a cone beam computed tomography (CBCT) imaging examination.

Filament: The spiral tungsten coil in the focusing cup of the cathode of a dental x-ray tube.

Film duplicator: A device that uses infrared and ultraviolet light to expose specially coated duplicating film for the purpose of making copies of intra- and extraoral film-based radiographs.

Film feed slot: Opening in an automatic film processor where the film is inserted for processing.

Film fog: An overall darkening or grainy appearance of a radiograph caused as film ages and/or by exposure to scatter radiation, excessive light, heat, and humidity, and chemical vapors.

Film hanger: Hanger or rack equipped with clips used to hold films during manual processing.

Film loop: An image receptor loop holder with a bitetab extension that wraps around an image receptor providing a surface for a patient to occlude on to stabilize the image receptor during a bitewing exposure.

Film mount: Plastic or cardboard holder with frames or windows that display dental radiographs for viewing.

Film packet: Intraoral dental radiographic film packaged in a moisture-proof outer plastic or paper wrap. May contain one or two films, wrapped in dark protective paper on either side, with a thin sheet of lead foil on the back side of the film(s).

Film recovery slot: Opening in an automatic film processing unit where the finished radiograph exits at the completion of the processing cycle.

Film speed: Sensitivity of a dental radiographic film to radiation exposure. Fast-film speed requires less radiation; slow film speed requires more radiation to produce an image.

Filter: Absorbing material, usually aluminum, placed in the path of a beam of radiation to remove a high percentage of low-energy (longer wavelength) x-rays.

Filtration: Selectively absorbing or screening out low-energy x-rays from the primary beam. *See* Added filtration, Inherent filtration, and Total filtration.

Fixer: The chemical solution used in film processing that removes all unexposed and any remaining undeveloped silver halide crystals from film emulsion to make an image permanently visible.

Flat panel detector (FPD): An image receptor used in cone beam computed tomography (CBCT) imaging.

Focal opacity: Descriptive term for the architecture of a radiopaque lesion that appears as a single entity.

Focal spot: Small area on the target on the anode toward which the electrons from the focusing cup of the cathode are directed. X-rays originate at the focal spot.

Focal trough/layer: The predetermined area between the x-ray source and the panoramic image receptor where anatomic structures will be imaged distinctly.

Focusing cup: A curved device around the cathode wire filament that is designed to focus the free electrons toward the tungsten target of the anode.

Foreign object: Item recorded on dental radiographs that does not represent normal physiologic structure; includes dental materials placed iatrogenically (purposefully for the treatment of pathology or a condition needing correcting), and objects placed accidentally, or as a result of trauma.

Foreshortened image: Refers to a distortion of a radiographic image in which the tooth structures appear shorter than the actual anatomical size. Often caused by excessive vertical angulation of the central rays of the x-ray beam.

Foreshortening: A radiographic image that appears shorter than normal.

FOV: *See* Field of view.

Frankfort plane: An imaginary plane or line from the orbital ridge (under the eye) to the acoustic meatus of the ear; an important landmark used to determine correct positioning for a panoramic radiograph.

Frequency: The number of crests of a wavelength passing a given point per second.

Fresh film test: Quality control test used to monitor the quality of each new box of radiographic dental film.

Full mouth series (survey): A set of 14 to 22 periapical and bitewing radiographs that records the entire dentition.

Furcation involvement: Bone loss between the roots of multirooted teeth.

Gelatin: Component of film emulsion in which halide crystals are suspended.

Genetic effect: Radiation effect that is passed on to future generations.

Geometric factors: Factors that relate to the relationships of angles, lines, points, or surfaces that contribute to the quality of radiographic image definition.

Ghost image: Mirror or second image of an anatomical structure or other object that is penetrated twice by the x-ray beam observed on a panoramic radiograph.

Gingivitis: Inflammation of the gingiva.

Glossopharyngeal air space: Open space posterior to the tongue that continues into the oral-pharyngeal (throat) region. Appears as a radiolucent shadow on a panoramic radiograph.

Gray (Gy): *Système Internationale* unit for measuring absorbed dose. One Gy equals 100 rads; 1000 milligrays equals 1 Gy.

Gray scale: Refers to the total number of shades of gray visible in a digital radiographic image.

Gray value: Number that corresponds to the amount of radiation received by a pixel within a digital sensor.

A computer uses this value to determine the shade of gray displayed on a computer monitor.

Gutta percha: An organic endodontic material used to fill pulp canals following a pulpectomy; appears slightly radiopaque.

Half-value layer (HVL): Thickness of a specified material that, when introduced into the path of a given beam of radiation, reduces the exposure by half.

Handheld x-ray device: Portable, battery-operated dental x-ray unit that a radiographer holds in place during exposure.

Hand hygiene: Refers to the need for handwashing with soap and water, and/or cleaning hands with an alcohol-based preparation for the purpose of reducing the number of viable microorganisms.

Hazardous waste: Waste materials that present a threat to community health or the environment.

Head positioner guides: Devices on panoramic and other extraoral dental imaging systems used to stabilize the head in the correct position during exposure.

Health Insurance Portability and Accountability Act (HIPAA): Federal law designed to provide patients with more control over how their personal health information is used and disclosed. A patient will usually be asked to sign a notice that indicates how their radiographs may be used and their privacy rights under this law.

Herringbone error: Refers to the image produced on a film-based radiograph that results when the packet is placed in the oral cavity backwards, causing the x-ray beam to penetrate the embossed pattern in the lead foil.

HIPAA: *See* Health Insurance Portability and Accountability Act.

Horizontal angulation: Refers to the direction of the dental ray machine tube head and position indicating device (PID), and the central rays of the x-ray beam in a horizontal plane. Incorrect horizontal angulation results in overlapping proximal structures.

Horizontal bone loss: Bone loss that occurs in a plane parallel to the cementoenamel junction (CEJ) of adjacent teeth.

HVL: *See* Half-value layer.

Hydroquinone: Developer solution agent that reduces (converts) exposed silver halide crystals within dental radiographic film emulsion to metallic silver. Slowly builds up black tones and contrast.

Hypersensitive gag reflex: An exaggerated or overly sensitive protective mechanism that naturally serves to clear the airway of obstruction.

Identification dot: Small, circular embossed mark on the corner of intraoral dental radiographic film. Used to determine the right and left sides when viewing radiographs.

Idiopathic: Of unknown original.

Image Gently®: Campaign organized by the Alliance for Radiation Safety in Pediatric Imaging and supported by numerous health care professional organizations to raise awareness for radiation safety and "as low as reasonably achievable" (ALARA) protocols for radiographic imaging of children.

Image receptor positioner (holder): Positioner used to stabilize an intraoral film packet, digital sensor, or phosphor plate in the oral cavity during exposure.

Impulse: Measure of radiation exposure time. There are 60 impulses per second.

Indicator ring: A ring or rectangle attached to an extension arm of an image receptor positioner used to assist in locating correct angles and points of entry, eliminating the need for precise patient head positioning.

Indirect theory: States that cell damage results indirectly when x-rays cause the formation of toxins such as hydrogen peroxide.

Informed consent: Permission given by a patient after being informed of the details of a radiographic examination, including the purpose of taking radiographs, benefits radiographs will supply, possible risks of radiation exposure, possible risks of refusing radiographs, and identification of the person who will perform the procedure.

Inherent filtration: Filtration built into a dental x-ray machine by the manufacturer; includes the glass wall of the x-ray tube, the insulating materials of the tube head, and the materials that seal the port.

Intensifying screens: A pair of plastic sheets coated with calcium tungstate or rare-earth fluorescent salt crystals positioned inside a cassette, used to expose film-based extraoral radiographs. When exposed to radiation, calcium tungstate and rare-earth screens produce blue and green light, respectively.

Interdental septa: Alveolar bone between adjacent teeth.

Interpersonal skills: Techniques that increase successful communication with others.

Interpretation: The ability to read and explain what is revealed by a radiographic image.

Interradicular: A descriptive radiographic term for the location of a lesion between teeth roots.

Intraoral: Inside the oral cavity.

Intraoral film: Dental radiographic film designed for use inside the oral cavity; includes periapical, bitewing, and occlusal radiographs.

Inverse square law: Rule that states that the intensity of radiation is inversely proportional to the square of the distance from the source of the radiation to the point of measurement.

Inverted Y: Radiographic landmark made up of the lateral wall of the nasal fossa and the anterior-medial wall of the maxillary sinus often observed near the canine-premolar region.

Ion: An electrically charged particle, either negative or positive.

Ion pair: A pair of ions, one positive and one negative.

Ionization: The formation of ion pairs.

Ionizing radiation: Radiation that is capable of producing ions.

Isometric triangle: A triangle with two sides equal in length and two identical angles opposite these two equal sides. Important geometric principle upon which the bisecting technique is based.

Kilovolt peak (kVp): The crest value in kilovolts of the potential difference of a pulsating dental x-ray machine generator.

Kinetic energy: Energy possessed by a mass because of its motion.

Labial mounting method: Arrangement of radiographs where the view is oriented as if standing in front of, and facing, a patient; achieved by positioning the embossed radiographic film dot in a convex position. Recommended over the lingual mounting method.

Lamina dura: A thin, hard layer of cortical bone that lines the dental alveolus. Appears as a thin, radiopaque line around the roots of the teeth.

Latent image: Invisible image produced when radiographic film is exposed to x-ray photons. Image remains stored by the silver halide crystals within the film emulsion until the film is processed.

Latent period: Time between exposure to radiation and the first clinically observable symptoms.

Lead/lead equivalent apron: Protective barrier made of lead or lead equivalent materials used to shield a patient from scatter radiation during radiographic exposures.

Lethal dose: Amount of radiation that is sufficient to cause the death of an organism.

Liable: To be legally obligated to make good any loss or damage that may occur as a result of treatment.

Light-tight: Securing an area against all sources of white light. Characteristic of a darkroom.

Line pair: Refers to the number of paired lines visible in 1 mm of a digital radiographic image. The more line pairs visible, the better the spatial resolution.

Lingual mounting method: Arrangement of radiographs where the view is oriented as if standing behind a patient; achieved by positioning the embossed radiographic film dot in a concave position. No longer a recommended mounting method.

Local contributing factor: Amalgam overhangs, poorly contoured crown margins, and calculus deposits, each of which attract and can lead to a buildup of bacterial pathogens that cause periodontal diseases.

Localization: Radiographic methods used to obtain a third dimension from two-dimensional radiographs for the purpose of determining whether an object is located on the facial (buccal) or lingual.

Localized bone loss: Bone loss that occurs in isolated areas.

Long-scale contrast: Low-contrast image, revealing more shades of gray, produced with a higher kilovoltage setting.

Lucent-opaque: A descriptive radiographic term for a mixed radiolucent and radiopaque lesion.

Mach band effect: A radiographic optical illusion that mimics decay; appears along the boundaries of sharp contrast, especially in areas of slight overlapping between adjacent teeth.

Malpractice: Improper practice that results when one is negligent.

Maryland bridge: Dental restorative treatment that consists of a pontic with one or two metal clasps or wings on one or both sides that are cemented or bonded to adjacent natural teeth.

Maxillofacial: Pertaining to the dental arches (maxilla and mandible) and other supporting facial structures of the head and neck region.

Maximum permissible dose (MPD): The dose equivalent of ionizing radiation that, in light of present knowledge, is not expected to cause detectable body damage to average persons at any point during their lifetime.

Mean tangent: Average point where several curved surfaces touch if a ruler is held against them. The labial or buccal surfaces of all teeth have their most prominent point toward the lips or the cheeks and curve toward the mesial or distal. A mean tangent would be established by using a small ruler or any straight edge (such as a tongue depressor) and attempting to align as many of the teeth as possible. Used to establish correct horizontal angulation, which requires that the central rays of the x-ray beam be directed at right angles to the mean tangent.

Mesiodistal overlap: When the projection angle of an x-ray beam is directed obliquely from mesial to distal resulting in overlapping error that appears more severe in the posterior region of the image.

Microbial aerosol: Suspension of microorganisms that may be capable of causing disease that is produced during normal breathing and speaking.

Microsievert (μSv): One millionth of a seivert. *See* Seivert.

Midsagittal plane: An imaginary vertical line or plane passing through the center of the body that divides it into a right and left half. Important orientation line in determining the ideal head position during radiographic exposures.

Milliampere (mA): One thousandth of an ampere. Measurement of the strength of an electric current that determines the number of electrons available at the filament inside the dental x-ray machine tube head.

Milliampere second (mAs): The relationship between the milliamperage and the exposure time in seconds. When one is increased, the other must be correspondingly decreased to maintain image density.

Mitosis: Cell division.

Modeling: Technique used to orient patients, especially children, to a radiographic procedure where an individual is given the opportunity to observe the procedure being performed on another, such as a sibling or parent. May help to alleviate fear of the unknown and gain patient cooperation.

Molecule: Chemical combination of two or more atoms that forms the smallest particle of a substance that retains the properties of that substance.

MPD: *See* Maximum permissible dose.

Multifocal: Descriptive radiographic term for multiple radiopaque lesions that appear to be joined or are in an overlapping relationship.

Multilocular: Descriptive radiographic term for a radiolucent lesion with more than one compartment that appears to be separated by radiopaque walls or septa.

Nasopharyngeal air space: Open space superior to the soft palate. Appears as a radiolucent shadow on a panoramic radiograph.

Negative angulation: Referring to dental radiographic techniques, the direction in which the x-ray tubehead and position indicating device (PID) and central rays of the x-ray beam are directed upward from a horizontal plane.

Negative shadows: Term given to the radiolucencies produced on a panoramic radiograph as a result of more radiation reaching the image receptor in the areas of air spaces. Negative shadows are shadows of "nothing."

Negligence: Failure to use a reasonable amount of care that results in injury or damage to another.

Neutron: One form of particulate radiation or subatomic particle. A neutron has no electric charge and has about the same mass as a proton.

Noise: The digital equivalent to film fog. An electrical disturbance that clutters a digital image reducing image clarity and contrast.

Nonverbal communication: Communication achieved without words. Includes gestures, facial expressions, body movement, and listening.

Occlusal plane: Anatomical plane between the maxillary and the mandibular teeth.

Occlusal radiograph: An intraoral radiograph that records the entire arch: maxilla or mandible. A large size 4 image receptor is positioned against the incisal or occlusal plane and held in place when a patient occludes. *See* Cross-sectional technique and Topographical technique.

Occlusal trauma: Excessive or repetitive force against the teeth that results in a response.

Occult disease: Disease that may exist without signs or symptoms, the presence of which is not apparent clinically, but detected via a diagnostic test, such as a radiograph.

Odontogenic: Pertaining to the development of teeth.

Opportunistic screening: Anomalies and lesions detected incidentally by a radiographic examination that was prescribed to assess another condition.

Optically stimulated luminescence (OSL) monitor: A personnel radiation monitor that uses crystals to absorb radiation. The crystals release energy during optical stimulation that is calculated by a computer for the purpose of determining the amount of radiation to which the device was exposed.

Oral radiography: Radiographic examinations of the oral and maxillofacial regions.

OSL: *See* Optically stimulated luminescence monitor.

Ossification: The pathological or abnormal conversion of soft tissues into bone.

Overdevelopment: Leaving a radiographic film in developer processing solution too long or using developer that is too warm. Overdevelopment results in a dark image.

Overexposure: Exposing an image receptor too long or using an inappropriately increased kilovoltage or milliaperage setting. Overexposure results in a dark image.

Overgloves: Plastic gloves used as a temporary protectant cover either for clean, dry hands or over patient treatment gloves.

Overhang: A restoration that is not contoured to the tooth properly.

Overlap: Refers to a distortion of the tooth image in which the structures of one tooth are superimposed over the structures of the adjacent tooth. Caused by incorrect horizontal angulation of the central beam and/or incorrect positioning of the image receptor in relation to the teeth of interest. *See* Distomesial and Mesiodistal overlap.

Oxidation: The process during which the chemicals of the developing and fixing solutions combine with oxygen and lose strength.

Palatoglossal air space: Open space between the tongue and palate. Appears as a radiolucent shadow on a panoramic radiograph.

Panoramic radiograph: Term meaning "wide view" used to describe an extraoral dental radiographic image that records the entire dentition and supporting structures of the maxilla and mandible.

Panoramic radiography: An extroral radiographic technique used to image the entire dentition and surrounding structures based on the principle of tomography; used to record images of structures within a selected plane of tissue while blurring structures outside the selected plane.

Paralleling technique: Intraoral radiographic technique that positions an image receptor parallel to the long axes of the teeth and directs the central rays of the x-ray beam perpendicular to both the long axes of the teeth and the image receptor.

Particulate radiation: Minute subatomic particles such as protons, electrons, and neutrons; also alpha and beta particles. These particles occupy space, have mass and weight, and, with the exception of neutrons, have an electrical charge.

Pathogen: A disease-causing microorganism.

Patient education: Informing patients about the benefits and value of a dental radiographic examination and providing information regarding radiation safety measures.

Patient relations: Establishment of a relationship between patient and radiographer that demonstrates an understanding of patient needs and an ability to respond in a manner that builds confidence and trust.

PDL: *See* Periodontal ligament.

Pediatric dentistry: Branch of dentistry that specializes in providing comprehensive preventive and therapeutic oral health care for children.

Penumbra: Partial shadow or fuzzy outline around a radiographic image.

Periapical radiograph: An intraoral radiograph that records the entire tooth or teeth and supporting tissues. *Peri* means "around" and *apical* refers to the root end of the tooth.

Pericoronal: Refers to a location around a tooth crown.

Periodontal ligament (PDL): Dense, strong fibrous tissues that attach a tooth to the lamina dura. Soft tissue is not visible radiographically; the PDL *space* is identified radiographically as a thin radiolucent outline between the lamina dura and the tooth root.

Periodontitis: Inflammation of the periodontium.

Periodontium: Tissues that invest and support the teeth (gingiva and alveolar bone).

Permanent teeth: Teeth that erupt after the primary teeth have been exfoliated (shed). Consists of 32 teeth—8 incisors, 4 canines, 8 premolars, and 12 molars.

Personal protective equipment (PPE): Clothing, masks, eyewear, and gloves worn by a radiographer as a protective barrier that prevents the transmission of infective microorganisms between oral health care practitioners and patients.

Personnel monitoring: The occasional or routine measuring of the amount of radiation to which a radiation worker may be exposed during a given period of time.

Photon: A quantum of energy. Both x-rays and gamma rays are photons.

Photostimulable phosphor (PSP): An indirect digital image receptor that replaces dental radiographic film with a polyester plate coated with a storage phosphor (europium activated barium fluorohalide) that when exposed to x-rays, *stores* energy until stimulated by a laser beam to produce a digital image.

PID: *See* Position indicating device.

Pixel: *Pix*, plural of picture and *el*, short for element are tiny dots representing discrete units of digital information that together constitute an image.

Point of entry: Predetermined spot or anatomical landmark on the surface of the face toward which the central rays of the x-ray beam are directed when aligning the dental x-ray machine tube head and position indicating device (PID) for the purpose of exposing intraoral radiographs.

Polychromatic: A term derived from the Greek meaning "having many colors." Used in dental radiography to describe the x-ray beam because it is composed of many different wavelengths.

Port: Opening in a dental x-ray tube head that is covered with a permanent seal of glass, beryllium, or aluminum through which x-rays exit. The port is opposite the window in an x-ray tube where the position indicating device (PID) attaches to the tube head.

Portal of entry/exit: A link in the chain of infection, portals are routes a pathogen takes to exit a reservoir and enter a susceptible host.

Position indicating device (PID): An open-ended, cylindrical or rectangular device attached to a dental x-ray machine tube head at the aperture used to direct the useful beam of radiation; available in different lengths.

Positive angulation: Referring to dental radiographic techniques, the direction in which the x-ray tube head and position indicating device (PID) and central rays of the x-ray beam are directed downward from a horizontal plane.

Post and core: Metal restorative material used in an endodontically treated tooth when support for a crown is needed; appears radiopaque.

Postmortem radiograph: An image exposed after death for identification of remains through comparison with available antemortem images.

PPE: *See* Personal protective equipment.

Primary radiation: The original, undeflected useful beam of radiation that emanates at the focal spot of an x-ray tube and emerges through the aperture of the tube head.

Primary teeth: Teeth that are exfoliated naturally. Consists of 20 teeth—8 incisors, 4 canines, and 8 molars.

Processing: The steps used to transform a latent image contained within radiographic film emulsion, into a permanent visible image. Steps include developing, rinsing, fixing, washing, and drying.

Processing tank: Stainless steel receptacle used to process dental radiographs; divided into compartments containing chemical solutions of developer and fixer, and water for rinsing and washing.

Professional appearance: Thoughtful selection of attire, attention to personal hygiene and grooming, and the adoption of mannerisms and speech that conveys competence.

Professionalism: Attitude projected that conveys skill and distinguishes a person as an expert.

Protected health-related information (PHI): Medical and dental information that can be identified with a patient that must be kept confidential.

Proton: A positive electrical charged subatomic particle contained in the nucleus of an atom.

Proximal surface: Where adjacent teeth contact each other in the arch. The mesial and distal surfaces are proximal surfaces.

PSP: *See* Photostimulable phosphor.

Psychogenic stimuli: Originating in the mind; important in managing a hypersensitive gag reflex.

Rad: Traditional unit for measuring absorbed dose: 100 rads equal 1 gray (Gy); 1 rad equals 0.01 Gy; 1000 millirads equal 1 rad.

Radiation: The emission and propagation of energy through space or through a material medium in the form of electromagnetic waves, particulate emissions such as alpha and beta particles, or rays of mixed and unknown types such as cosmic rays. Radiation used for oral health care examinations is capable of producing ions directly or indirectly by interaction with matter.

Radiation worker: A person who works with or near ionizing radiation or equipment that produces ionizing radiation.

Radiator: A large mass of copper connected to the anode terminal that functions to dissipate excess heat produced during energy exchange when electrons are converted into x-rays.

Radioactivity: The process whereby certain unstable elements undergo spontaneous disintegration (decay). The process is accompanied by emissions of one or more types of radiation and generally results in the formation of a new isotope.

Radiograph: Term given to a film-based or digital image produced by exposure to x-rays for the purpose of assessing, diagnosing, and evaluating a condition or treatment intervention.

Radiography: The making of radiographs by exposing an image receptor to ionizing radiation.

Radiology: The study of radiation and the techniques and technology used to produce radiographic images.

Radiolucent: The dark or black portion of a radiographic image, representing structures that lack density, permitting the passage of x-rays with little or no resistance.

Radiolysis of water: Ionization can dissociate water within a cell into hydrogen and hydroxyl radicals that have the potential to recombine into new chemicals such as hydrogen peroxide. These new chemicals act as toxins, causing cellular dysfunction. Considered an indirect effect of radiation exposure.

Radiopaque: The light or white/clear portion of a radiographic image, representing dense structures that resist the passage of x-rays.

Radioresistant: Refers to a substance or tissue that is not easily injured by ionizing radiation.

Radiosensitive: Refers to a substance or tissue that is relatively susceptible to injury by ionizing radiation.

Rare-earth phosphors: Lanthanum (La) and gadolinium (Gd) salt crystals used in intensifying screens that fluoresce and emit energy in the form of green light when x-rays are absorbed.

Reconstruction: Computer-assisted mechanism used to combine all slice data obtained by a cone beam computed tomography (CBCT) examination into a three-dimensional image.

Reference film: A radiograph processed under ideal conditions that is used to compare subsequent films for the purpose of monitoring dental radiographic processing solutions.

Rem: Traditional unit for measuring dose equivalent: 100 rem equals 1 sievert (Sv); 1 rem equals 0.01 Sv; 1000 millirems equal 1 rem.

Reservoir: A link in the chain of infection where sufficient numbers of pathogens exist to initiate infection.

Respiratory hygiene: Steps taken to prevent transmission of respiratory pathogens; includes cough etiquette, providing tissues and/or masks to contain respiratory secretions, and performing hand hygiene when in contact with respiratory secretions.

Retake policy: Established protocol upon which to base a decision to retake an undiagnostic radiograph.

Retake radiograph: A second radiograph that must be taken after the first image is deemed undiagnostic.

Retention pin: Metal pin used to support a dental restoration; appears radiopaque.

Roentgen (R): Traditional unit measurement of radiation exposure. Defined as the amount of x-radiation or gamma radiation that will produce an electric charge of 0.000258 coulomb per kilogram of dry air at standard atmospheric conditions and 0°C.

Roentgen ray: Term given to x-rays by scientists following its discovery by Wilhelm Conrad Roentgen in 1895 after his findings were reported and published. The term was eventually replaced with the term *x-ray*.

Roentgenograph: Term given to the image Wilhelm Conrad Roentgen produced on photosensitive film in 1895. The term was eventually replaced with the term *radiograph*.

Roller transport system: Motor-driven gears or belts that propel dental radiographic films through the developer, fixer, water, and drying compartments of an automatic processor.

Rule of isometry: Geometric theorem that is the basis for the bisecting technique; stating that two triangles with two equal angles and a common side are equal (isometric) triangles.

Safelight: Special filtered darkroom light that provides enough visibility to perform the steps of film processing without diminishing the quality of the film.

Safelight filter: Removes short wavelengths in the blue-green region of visible light allowing only longer wavelength red-orange light to pass through, for the purpose of illuminating a darkroom without fogging film.

Safety Data Sheets (SDS): Formally called Material and Safety Data Sheets (MSDS), documentation available from manufacturers of chemical products that provide information regarding the properties and the potential health effects of using a product.

Sagittal plane: Anatomical plane that divides an area of interest into right and left slices of data in the vertical dimension.

Scatter correction algorithm: Computer-assisted software that reconstructs image data captured during a cone beam computed tomography (CBCT) examination to produce enhanced two- and three-dimensional digital radiographic images.

Scatter radiation: Radiation that has been deflected from its path and scattered in all directions by impact during its passage through matter.

Screen film: Extraoral dental radiographic film used in conjunction with a cassette and a pair of intensifying screens. Produces an image as a result of exposure to both radiation and green, blue, and violet light that is emitted when radiation strikes intensifying screen phosphors.

Secondary radiation: Emitted by any matter irradiated with x-rays. Created at the instant the primary beam interacts with matter and gives off some of its energy, forming new and less powerful wavelengths. Often referred to as scatter radiation.

Selection criteria: Guidelines developed by an expert panel of health care professionals to assist in deciding when, what type, and how many radiographs should be prescribed for specific conditions.

Selective reduction: The method by which film processing developing agents separate or remove the unexposed, nonmetallic elements from a film emulsion, and leave the exposed metallic silver intact. The temperature of, and the time the film is left in, the developer must be within a precise range for selective reduction to produce an acceptable radiographic image.

Self-determination: The legal right of an individual to make choices concerning health care treatment.

Sensor: An image receptor based on charge-coupled device (CCD) or complementary metal oxide semiconductor active pixel sensor (CMOS-APS) technology, containing an electronic chip, made up of a grid of x-ray or light-sensitive cells (pixels) that convert x-rays into an electronic signal that is sent to a computer that will produce a digital radiographic image.

Shadow casting: Principle that x-rays cast shadows of images onto an image receptor, producing a radiographic image of the dentition and supporting structures.

Short-scale contrast: High-contrast image, revealing less shades of gray, produced with a lower kilovoltage setting.

"Show-Tell-Do": Technique used to orient a patient, especially a child, to the radiographic procedure to help to alleviate fear of the unknown and gain patient cooperation. Consists of a demonstration of the equipment use prior to performing the examination.

Sievert (Sv): *Système Internationale* unit for measuring the dose equivalent: 1 sievert equals 100 rem. *See* Microsievert.

Silver halide crystals: Radiation-sensitive compounds of approximately 90 to 99 percent bromine and 1 to 10 percent silver iodide that make up dental radiographic film emulsion. When exposed to x-rays, silver halide crystals retain the latent image.

Silver point: Endodontic filling material used to fill pulp canals following a pulpectomy; appears radiopaque.

Silver thiosulphate complex: A stable form of silver found in radiographic fixer as a result of the removal of unexposed and undeveloped silver halide crystals from the emulsion of radiographic film.

Slice data: Cone beam computed tomography (CBCT) images that are reconstructed into three anatomical planes—sagittal, coronal, and axial—for viewing and interpretation on a computer monitor.

S.L.O.B. rule: Stands for "same on lingual opposite on buccal." Used in localization techniques to determine the facial (buccal) or lingual position of objects. Rule states that if an object appears to move in the same direction as the horizontal or vertical shift of the tube, then the object is located on the lingual. Conversely, if the object appears to move in the opposite direction of the shift of the tube, then the object is located on the buccal.

Sodium thiosulfate: Chemical of the fixer solution that together with the ammonium thiosulfate removes the unexposed and any remaining undeveloped silver halide crystals.

Solarized emulsion: One side of duplicating film that responds to infrared and ultraviolet light by getting lighter with longer exposure time, and darker with shorter exposure time.

Solid state: Specifically means, no moving parts. Refers to digital radiographic image sensors, based on charge-coupled device (CCD) or complementary metal oxide semiconductor active pixel sensor (CMOS-APS) technology.

Somatic effect: When radiation affects all body cells except the reproductive cells.

Spatial resolution: The discernable separation of closely adjacent image details that contributes to image sharpness determined by the number and size of pixels and measured in line pairs.

Spatter: A heavier concentration of microbial aerosols such as visible particles from a cough or sneeze.

Speech reading: Method of lip reading used by an individual with a hearing impairment.

Standard precautions: A practice of care to protect persons from pathogens spread via blood or any other body fluid, excretion, or secretion (except sweat). All-inclusive term that has replaced universal precautions, where the focus was on blood-borne pathogens.

Statute of limitations: Time period during which a person may bring a legal malpractice action against another person.

Step-down transformer: Electromagnetic device inside a dental x-ray machine that decreases voltage from a wall outlet to approximately 5 V, just enough to heat the filament and form an electron cloud for the production of x-rays.

Step-up transformer: Electromagnetic device inside a dental x-ray machine that increases voltage from a wall outlet to approximately 50–100 kVp to propel electrons toward the target for the production of x-rays.

Step-wedge: A device consisting of increasing increments of an absorbing material. A radiographic exposure made with a step-wedge is used to determine the amount of radiation reaching an image receptor through each of the increments. Measurements of radiographic image density may be used to evaluate the intensity and penetrative power of the radiation.

Sterilization: Aseptic treatment, autoclaving, or dry heat processes that result in the total destruction of spores and disease-producing microorganisms.

Stochastic effect: When a biological response is based on the probability of occurrence rather than the severity of the change.

Storage phosphor: Europium activated barium fluorohalide coating on a photostimulable phosphor (PSP) plate that captures and "stores" x-ray energy similar to the way silver halide crystals within radiographic film emulsion store a latent image. A scanning device is used to release the stored energy converting it to a radiographic image displayed on a computer monitor.

Streaking artifact: An artifact sometimes present on a cone beam computed tomography (CBCT) image that appears as radiolucent distorted lines usually occurring between two adjacent objects, usually large metallic restorations, of high density.

Supernumerary: Extra; often used to describe extra teeth not normally a part of the dentition; or an additional tooth root not part of normal tooth morphology.

Surface barrier: Plastic wrap or other impervious material used to cover those surfaces most likely to be contaminated during a radiographic procedure, especially surfaces that are difficult to clean and disinfect.

Susceptible host: A link in the chain of infection where an unvaccinated individual, or an individual with a weakened immune system, will be prone to infection.

Tactile stimuli: Originating from touch; important in managing a hypersensitive gag reflex.

Target: A tungsten plate embedded in a copper bar on the anode side of an x-ray tube that faces the focusing cup of the cathode; set at a 20-degree angle to direct most of the x-rays produced in the direction of the port.

Target lesion: Descriptive radiographic term for a focal opacity that presents with a radiolucent ringlike outline.

Thermionic emission: The release of electrons when a material such as tungsten is heated to incandescence. Electrons are boiled off from a cathode filament in an x-ray tube when electric current is passed through it.

Thermoluminescent dosimeter (TLD): A personnel radiation monitor that uses crystalline compounds to absorb radiation. The crystals release light energy when heated that is calculated by a computer for the purpose of determining the amount of radiation to which the device was exposed.

Thyroid collar: An attached or detachable supplemental protective barrier made of lead or lead equivalent materials used to shield the thyroid gland from scatter radiation during radiographic exposures.

Time-temperature: Principle of dental radiographic film processing where the length of time a film stays in the developer solution depends on the temperature of the developer solution. A low temperature requires an increased developing time; a high temperature requires a decreased developing time to produce an acceptable radiographic image.

TLD: *See* Thermoluminescent dosimeter.

Tomography: The basic principle of panoramic imaging, where structures located within a selected plane of tissue will be recorded with relative clarity, while structures outside the selected plane will appear less visible.

Topographical technique: Occlusal radiographic technique based on the bisecting technique, where the central rays of the x-ray beam are directed through the apices of the teeth perpendicularly toward the bisector to produce an image.

Torus mandibularis (lingual torus): Benign tumor detected as a hard, bony protuberance on the lingual surface of the mandible.

Torus palatinus (palatal torus): Benign tumor detected as a hard, bony protuberance on the midline of the maxilla.

Total filtration: The combination of inherent and added filtration. Many state radiation safety regulations require a total filtration of 2.5 mm of aluminum equivalent for dental x-ray machines operating at or above 70 kVp.

Trabeculae: Interconnected bars or plates that form a multitude of various-sized mixed radiolucent-radiopaque honeycomb compartments of cancellous bone.

Trajectory: Path the x-ray beam takes during cone beam computed tomography (CBCT) exposure.

Transfer box: A light-tight box used to keep exposed photostimulable phosphor (PSP) plates protected from prolonged white light exposure until ready for the scanning step.

Transitional (mixed) dentition: Having both primary and permanent teeth present in the oral cavity; condition usually exists between 6 and 12 years of age.

Transmission: A link in the chain of infection that includes direct contact with pathogens in open lesions, blood, saliva, or respiratory secretions; and with airborne contaminants present in aerosols of oral and respiratory fluids; or by indirect contact with contaminated objects such as radiographic equipment.

Triangulation: Widening of the periodontal ligament (PDL) space at the crest of interproximal bone.

Tube head: Protective metal covering that contains an x-ray tube, high-voltage and low-voltage transformers, and insulating oil; attached to a flexible extension arm by a yoke; positioning indicating device (PID) attaches to the tube head at the port.

Underdevelopment: Not leaving a radiographic film in developer processing solution long enough or using developer that is old, weak, or too cool. Underdevelopment results in a light image.

Underexposure: Not exposing a radiographic image receptor long enough or using an inappropriately decreased kilovoltage or milliaperage setting. Underexposure results in a light image.

Unilocular: Descriptive radiographic term for a radiolucent lesion that is not compartmentalized, but appears as a single radiolucent part.

Universal precautions: A single infection control standard based on research that has demonstrated that human blood and all other body fluids, including saliva, are potentially infectious for blood-borne diseases, and that all patients have the potential to be a risk for transmitting blood-borne infection.

Useful beam: That part of the primary beam permitted to emerge from the dental x-ray machine tube head; limited by the port, collimator, and lead-lined position indicating device (PID).

Velocity: Property exhibited by electromagnetic radiation that refers to the speed of a wave as it travels through space. In a vacuum, all electromagnetic radiations travel at the speed of light (186,000 miles/sec or 3×10^8 m/sec).

Verbal communication: Using words to exchange information between two or more persons.

Vertical angulation: Refers to the direction of the dental ray machine tube head and position indicating device (PID), and the central rays of the x-ray beam in a vertical (up and down) plane. *See* Negative angulation and Positive angulation.

Vertical bitewing radiograph: Bitewing radiograph placed in the oral cavity with the long dimension of the image receptor positioned vertically. Records more information in the vertical dimension, especially useful when the area of interest is the periodontium.

Vertical (angular) bone loss: Alveolar crest that is reduced in a vertical direction creating angular defects.

View box: Device with a light source illuminator behind an opaque glass used to view dental radiographs.

Voxel (volume element): Similar to a pixel, *vol* is short for volume and *el* is short for element; captures digital data during cone beam computed tomography (CBCT) exposure producing a three-dimensional image.

Waste stream: The collective flow of waste materials beginning at the point of discard, through waste treatments, to the final disposition of the material.

Wavelength: The distance from the crest, or top, of one electromagnetic wave to the crest of the next; determines the penetration ability of the radiation.

Wet reading: Viewing a radiograph when a diagnosis is needed quickly under white light conditions after two or three minutes of fixation. Following a wet reading, film must be returned to the fixer to complete processing.

Working radiograph: A film that is rapidly processed with special chemistry when information is needed quickly, such as during endodontic procedures. Working radiographs are not permanent images due to short developing and fixing times, and minimal washing.

X-ray: Ionizing radiation of minute bundles of pure electromagnetic energy with the ability to penetrate materials and tissues and record shadow images on photographic film, phosphor plates, and digital sensors.

X-ray film: Photographic film especially adapted in size, emulsion, speed, and packaging for producing examinations of the oral and maxillofacial regions.

X-ray tube: Electronic tube located in the dental x-ray machine tube head that generates x-rays.

Yoke: Curved portion of a dental x-ray machine that connects the tube head to the extension arm, allowing the tube head to be positioned vertically and horizontally.

INDEX

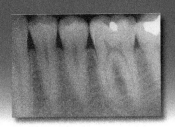

Note: Page numbers followed by *f* and *t* indicate figures and tables, respectively. Boxes are indicated by *b*.